W0049891

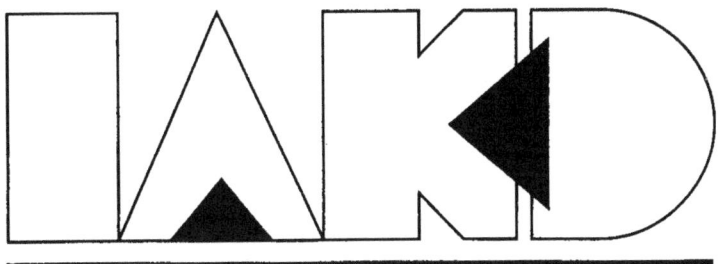

The Immunoassay Kit Directory

Managing Editors
Dr Elizabeth Naysmith
Dr Jane Kent
Kluwer Academic Publishers
Edinburgh
Scotland

Consulting Editor
Professor Keith James
Department of Surgery
University of Edinburgh
Edinburgh
Scotland

Editorial Assistants
Linda Thomas
Jenny Kellett
Kluwer Academic Publishers, Lancaster

Series B: Infectious Diseases

Editor-in-Chief
Dr Hugh Young
Department of Medical Microbiology
University of Edinburgh
Edinburgh
Scotland

Editorial Advisory Board
A Linde, Stockholm, Sweden
D J Merry, Adelaide, Australia
A Rodriguez Torres, Valladolid, Spain
J Orfila, Amiens, France

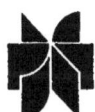

Springer Science+Business Media

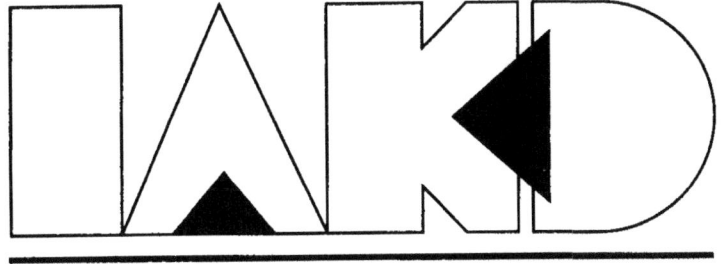

The Immunoassay Kit Directory

Series B: Infectious Diseases

Volume 1: Part 1
Genitourinary Infections
November 1994

Guest Editors
Dr Hugh Young
Dr Marie Ogilvie
Department of Medical Microbiology
University of Edinburgh
Edinburgh
Scotland

Springer Science+Business Media

ISSN 1381-5067

The Immunoassay Kit Directory

Series B: Infectious Diseases

SUBSCRIPTION INFORMATION

The subscription price for Volume 1 (three parts) is:

US$ 490 / Dfl. 850 inclusive of shipping and handling

COPYRIGHT

© 1994 by Springer Science+Business Media New York

Originally published by Kluwer Academic Publishers in 1994.

All rights reserved. No part of this publication may be reproduced, stored in a retrieval system, or transmitted in any form or by any means, electronic, mechanical, photocopying, recording or otherwise, without prior permission from the publishers, Kluwer Academic Publishers, PO Box 55, Lancaster, LA1 1PE, United Kingdom

Published in the United Kingdom by Kluwer Academic Publishers bv, PO Box 55, Lancaster, LA1 1PE UK

ISBN 978-0-7923-8811-1   ISBN 978-94-017-5080-6 (eBook)
DOI 10.1007/978-94-017-5080-6

ISSN: 1381-5067

CONTENTS

(continued overleaf)

ABOUT THIS PUBLICATION

Introduction

This is a new series of the Immunoassay Kit Directory and deals with commercially available immunoassay kits in the area of infectious diseases. A companion publication, Series A: Clinical Chemistry, was started some years ago and is now in its third volume.

The aim of the publication is to provide a comprehensive, independent and easy-to-use reference source on the large and growing number of kits currently on the market for the diagnosis of clinically important infectious diseases.

Detailed information about each kit is provided; over 19 different major parameters are listed in a consistent manner to allow for easy comparison.

Each organism begins with a short introduction written by the guest editors. There are also review articles of relevance to the current issue.

Full details of the manufacturers and distributors are also included as well as several indexes.

Each volume of Series B will initially consist of three parts:

    Part 1:   Genitourinary Infections
    Part 2:   Respiratory Infections
    Part 3:   Enteric and other infections

Where appropriate, some organisms may be represented in more than one part.

About this part – Genitourinary Infections

This, the first part of the Volume, covers kits for organisms that infect the genitourinary system or use this as a route of infection.

How is the publication organised?

The main body of the publication consists of the immunoassay kit entries. These are ranked as follows:

Alphabetically by organism, first by antigen detection and then by antibody detection. Antigen detection kits are then ranked alphabetically by assay type and then by manufacturer. Antibody detection kits are ranked first by assay type, second by antibody class and third by manufacturer.

Thus entries for *Chlamydia trachomatis* will be sorted as shown below.

Chlamydia trachomatis
1. Antigen detection
    EIA (non-competitive), by manufacturer
    Immunochromatographic assay, by manufacturer
    Immunofluorescence assay (direct), by
        manufacturer

2. Antibody detection
    EIA (non-competitive)
        *Total or non-specified Ab class, by
            manufacturer*
        IgA, by manufacturer
        IgG, by manufacturer
        IgM, by manufacturer
    Immunofluorescence assay (direct)
        *Total or non-specified Ab class, by
            manufacturer*
        IgG, by manufacturer
        IgM, by manufacturer

Virus types

Viruses such as human immunodeficiency virus, herpes simplex virus and human T-cell lymphotropic virus can be differentiated by type. The grouping of assay kits in relation to type has been defined as follows:

Human immunodeficiency virus:
Kits listed under this heading will detect antigen/antibody from either or both HIV-1 and HIV-2 but cannot distinguish between them (or give no details of specificity).

Human immunodeficiency virus (HIV-1):
Kits listed under this heading will detect only HIV-1 antigens or antibodies.

Human immunodeficiency virus (HIV-1 and HIV-2):
Kits listed under this heading will detect and differentiate between antigen or antibody to HIV-1 and HIV-2 separately by parallel use of specific antibody conjugates or antigens.

© *KLUWER ACADEMIC PUBLISHERS 1994, ISSN 1381-5067*

Human immunodeficiency virus (HIV-2): Kits listed under this heading will detect only HIV-2 antigens or antibodies.

The grouping for HSV and HTLV is defined in a similar way.

Two main indexes are provided at the back of the Directory to cross-reference many of these parameters. Firstly, an index by manufacturer, assay type, antibody/antigen detection and microorganism; secondly, by assay type, microorganism, antibody/antigen detection and manufacturer.

How frequently will the information be revised?

We will be revising the database of information that we are compiling on an on-going basis. Each major part of the directory, such as this part on Genitourinary infections will be revised on a roughly annual basis.

How is the information collected?

Information about what kits are available has been gathered by a variety of means:
> Direct contact with manufacturers
> Research by the editorial board
> Exhibitions and conferences

Whilst most manufacturers have been extremely helpful in giving us information there have been a very small number who, for one reason or another, have not supplied information. We hope that with the establishment of the directory they will feel that they are now able to contribute.

No charge has been made to manufacturers for the inclusion of information.

What parameters have been used to select kits?

The basic parameter for the inclusion of a kit in the directory is that it should be readily available to the average user on an international basis. Having said this, however, it may be that, because of regulatory or other restrictions, certain kits are available only in certain countries. Contact with the manufacturer will, we hope, clarify the availability and we would be grateful for any feedback that users can give us on this matter.

Information about the kits themselves has been compiled by contacting manufacturers for detailed information, often in the form of kit inserts. This has then been carefully edited and checked by the editorial staff to compile the basic entries that form the body of the directory. Manufacturers have then had the opportunity to see at least one set of proofs.

The parameters that have been used are shown in detail in the definitions section of the directory.

Haemagglutination assays have not been included.

How can the user help?

This publication aims to be of practical use to the users of kits. We carried out extensive market research to define more closely the needs of the target audience and some of the results of this have been incorporated into the publication you now hold.

We very much would like to continue to incorporate the views and needs of users into the publication. Please feel free to contact us here with any comments at all, good or bad, about the publication. Letters to the Editor will be published. We will always welcome information about kits and their manufacturers that we may have overlooked.

What further developments will there be?

Now that Series A (Clinical Chemistry) is established and Series B (Infectious Diseases) is underway we already have plans for similar series to deal with other major areas of clinical practice and bio-medical research such as haematology, immunology and oncology.

A Final Note . . .

Many people have assisted in the preparation of the Directory and I would like to thank, in addition to those acknowledged on the first page, the following: the manufacturers of kits who have kindly and generously provided us with information on their products; Dr Jan Boyd who assisted in the analysis of kit inserts; and Dr Marian Bain and Dr Sadhana Yellamanchili who assisted in the collection and analysis of material in the early stages.

Dr Peter L Clarke

Kluwer Academic Publishers, Lancaster

November 1994

Related Publications

Series A: Clinical Chemistry

Following a similar approach to Series B, the Clinical Chemistry Series of the Immunoassay Kit Directory is a comprehensive source of information on commercially available kits.

Now in its third volume, there are five parts covering:

 Peptide Hormones
 Steroid and Thyroid Hormones
 Proteins and Tumour Markers
 Drugs; Eicosanoids: Second
  Messengers
 Equipment

For further information on this series please contact the publisher.

© *KLUWER ACADEMIC PUBLISHERS 1994, ISSN 1381-5067*

IMPORTANT ANNOUNCEMENT

Whilst every care has been made to ensure the accuracy of information contained in this publication the publishers cannot accept responsiblity for any errors contained herein or occurring as a result of the use of the information in any way. The inclusion or otherwise of information concerning a commercially available product or service is not intended to be an endorsement or otherwise of that product.

INFORMATION TO MANUFACT- URERS OF IMMUNOASSAY KITS

For further information on the inclusion of kits in forthcoming issues of the *Immunoassay Kit Directory* please contact:
    Dr Elizabeth Naysmith,
    Managing Editor,
    The Immunoassay Kit Directory

at the following address:
    Department of Surgery
    University Medical School
    Teviot Place
    Edinburgh EH8 9AG,
    United Kingdom
    Telefax 0131 667 0804

Or via our office in North America:
    Kluwer Academic Publishers
    101 Philip Drive
    Assinippi Park
    Norwell, MA 02061
    USA
    Telefax (617) 871 6528

© *KLUWER ACADEMIC PUBLISHERS 1994, ISSN 1381-5067*

REVIEW ARTICLE

Immunoassays in medical microbiology: general aspects

M.M. Ogilvie and H. Young

Department of Medical Microbiology, Edinburgh University Medical School, Teviot Place, Edinburgh EH8 9AG

Medical Microbiology laboratories aim to support the diagnosis, prevention and treatment of infectious diseases both in the hospital and in the community, and to provide surveillance data on the occurrence of certain infections or the level of immunity in a general population. The organisation of such work follows a variety of arrangements in different countries [1], with generalist or monospecialty accredited pathologists (medical and scientist), trained laboratory technical staff, and laboratory assistants, being employed in small district hospital laboratories, large national or regional centres, private laboratories, or separately in the microbiology section of Blood Transfusion Services. Systems for the accreditation of laboratories undertaking such diagnostic work [2] are in place in a great many countries, and include documentation and inspection to ascertain that appropriately qualified staff lead and provide the service. External quality assessment schemes are used to monitor the performance of a wide variety of investigations, including immunoassays [3].

Over the last twenty five years immunoassays have become an ever increasing proportion of the investigations performed in microbiology laboratories, significantly so in virology, and to a lesser extent in bacteriology, parasitology and mycology. The traditional biological assays which rely on observation of cultural characteristics such as colony appearance and cytopathic effects are not necessarily replaced, since isolates are often required for further studies such as typing or sensitivity testing. In modern clinical management, rapid diagnosis is crucial to early treatment and infection control, and for the safe supply of donor blood or organs standardised sensitive screening assays are essential. Culture methods however are still the most specific and sometimes the most sensitive reference (the 'gold standard') when comparing the performance of assays. The advances in nucleic acid detection methods, in particular the amplification of DNA by the polymerase chain reaction (PCR) from even one single genome, have revolutionised direct diagnosis of infection [4]. The initial introductions of this technique into service laboratories have tended to be for agents that are difficult to detect by other methods, such as the viruses HIV, hepatitis C, human papilloma, or are slow to grow in culture, such as mycobacteria, toxoplasma, cytomegalovirus. The practicalities and cost of extraction of nucleic acids, amplification and detection, with the necessary separation of different stages of the work to prevent DNA contamination in this exquisitely sensitive procedure, have delayed widespread routine use. However it is likely that for direct detection of organisms, particularly when quantitative assays in an automated format are available, PCR or a similar nucleic acid based assay will become the new gold standard. For the present, many immunoassays are providing rapid, sensitive and specific results of antigen or antibody detection pertinent to the management of infection.

Immunofluorescence (IF) has a longer history in routine use than many other immunoassays, especially in regard to early direct diagnosis of respiratory virus infections following the pioneering work of Gardner and McQuillin [5] in Newcastle, England. Specificity of assays and the range available improved greatly with the development of monoclonal antibodies reacting with defined epitopes. Pools of monoclonal antibodies may be employed for a single virus or bacterial species, covering different epitopes to minimise problems of strain variation, or to screen for any one of a range of viruses, for instance in the centrifugation-enhanced 'shell vial' technique for respiratory viruses [6]. The IF methods are still very important in rapid direct detection of infected cells in virology, or organisms (*Pneumocystis carinii*), particularly for single samples or small numbers of investigations. The sensitivity of immunofluoresence for antibody determination has been very useful over the years, but more sensitive and less subjective measurements of antibody are now appropriate. Methods which can be readily automated are also preferred for large scale screening for antibody or antigen.

Immunoassays vary in sensitivity and specificity, as do all laboratory investigations. The inherent sensitivity (percentage of true positives shown as positive) and specificity (percentage of true negatives shown as negative) are features of the test product. However, in the clinical setting the usefulness of a test depends on the predictive values of the results and these vary with the prevalence of the disease concerned in the population under study. For example, with a prevalence of 1% (not uncommon in a screening situation) a test with a specificity of 95% would result in only 17 correct positive results out of every 100 positives, i.e. 83 out of 100 would be false positives: a specificity of 99% would result in half the positive results being false positives whilst a specificity of 99.9% would produce only 1 false positive in every 10 positive results (Figure 1a). Therefore in screening low prevalence populations a test with high specificity is required in order to reduce the burden of confirmatory testing of positive results which turn out to be false. As shown in Figure 1a, as the prevalence increases so does the positive predictive value such that at a disease prevalence of 50% a test kit with a specificity of 95% would give only 5 false positive out of every 100 positive results.

The opposite situation occurs in the case of the negative predictive value which decreases as the disease prevalence increases (Figure 1b) – this is because more

true positives means fewer true negatives but more false negatives. The actual number of false negatives is related to the sensitivity of the test. For example in a population with a disease prevalence of 1% a test with a sensitivity of 95% gives a negative predictive value of 99.95% and would result in 5 false negatives per 10,000 negative results: a sensitivity of 99% gives a negative predictive value of 99.99% (1 false negative per 10,000 negative results) while a sensitivity of 99.9% gives a negative predictive value of 99.999% (1 false negative per 100,000 negative results).

Clearly a knowledge of the positive and negative predictive values is required to determine the accuracy of a test in a particular situation [7]. Unfortunately sensitivity usually shows an inverse correlation with specificity and taking account of the disease prevalence a balance must be drawn between these characteristics to minimise the number of infections likely to be missed while at the same time ensuring that the number of confirmatory tests required is not too high. However, in blood donor screening, although the disease prevalence is low, false negative results are critical and in this situation a relatively large proportion of unproductive confirmatory tests must be accepted. Although occasional false negative results may not be considered quite so important in other situations (e.g. screening for sexually transmitted diseases) samples which are non-reactive in screening immunoassays are generally not subjected to repeated or alternative assays (unless there are other grounds for suspicion of infection) so it is important that screening tests have as high a sensitivity as possible in keeping with a level of specificity compatible with an acceptable level of confirmatory testing. A confirmatory test (unless involving a specific blocking reaction) should generally be of a different format from the screening test and be of equivalent or higher sensitivity to minimise the number of true positives that will not be confirmed. Because the disease

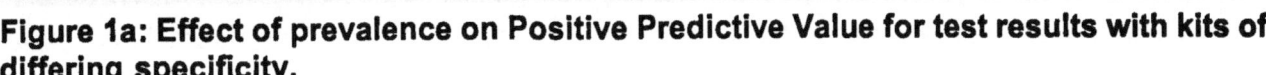

Figure 1a: Effect of prevalence on Positive Predictive Value for test results with kits of differing specificity.

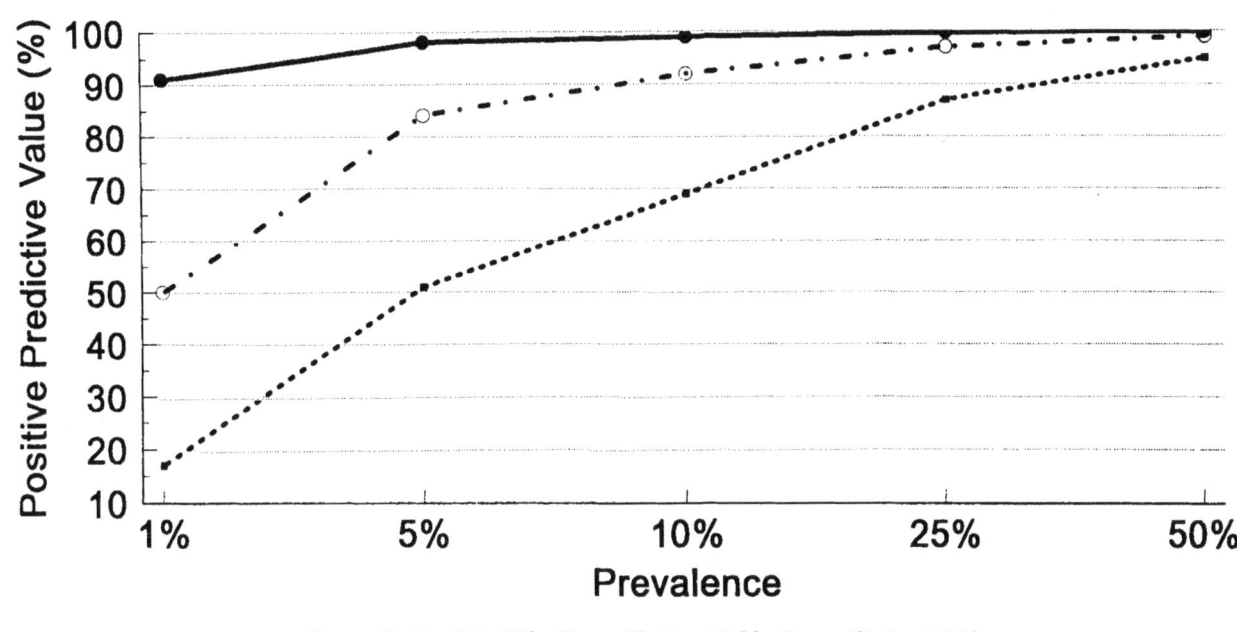

Figure 1b: Effect of prevalence on Negative Predictive Value for test results with kits of differing sensitivity.

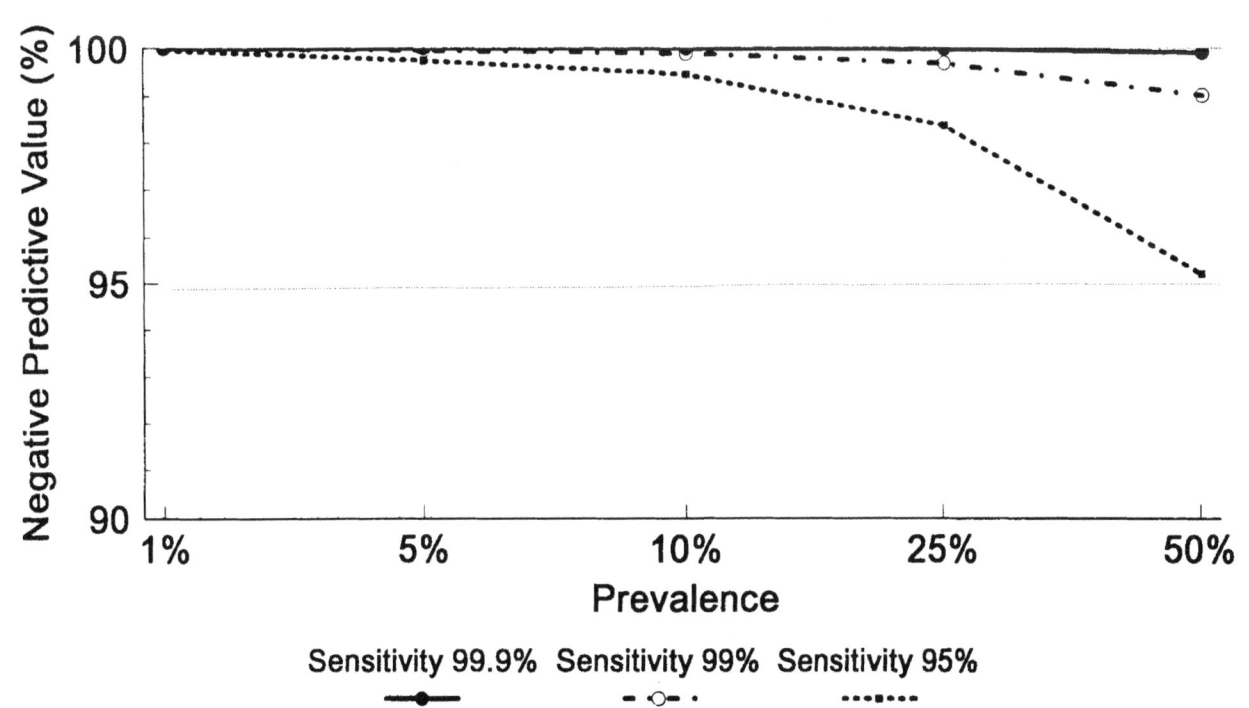

prevalence has been increased by screening, a useful confirmatory test need not necessarily be of overall higher specificity but it is important that it does not show the same pattern of false reactivity as the screening test. For example, as discussed above, at a disease prevalence of 1% a test with a specificity of 99% has a positive predictive value of 50%. When this group of sera is taken for confirmatory testing the disease prevalence has therefore increased to 50% and a confirmatory test with a specificity of 99% (the same as the screening test) will give a positive predictive value of 99% resulting in only 1 false positive per 100 positive confirmatory tests.

Reactivity in a screening assay requires to be confirmed by additional testing of the same sample and in some circumstances by examination of a second sample. In the context of sexually transmitted disease, confirmation (or use of a test which does not produce false positives, such as culture) is important because of the implications for contact tracing and investigation.

Screening immunoassays are available in a confusing multitude of formats, based on different antigen or antibody sources and utilising a variety of detection systems. The enzyme label has largely superseded the radioactive one for routine use, on grounds of safety, longer shelf life and acceptable sensitivity, particularly when amplified detection systems are used. The developments in molecular biology have made it possible to produce proteins expressed from recombinant DNA in various systems (bacteria, yeasts, insect cells and others), or to manufacture synthetic oligopeptides. These defined antigens are incorporated in a huge range of assays, and play a significant role in the daily screening for antibodies to HIV1/2, for instance. Hepatitis C virus assays are unique in that no native antigens have been available, but, since the virus was obtained by molecular cloning, an increasing number of structural or non-structural antigens have been expressed or synthesised. The careful choice of antigens to be

included in a screening assay is essential to detection of infections at different stages or where more than one strain of virus may be responsible.

Confirmatory tests for antigen (such as for *C. trachomatis*) may be assays of the same format as the screen using simple blocking (neutralisation) with a monoclonal antibody. More complex assays have come into general use in referral centres offering confirmation of the presence of antibodies to HIV or hepatitis C. Originally the HIV antibody tests were based on infected cell or viral lysate preparations, and the transfer of viral proteins, separated by electrophoresis in a gel, to a membrane (Western blot) enabled reactions with individual viral proteins to be ascertained. Variations on this method of presenting viral proteins separated by size are commercially available for a range of viruses and bacteria as standardised strips. Hepatitis C virus posed the necessity to use totally recombinant proteins (or some synthetic peptides) in an equivalent test format so that antibodies to a range of viral antigens could be detected, hence the recombinant immunoblot (RIBA) or line assays, with the proteins applied directly to the membranes. Detailed guidelines on the interpretation of the results obtained with HIV immunoblotting are published [8].

The introduction of automation for immunoassay procedures in medical microbiology is now proceeding apace, although far behind that in clinical biochemistry. Cost-effective, labour saving methods are valuable, particularly where a rapid turn around time provides the clinician with the relevant result in time to influence patient care [9]. The need for continuing medical and scientific supervision of the choice, application and interpretation of these methods is even greater than when 'catch-all' methods based on culture were the norm. Simultaneously, there is a great expansion in simple rapid tests which can be carried out without any but the most basic equipment, ideal for field use, or near-patient testing. Provision and supervision of such tests should be in conjunction with an accredited laboratory, where advice on safe handling, limitations of the tests and confirmatory or further investigations can be obtained [10].

This first part of the Immunoassay Kit Directory Series B on Infectious Diseases is devoted to Genitourinary Infections. The range of infections included are summarised

in Table 1. The majority of these infections were chosen on the basis that they are frequently or occasionally transmitted through sexual contact [11], and that immunoassay kits were available for detection of the infection. Some of these infections are thought of almost exclusively as sexually transmitted disease (gonorrhoea and syphilis) while others are recognised as having a significant blood-borne spread also

Table 1   Genitourinary Infection: *pathogens included in Series B Part 1 of the Immunoassay Kit Directory

Pathogen	Main clinical presentations	Common or serious sequelae
Chlamydia trachomatis (serovars D–K)	Urethritis, cervitis	Neonatal infection; pelvic inflammatory disease, ectopic pregnancy, infertility, arthritis
Cytomegalovirus	Primary infection usually sub-clinical; occasional mononucleosis	Congenital infection; in immuno-compromised – colitis, pneumonitis, retinitis, hepatitis
Hepatitis A virus	Hepatitis	
Hepatitis B virus	Hepatitis	Chronic hepatitis, cirrhosis, hepatocellular carcinoma
Hepatitis C virus	Hepatitis	Chronic hepatitis, cirrhosis, hepatocellular carcinoma
Hepatitis D virus	Hepatitis (simultaneous HBV required)	Chronic hepatitis, cirrhosis
Herpes simplex virus	Ulcers/vesicles – lower genital tract; mouth or pharynx; skin	Recurrent episdoes; neonatal infection
Human immuno-deficiency virus	Immunodeficiency	AIDS
Human T-cell lympho-tropic virus	Leukaemia, lymphoma, tropical spastic paresis	
Neisseria gonorrhoeae	Urethritis, cervicitis	Neonatal infection, pelvic inflammatory disease, ectopic pregnancy, infertility, disseminated infection
Streptococcus haemolytic group B (Streptococcus agalactiae)	Asymptomatic carriage common in genital and gastrointestinal tracts of adults	Septicaemia and meningitis in newborn; post-partum septicaemia
Treponema pallidum	Syphilis	Congenital infection; neurological and cardiovascular disease
Urinary tract pathogens	Urinary tract infection frequency and/or dysuria	Pyelonephritis

*(Adapted from reference 11). Information was sought on kits for Candida albicans, Gardnerella vaginalis, Haemophilus ducreyi, human papilloma virus and Trichomonas vaginalis. Although a few kits were available for C. albicans they were for use in systemic infection.

© KLUWER ACADEMIC PUBLISHERS 1994, ISSN 1381-5067

(HIV). In some cases, spread by sexual contact is much less important in transmission than other means of exposure (hepatitis A), or is still not clearly confirmed as a mode of spread (hepatitis C).

References

1. Medical and scientific staffing of National Health Service pathology laboratories. London: Royal College of Pathologists, 1992.

2. Advisory Task Force on Standards to the Audit Steering Committee of the Royal College of Pathologists. Pathology department accreditation in the United Kingdom: a synopsis. Journal of Clinical Pathology 1991; 44: 798–802.

3. Snell JJS, Farrell ID, Roberts C, eds. Quality Control: Principles and practice in the microbiology laboratory. London: Public Health Laboratory Service, 1991.

4. Persing DH. Polymerase chain reaction: trenches to benches. Journal of Clinical Microbiology 1991; 29: 1287–1295.

5. Gardner PS, McQuillin J. Rapid virus diagnosis. Application of immunofluorescence, 2nd edition. London: Butterworths, 1980.

6. Schirm J, Dirk SL, Pastoor GW, et al. Rapid detection of respiratory viruses using mixtures of monoclonal antibodies on shell vial cultures. Journal of Medical Virology 1992; 38: 147–151.

7. Washington JA, Doern GV. Assessment of new technology. In: Balows A, Hausler WJ, Herrmann KL, Isenberg HD, Shadomy HJ, eds. Manual of Clinical Microbiology, 5th edition. Washington DC: American Society for Microbiology, 1991: 44–48.

8. Consortium for retrovirus serology standardization. Serological diagnosis of human immunodeficiency virus infection by Western blot testing. Journal of the American Medical Association. 1988; 260: 674–679.

9. Hosein IK, Duerden BI. Introducing rapid methods in the diagnostic laboratory. Reviews in Medical Microbiology 1994; 5: 39–45.

10. Hurley R, and the Joint Working Group on Quality Assurance. Guidelines on the control of Near-Patient Tests (NPT) and procedures performed on patients by non-pathology staff. The Bulletin of the Royal College of Pathologists (London) 1993; 81: 22–23.

11. Catchpole MA. Sexually transmitted diseases in England and Wales; 1981–1990 Communicable Disease Report 1992; 2: R1–R7.

ABBREVIATIONS AND DEFINITIONS

List of Abbreviations

Ab	antibody
ABTS	2,2-azinobis (3-ethylbenzothiazoline-6-sulphonic acid), diammonium salt
Ag	antigen
AHIg	anti-human immunoglobulin
AHIgA	anti-human immunoglobulin A
AHIgG	anti-human immunoglobulin G
AHIgM	anti-human immunoglobulin M
AMIgG	anti-murine immunoglobulin G
ampl	amplified
AP	alkaline phosphatase
ARIg	anti-rabbit immunoglobulin
ARIgG	anti-rabbit immunoglobulin G
BCIP	5-bromo-4-chloro-3-indolyl phosphate
CMV	Cytomegalovirus
CoA	coagglutination
CSF	cerebrospinal fluid
EDTA	ethylene diamine tetraacetic acid
EIA	enzyme immunoassay
Fab	fragment antigen binding
Fc	fragment crystallisable
FITC	fluorescein isothiocyanate
GBS	Group B beta-haemolytic streptococci
HAV	Hepatitis A virus
HBs	Hepatitis B virus surface antigen
HBc	Hepatitis B virus core antigen
HBe	Hepatitis B virus e antigen
HCV	Hepatitis C virus
HD	Hepatitis D antigen
HDV	Hepatitis D virus
HIV	human immunodeficiency virus
HRP	horseradish peroxidase
HSV	Herpes simplex virus
HTLV	human T cell lymphotropic virus
IFA	immunfluorescent antibody
Ig	immunoglobulin
IgA	immunoglobulin A
IgG	immunoglobulin G
IgM	immunoglobulin M
LPS	lipopolysaccharide
MAb	monoclonal antibody
MEM	Minimum Essential Medium
4-MP	4-methylumbelliferyl phosphate
NA	not applicable
NAD	nicotinamide adenine dinucleotide
NADP	nicotinamide adenine dinucleotide phosphate
NBT	nitroblue tetrazolium
Neg	negative
OD	optical density
OPD	O-phenylenediamine
PAb	polyclonal antibody
PBS	phosphate buffered saline
PMP	phenolphthalein monophosphate
PNP	p-nitrophenyl phosphate
POD	peroxidase
Pos	positive
RBC	red blood cells
rec	recombinant
RF	rheumatoid factor
RIA	radioimmunoassay
RITC	rhodamine isothiocyanate
RT	room temperature
staph	staphylococcus
strep	streptococcus
strept	streptavidin
syn	synthetic
temp	temperature
TMB	tetramethylbenzidine
TmpA	*Treponema pallidum* recombinant antigen (TpN44.5(a))
WB	Western blot
g	goat
gp	guinea pig
h	human
m	mouse
p	pig
r	rabbit
sh	sheep
hr	hours
min	minutes
sec	seconds
γ	gamma

Outline of kit descriptions and definition of headings

Each entry is introduced by the full name of the organism and is followed by a statement indicating whether the assay detects antigen and/or antibody. Assays which detect both antigen and antibody are entered and indexed under both antigen and antibody with appropriate cross-reference. For antibody detection the class(es) of immunoglobulin(s) to be detected are stated. For antigen detection the assay is for clinical specimens unless stated otherwise. The primary manufacturer and the catalogue number of the smallest kit available is given.

Definitions of headings

Summary: A schematic representation of the assay system showing the component being measured (**Ab** or **Ag**) in bold. This is presented in a linear form beginning with the solid phase but it does not necessarily represent the actual sequence of reactions – in a competitive assay the analyte and the competitor are placed above and below the line, e.g.

$$[Well\text{-}Ag]\text{–}\textbf{Ab}\text{–}[AHIgG\text{-}AP]\text{–}[PMP]\text{–}A_{550}$$

$$[Well\text{-}Ag]\text{–}\textbf{Ab}\text{–}[AHIgG\text{-}FITC]\text{–}fluorescence$$

$$\left.\begin{array}{c}\textbf{Ab}\\ [Bead\text{-}Ab]\end{array}\right\}[Ag]\text{–}[Ab\text{-}^{125}I]\text{–}radioactivity$$

Assay type: The assay type is written in full apart from enzyme immunoassay and radioimmunoassay which are abbreviated to EIA and RIA. These assays are also designated as competitive or non-competitive and whenever appropriate as amplified. The assay types and their corresponding detection systems are given in Table 1.

Detection: A description of the method used to measure the result of the assay, e.g. colorimetric, luminometric, radioisotopic, fluorometric, fluorescence microscopy, visual.

Format: The physical format in which the assay is presented, e.g. 'microtitre well Ab coated' or 'slide well Ag coated'.

Sample type: The samples recommended for use with the kit, e.g. plasma, serum. If heat inactivation of serum is not recommended this is cited as 'serum (do not heat inactivate)'.

Sample pre-treatment: Treatment performed on the sample before performing the assay, e.g. extracting antigen from swab, removal of IgG. Dilution of the sample is not considered as pre-treatment.

Sample volume: The volume of sample required to perform a single estimate. Diluent volume, where recommended is shown in parenthesis, e.g. 10 μl (+ 500 μl diluent) otherwise the recommended dilution is given, e.g. '20 μl of 1:10 dilution'.

Number of tests: The number of tests for the smallest kit followed by the number of tests for any larger kit(s), e.g. 96; 960.

Controls - standards run in assay: The number and type of controls and calibrators/standards run in assay, e.g.

Controls: Neg(1), Low Pos(2), High Pos(1)

Standards: Neg(1), Low Pos(1), High Pos(1)

Calibrators: Neg(1), Mid Pos(1), High Pos(1)

Incubation: A summary of the incubation steps giving time in hours and minutes and temperatures in °C or room temperature (RT), e.g.

2 hr (RT) + 18-22 hr (RT) + 15 min (45°C)

Washes: The total number of washing cycles. If there is a preliminary plate wash this is also mentioned, e.g. '3 (+ preliminary plate wash)'

Antibodies, antigens and labelled components: The antibodies, antigens and labelled components included in the kit. The type of antibody - polyclonal (PAb) or monoclonal (MAb), the source of the antibody or antigen and the phase to which it is bound are stated if known, e.g.

Anti-chlamydia PAb(r) bound to particles

CMV (AD 169) bound to well

Anti-HAV PAb (h) ^{125}I labelled

Anti-human IgG MAb (m) biotinylated

Streptavidin HRP conjugated

Substrate: The substrate of the conjugate, e.g. OPD

Controls - standards supplied: A description of the controls and calibrators/standards supplied with the kit, e.g.

Controls: Neg, Low Pos, High Pos (human serum)

Calibrators: 4 with assigned titre values (human serum)

Additional reagents required: Any reagents required for the assay but not provided with the kit, e.g. 'controls/calibrators not supplied but available separately', 'H_2SO_4 stop solution' - common materials such as distilled water, saline and simple buffers such as Tris, PBS etc. are excluded.

Special equipment required: Dedicated equipment that is *essential* to the performance of the assay, e.g. 'FIAX fluorometer'. Equipment designed by the manufacturer for optional use in the assay may be listed as such, e.g. 'automated system and software (optional)'.

Scoring/comments and interpretation: General comment on whether equivocal/grey zones are recognised, if repeat or supplemental testing is recommended by the manufacturer, options available for quantitative testing and/or comparing acute and convalescent sera.

Number of references: The number of references given in the kit insert: these do not always include references giving performance data of the product itself.

Notes: Additional points of potential relevance to the kit used, e.g. kits designated 'for research use only'; certain types of swab unsuitable; recommended use of different incubation procedures; cross-reference to the appropriate section for kits detecting both antigen and antibody; etc.

Information not included

There are several parameters (outlined below) that, after careful consideration, we did not include. Although these are of interest it was not feasible to include them in a directory of this type.

Cost: The list price often bears little relationship to the discounted price paid by many laboratories. In addition list prices vary from country to country, supplier to supplier, and are subject to frequent change.

Sensitivity and specificity: These parameters are often quoted in product inserts but profound variation in the nature of the populations evaluated, the number of samples tested and the diversity of comparative methods make unqualified comparisons relatively meaningless and possibly misleading. In addition, as pointed out in the introductory article, the true utility of a test is given by the predictive value which is dependent on the prevalence of infection in the population being screened/tested.

Time to run tests: This can vary depending on pre-treatment, sample dilution, number of controls/ standards and tests per batch, number and nature of wash cycles and the number and length of incubation stages. As the number and length of incubation stages is usually the most significant influence on assay running time a minimum comparative value for the time to run tests can be obtained from the details given in the **Incubation** field. If the number of wash cycles (**Washes** field) is also taken into account a more accurate estimate of the overall time required to run tests can be obtained.

Table 1 Assay types and corresponding detection systems

Assay type	Detection system(s)
EIA (competitive) EIA (non-competitive) EIA (non-competitive) amplified	Colorimetric (occasionally visual, fluorometric or light microscopy)
Immunofluorescence assay (direct) Immunofluorescence assay (indirect)	Fluorometric or Fluorescence microscopy
Luminometric assay (competitive) Luminometric assay (non-competitive)	Luminometric
RIA (competitive) RIA (non-competitive)	Radioisotopic
Immunoblot assay Immunochromatographic assay Particle agglutination assay Particle agglutination assay (coagglutination)	Visual (occasionally colorimetric)

Haemagglutination assays have not been included nor have simple flocculation/agglutination assays such as VDRL and RPR tests used in syphilis serology.

© *KLUWER ACADEMIC PUBLISHERS 1994, ISSN 1381-5067*

STOP PRESS

The following information became available at too late a stage to include as full entries in the directory:

Abbott Laboratories

(For address see main index)

IMX® Chlamydia	2208
IMX® HCV	3A99
IMX® CMV-M	2209
IMX® HIV 1/2 3rd GEN	2291
Anti-Delta RIA	1009.22
AUSAB® EIA	9006.24
AUSAB® RIA	7554.24
CMV Total	5163.24
CMV M	3739.22
HAVAB® EIA	7895.24
HAVAB® M EIA	9843.24
HBE RIA	1237.24
HIVAG MONOCLONAL	1AO1.24
HTLV EIA	3077.24
HCV 2nd GEN KIT	4A14.24
HIV 1/2 TEST PACK	1ABS 21

Clark Laboratories Inc

(For address see main index)

Infectious disease ELISA kits:

Chlamydia trachomatis IgG	2306200*
Chlamydia trachomatis IgA	2306230*
Cytomegalovirus IgG, A, M	2305270*
Cytomegalovirus IgG	2305200
Cytomegalovirus IgM	2305250
Herpes Simplex 1 IgG	2305400
Herpes Simplex 1 IgM	2305450*
Herpes Simplex 2 IgG	2305500
Herpes Simplex 2 IgM	2305550*
TPA (Syphillis) IgG	2306300*

*At the time of printing, product is for export or 'Research Use Only'

Please call Clark Laboratories for latest FDA market release status

Labsystems Oy

(For address see main index)

HSV 1+2 IgM EIA	61.10.420
HSV-1 IgG EIA	61.10.400

Mast Diagnostics

(for address see main index)

MASTAZYME® - Syphilis	EIA 601

© *KLUWER ACADEMIC PUBLISHERS 1994, ISSN 1381-5067*

FULL CONTENTS LISTING

Chlamydia trachomatis

Cytomegalovirus

Antibody detection (IgM)	EIA (non-competitive)	Bouty Diagnostici	56
Antibody detection (IgM)	EIA (non-competitive)	Centocor Inc	56
Antibody detection (IgM)	EIA (non-competitive)	Chimica Diagnostica	57
Antibody detection (IgM)	EIA (non-competitive)	Diamedix Corporation	57
Antibody detection (IgM)	EIA (non-competitive)	E. Merck	58
Antibody detection (IgM)	EIA (non-competitive)	Eurogenetics	58
Antibody detection (IgM)	EIA (non-competitive)	Gamma SA	59
Antibody detection (IgM)	EIA (non-competitive)	Gull Laboratories	59
Antibody detection (IgM)	EIA (non-competitive)	Human GmbH	60
Antibody detection (IgM)	EIA (non-competitive)	IFCI Clone Systems	60
Antibody detection (IgM)	EIA (non-competitive)	Incstar	61
Antibody detection (IgM)	EIA (non-competitive)	International Immunodiagnostics	61
Antibody detection (IgM)	EIA (non-competitive)	Laboratoire Eurobio	62
Antibody detection (IgM)	EIA (non-competitive)	Labsystems Oy	62
Antibody detection (IgM)	EIA (non-competitive)	Medac Diagnostika	63
Antibody detection (IgM)	EIA (non-competitive)	Melotec S.A.	63
Antibody detection (IgM)	EIA (non-competitive)	Menarini Diagnostics	64
Antibody detection (IgM)	EIA (non-competitive)	Murex Diagnostics Limited	64
Antibody detection (IgM)	EIA (non-competitive)	Organon Teknika NV	65
Antibody detection (IgM)	EIA (non-competitive)	Radim	65
Antibody detection (IgM)	EIA (non-competitive)	Roche Diagnostic Systems	66
Antibody detection (IgM)	EIA (non-competitive)	Savyon Diagnostics Ltd	66
Antibody detection (IgM)	EIA (non-competitive)	Schiapparelli Biosystems Inc	67
Antibody detection (IgM)	EIA (non-competitive)	Sigma Diagnostics	67
Antibody detection (IgM)	EIA (non-competitive)	Sigma Diagnostics	68
Antibody detection (IgM)	EIA (non-competitive)	Sorin Biomedica	68
Antibody detection (IgM)	EIA (non-competitive)	United Biotech Inc	69
Antibody detection (IgM)	EIA (non-competitive)	Zeus Scientific Inc	69
Antibody detection (IgG)	Immunoblot assay	Gen Bio	70
Antibody detection (IgG)	Immunoblot assay	Gen Bio	70
Antibody detection	Immunofluorescence assay (indirect)	Gull Laboratories	71
Antibody detection	Immunofluorescence assay (indirect)	Incstar	71
Antibody detection (IgG)	Immunofluorescence assay (indirect)	Amico Laboratories Inc	72
Antibody detection (IgG)	Immunofluorescence assay (indirect)	Bion Enterprises Ltd	72
Antibody detection (IgG)	Immunofluorescence assay (indirect)	Biowhittaker	73
Antibody detection (IgG)	Immunofluorescence assay (indirect)	Gen Bio	73
Antibody detection (IgG)	Immunofluorescence assay (indirect)	Schiapparelli Biosystems Inc	74
Antibody detection (IgG)	Immunofluorescence assay (indirect)	Stellar Bio Systems Inc	74
Antibody detection (IgG)	Immunofluorescence assay (indirect)	Zeus Scientific Inc	75
Antibody detection (IgM)	Immunofluorescence assay (indirect)	Amico Laboratories Inc	75
Antibody detection (IgM)	Immunofluorescence assay (indirect)	Gen Bio	76
Antibody detection (IgM)	Immunofluorescence assay (indirect)	Gull Laboratories	76
Antibody detection (IgM)	Immunofluorescence assay (indirect)	Schiapparelli Biosystems Inc	77
Antibody detection	Particle agglutination assay	Becton Dickinson	77

Hepatitis A virus

			page
Antigen detection	EIA (non-competitive)	Organon Teknika NV	79
Antibody detection	EIA (competitive)	Abbott Laboratories	79
Antibody detection	EIA (competitive)	ADI Diagnostics	80
Antibody detection	EIA (competitive)	Boehringer Mannheim	80
Antibody detection	EIA (competitive)	Laboratoire Eurobio	81
Antibody detection	EIA (competitive)	Murex Diagnostics Limited	81
Antibody detection	EIA (competitive)	Organon Teknika NV	82
Antibody detection	EIA (competitive)	Roche Diagnostic Systems	82
Antibody detection	EIA (competitive)	Schiapparelli Biosystems Inc	83
Antibody detection	EIA (competitive)	Sorin Biomedica	83
Antibody detection	EIA (competitive)	Syva Company	84

Antibody detection (IgG)	EIA (non-competitive)	Amico Laboratories Inc	84
Antibody detection (IgM)	EIA (non-competitive)	Abbott Laboratories	85
Antibody detection (IgM)	EIA (non-competitive)	ADI Diagnostics	85
Antibody detection (IgM)	EIA (non-competitive)	Amico Laboratories Inc	86
Antibody detection (IgM)	EIA (non-competitive)	bioMerieux	86
Antibody detection (IgM)	EIA (non-competitive)	Boehringer Mannheim	87
Antibody detection (IgM)	EIA (non-competitive)	Laboratoire Eurobio	87
Antibody detection (IgM)	EIA (non-competitive)	Murex Diagnostics Limited	88
Antibody detection (IgM)	EIA (non-competitive)	Organon Teknika NV	88
Antibody detection (IgM)	EIA (non-competitive)	Roche Diagnostic Systems	89
Antibody detection (IgM)	EIA (non-competitive)	Schiapparelli Biosystems Inc	89
Antibody detection (IgM)	EIA (non-competitive)	Sorin Biomedica	90
Antibody detection (IgM)	EIA (non-competitive)	Syva Company	90
Antibody detection (IgM)	Luminometric immunoassay (non-competitive)	Kodak Clinical Diagnostics	91
Antibody detection	RIA (competitive)	Abbott Laboratories	91
Antibody detection	RIA (competitive)	Sorin Biomedica	92
Antibody detection (IgM)	RIA (non-competitive)	Abbott Laboratories	92
Antibody detection (IgM)	RIA (non-competitive)	Sorin Biomedica	93

Hepatitis B virus (core antigen)

page

Antibody detection	EIA (competitive)	Abbott Laboratories	95
Antibody detection	EIA (competitive)	Abbott Laboratories	95
Antibody detection	EIA (competitive)	ADI Diagnostics	96
Antibody detection	EIA (competitive)	Behringwerke AG	96
Antibody detection	EIA (competitive)	bioMerieux	97
Antibody detection	EIA (competitive)	Boehringer Mannheim	97
Antibody detection	EIA (competitive)	IFCI Clone Systems	98
Antibody detection	EIA (competitive)	Labsystems Oy	98
Antibody detection	EIA (competitive)	Melotec S.A.	99
Antibody detection	EIA (competitive)	Murex Diagnostics Limited	99
Antibody detection	EIA (competitive)	Organon Teknika NV	100
Antibody detection	EIA (competitive)	Organon Teknika NV	100
Antibody detection	EIA (competitive)	Radim	101
Antibody detection	EIA (competitive)	Randox Laboratories Ltd	101
Antibody detection	EIA (competitive)	Roche Diagnostic Systems	102
Antibody detection	EIA (competitive)	Sanofi Diagnostics Pasteur	102
Antibody detection	EIA (competitive)	Schiapparelli Biosystems Inc	103
Antibody detection	EIA (competitive)	Sorin Biomedica	103
Antibody detection	EIA (competitive)	Sorin Biomedica	104
Antibody detection	EIA (competitive)	Syva Company	104
Antibody detection	EIA (competitive)	VEDA-LAB	104
Antibody detection (IgM)	EIA (non-competitive)	Abbott Laboratories	105
Antibody detection (IgM)	EIA (non-competitive)	Abbott Laboratories	105
Antibody detection (IgM)	EIA (non-competitive)	ADI Diagnostics	106
Antibody detection (IgM)	EIA (non-competitive)	Behringwerke AG	106
Antibody detection (IgM)	EIA (non-competitive)	bioMerieux	107
Antibody detection (IgM)	EIA (non-competitive)	Boehringer Mannheim	107
Antibody detection (IgM)	EIA (non-competitive)	IFCI Clone Systems	108
Antibody detection (IgM)	EIA (non-competitive)	Labsystems Oy	108
Antibody detection (IgM)	EIA (non-competitive)	Murex Diagnostics Limited	109
Antibody detection (IgM)	EIA (non-competitive)	Organon Teknika NV	109
Antibody detection (IgM)	EIA (non-competitive)	Radim	110
Antibody detection (IgM)	EIA (non-competitive)	Randox Laboratories Ltd	110
Antibody detection (IgM)	EIA (non-competitive)	Roche Diagnostic Systems	111
Antibody detection (IgM)	EIA (non-competitive)	Sanofi Diagnostics Pasteur	111
Antibody detection (IgM)	EIA (non-competitive)	Schiapparelli Biosystems Inc	112

Antibody detection (IgM)	EIA (non-competitive)	Sorin Biomedica	112
Antibody detection (IgM)	EIA (non-competitive)	Sorin Biomedica	113
Antibody detection (IgM)	EIA (non-competitive)	Syva Company	113
Antibody detection	Luminometric immunoassay (competitive)	Kodak Clinical Diagnostics	114
Antibody detection (IgM)	Luminometric immunoassay (non-competitive)	Kodak Clinical Diagnostics	114
Antibody detection	RIA (competitive)	Abbott Laboratories	115
Antibody detection	RIA (competitive)	Radim	115
Antibody detection	RIA (competitive)	Sorin Biomedica	116
Antibody detection (IgM)	RIA (non-competitive)	Abbott Laboratories	116
Antibody detection (IgM)	RIA (non-competitive)	Radim	117
Antibody detection (IgM)	RIA (non-competitive)	Sorin Biomedica	117

Hepatitis B virus (e antigen)

			page
Antigen detection	EIA (non-competitive)	Abbott Laboratories	118
Antigen detection	EIA (non-competitive)	Abbott Laboratories	118
Antigen detection	EIA (non-competitive)	ADI Diagnostics	119
Antigen detection	EIA (non-competitive)	Behringwerke AG	119
Antigen detection	EIA (non-competitive)	Boehringer Mannheim	120
Antigen detection	EIA (non-competitive)	IFCI Clone Systems	120
Antigen detection	EIA (non-competitive)	Melotec S.A.	121
Antigen detection	EIA (non-competitive)	Organon Teknika NV	121
Antigen detection	EIA (non-competitive)	Radim	122
Antigen detection	EIA (non-competitive)	Randox Laboratories Ltd	122
Antigen detection	EIA (non-competitive)	Sanofi Diagnostics Pasteur	123
Antigen detection	EIA (non-competitive)	Schiapparelli Biosystems Inc	123
Antigen detection	EIA (non-competitive)	Sorin Biomedica	124
Antigen detection	EIA (non-competitive)	Sorin Biomedica	124
Antigen detection	EIA (non-competitive)	Syva Company	125
Antigen detection	EIA (non-competitive)	VEDA-LAB	125
Antigen detection	RIA (non-competitive)	Radim	126
Antigen detection	RIA (non-competitive)	Sorin Biomedica	126
Antigen and antibody detection	EIA (non-competitive)	Murex Diagnostics Limited	127
Antigen and antibody detection	Luminometric immunoassay (non-competitive)	Kodak Clinical Diagnostics	127
Antibody detection	EIA (competitive)	Abbott Laboratories	128
Antibody detection	EIA (competitive)	Abbott Laboratories	128
Antibody detection	EIA (competitive)	ADI Diagnostics	129
Antibody detection	EIA (competitive)	Behringwerke AG	129
Antibody detection	EIA (competitive)	Boehringer Mannheim	130
Antibody detection	EIA (competitive)	IFCI Clone Systems	130
Antibody detection	EIA (competitive)	Melotec S.A.	131
Antibody detection	EIA (competitive)	Organon Teknika NV	131
Antibody detection	EIA (competitive)	Radim	132
Antibody detection	EIA (competitive)	Randox Laboratories Ltd	132
Antibody detection	EIA (competitive)	Roche Diagnostic Systems	133
Antibody detection	EIA (competitive)	Sanofi Diagnostics Pasteur	133
Antibody detection	EIA (competitive)	Schiapparelli Biosystems Inc	134
Antibody detection	EIA (competitive)	Sorin Biomedica	134
Antibody detection	EIA (competitive)	Sorin Biomedica	135
Antibody detection	EIA (competitive)	Syva Company	135
Antibody detection	EIA (competitive)	VEDA-LAB	136
Antibody detection	RIA (competitive)	Radim	136
Antibody detection	RIA (competitive)	Sorin Biomedica	137

Hepatitis B virus (surface antigen)

			page
Antigen detection	EIA (non-competitive)	Abbott Laboratories	137
Antigen detection	EIA (non-competitive)	Abbott Laboratories	138
Antigen detection	EIA (non-competitive)	ADI Diagnostics	138
Antigen detection	EIA (non-competitive)	Behringwerke AG	139
Antigen detection	EIA (non-competitive)	BIOKIT SA	139
Antigen detection	EIA (non-competitive)	bioMerieux	140
Antigen detection	EIA (non-competitive)	Biotest Diagnostics	140
Antigen detection	EIA (non-competitive)	Boehringer Mannheim	141
Antigen detection	EIA (non-competitive)	Genetic Systems Corporation/Sanofi Diagnostics Pasteur	141
Antigen detection	EIA (non-competitive)	Human GmbH	142
Antigen detection	EIA (non-competitive)	Labsystems Oy	142
Antigen detection	EIA (non-competitive)	Melotec S.A.	143
Antigen detection	EIA (non-competitive)	Melotec S.A.	143
Antigen detection	EIA (non-competitive)	Mitsui Pharmaceuticals Inc	144
Antigen detection	EIA (non-competitive, amplified)	Murex Diagnostics Limited	144
Antigen detection	EIA (non-competitive)	Murex Diagnostics Limited	145
Antigen detection	EIA (non-competitive)	Omega Diagnostics Ltd	145
Antigen detection	EIA (non-competitive)	Organon Teknika NV	146
Antigen detection	EIA (non-competitive)	Organon Teknika NV	146
Antigen detection	EIA (non-competitive)	Radim	147
Antigen detection	EIA (non-competitive)	Randox Laboratories Ltd	147
Antigen detection	EIA (non-competitive)	Roche Diagnostic Systems	148
Antigen detection	EIA (non-competitive)	Sanofi Diagnostics Pasteur	148
Antigen detection	EIA (non-competitive)	Schiapparelli Biosystems Inc	149
Antigen detection	EIA (non-competitive)	Sorin Biomedica	149
Antigen detection	EIA (non-competitive)	Sorin Biomedica	150
Antigen detection	EIA (non-competitive)	Sorin Biomedica	150
Antigen detection	EIA (non-competitive)	Syva Company	151
Antigen detection	EIA (non-competitive)	United Biotech Inc	151
Antigen detection	EIA (non-competitive)	VEDA-LAB	152
Antigen detection	Immunochromatographic assay	Chembio Diagnostic Systems Inc	152
Antigen detection	Immunochromatographic assay	Savyon Diagnostics Ltd	153
Antigen detection	Luminometric immunoassay (non-competitive)	Kodak Clinical Diagnostics	153
Antigen detection	Particle RBC agglutination assay	Agen Biomedical Ltd	154
Antigen detection	Particle agglutination assay	Human GmbH	154
Antigen detection	Particle agglutination assay	Omega Diagnostics Ltd	155
Antigen detection	Particle agglutination assay	VEDA-LAB	155
Antigen detection	RIA (non-competitive)	Radim	156
Antigen detection	RIA (non-competitive)	Sorin Biomedica	156
Antibody detection	EIA (non-competitive)	Abbott Laboratories	157
Antibody detection	EIA (non-competitive)	ADI Diagnostics	157
Antibody detection	EIA (non-competitive)	Behringwerke AG	158
Antibody detection	EIA (non-competitive)	Boehringer Mannheim	158
Antibody detection	EIA (non-competitive)	Melotec S.A.	159
Antibody detection	EIA (non-competitive)	Mitsui Pharmaceuticals Inc	159
Antibody detection	EIA (non-competitive, amplified)	Murex Diagnostics Limited	160
Antibody detection	EIA (non-competitive)	Organon Teknika NV	160
Antibody detection	EIA (non-competitive)	Randox Laboratories Ltd	161
Antibody detection	EIA (non-competitive)	Roche Diagnostic Systems	161
Antibody detection	EIA (non-competitive)	Roche Diagnostic Systems	162
Antibody detection	EIA (non-competitive)	Sanofi Diagnostics Pasteur	162
Antibody detection	EIA (non-competitive)	Schiapparelli Biosystems Inc	163
Antibody detection	EIA (non-competitive)	Sorin Biomedica	163
Antibody detection	EIA (non-competitive)	Sorin Biomedica	164
Antibody detection	EIA (non-competitive)	Sorin Biomedica	164

Antibody detection	EIA (non-competitive)	Syva Company	165
Antibody detection	EIA (non-competitive)	VEDA-LAB	165
Antibody detection	Luminometric immunoassay (non-competitive)	Kodak Clinical Diagnostics	166
Antibody detection	RIA (non-competitive)	Radim	166
Antibody detection	RIA (non-competitive)	Sorin Biomedica	167

Hepatitis C virus

page

Antibody detection (IgG)	EIA (non-competitive)	Boehringer Mannheim	169
Antibody detection (IgG)	EIA (non-competitive)	Innogenetics SA	169
Antibody detection (IgG)	EIA (non-competitive)	Melotec S.A.	170
Antibody detection (IgG)	EIA (non-competitive)	Murex Diagnostics Limited	170
Antibody detection (IgG)	EIA (non-competitive)	Sanofi Diagnostics Pasteur	171
Antibody detection (IgG)	EIA (non-competitive)	Sorin Biomedica	171
Antibody detection	Immunoblot assay	Innogenetics SA	172

Hepatitis D virus

page

Antigen detection	EIA (non-competitive)	Cambridge Biotech Corporation	174
Antigen detection	EIA (non-competitive)	Murex Diagnostics Limited	174
Antigen detection	EIA (non-competitive)	Organon Teknika NV	175
Antigen detection	EIA (non-competitive)	Sanofi Diagnostics Pasteur	175
Antigen detection	EIA (non-competitive)	Sorin Biomedica	176
Antigen detection	RIA (non-competitive)	Sorin Biomedica	176
Antibody detection	EIA (competitive)	Abbott Laboratories	177
Antibody detection	EIA (competitive)	Cambridge Biotech Corporation	177
Antibody detection	EIA (competitive)	Murex Diagnostics Limited	178
Antibody detection	EIA (competitive)	Organon Teknika NV	178
Antibody detection	EIA (competitive)	Sanofi Diagnostics Pasteur	179
Antibody detection	EIA (competitive)	Sorin Biomedica	179
Antibody detection	EIA (competitive)	Sorin Biomedica	180
Antibody detection (IgM)	EIA (non-competitive)	Cambridge Biotech Corporation	180
Antibody detection (IgM)	EIA (non-competitive)	Murex Diagnostics Limited	181
Antibody detection (IgM)	EIA (non-competitive)	Sanofi Diagnostics Pasteur	181
Antibody detection (IgM)	EIA (non-competitive)	Sorin Biomedica	182
Antibody detection	RIA (competitive)	Sorin Biomedica	182
Antibody detection (IgM)	RIA (non-competitive)	Sorin Biomedica	183

Herpes simplex virus

page

Antigen detection	EIA (non-competitive, amplified)	Dako A/S	185
Antigen detection	EIA (non-competitive)	Kodak Clinical Diagnostics	185
Antigen detection	EIA (non-competitive, amplified)	Murex Diagnostics Limited	186
Antigen detection	EIA (non-competitive)	Savyon Diagnostics Ltd	186
Antigen detection	Immunofluorescence assay (direct)	Baxter Diagnostics Inc (Bartels Division)	187
Antigen detection	Immunofluorescence assay (direct)	Syva Company	187
Antibody detection (IgG)	EIA (non-competitive)	Amico Laboratories Inc	188
Antibody detection (IgG)	EIA (non-competitive)	Behringwerke AG	188
Antibody detection (IgG)	EIA (non-vompetitive)	Biowhittaker	189
Antibody detection (IgG)	EIA (non-competitive)	Biowhittaker	189
Antibody detection (IgG)	EIA (non-competitive)	Laboratoire Eurobio	190
Antibody detection (IgG)	EIA (non-competitive)	Menarini Diagnostics	190
Antibody detection (IgM)	EIA (non-competitive)	Amico Laboratories Inc	191
Antibody detection (IgM)	EIA (non-competitive)	Behringwerke AG	191
Antibody detection (IgM)	EIA (non-competitive)	Bio-Stat Diagnostics	192

Antibody detection (IgM)	EIA (non-competitive)	E. Merck	192
Antibody detection (IgM)	EIA (non-competitive)	Eurogenetics	193
Antibody detection (IgM)	EIA (non-competitive)	Gamma SA	193
Antibody detection (IgM)	EIA (non-competitive)	Human GmbH	194
Antibody detection (IgM)	EIA (non-competitive)	Laboratoire Eurobio	194
Antibody detection (IgM)	EIA (non-competitive)	Menarini Diagnostics	195
Antibody detection (IgM)	EIA (non-competitive)	Radim	195
Antibody detection (IgM)	EIA (non-competitive)	Schiapparelli Biosystems Inc	196
Antibody detection (IgG)	Immunoblot assay	Gen Bio	196
Antibody detection (IgG)	Immunoblot assay	Gen Bio	197
Antibody detection	Immunofluorescence assay (indirect)	Gull Laboratories	197
Antibody detection (IgG)	Immunofluorescence assay (indirect)	Amico Laboratories Inc	198
Antibody detection (IgM)	Immunofluorescence assay (indirect)	Amico Laboratories Inc	198
Antibody detection (IgM)	Immunofluorescence assay (indirect)	Gull Laboratories	199

Herpes simplex virus (HSV-1)
page

Antigen detection	EIA (non-competitive)	Bio-Stat Diagnostics	199
Antibody detection (IgG)	EIA (non-competitive)	Biologische Analysensystem GmbH	200
Antibody detection (IgG)	EIA (non-competitive)	Cambridge Biotech Corporation	200
Antibody detection (IgG)	EIA (non-competitive)	Chimica Diagnostica	201
Antibody detection (IgG)	EIA (non-competitive)	Diamedix Corporation	201
Antibody detection (IgG)	EIA (non-competitive)	E. Merck	202
Antibody detection (IgG)	EIA (non-competitive)	Eurogenetics	202
Antibody detection (IgG)	EIA (non-competitive)	Gamma SA	203
Antibody detection (IgG)	EIA (non-competitive)	Human GmbH	203
Antibody detection (IgG)	EIA (non-competitive)	Immunobiological Laboratories	204
Antibody detection (IgG)	EIA (non-competitive)	Incstar	204
Antibody detection (IgG)	EIA (non-competitive)	International Immunodiagnostics	205
Antibody detection (IgG)	EIA (non-competitive)	Melja Diagnostik GmbH	205
Antibody detection (IgG)	EIA (non-competitive)	Melotec S.A.	206
Antibody detection (IgG)	EIA (non-competitive)	Radim	206
Antibody detection (IgG)	EIA (non-competitive)	Schiapparelli Biosystems Inc	207
Antibody detection (IgG)	EIA (non-competitive)	Sigma Diagnostics	207
Antibody detection (IgG)	EIA (non-competitive)	United Biotech Inc	208
Antibody detection (IgM)	EIA (non-competitive)	Baxter Diagnostics Inc (Bartels Division)	208
Antibody detection (IgM)	EIA (non-competitive)	Biologische Analysensystem GmbH	209
Antibody detection (IgM)	EIA (non-competitive)	Cambridge Biotech Corporation	209
Antibody detection (IgM)	EIA (non-competitive)	Chimica Diagnostica	210
Antibody detection (IgM)	EIA (non-competitive)	Gull Laboratories	210
Antibody detection (IgM)	EIA (non-competitive)	Immunobiological Laboratories	211
Antibody detection (IgM)	EIA (non-competitive)	International Immunodiagnostics	211
Antibody detection (IgM)	EIA (non-competitive)	Melja Diagnostik GmbH	212
Antibody detection (IgM)	EIA (non-competitive)	Melotec S.A.	212
Antibody detection (IgM)	EIA (non-competitive)	United Biotech Inc	213
Antibody detection	Immunofluorescence assay (indirect)	Incstar	213
Antibody detection (IgG)	Immunofluorescence assay (indirect)	Bion Enterprises Ltd	214
Antibody detection (IgG)	Immunofluorescence assay (indirect)	Biowhittaker	214
Antibody detection (IgG)	Immunofluorescence assay (indirect)	Gen Bio	215
Antibody detection (IgG)	Immunofluorescence assay (indirect)	Schiapparelli Biosystems Inc	215
Antibody detection (IgG)	Immunofluorescence assay (indirect)	Zeus Scientific Inc	216
Antibody detection (IgM)	Immunofluorescence assay (indirect)	Gen Bio	216

Herpes simplex virus (HSV-1 and HSV-2)
page

Antigen detection	Immunofluorescence assay (direct)	Baxter Diagnostics Inc (Bartels Division)	217

Antigen detection	Immunofluorescence assay (direct)	Dako A/S	217
Antigen detection	Immunofluorescence assay (direct)	Syva Company	218
Antigen detection	Immunofluorescence assay (direct)	Syva Company	218
Antibody detection (IgG)	EIA (non-competitive)	Biowhittaker	219
Antibody detection (IgG)	EIA (non-competitive)	Biowhittaker	219
Antibody detection (IgG)	EIA (non-competitive)	Zeus Scientific Inc	220
Antibody detection (IgM)	EIA (non-competitive)	Zeus Scientific Inc	220

Herpes simplex virus (HSV-2)
page

Antigen detection	EIA (non-competitive)	Bio-Stat Diagnostics	221
Antibody detection (IgG)	EIA (non-competitive)	Baxter Diagnostics Inc (Bartels Division)	221
Antibody detection (IgG)	EIA (non-competitive)	Bio-Stat Diagnostics	222
Antibody detection (IgG)	EIA (non-competitive)	Biologische Analysensystem GmbH	222
Antibody detection (IgG)	EIA (non-competitive)	Cambridge Biotech Corporation	223
Antibody detection (IgG)	EIA (non-competitive)	Chimica Diagnostica	223
Antibody detection (IgG)	EIA (non-competitive)	Diamedix Corporation	224
Antibody detection (IgG)	EIA (non-competitive)	E. Merck	224
Antibody detection (IgG)	EIA (non-competitive)	Eurogenetics	225
Antibody detection (IgG)	EIA (non-competitive)	Gamma SA	225
Antibody detection (IgG)	EIA (non-competitive)	Gull Laboratories	226
Antibody detection (IgG)	EIA (non-competitive)	Human GmbH	226
Antibody detection (IgG)	EIA (non-competitive)	Immunobiological Laboratories	227
Antibody detection (IgG)	EIA (non-competitive)	Incstar	227
Antibody detection (IgG)	EIA (non-competitive)	International Immunodiagnostics	228
Antibody detection (IgG)	EIA (non-competitive)	Melja Diagnostik GmbH	228
Antibody detection (IgG)	EIA (non-competitive)	Melotec S.A.	229
Antibody detection (IgG)	EIA (non-competitive)	Radim	229
Antibody detection (IgG)	EIA (non-competitive)	Schiapparelli Biosystems Inc	230
Antibody detection (IgG)	EIA (non-competitive)	Sigma Diagnostics	230
Antibody detection (IgG)	EIA (non-competitive)	United Biotech Inc	231
Antibody detection (IgM)	EIA (non-competitive)	Biologische Analysensystem GmbH	231
Antibody detection (IgM)	EIA (non-competitive)	Cambridge Biotech Corporation	232
Antibody detection (IgM)	EIA (non-competitive)	Chimica Diagnostica	232
Antibody detection (IgM)	EIA (non-competitive)	Gull Laboratories	233
Antibody detection (IgM)	EIA (non-competitive)	Immunobiological Laboratories	233
Antibody detection (IgM)	EIA (non-competitive)	International Immunodiagnostics	234
Antibody detection (IgM)	EIA (non-competitive)	Melja Diagnostik GmbH	234
Antibody detection (IgM)	EIA (non-competitive)	Melotec S.A.	235
Antibody detection (IgM)	EIA (non-competitive)	United Biotech Inc	235
Antibody detection	Immunofluorescence assay (indirect)	Incstar	236
Antibody detection (IgG)	Immunofluorescence assay (indirect)	Bion Enterprises Ltd	236
Antibody detection (IgG)	Immunofluorescence assay (indirect)	Gen Bio	237
Antibody detection (IgG)	Immunofluorescence assay (indirect)	Schiapparelli Biosystems Inc	237
Antibody detection (IgG)	Immunofluorescence assay (indirect)	Zeus Scientific Inc	238
Antibody detection (IgM)	Immunofluorescence assay (indirect)	Gen Bio	238

Human immunodeficiency virus
page

Antigen detection	EIA (non-competitive)	Innogenetics SA	240
Antibody detection	EIA (competitive)	Organon Teknika NV	240
Antibody detection	EIA (non-competitive)	Abbott Laboratories	241
Antibody detection	EIA (non-competitive)	Behringwerke AG	241
Antibody detection	EIA (non-competitive)	Cambridge Biotech Corporation	242
Antibody detection	EIA (non-competitive)	Genetic Systems Corporation/Sanofi Diagnostics Pasteur	242
Antibody detection	EIA (non-competitive, amplified)	Murex Diagnostics Limited	243

Human immunodeficiency virus (HIV-1)

Human immunodeficiency virus (HIV-1 and HIV-2)

Human immunodeficiency virus (HIV-2)

Chlamydia trachomatis serovars D-K (oculogenital chlamydial infection)

Natural history

Chlamydia are obligate intracellular bacteria depending on eukaryotic cells for energy and replicating within endosomal vacuoles (inclusion bodies). The species *C. trachomatis* is a cause of ocular and genital tract infections. Serovars A-C cause blinding trachoma, serovars L_1-L_3 cause the sexually-transmitted condition lymphogranuloma venereum; both diseases are seldom encountered in the West. Serovars D-K infect columnar and transitional epithelial cells, causing the commonest of all sexually-transmitted infections. Urethritis in males, cervicitis or occasionally urethritis in females are presenting features, however many infections are asymptomatic and likely to go untreated unless specifically sought in at-risk groups/contacts. Complications are related to persistence, reinfections and hypersensitivity; upper genital tract disease (pelvic inflammatory disease) is common in untreated cases, and scarring can lead to infertility or ectopic pregnancy; acute epididymitis and reactive arthritis are also found. Half the neonates exposed to genital chlamydia at birth develop conjunctivitis approximately 5–12 days later; a pneumonitis may follow. Acute follicular conjunctivitis caused by *C. trachomatis* D-K is quite common in the sexually active young adult. Another species, *C. pneumoniae*, is a common cause of human respiratory tract infection. psittaci of avian origin occasionally infects humans, and rarely systemic infection with ovine *C. psittaci* causes abortion in women.

Diagnosis and markers

Isolation of *C. trachomatis* has been the gold standard for detection, but is not 100% sensitive in all conditions. Isolation is however dependent on cell culture and is not widely available. Detection of chlamydial ribosomal RNA is used increasingly, but nucleic acid amplification by PCR is the most sensitive method. Immunofluorescence (IF) is used for direct detection; an experienced observer can detect 2–5 chlamydia elementary bodies (EBs) in cellular smears or in centrifuged deposit from samples, using fluorescent-labelled monoclonal antibody. Antibody may be genus-specific, detecting common lipopolysaccharide (LPS), or specific for *C. trachomatis* major outer membrane protein (MOMP). Enzyme immuno-assays for antigen are suitable for batch testing and are less subjective than IF; however confirmation of reactive samples with a blocking (neutralisation) assay or IF is advised. Assays detecting LPS are more sensitive than those for EBs since free LPS is also measured. Chlamydial serology has been largely based on indirect immunofluorescence. Methods using whole inclusion bodies (WIF) detect predominantly genus-specific and some species-specific antibody, whilst microimmunofluorescence (MIF) based on dots of EBs can reveal antibody to different species and groups of serovars. Expertise in reading and interpretation of the results is required. EIAs based on infected cells or EB preparations as antigen detect cross-reacting antibodies. Recombinant or synthetic antigen based assays have been used experimentally, and chlamydia-specific rLPS based assays are now available. Serology is not appropriate for diagnosis of acute lower genital tract infections, when the organism should be identified; its place lies in the investigation of complications.

Comment

Antigen or nucleic acid detection will reveal non-viable organisms. For the male patient, a less invasive sampling method than endourethral swabbing is welcomed. Urine samples ("first catch") have proved useful, with the centrifuged deposit being examined by IF or EIA.

Reference

Centers for Disease Control. Recommendations for the prevention and management of *Chlamydia trachomatis* infection. Morbidity and Mortality Weekly Reports. 1993;42(RR-12):1–36.

© KLUWER ACADEMIC PUBLISHERS 1994, ISSN 1381-5067

Chlamydia trachomatis
ANTIGEN DETECTION

Manufacturer: Abbott Laboratories
Cat. No./Trade name: 1803/CHLAMYDIAZYME®
Diagnostic Kit

SUMMARY

[Bead-Chlamydiazyme]–**Ag**–[Ab]–[ARIgG-HRP]–[OPD]–
A_{492}

Assay type: EIA (non-competitive)
Detection: Colorimetric A_{492}
Format: Reaction well, CHLAMYDIAZYME® coated bead
Sample type: Swabs: urethral (male), endocervical,
    conjunctival and nasopharyngeal (neonates)
Sample pre-treatment:
    Swabs: Swab + 1 ml diluent (10-15 min); vortex
    Urine: Centrifuge 20 ml; pellet + 1 ml diluent; vortex
Sample volume: 200 µl of treated sample
Number of tests: 100, 500
Controls - standards run in assay:
    Controls: Neg (3), Pos (1)
Incubation:
    1 hr (37°C) + 1 hr (37°C) + 1 hr (37°C) + 30 min (RT)
Washes: 3

CONTENTS

Antibodies, antigens, labelled components:
    CHLAMYDIAZYME® bound to bead
    Anti-C. trachomatis Ab (r)
    Anti-rabbit IgG Ab (g) HRP conjugated
Substrate: OPD, H_2O_2
Controls - standards supplied:
    Controls: Neg and Pos
Additional reagents:
    None
Special equipment required:
    None

INTERPRETATION

Comments on interpretation:
    Classification of results is according to cut-off; no further
        testing
    This assay can be used to determine a patient's
        response to antibiotic therapy
No. of references: 20

NOTES

110302.0

Use only STD-EZE (female), STD-PEN (male) swabs
    provided

Chlamydia trachomatis
ANTIGEN DETECTION

Manufacturer: Baxter Diagnostics Inc (Bartels Division)
Cat. No./Trade name: B1029-400/Chlamydia EIA Kit

SUMMARY

[Well-treated]–**Ag**–[Ab]–[AMIgG-HRP]–[TMB]–A_{450}

Assay type: EIA (non-competitive)
Detection: Colorimetric A_{450}
Format: Microtitre well, treated to bind Chlamydia antigen
Sample type: Swabs: urogenital and ocular in transport
    medium
Sample pre-treatment:
    Vortex, heat 10 min (100°C), cool, revortex before testing
Sample volume: 200 µl of extracted specimen
Number of tests: 96
Controls - standards run in assay:
    Controls: Neg (2), Pos (1)
Incubation:
    1 hr (37°C) + 20 min (RT)
Washes: 1

CONTENTS

Antibodies, antigens, labelled components:
    Microtitre wells treated to bind Chlamydia antigen*
    Anti-C. trachomatis LPS Ab (m)
    Anti-murine IgG Ab (sh) HRP conjugated
Substrate: TMB, H_2O_2
Controls - standards supplied:
    Controls: Neg and Pos
Additional reagents:
    Chlamydia EIA transport medium
Special equipment required:
    None

INTERPRETATION

Comments on interpretation:
    Classification of samples is according to cut-off; no
        further testing
No. of references: 6

NOTES

110568.0

*Treatment of microtitre wells not specified

Chlamydia (*C. trachomatis, C. psittaci, C. pneumoniae*)
ANTIGEN DETECTION

Manufacturer: Behringwerke AG
Cat. No./Trade name: OWUG/Enzygnost® Chlamydia (Ag)

SUMMARY

[Well-treated]–**Ag**–[MAb]–[AMIgG-HRP]–[TMB]–A_{450}

Assay type: EIA (non-competitive)
Detection: Colorimetric A_{450}
Format: Microtitre well, pre-treated to bind Chlamydia
Sample type: Male urethral, female endocervical and ophthalmic specimens
Sample pre-treatment:
    Boil (10 min)
Sample volume: 200 µl
Number of tests: 96
Controls - standards run in assay:
    Controls: Neg (2), Pos (1)
Incubation:
    1 hr (37°C) + 20 min (RT)
Washes: 1

CONTENTS

Antibodies, antigens, labelled components:
    Anti-chlamydia MAb (m)
    Anti-murine IgG (sh) HRP conjugated
Substrate: TMB, H_2O_2
Controls - standards supplied:
    Controls: Neg (transport medium) and Pos
Additional reagents:
    Sample collection and transport kit
Special equipment required:
    Behring ELISA processor (optional)

INTERPRETATION

Comments on interpretation:
    Equivocal: within cut-off and cut-off + 0.05 absorbance units; retest to confirm
No. of references: 0

NOTES

110458.0

Chlamydia
ANTIGEN DETECTION

Manufacturer: bioMerieux
Cat. No./Trade name: 30101/VIDAS CHLAMYDIA (CHL)

SUMMARY

[Solid phase]–**Ag**–[MAb]–[AMIg-AP]–[4-MP]–
fluorescence

Assay type: EIA (non-competitive)
Detection: Fluorometric
Format: Solid phase receptacle (SPR), and reagent strip
Sample type: Endocervical and male urethral swabs, male urine*
Sample pre-treatment:
    Boil sample with treatment reagent 15-30 min
Sample volume: 350 µl minimum
Number of tests: 60
Controls - standards run in assay:
    Controls: Neg (1), Pos (1)
    Standard: (1)
Incubation:
    Automated - total time 2 hr
Washes: Automated

CONTENTS

Antibodies, antigens, labelled components:
    Anti-chlamydia MAb (m)
    Anti-murine Ig PAb (g) AP conjugated
Substrate: 4-MP
Controls - standards supplied:
    Controls: Neg (buffer) and Pos (Ag)
    Standard: Buffer
Additional reagents:
    VIDAS Chlamydia collection kit
Special equipment required:
    Vitek Immunodiagnostic assay system (VIDAS)

INTERPRETATION

Comments on interpretation:
    Sample reactivity is calculated automatically and classification is according to cut-off
    Equivocal: retest to confirm
    Invalid: retest original or fresh specimen
No. of references: 0

NOTES

110480.0

*Use VIDAS Chlamydia specimen collection kit (30515)

Chlamydia trachomatis (and C. psittaci)
ANTIGEN DETECTION

Manufacturer: Boule Diagnostics AB
Cat. No./Trade name: 10-9142-12/Phadebact® Chlamydia EIA

SUMMARY

[Well-treated]–**Ag**–[Mab-AP]–[PNP]–A_{405}

Assay type: EIA (non-competitive)
Detection: Colorimetric A_{405}
Format: Microtitre well, able to absorb Chlamydia antigen
Sample type: Swabs: endocervical, urethral
Sample pre-treatment:
    Add diluent to tube, incubate 10-15 min (RT), vortex (1 min), boil 10-15 min, cool, re-vortex
Sample volume: 100 µl of prepared sample
Number of tests: 96
Controls - standards run in assay:
    Controls: Neg (3), Pos (1)
Incubation:
    30 min (37°C) + 45 min (37°C) + 1 hr (37°C)
Washes: 1

CONTENTS

Antibodies, antigens, labelled components:
    Microtitre wells able to absorb Chlamydia antigens*
    Anti-Chlamydia trachomatis MAb (m) AP conjugated
Substrate: PNP
Controls - standards supplied:
    Controls: Neg, Pos (inactivated Chlamydia organisms)
Additional reagents:
    None
Special equipment required:
    Phadebact® Chlamydia EIA Urethra and Phadebact® Chlamydia EIA Cervix Collection Kits

INTERPRETATION

Comments on interpretation:
    Classification of samples is according to cut-off; no further testing
No. of references: 7

NOTES

110565.0

*Treatment of wells not specified

Chlamydia trachomatis
ANTIGEN DETECTION

Manufacturer: Cellabs Pty Ltd
Cat. No./Trade name: /CHLAMYDIA CELISA

SUMMARY

[Well-treated]–**Ag**–[MAb]–[AMIg-HRP]–[TMB]–A_{450}

Assay type: EIA (non-competitive)
Detection: Colorimetric A_{450}
Format: Microtitre well, treated to bind to Chlamydia LPS Ag
Sample type: Swabs: male urethra, cervical, first void male urine in CELISA transport medium
Sample pre-treatment:
    Vortex, remove swab, boil (15 min), revortex before testing
Sample volume: 100 µl
Number of tests: 96
Controls - standards run in assay:
    Controls: Neg (2), Pos (1)
Incubation:
    30 min (37°C) + 30 min (37°C) + 30 min (37°C) + 10 min (RT)
Washes: 2

CONTENTS

Antibodies, antigens, labelled components:
    Microtitre well treated to bind Chlamydia LPS Ag
    Anti-Chlamydia LPS MAb (m)
    Anti-murine Ig HRP conjugated
Substrate: TMB
Controls - standards supplied:
    Controls: Neg and Pos
Additional reagents:
    None
Special equipment required:
    Chlamydia CELISA specimen transport medium vials

INTERPRETATION

Comments on interpretation:
    Equivocal: between cut-off and Neg control mean x 3; retest (sample to be boiled again)
    Positive results can be verified using slide preparation and chlamydia IF test reagent (included in kit)
No. of references: 6

NOTES

110140.0

Chlamydia trachomatis
ANTIGEN DETECTION

Manufacturer: Dako A/S
Cat. No./Trade name: K6001/IDEIA® Chlamydia

SUMMARY

[Well-MAb]–**Ag**–[MAb-AP]–[NADP + ampl]–A_{492}

Assay type: EIA (non-competitive, amplified)
Detection: Colorimetric A_{492}
Format: Microtitre well, Ab coated
Sample type: Swabs (+1 ml transport medium); male urethral, endocervix, ophthalmic; male urine
Sample pre-treatment:
  Swabs: vortex (15 sec); boil (15 min); cool; vortex (15 sec)
  Urine: centrifuge; resuspend deposit in 1 ml transport medium, vortex (15 sec); boil (15 min); cool; vortex (15 sec)
Sample volume: 200 µl
Number of tests: 96, 192
Controls - standards run in assay:
  Controls: Neg (3), Pos (1)
Incubation:
  Standard: 2 hr (RT) + 1 hr (RT) + 40 min (RT) + 10 min (RT)
  Overnight: 16 hr (RT) + 1 hr (RT) + 40 min (RT) + 10 min (RT)
  Rapid: 1 hr (37°C) + 20 min (37°C) + 10 min (37°C)*
Washes: 1

CONTENTS

Antibodies, antigens, labelled components:
  Anti-Chlamydia MAb bound to well
  Anti-Chlamydia MAb (Fab') AP conjugated
Substrate: NADP + amplifier
Controls - standards supplied:
  Controls: Neg and Pos
Additional reagents:
  None
Special equipment required:
  Chlamydia Specimen Collection Kit (optional)

INTERPRETATION

Comments on interpretation:
  Equivocal: within cut-off ±0.015; retest or test fresh sample
  IDEIA Chlamydia Confirmatory Test may be used to confirm reactive samples
  Visual interpretation is possible
No. of references: 13

NOTES

110002.0

*All incubation procedures are of equivalent performance
All 37°C incubations performed with shaking

Chlamydia trachomatis*
ANTIGEN DETECTION

Manufacturer: International Mycoplasma
Cat. No./Trade name: 11060/CHLAMYFAST®

SUMMARY

[Membrane-treated]–**Ag**–[MAb-POD]–[substrate]–
red spot

Assay type: EIA (non-competitive)
Detection: Visual
Format: Test cell, membrane treated to bind chlamydia LPS
Sample type: Endocervical, urethral and ophthalmic swabs; urine
Sample pre-treatment:
  Sample extraction (4 min)
Sample volume: Not specified
Number of tests:
Controls - standards run in assay:
  Controls: Neg integral (1), Pos integral (1)
Incubation:
  2 min (RT) + 3 min (RT)
Washes: 2

CONTENTS

Antibodies, antigens, labelled components:
  Membrane treated to bind chlamydia LPS
  Anti-chlamydia LPS MAb POD conjugated
Substrate: Not specified
Controls - standards supplied:
  Controls: Neg and Pos (integral controls bound to membrane)
Additional reagents:
  None
Special equipment required:
  Workstation (Cat no. 11901) (optional)

INTERPRETATION

Comments on interpretation:
  Positive: pink/red colour in test well on membrane.
    Further details not specified
No. of references: 4

NOTES

110673.0

*This kit also detects C. pneumoniae (TWAR strain) and C. psittaci and is not specific for C. trachomatis

Chlamydia trachomatis
ANTIGEN DETECTION

Manufacturer: Kodak Clinical Diagnostics
Cat. No./Trade name: 193 7804/KODAK SURECELL® Chlamydia Test Kit

SUMMARY

[Membrane-treated]–**Ag**–[MAb-HRP]–[dye]–pink dot

Assay type: EIA (non-competitive)
Detection: Visual
Format: Test cell, membrane treated to bind Chlamydia Ag
Sample type: Swabs* (cervical, urethral, ocular), male urine cervical cytology brush
Sample pre-treatment:
Sample extraction: tubes and reagents provided. Urine may require centrifugation
Sample volume: Not specified
Number of tests: 10, 25, 100
Controls - standards run in assay:
Controls: Neg (1), Integral Pos (1)
Incubation:
Read results 3 min after adding the final reagent (dye) to wells
Washes: 2

CONTENTS

Antibodies, antigens, labelled components:
Anti-Chlamydia MAb HRP conjugated
Substrate:
Controls - standards supplied:
Controls: Neg control conjugate, Integral Pos (Chlamydia Ag bound to membrane in Pos control well)
Additional reagents:
None
Special equipment required:
None

INTERPRETATION

Comments on interpretation:
Negative: colour in sample well equal to colour in Neg control well
Positive: red/pink colour in the sample well greater than the colour in the Neg control well
Invalid: strong red/pink colour in Neg control well and sample well or no colour in Pos control well; repeat test
No. of references: None

NOTES

110661.0

*It is preferable to use special swabs provided. Do not use calcium alginate swabs

Chlamydia trachomatis
ANTIGEN DETECTION

Manufacturer: Labsystems Oy
Cat. No./Trade name: 61 08 350/CHLAMYDIA AG EIA KIT

SUMMARY

[Well-treated]–**Ag**–[MAb-HRP]–[TMB]–A_{450}

Assay type: EIA (non-competitive)
Detection: Colorimetric A_{450}
Format: Microtitre well, treated to bind Chlamydia LPS
Sample type: Urethral and endocervical swabs
Sample pre-treatment:
Vortex, heat 15 min (95-100°C), cool, revortex before use
Sample volume: 200 µl
Number of tests: 96
Controls - standards run in assay:
Controls: Neg (3), Pos (2)
Incubation:
1 hr (37°C) + 1 hr (37°C) + 30 min (RT)
Washes: 1

CONTENTS

Antibodies, antigens, labelled components:
Anti-chlamydial LPS MAb HRP conjugated
Substrate: TMB, H_2O_2
Controls - standards supplied:
Controls: Neg (transport medium), Pos (C. trachomatis)
Additional reagents:
H_2SO_4
Special equipment required:
LABSYSTEMS Chlamydia Ag Specimen Collection Kit (Cat no. 60 00 035)
Auto-EIA II Analyzer (optional)

INTERPRETATION

Comments on interpretation:
Classification of samples is according to cut-off; no further testing
No. of references: 8

NOTES

110535.0

Chlamydia trachomatis
ANTIGEN DETECTION

Manufacturer: Mast Diagnostics Ltd
Cat. No./Trade name: /MASTAZYME® Chlamydia

SUMMARY

[Well-treated]–Ag–[Ab-HRP]–[TMB]–A_{450}

Assay type: EIA (non-competitive)
Detection: Colorimetric A_{450}
Format: Microtitre well, treated to bind Chlamydia Ag
Sample type: Swabs: urogenital in transport medium vial
Sample pre-treatment:
  Boil (10 min)
Sample volume:
Number of tests: 96
Controls - standards run in assay:
  Controls: Neg (1), Pos (1)
Incubation:
  1 hr (37°C) + 20 min (RT)
Washes: 1

CONTENTS

Antibodies, antigens, labelled components:
  Microtitre well treated to bind Chlamydia Ag
  Anti-Chlamydia trachomatis LPS MAb (m) HRP
    conjugated
Substrate: TMB
Controls - standards supplied:
  Controls: Neg and Pos
Additional reagents:
  None
Special equipment required:
  None

INTERPRETATION

Comments on interpretation:
  Classification of sample is according to cut-off; no further
    testing
No. of references: 0

NOTES

110324.0

Swabs must be Dacron® tipped and wooden shafts avoided
Transport medium vial provided

Chlamydia trachomatis
ANTIGEN DETECTION

Manufacturer: Murex Diagnostics Limited
Cat. No./Trade name: WZ04/Wellcozyme Chlamydia

SUMMARY

[Well-MAb]–Ag–[MAb-AP]–[NADP–ampl]–A_{492}

Assay type: EIA (non-competitive, amplified)
Detection: Colorimetric A_{492}
Format: Microtitre well, Ab coated
Sample type: Swabs: (urethra, endocervical)
Sample pre-treatment:
  Swabs: add extraction buffer, vortex (15 sec), boil to
    release antigen (4 min), cool, vortex (10 sec)
Sample volume: 150 µl
Number of tests: 96
Controls - standards run in assay:
  Controls: Neg (3), Pos (2)
Incubation:
  2 hr (37°C) + 30 min (37°C) + 10 min (RT)
Washes: 1

CONTENTS

Antibodies, antigens, labelled components:
  Anti-Chlamydia LPS MAb (m) bound to well
  Anti-Chlamydia LPS MAb (m) AP conjugated
Substrate: NADP + amplifier
Controls - standards supplied:
  Controls: Neg (diluted extraction buffer) and Pos
Additional reagents:
  H_2SO_4
Special equipment required:
  Chlamydia specimen collection kit (optional)
  Wellcozyme microwell plate washing system (optional)
  Wellcozyme microwell plate reader system (optional)

INTERPRETATION

Comments on interpretation:
  Neg and Pos samples are classified according to cut-off
    but where sample OD lies within cut-off and cut-off
    +0.4; retest or confirm using Wellcozyme Chlamydia
    neutralization test
No. of references: 6

NOTES

110173.0

Chlamydia (C. trachomatis, C. psittaci, C. pneumoniae)
ANTIGEN DETECTION

Manufacturer: Sanofi Diagnostics Pasteur
Cat. No./Trade name: 31003/PATHFINDER® CHLAMYDIA MICROPLATE

SUMMARY

[Well-Ab]–**Ag**–[Ab]–[Ab-HRP]–[OPD]–$A_{492/620}$

Assay type: EIA (non-competitive)
Detection: Colorimetric $A_{492/620}$
Format: Microtitre well, Ab coated
Sample type: Swabs: (urethral, cervical); endocervical brush specimens*
Sample pre-treatment:
   Sample extraction (10 min incubation)
Sample volume: 100 µl
Number of tests: 96
Controls - standards run in assay:
   Controls: Neg (3), Pos (1)
Incubation:
   a) 1 hr (RT) + 1 hr (RT) + 1 hr (RT) + 30 min (RT)
   b) 30 min (26°C) + 30 min (26°C) + 30 min (26°C) all in shaker-incubator + 30 min (RT)
Washes: 1

CONTENTS

Antibodies, antigens, labelled components:
   Anti-chlamydia MAb (m) bound to well
   Anti-chlamydia PAb
   PAb HRP conjugated (non-specified)
Substrate: OPD
Controls - standards supplied:
   Controls: Neg and Pos
Additional reagents:
   None
Special equipment required:
   None

INTERPRETATION

Comments on interpretation:
   Classification of samples is according to cut-off; no further testing
No. of references: 21

NOTES

110258.0

*Collection kits available

Chlamydia trachomatis*
ANTIGEN DETECTION

Manufacturer: Shield Diagnostics
Cat. No./Trade name: FCHL/100/AntigEnz Chlamydia

SUMMARY

[Well-treated]–**Ag**–[MAb]–[AMIgG-HRP]–[TMB]–A_{450}

Assay type: EIA (non-competitive)
Detection: Colorimetric A_{450}
Format: Microtitre well, treated to bind Chlamydia LPS Ag
Sample type: Swabs: endocervical, male urethra, ophthalmic in transport medium; male urine
Sample pre-treatment:
   Swabs: vortex, heat 10 min (100°C), cool
   Male urine: vortex, centrifuge 20 min, resuspend in transport medium, vortex, heat 10 min (100°C), cool
Sample volume: 200 µl of extract
Number of tests: 96
Controls - standards run in assay:
   Controls: Neg (2), Pos (1)
Incubation:
   1 hr (37°C) + 20 min (RT)
Washes: 1

CONTENTS

Antibodies, antigens, labelled components:
   Microtitre well treated to bind Chlamydia (LPS)
   Anti-Chlamydia MAb (m)
   Anti-murine IgG Ab (s) HRP conjugated
Substrate: TMB
Controls - standards supplied:
   Controls: Neg and Pos
Additional reagents:
   None
Special equipment required:
   Female endocervical swabs (Cat. no. E512)
   Male urethral swabs (Cat. no. E511)

INTERPRETATION

Comments on interpretation:
   Grey zone: within cut-off and cut-off + 0.05; retest or confirm with AntigEnz Chlamydia Confirmatory Test (Cat. no. FCHL300)
   Positive: > cut-off + 0.05 and confirmed by AntigEnz Chlamydia Confirmatory Test
No. of references: 6

NOTES

110668.0

*This assay does not differentiate between C. trachomatis, C. psittaci and C. pneumoniae

Chlamydia trachomatis
ANTIGEN DETECTION

Manufacturer: Sigma Diagnostics
Cat. No./Trade name: SIA 115-A/SIA Chlamydia kit

SUMMARY

[Well-MAb]–**Ag**–[Ab]–[ARIgG-HRP]–[OPD]–A_{492}

Assay type: EIA (non-competitive)
Detection: Colorimetric A_{492}
Format: Microtitre well, Ab coated
Sample type: Swabs: (male urethral; endocervical)
Sample pre-treatment:
    Sample swab extraction (10 minutes)
Sample volume: 100 µl
Number of tests: 96
Controls - standards run in assay:
    Controls: Neg (3), Pos (1)
Incubation:
    1 hr (RT) + 1 hr (RT) + 1 hr (RT) + 30 min (RT)
Washes: 1

CONTENTS

Antibodies, antigens, labelled components:
    Anti-C. trachomatis MAb (m) bound to well
    Anti-C. trachomatis PAb (r)
    Anti-rabbit IgG PAb (g) HRP conjugated
Substrate: OPD; H_2O_2
Controls - standards supplied:
    Controls: Neg and Pos
Additional reagents:
    None
Special equipment required:
    Sigma Diagnostics collection swab pack
    Sigma EIA microwell or strip reader (optional)

INTERPRETATION

Comments on interpretation:
    Sample reactivity is calculated automatically and
        classification is according to cut-off; no further testing
No. of references: 18

NOTES

110117.0

Chlamydia trachomatis
ANTIGEN DETECTION

Manufacturer: Syva Company
Cat. No./Trade name: 8H709UL/MicroTrak® II
Chlamydia EIA

SUMMARY

[Well-treated]–**Ag**–[Ab]–[ARIgG-HRP]–[TMB]–$A_{450/630}$

Assay type: EIA (non-competitive)
Detection: Colorimetric $A_{450/630}$
Format: Microtitre well
Sample type: Swabs: (male urethral, endocervical,
    conjunctival); urine (males)
Sample pre-treatment:
    Extract swabs or urine pellet with specimen treatment
        solution (15 min, 100°C)
Sample volume: 100 µl
Number of tests: 96
Controls - standards run in assay:
    Controls: Neg (3), Pos (1)
Incubation:
    1 hr 30 min (37°C) + 30 min (37°C) + 30 min (37°C)
Washes: 2

CONTENTS

Antibodies, antigens, labelled components:
    Anti-C. trachomatis LPS PAb (r)
    Anti-rabbit IgG PAb (g) HRP conjugated
Substrate: TMB, H_2O_2
Controls - standards supplied:
    Controls: Neg, Pos (elementary bodies)
Additional reagents:
    MicroTrak® II EIA universal reagents (8K209UL)
Special equipment required:
    Syva MicroTrak® Chlamydia EIA specimen collection kit
    MicroTrak® EIA 96-well dry bath system, autowasher,
        autoreader
    Syva Microtrack® XL system

INTERPRETATION

Comments on interpretation:
    Positive: ≥ cut-off and confirmed by cell culture or
        fluorescent antibody staining
No. of references: 17

NOTES

110054.0

© KLUWER ACADEMIC PUBLISHERS 1994, ISSN 1381-5067

Chlamydia trachomatis
ANTIGEN DETECTION

Manufacturer: Chembio Diagnostic Systems Inc
Cat. No./Trade name: CH101/Chlamydia STAT-PAK

SUMMARY

[Membrane-Ab]–**Ag**–[MAb-gold]–rose band

Assay type: Immunochromatographic assay
Detection: Visual
Format: Testcard, Ab coated membrane
Sample type: Swabs: endocervical, urethral; male urine
Sample pre-treatment:
   Swab: immerse swab in extraction reagent, incubate RT (10-15 min)
   Urine: centrifuge, resuspend sediment in extraction reagent
Sample volume: 7 drops of extract
Number of tests: 20, 40
Controls - standards run in assay:
   Controls: Neg (1), Pos (1)*
   Integral control (1)
Incubation:
   Read results 10-20 min after adding extract to sample window of test card
Washes:

CONTENTS

Antibodies, antigens, labelled components:
   Anti-Chlamydia (LPS) PAb (r) bound to membrane (test well)
   Anti-Chlamydia (LPS) MAb (m) colloidal gold labelled (absorbent pad)
   Anti-murine Ab (g) (control well)
Substrate:
Controls - standards supplied:
   Controls: Pos
Additional reagents:
   None
Special equipment required:
   Chembio workstation (optional)

INTERPRETATION

Comments on interpretation:
   Negative: rose coloured band in control well, and no rose coloured band in test well
   Positive: rose coloured band in control well and distinct rose coloured band in test well
   Inconclusive: no rose coloured band in control well. Test a fresh specimen or repeat if present specimen less than 1 hr old
No. of references: 5

NOTES

110601.0

*Run controls at least once per day using the Pos control provided and a sterile swab for the Neg control

Chlamydia trachomatis
ANTIGEN DETECTION

Manufacturer: Savyon Diagnostics Ltd
Cat. No./Trade name: CHLAMYDIA MEMBRANE TEST

SUMMARY

[Membrane-Ab]–**Ag**–[MAb-gold]–pink line

Assay type: Immunochromatographic assay
Detection: Visual
Format: Test slide unit, Ab coated membrane
Sample type: Swabs: endocervical, urethral*, male urine
Sample pre-treatment:
   Extraction of swab with reagents provided, incubate 10-15 min (RT)
   Urine: centrifuge, resuspend sediment in extraction solution
Sample volume: 7 drops of extracted material
Number of tests: 20
Controls - standards run in assay:
   Batch controls: Pos (1)
   Integral reagent control (1)
Incubation:
   Result read 10-20 min after addition of patient sample to slide unit
Washes: NA

CONTENTS

Antibodies, antigens, labelled components:
   Anti-chlamydia PAb bound to membrane (test window)
   Anti-murine Ig Ab (g) bound to membrane (reagent control window)
   Anti-chlamydia MAb colloidal gold labelled (in absorbent pad)
Substrate:
Controls - standards supplied:
   Controls: Pos
   Integral reagent control bound to membrane
Additional reagents:
   None
Special equipment required:
   None

INTERPRETATION

Comments on interpretation:
   Negative: pink line in control window, no line in test window
   Inconclusive: no line in control window; repeat with fresh unit using same or fresh sample
   Positive: pink line in control window and test window
No. of references: 5

NOTES

110358.0

*Special swabs and transport tubes provided with kit

© KLUWER ACADEMIC PUBLISHERS 1994, ISSN 1381-5067

Chlamydia trachomatis
ANTIGEN DETECTION

Manufacturer: Unipath Limited
Cat. No./Trade name: /CLEARVIEW CHLAMYDIA

SUMMARY

[Unit-latex-MAb]–**Ag**–[MAb-detector]–visible line

Assay type: Immunochromatographic assay
Detection: Visual
Format: Test unit, latex particle Ab coated
Sample type: Endocervical swab
Sample pre-treatment:
  Heat swabs with extraction buffer for 10-15 min (80°C)
Sample volume: 5 drops of extracted volume
Number of tests: 20
Controls - standards run in assay:
  Controls: Neg (1), Pos (1)
  Integral reagent control: (1)
Incubation:
  Read test 15 min after adding extracted suspension to sample window (strong Pos may give quicker result)
Washes: 0

CONTENTS

Antibodies, antigens, labelled components:
  Anti-Chlamydia LPS MAb (m) bound to latex (sample window)
  Anti-murine Ab (r) (control window)
  Anti-Chlamydia LPS MAb (m) detector conjugated (result window)
Substrate:
Controls - standards supplied:
  Controls: Pos
  Integral reagent control bound to control window of test unit)
Additional reagents:
  Neg control: sterile clearview Chlamydia swab
Special equipment required:
  Clearview Chlamydia Female Specimen Collection Kit (120068)
  Clearview workstation (optional)

INTERPRETATION

Comments on interpretation:
  Negative: no line in result window and a line in control window. Confirm by culture if symptoms persist
  Positive: a line in result window and a line in control window
  Unsatisfactory: no line in control or result window; repeat with a fresh test unit
No. of references: 3

NOTES

110142.0

Chlamydia trachomatis
ANTIGEN DETECTION

Manufacturer: Baxter Diagnostics Inc (Bartels Division)
Cat. No./Trade name: B1029-84/Chlamydia Monoclonal FA Direct Smear Kit

SUMMARY

[Slide]–**Ag**–[MAb-FITC]–fluorescence

Assay type: Immunofluorescence assay (direct)
Detection: Visual
Format: Slide well
Sample type: Swabs: urethral, cervical
Sample pre-treatment:
  Apply swab to slide well, air dry, fix with acetone
Sample volume: 1 swab
Number of tests: 100-150
Controls - standards run in assay:
  Controls: Neg (1), Pos (1)
Incubation:
  30 min (37°C)
Washes: 1

CONTENTS

Antibodies, antigens, labelled components:
  Anti-C. trachomatis LPS MAb (m) FITC conjugated
Substrate:
Controls - standards supplied:
  Controls: Neg, Pos (Ag coated slides with Neg and Pos wells)
Additional reagents:
  None
Special equipment required:
  None

INTERPRETATION

Comments on interpretation:
  Negative: at least 3 columnar epithelial cells per field and no fluorescence
  Positive: bright green fluorescent elementary bodies or initial bodies
  Inadequate: less than 3 intact columnar cells per field and no fluorescence
No. of references: 3

NOTES

110567.0

Chlamydia trachomatis
ANTIGEN DETECTION

Manufacturer: Cellabs Pty Ltd
Cat. No./Trade name: /CHLAMYDIA-CEL IF TEST

SUMMARY

[Slide well]–**Ag**–[MAb-FITC]–fluorescence

Assay type: Immunofluorescence assay (direct)
Detection: Fluorescence microscopy
Format: Slide well
Sample type: Swabs: urethral (male), cervical, ocular, respiratory
Sample pre-treatment:
  Apply swabs to slide, dry, fix
Sample volume:
Number of tests: 50
Controls - standards run in assay:
  Controls: Pos (1)
Incubation:
  30 min (37°C)
Washes: 1

CONTENTS

Antibodies, antigens, labelled components:
  Anti-Chlamydia trachomatis MAb FITC conjugated
Substrate:
Controls - standards supplied:
  Controls: Pos (slide-fixed mammalian cells with elementary bodies and reticular bodies)
Additional reagents:
  Methanol
Special equipment required:
  None

INTERPRETATION

Comments on interpretation:
  Negative: at least 10 columnar cells and < 10 fluorescent chlamydial bodies
  Positive: ≥ 10 fluorescent chlamydial bodies
No. of references: 10

NOTES

110141.0

Chlamydia trachomatis
ANTIGEN DETECTION

Manufacturer: Dako A/S
Cat. No./Trade name: K6101/IMAGEN® Chlamydia

SUMMARY

[Slide well/monolayer]–**Ag**–[MAb-FITC]–fluorescence

Assay type: Immunofluorescence assay (direct)
Detection: Fluorescence microscopy
Format: Slide well
Sample type: Swabs: male urethra, cervix, conjunctiva; cell culture
Sample pre-treatment:
  Swabs: roll on slide, dry, fix
  Cell culture: drain fluid, fix monolayer
Sample volume:
Number of tests: 50
Controls - standards run in assay:
  Controls: Pos (1)
Incubation:
  15 min (37°C)
Washes: 1

CONTENTS

Antibodies, antigens, labelled components:
  Anti-chlamydia MAb (m) FITC conjugated
Substrate:
Controls - standards supplied:
  Controls: Pos (control slide x 2)
Additional reagents:
  Acetone
Special equipment required:
  Teflon coated microscope slides with wells
  IMAGEN® chlamydia collection kit (optional)

INTERPRETATION

Comments on interpretation:
  Clinical Specimens:
  Negative: counterstained cells and no fluorescent elementary bodies
  Positive: ≥ 10 fluorescent chlamydial elementary bodies
  Cell Culture:
  Positive: ≥ 1 fluorescent intracellular chlamydial inclusion
No. of references: 13

NOTES

110006.0

© *KLUWER ACADEMIC PUBLISHERS 1994, ISSN 1381-5067*

Chlamydia trachomatis
ANTIGEN DETECTION

Manufacturer: Orion Diagnostica
Cat. No./Trade name: 67255/CHLAMYSET® ANTIGEN FA

SUMMARY

[Slide]–**Ag**–[MAb-FITC]–fluorescence

Assay type: Immunofluorescence assay (direct)
Detection: Fluorescence microscopy
Format: Slide well
Sample type: Swabs: cervix, male urethra, ocular
Sample pre-treatment:
    Apply swabs to slide, dry, fix
Sample volume: 1 swab
Number of tests: 30
Controls - standards run in assay:
    Controls: reference slides: Neg (1), Pos (1)
Incubation:
    15 min (RT)
Washes: 1

CONTENTS

Antibodies, antigens, labelled components:
    Anti-Chlamydia trachomatis MAb (m) FITC conjugated
Substrate:
Controls - standards supplied:
    Controls: reference slides: Neg and Pos
Additional reagents:
    Methanol or acetone
Special equipment required:
    None

INTERPRETATION

Comments on interpretation:
    Negative: red stained cellular background, no bright
        green fluorescent elementary bodies
    Positive: ≥ 10 bright green fluorescent elementary
        bodies on a red stained cellular background
No. of references: 8

NOTES

110151.0

Chlamydia trachomatis
ANTIGEN DETECTION

Manufacturer: Shield Diagnostics
Cat. No./Trade name: FICH 100/DetectIF Chlamydia

SUMMARY

[Slide]–**Ag**–[Ab-FITC]–fluorescence

Assay type: Immunofluorescence assay (direct)
Detection: Fluorescence microscopy
Format: Slide
Sample type: Swabs: urethral, cervical, ophthalmic
Sample pre-treatment:
    Apply swabs to slide, fix with acetone
Sample volume: One swab
Number of tests: 60
Controls - standards run in assay:
    Controls: Neg (1), Pos (1)
Incubation:
    15 min (37°C)
Washes: 1

CONTENTS

Antibodies, antigens, labelled components:
    Anti-C. trachomatis Ab FITC conjugated
Substrate:
Controls - standards supplied:
    Controls: Neg and Pos (slides)
Additional reagents:
    None
Special equipment required:
    None

INTERPRETATION

Comments on interpretation:
    Negative: no fluorescence seen
    Positive: fluorescence seen
No. of references: None

NOTES

110580.0

Chlamydia trachomatis
ANTIGEN DETECTION

Manufacturer: Syva Company
Cat. No./Trade name: 8H019/MicroTrak® Chlamydia trachomatis culture confirmation test

SUMMARY

[Slide–**Ag**]–[MAb-FITC]–fluorescence

Assay type: Immunofluorescence assay (direct)
Detection: Fluorescence microscopy
Format: Slide well specimen coated
Sample type: Infected tissue culture cells
Sample pre-treatment:
  Ethanol fix monolayers (1-10 min)
Sample volume:
Number of tests: 85
Controls - standards run in assay:
  Controls: Neg (1), Pos (1)
Incubation:
  30 min (37°C)
Washes: 1

CONTENTS

Antibodies, antigens, labelled components:
  Anti-C. trachomatis MAb FITC conjugated
Substrate:
Controls - standards supplied:
  None
Additional reagents:
  Pos and Neg controls
Special equipment required:
  None

INTERPRETATION

Comments on interpretation:
  Positive: fluorescent staining of inclusion bodies
No. of references: 36

NOTES

110523.0

Chlamydia trachomatis
ANTIGEN DETECTION

Manufacturer: Syva Company
Cat. No./Trade name: 8H149/MicroTrak® Chlamydia trachomatis direct specimen test

SUMMARY

[Slide]–**Ag**–[MAb-FITC]–fluorescence

Assay type: Immunofluorescence assay (direct)
Detection: Fluorescence microscopy
Format: Slide well specimen coated
Sample type: Swabs: male urethral, endocervical, rectal, conjunctival, nasopharyngeal); cytobrush (endocervical)
Sample pre-treatment:
  Methanol fix air-dried smear (5 min)
Sample volume:
Number of tests: 60
Controls - standards run in assay:
  Controls: Neg (1), Pos (1)
Incubation:
  15 min (RT)
Washes: 1

CONTENTS

Antibodies, antigens, labelled components:
  Anti-C. trachomatis MAbs FITC conjugated
Substrate:
Controls - standards supplied:
  None
Additional reagents:
  Controls: Neg and Pos slides supplied separately (Cat. no. 8H199)
Special equipment required:
  Syva MicroTrak® Chlamydia trachomatis specimen collection kits (Cat. no. 8H169)

INTERPRETATION

Comments on interpretation:
  Positive: fluorescent staining of extra-cellular elementary bodies
No. of references: 44

NOTES

110524.0

© KLUWER ACADEMIC PUBLISHERS 1994, ISSN 1381-5067

Chlamydia trachomatis
ANTIBODY DETECTION

Manufacturer: Savyon Diagnostics Ltd
Cat. No./Trade name: 011-01-144/IPAzyme® Chlamydia

SUMMARY

[Slide-Ag]–**Ab**–[AHIgG/IgA-HRP]–[substrate]–blue
precipitate

Assay type: EIA (non-competitive)
Detection: Light microscopy
Format: Slide well, Ag coated
Sample type: Serum
Sample pre-treatment:
   None
Sample volume: IgG: 10 μl (of a 1:64 and 1:128 dilution)
   IgA: 10 μl (of a 1:16 dilution)
Number of tests: 144
Controls - standards run in assay:
   Controls: Neg (1), Pos IgG (1), Pos IgA (1)
Incubation:
   45 min (37°C) + 45 min (37°C) + 15 min (RT)
Washes: 3

CONTENTS

Antibodies, antigens, labelled components:
   C trachomatis Ag bound to slide well
   Anti-human IgG Ab (r) HRP conjugated
   Anti-human IgA Ab (r) HRP conjugated
Substrate: Not specified
Controls - standards supplied:
   Controls: Neg, Pos (for anti-Chlamydia IgG Ab) and Pos
      (for anti-Chlamydia IgA Ab) (human serum)
Additional reagents:
   None
Special equipment required:
   None

INTERPRETATION

Comments on interpretation:
   Negative: no blue precipitate in cells
   Positive: blue precipitate in infected cells
No. of references: 33

NOTES

110593.0

Chlamydia trachomatis
ANTIBODY DETECTION (IgA)

**Manufacturer: Biologische
Analysensytem GmbH**
Cat. No./Trade name: 5280/BAG - Chlamydia - EIA - A

SUMMARY

[Well-Ag]–**Ab**–[AHIgA-HRP]–[TMB]–A_{450}

Assay type: EIA (non-competitive)
Detection: Colorimetric A_{450}
Format: Microtitre well, Ag coated
Sample type: Serum
Sample pre-treatment:
   None
Sample volume: 10 μl (+ 1 ml diluent)
Number of tests: 96
Controls - standards run in assay:
   Controls: Neg (1), Cut-off (2), Pos (1)
Incubation:
   30 min (RT) + 30 min (RT) + 10 min (RT)
Washes: 2

CONTENTS

Antibodies, antigens, labelled components:
   Chlamydia trachomatis Ag bound to well
   Anti-human IgA Ab (sh) HRP conjugated
Substrate: TMB
Controls - standards supplied:
   Controls: Neg, Pos and Cut-off
Additional reagents:
   None
Special equipment required:
   None

INTERPRETATION

Comments on interpretation:
   Equivocal: within cut-off ± 10%; retest to confirm
No. of references: 0

NOTES

110643.0

© *KLUWER ACADEMIC PUBLISHERS 1994, ISSN 1381-5067*

Chlamydia trachomatis
ANTIBODY DETECTION (IgA)

Manufacturer: Eurogenetics
Cat. No./Trade name: /Eurogenetics® Chlamydia IgA ELISA

SUMMARY

$$[Well-Ag]-Ab-[AHIgA-POD]-[OPD]-A_{492}$$

Assay type: EIA (non-competitive)
Detection: Colorimetric A_{492}
Format: Microtitre well, Ag coated
Sample type: Serum
Sample pre-treatment:
    None
Sample volume: 100 µl of 1:300 dilution x 2
Number of tests: 96
Controls - standards run in assay:
    Controls: Neg (2), Pos (2)
Incubation:
    1 hr (37°C) + 30 min (37°C) + 20 min (RT)
Washes: 2 (+ preliminary plate wash)

CONTENTS

Antibodies, antigens, labelled components:
    Chlamydia Ag bound to wells
    Anti-human IgA Ab POD conjugated
Substrate: OPD, H_2O_2
Controls - standards supplied:
    Controls: Neg and Pos (human serum)
Additional reagents:
    None
Special equipment required:
    Eurogenetics Microtitre plate reader (or similar)

INTERPRETATION

Comments on interpretation:
    Equivocal: within cut-off + 0.1; retest a fresh sample
No. of references: 11

NOTES

110005.0

Chlamydia trachomatis
ANTIBODY DETECTION (IgA)

Manufacturer: Medac Diagnostika
Cat. No./Trade name: 490/Chlamydia IgA rELISA medac

SUMMARY

$$[Well-Ag]-Ab-[AHIgA-POD]-[ABTS]-A_{405}$$

Assay type: EIA (non-competitive)
Detection: Colorimetric A_{405}
Format: Microtitre well, Ag coated
Sample type: Serum
Sample pre-treatment:
    None
Sample volume: 10 µl (+490 µl diluent)*
Number of tests: 96
Controls - standards run in assay:
    Controls: Neg (2) and Pos (2)
Incubation:
    1 hr (37°C) + 1 hr (37°C) + 30 min (37°C)
Washes: 2 (+ preliminary plate wash)

CONTENTS

Antibodies, antigens, labelled components:
    rec Chlamydia LPS bound to well
    Anti-human IgA Ab POD conjugated
Substrate: ABTS, H_2O_2
Controls - standards supplied:
    Controls: Neg and Pos (serum)
Additional reagents:
    None
Special equipment required:
    None

INTERPRETATION

Comments on interpretation:
    Grey zone: within cut-off ± 10%; retest in parallel with a
        fresh specimen in 14 days
    Positive: > cut-off + 10%; interpret with reference to
        IgG, clinical picture and further diagnostic parameters
No. of references: 7

NOTES

110003.0

*Samples assayed in duplicate

© KLUWER ACADEMIC PUBLISHERS 1994, ISSN 1381-5067

Chlamydia
ANTIBODY DETECTION (IgA)

Manufacturer: Radim
Cat. No./Trade name: K4CA/CHLAMYDIA IgA EIA WELL

SUMMARY

[Well-Ag]–**Ab**–[AHIgA-HRP]–[TMB]–A_{450}

Assay type: EIA (non-competitive)
Detection: Colorimetric A_{450}
Format: Microtitre well, Ag coated
Sample type: Serum or plasma
Sample pre-treatment:
   None
Sample volume: 100 µl of 1:300 dilution x 2
Number of tests: 96
Controls - standards run in assay:
   Controls: Neg (2), Pos (2), cut-off (2)
Incubation:
   1 hr (37°C) + 30 min (37°C) + 10 min (37°C) or 15 min (RT)
Washes: 2

CONTENTS

Antibodies, antigens, labelled components:
   Chlamydia Ag (L2) bound to well
   Anti-human IgA HRP conjugated
Substrate: TMB, H_2O_2
Controls - standards supplied:
   Controls: Neg, Pos, cut-off (serum)
Additional reagents:
   None
Special equipment required:
   None

INTERPRETATION

Comments on interpretation:
   Grey area: within cut-off value ±10%; retest to confirm
No. of references: 4

NOTES

110451.0

Chlamydia trachomatis
ANTIBODY DETECTION (IgA)

Manufacturer: Schiapparelli Biosystems Inc
Cat. No./Trade name: 5772951/CHLAMYDIA IgA ELISA SYSTEM

SUMMARY

[Well-Ag]–**Ab**–[AHIgA-HRP]–[OPD]–A_{492}

Assay type: EIA (non-competitive)
Detection: Colorimetric A_{492}
Format: Microtitre well, Ag coated
Sample type: Serum (do not heat inactivate)
Sample pre-treatment:
   None
Sample volume: 100 µl of 1:300 dilution x 2
Number of tests: 96
Controls - standards run in assay:
   Controls: Neg (2), Pos (2)
Incubation:
   1 hr (37°C) + 30 min (37°C) + 10 min (37°C)
Washes: 3

CONTENTS

Antibodies, antigens, labelled components:
   C. trachomatis specific Ag bound to well
   Anti-human IgA Ab (g) HRP conjugated
Substrate: OPD, H_2O_2
Controls - standards supplied:
   Controls: Neg and Pos (human serum)
Additional reagents:
   None
Special equipment required:
   None

INTERPRETATION

Comments on interpretation:
   Doubtful range: within cut-off value and cut-off + 0.100; retest to confirm
No. of references: 4

NOTES

110422.0

© KLUWER ACADEMIC PUBLISHERS 1994, ISSN 1381-5067

Chlamydia
ANTIBODY DETECTION (IgG)

Manufacturer: Amico Laboratories Inc
Cat. No./Trade name: 5400G/AMIZYME® Chlamydia IgG

SUMMARY

[Well-Ag]–**Ab**–[AHIgG-HRP]–[ABTS]–A_{405}

Assay type: EIA (non-competitive)
Detection: Colorimetric A_{405} and visual
Format: Microtitre well, Ag coated
Sample type: Serum
Sample pre-treatment:
    None
Sample volume: 5 µl (+245 µl diluent)
Number of tests: 96
Controls - standards run in assay:
    Controls: Neg (1), Pos (1)
    Calibrator: (1)
Incubation:
    25 min (RT) + 25 min (RT) + 25 min (RT)
Washes: 2

CONTENTS

Antibodies, antigens, labelled components:
    Chlamydial antigens (L2 strain 434) bound to well
    Anti-human IgG Ab (g) HRP conjugated
Substrate: ABTS
Controls - standards supplied:
    Controls: Neg and Pos
    Calibrator: (1) with assigned value
Additional reagents:
    None
Special equipment required:
    None

INTERPRETATION

Comments on interpretation:
    Equivocal: within 81-99 U/ml; retest
    Repeatably equivocal: Retest a fresh sample
No. of references: 14

NOTES

110292.0

Chlamydia trachomatis
ANTIBODY DETECTION (IgG)

Manufacturer: Biologische Analysensytem GmbH
Cat. No./Trade name: 5281/BAG - Chlamydia - EIA - G

SUMMARY

[Well-Ag]–**Ab**–[AHIgG-HRP]–[TMB]–A_{450}

Assay type: EIA (non-competitive)
Detection: Colorimetric A_{450}
Format: Microtitre well, Ag coated
Sample type: Serum
Sample pre-treatment:
    None
Sample volume: 10 µl (+1 ml diluent)
Number of tests: 96
Controls - standards run in assay:
    Controls: Neg (1), Cut-off (2), Pos (1)
Incubation:
    30 min (RT) + 30 min (RT) + 10 min (RT)
Washes: 2

CONTENTS

Antibodies, antigens, labelled components:
    Chlamydia trachomatis Ag bound to well
    Anti-human IgG Ab (sh) HRP conjugated
Substrate: TMB
Controls - standards supplied:
    Controls: Neg, Pos and Cut-off
Additional reagents:
    None
Special equipment required:
    None

INTERPRETATION

Comments on interpretation:
    Equivocal: within cut-off ± 10%; retest to confirm
No. of references: 0

NOTES

110644.0

© KLUWER ACADEMIC PUBLISHERS 1994, ISSN 1381-5067

Chlamydia trachomatis
ANTIBODY DETECTION (IgG)

Manufacturer: Biowhittaker
Cat. No./Trade name: 30-660 U/Chlamydelisa II

SUMMARY

[Well-Ag]–**Ab**–[AHIgG-AP]–[PMP]–A_{550}

Assay type: EIA (non-competitive)
Detection: Colorimetric A_{550}
Format: Microtitre well, Ag coated
Sample type: Serum (do not heat inactivate)
Sample pre-treatment:
    None
Sample volume: 10 µl (+200 µl diluent)
Number of tests: 192
Controls - standards run in assay:
    Controls: Neg (1), Pos (1)
    Calibrators: (3)
Incubation:
    45 min (RT) + 45 min (RT) + 45 min (RT)
Washes: 2 (+ preliminary plate wash)

CONTENTS

Antibodies, antigens, labelled components:
    Chlamydia Ag (LGVII) bound to well
    Anti-human IgG Ab AP conjugated
Substrate: PMP
Controls - standards supplied:
    Controls: Pos and Neg (human serum).
    Calibrators: Neg, mid-Pos, high-Pos (human) with
        assigned Chlamydelisa values
Additional reagents:
    None
Special equipment required:
    None

INTERPRETATION

Comments on interpretation:
    Equivocal: Chlamydelisa value 0.16-0.17: retest to
        confirm
    Repeatably equivocal: retest with an alternative method
        or repeat with a fresh sample
    A critical ratio can be calculated to compare acute and
        convalescent sera
No. of references: 4

NOTES

110180.0

Chlamydia
ANTIBODY DETECTION (IgG)

Manufacturer: E. Merck
Cat. No./Trade name: 14083/Chlamydia IgG MAGIA®

SUMMARY

[Particle-Ag]–**Ab**–[AHIgG-AP]–[Substrate]–A_{405}

Assay type: EIA (non-competitive)
Detection: Colorimetric A_{405}
Format: Cuvette, Ag coated particles (magnetisable)
Sample type: Serum
Sample pre-treatment:
    None
Sample volume: 10 µl
Number of tests: 100
Controls - standards run in assay:
    Bought separately
Incubation:
    15 min (RT) + 15 min (RT) (automated system)
Washes: 2 (automated system)

CONTENTS

Antibodies, antigens, labelled components:
    Chlamydia antigens* bound to particles (magnetisable)
    Anti-human IgG Ab AP conjugated
Substrate: Bought separately
Controls - standards supplied:
    Bought separately
Additional reagents:
    Particle wash and system solutions (Cat. no. 14097,
        14096)
    Substrate (Cat. no. 14095)
    Calibrators (Cat. no. 14090 & 14092)
    Anti-foam (Cat. no. 14098)
Special equipment required:
    MAGIA 7000 Immunoanalyzer (Cat. no. 14011)
    Reaction cuvettes (Cat. no. 14085)

INTERPRETATION

Comments on interpretation:
    Sample concentration is calculated automatically
No. of references: 2

NOTES

110319.0

MAGIA® test Chlamydia IgG is linear up to 450 units
*LPS specific to C. trachomatis and C. psittaci and MOMP
    specific to C. trachomatis

© KLUWER ACADEMIC PUBLISHERS 1994, ISSN 1381-5067

Chlamydia trachomatis (and C. psittaci)
ANTIBODY DETECTION (IgG)

Manufacturer: E. Merck/Biotrol
Cat. No./Trade name: A 08320/CHLAMYDIA ELISA TEST G

SUMMARY

[Bead-Ag]–**Ab**–[AHIgG-AP]–[PNP]–A_{492}

Assay type: EIA (non-competitive)
Detection: Colorimetric A_{492}
Format: Tray/tube, Ag coated bead
Sample type: Serum
Sample pre-treatment:
    None
Sample volume: 50 µl (of 1:101 dilution) x 2
Number of tests: 100
Controls - standards run in assay:
    Controls: Neg (2)
    Standards: (8)
Incubation:
    1 hr (RT) with shaking + 1 hr (RT) with shaking + 30 min (37°C)
Washes: 2

CONTENTS

Antibodies, antigens, labelled components:
    Chlamydia Ag bound to bead (antigens common to C. trachomatis and C. psittaci)
    Anti-human IgG Ab AP conjugated
Substrate: PNP
Controls - standards supplied:
    Controls: Neg (human serum)
    Standards: 4 with defined EIA values
Additional reagents:
    None
Special equipment required:
    None

INTERPRETATION

Comments on interpretation:
    This is a quantitative assay
No. of references: 9

NOTES

110539.0

It is recommended that a test for Ag also be performed (Chlamydia Direct Test IF - Cat no. A 08300)

Chlamydia trachomatis
ANTIBODY DETECTION (IgG)

Manufacturer: Eurogenetics
Cat. No./Trade name: /EUROGENETICS® Chlamydia IgG ELISA

SUMMARY

[Well-Ag]–**Ab**–[AHIgG-POD]–[OPD]–A_{492}

Assay type: EIA (non-competitive)
Detection: Colorimetric A_{492}
Format: Microtitre well, Ag coated
Sample type: Serum
Sample pre-treatment:
    None
Sample volume: 100 µl of 1:300 dilution x 2
Number of tests: 96
Controls - standards run in assay:
    Controls: Neg (2), Pos (2)
Incubation:
    1 hr (37°C) + 30 min (37°C) + 20 min (RT)
Washes: 2 (+ preliminary plate wash)

CONTENTS

Antibodies, antigens, labelled components:
    Chlamydia Ag bound to wells
    Anti-human IgG Ab POD conjugated
Substrate: OPD, H_2O_2
Controls - standards supplied:
    Controls: Neg and Pos (human serum)
Additional reagents:
    None
Special equipment required:
    Eurogenetics Microtitre plate reader (or similar)

INTERPRETATION

Comments on interpretation:
    Equivocal: within cut-off + 0.1; retest a fresh sample
No. of references: 11

NOTES

110001.0

Chlamydia trachomatis
ANTIBODY DETECTION (IgG)

Manufacturer: Labsystems Oy
Cat. No./Trade name: 61 08 201/CHLAMYDIA IgG EIA KIT

SUMMARY

[Well-Ag]–**Ab**–[AHIgG-AP]–[PNP]–A$_{405}$

Assay type: EIA (non-competitive)
Detection: Colorimetric A$_{405}$
Format: Microtitre well, Ag coated
Sample type: Serum
Sample pre-treatment:
   None
Sample volume: 100 µl x 2
Number of tests: 96
Controls - standards run in assay:
   Controls: Neg (2), Pos (2)
Incubation:
   1 hr (37°C) + 1 hr (37°C) + 30 min (37°C)
Washes: 2

CONTENTS

Antibodies, antigens, labelled components:
   C. trachomatis bound to well
   Anti-human IgG PAb (sh) AP conjugated
Substrate: PNP
Controls - standards supplied:
   Controls: Neg and Pos (human serum)
Additional reagents:
   NaOH
Special equipment required:
   Auto-EIA II Analyzer (optional)
   MICROSTRIP® Reader (optional)

INTERPRETATION

Comments on interpretation:
   This is a quantitative assay
No. of references: 21

NOTES

110536.0

Chlamydia trachomatis
ANTIBODY DETECTION (IgG)

Manufacturer: Medac Diagnostika
Cat. No./Trade name: 480/Chlamydia IgG rELISA medac

SUMMARY

[Well-Ag]–**Ab**–[AHIgG-POD]–[ABTS]–A$_{405}$

Assay type: EIA (non-competitive)
Detection: Colorimetric A$_{405}$
Format: Microtitre well, Ag coated
Sample type: Serum
Sample pre-treatment:
   None
Sample volume: 5 µl (+ 495 µl diluent)*
Number of tests: 96
Controls - standards run in assay:
   Controls: Neg (2), Pos (2)
Incubation:
   1 hr (37°C) + 1 hr (37°C) + 30 min (37°C)
Washes: 2 (+ preliminary plate wash)

CONTENTS

Antibodies, antigens, labelled components:
   rec Chlamydia LPS bound to well
   Anti-human IgG Ab POD conjugated
Substrate: ABTS, H$_2$O$_2$
Controls - standards supplied:
   Controls: Neg and Pos (serum)
Additional reagents:
   None
Special equipment required:
   None

INTERPRETATION

Comments on interpretation:
   Grey zone: within cut-off ± 10%; retest in parallel with fresh specimen in 14 days
   Positive: > cut-off + 10%; interpret with reference to IgA, clinical picture and further diagnostic parameters
No. of references: 7

NOTES

110004.0

*Samples assayed in duplicate

Chlamydia trachomatis
ANTIBODY DETECTION (IgG)

Manufacturer: Melotec S.A.
Cat. No./Trade name: MCTG/MELOTEST CHLAMYDIA IgG

SUMMARY

[Well-Ag]–**Ab**–[AHIgG-HRP]–[TMB]–A_{450}

Assay type: EIA (non-competitive)
Detection: Colorimetric A_{450}
Format: Microtitre well, Ag coated
Sample type: Serum, plasma
Sample pre-treatment:
    None
Sample volume: 10 µl (+ 190 µl diluent)
Number of tests: 96
Controls - standards run in assay:
    Controls: Neg (1), low Pos (2), high Pos (1)
Incubation:
    20 min (RT) + 20 min (RT) + 10 min (RT)
Washes: 2

CONTENTS

Antibodies, antigens, labelled components:
    C. trachomatis Ag bound to well
    Anti-human IgG Ab HRP conjugated
Substrate: TMB, H_2O_2
Controls - standards supplied:
    Controls: Neg, low Pos, high Pos (human serum)
Additional reagents:
    None
Special equipment required:
    None

INTERPRETATION

Comments on interpretation:
    Equivocal: ratio of OD of sample to low Pos control is
        within range 0.9 to 1.1; retest fresh sample
    Repeatably equivocal: retest fresh sample in 4-6 weeks
No. of references: 8

NOTES

110053.0

Chlamydia trachomatis
ANTIBODY DETECTION (IgG)

Manufacturer: Menarini Diagnostics
Cat. No./Trade name: M6358/CHLAMYDIA IgG

SUMMARY

[Well-Ag]–**Ab**–[AHIgG-AP]–[PNP]–A_{405}

Assay type: EIA (non-competitive)
Detection: Colorimetric A_{405}
Format: Microtitre well, Ag coated
Sample type: Serum
Sample pre-treatment:
    None
Sample volume: 100 µl (of a 1:100 dilution) x 2
Number of tests: 96
Controls - standards run in assay:
    Controls: Neg (2), Pos (2)
Incubation:
    1 hr (37°C) + 1 hr (37°C) + 1 hr (37°C)
Washes: 2

CONTENTS

Antibodies, antigens, labelled components:
    C. trachomatis bound to well
    Anti-human IgG Ab AP conjugated
Substrate: PNP
Controls - standards supplied:
    Controls: Neg and Pos (serum)
Additional reagents:
    None
Special equipment required:
    Not specified

INTERPRETATION

Comments on interpretation:
    Not specified
No. of references: 0

NOTES

110356.0

© *KLUWER ACADEMIC PUBLISHERS 1994, ISSN 1381-5067*

Chlamydia
ANTIBODY DETECTION (IgG)

Manufacturer: Radim
Cat. No./Trade name: K4CG/CHLAMYDIA IgG

SUMMARY

[Well-Ag]–**Ab**–[AHIgG-HRP]–[TMB]–A_{450}

Assay type: EIA (non-competitive)
Detection: Colorimetric A_{450}
Format: Microtitre well, Ag coated
Sample type: Serum or plasma
Sample pre-treatment:
  None
Sample volume: 100 µl of 1:300 dilution x 2
Number of tests: 96
Controls - standards run in assay:
  Controls: Neg (2), Pos (2), cut-off (2)
Incubation:
  1 hr (37°C) + 30 min (37°C) + 10 min (37°C) or 15 min
    (RT)
Washes: 2

CONTENTS

Antibodies, antigens, labelled components:
  Chlamydia Ag (L2) bound to well
  Anti-human IgG HRP conjugated
Substrate: TMB, H_2O_2
Controls - standards supplied:
  Controls: Neg, Pos, cut-off (serum)
Additional reagents:
  None
Special equipment required:
  None

INTERPRETATION

Comments on interpretation:
  Grey area: within cut-off value ±10%; retest to confirm
No. of references: 11

NOTES

110450.0

Chlamydia trachomatis
ANTIBODY DETECTION (IgG)

Manufacturer: Schiapparelli Biosystems Inc
Cat. No./Trade name: 5772950/CHLAMYDIA IgG ELISA SYSTEM

SUMMARY

[Well-Ag]–**Ab**–[AHIgG-HRP]–[OPD]–A_{492}

Assay type: EIA (non-competitive)
Detection: Colorimetric A_{492}
Format: Microtitre well, Ag coated
Sample type: Serum (do not heat inactivate)
Sample pre-treatment:
  None
Sample volume: 100 µl of 1:300 dilution x 2
Number of tests: 96
Controls - standards run in assay:
  Controls: Neg (2), Pos (2)
Incubation:
  1 hr (37°C) + 30 min (37°C) + 10 min (37°C)
Washes: 3

CONTENTS

Antibodies, antigens, labelled components:
  C. trachomatis specific Ag bound to well
  Anti-human IgG Ab (g) HRP conjugated
Substrate: OPD, H_2O_2
Controls - standards supplied:
  Controls: Neg and Pos (human serum)
Additional reagents:
  None
Special equipment required:
  None

INTERPRETATION

Comments on interpretation:
  Doubtful range: within cut-off value and cut-off + 0.100;
    retest to confirm
No. of references: 9

NOTES

110421.0

© *KLUWER ACADEMIC PUBLISHERS 1994, ISSN 1381-5067*

Chlamydia
ANTIBODY DETECTION (IgM)

Manufacturer: Amico Laboratories Inc
Cat. No./Trade name: 5400M/AMIZYME® Chlamydia IgM

SUMMARY

[Well-Ag]–**Ab**–[AHIgM-HRP]–[ABTS]–A_{405}

Assay type: EIA (non-competitive)
Detection: Colorimetric A_{405} and visual
Format: Microtitre well, Ag coated
Sample type: Serum
Sample pre-treatment:
　None
Sample volume: 5 µl (+450 µl diluent)
Number of tests: 96
Controls - standards run in assay:
　Controls: Neg (1), Pos (1)
　Calibrator: (1)
Incubation:
　25 min (RT) + 25 min (RT) + 25 min (RT)
Washes: 2

CONTENTS

Antibodies, antigens, labelled components:
　Chlamydial antigens (L2 strain 434) bound to well
　Anti-human IgM Ab HRP conjugated
Substrate: ABTS
Controls - standards supplied:
　Controls: Neg and Pos
　Calibrator
Additional reagents:
　None
Special equipment required:
　None

INTERPRETATION

Comments on interpretation:
　Equivocal:　51-89 U/ml; retest
　Repeatably equivocal: test a fresh sample
No. of references: 14

NOTES

110293.0

Chlamydia trachomatis
ANTIBODY DETECTION (IgM)

Manufacturer: Biologische Analysensytem GmbH
Cat. No./Trade name: 5282/BAG - Chlamydia - EIA - M

SUMMARY

[Well-Ag]–**Ab**–[AHIgM-HRP]–[TMB]–A_{450}

Assay type: EIA (non-competitive)
Detection: Colorimetric A_{450}
Format: Microtitre well, Ag coated
Sample type: Serum
Sample pre-treatment:
　None
Sample volume: 10 µl (+1 ml diluent)
Number of tests: 96
Controls - standards run in assay:
　Controls: Neg (1), Cut-off (2), Pos (1)
Incubation:
　30 min (RT) + 30 min (RT) + 10 min (RT)
Washes: 2

CONTENTS

Antibodies, antigens, labelled components:
　Chlamydia trachomatis Ag bound to well
　Anti-human IgM Ab (sh) HRP conjugated
Substrate: TMB
Controls - standards supplied:
　Controls: Neg, Pos and Cut-off
Additional reagents:
　None
Special equipment required:
　None

INTERPRETATION

Comments on interpretation:
　Equivocal: within cut-off ± 10%; retest to confirm
No. of references: 0

NOTES

110645.0

Chlamydia trachomatis
ANTIBODY DETECTION (IgM)

Manufacturer: Medac Diagnostika
Cat. No./Trade name: 485/Chlamydia IgMr ELISA medac

SUMMARY

[Well-Ag]–**Ab**–[AHIgM-POD]–[ABTS]–A_{405}

Assay type: EIA (non-competitive)
Detection: Colorimetric A_{405}
Format: Microtitre well, Ag coated
Sample type: Serum
Sample pre-treatment:
    IgG/RF absorption
Sample volume: 10 μl (+130 μl diluent)*
Number of tests: 96
Controls - standards run in assay:
    Controls: Neg (2), Pos (2)
Incubation:
    1 hr (37°C) + 1 hr (37°C) + 30 min (37°C)
Washes: 2 (+ preliminary plate wash)

CONTENTS

Antibodies, antigens, labelled components:
    rec Chlamydia LPS bound to well
    Anti-human IgM Ab POD conjugated
Substrate: ABTS, H_2O_2
Controls - standards supplied:
    Controls: Neg and Pos (serum)
Additional reagents:
    None
Special equipment required:
    None

INTERPRETATION

Comments on interpretation:
    Grey zone: within cut-off ± 15%; retest in parallel with fresh specimen in 7 days
    Positive: > cut-off + 15%; interpret with reference to IgA, IgG clinical picture and further diagnostic parameters
No. of references: 9

NOTES

110648.0

*Samples assayed in duplicate

Chlamydia trachomatis
ANTIBODY DETECTION (IgM)

Manufacturer: Savyon Diagnostics Ltd
Cat. No./Trade name: 012-02-096/IPAzyme® Chlamydia TRUEIgM®

SUMMARY

[Slide-Ag]–**Ab**–[AHIgM-HRP]–[substrate]– dark blue precipitate

Assay type: EIA (non-competitive)
Detection: Light microscopy
Format: Slide well, Ag coated
Sample type: Serum
Sample pre-treatment:
    IgG/RF strip treatment of samples and controls: add stripping solution, vortex, incubate 30 min (0-4°C), add strip/stop reagent, vortex, centrifuge
Sample volume: 50 μl supernatant (+150 μl diluent)
Number of tests: 96
Controls - standards run in assay:
    Controls: Neg (1), Pos (2)
Incubation:
    2 hr (37°C) + 45 min (37°C) + 10 min (RT)
Washes: 3

CONTENTS

Antibodies, antigens, labelled components:
    C. trachomatis bound to slide well
    Anti-human IgM Ab HRP conjugated
Substrate: Not specified
Controls - standards supplied:
    Controls: Neg and Pos (human serum)
Additional reagents:
    None
Special equipment required:
    None

INTERPRETATION

Comments on interpretation:
    Negative: (-) no dark blue precipitate in any cells. If (±) precipitate in some cells; retest a fresh sample
    Positive: (+) presence of dark blue precipitate in approx 25% of cells on slide
    Invalid: dark blue precipitate in all cells
No. of references: 28

NOTES

110592.0

© *KLUWER ACADEMIC PUBLISHERS 1994, ISSN 1381-5067*

*Chlamydia trachomatis**
ANTIBODY DETECTION (IgM)

Manufacturer: Savyon Diagnostics Ltd
Cat. No./Trade name: 112-01-096/SeroELISA®
Chlamydia TRUEIgM®

SUMMARY

[Well-Ag]–**Ab**–[AHIgM-HRP]–[substrate]–A_{450}

Assay type: EIA (non-competitive)
Detection: Colorimetric A_{450}
Format: Microtitre well, Ag coated
Sample type: Serum
Sample pre-treatment:
 IgG/RF strip-treatment of samples and controls: add
  stripping solution, vortex, incubate 30 min (4°C), add
  strip-stop reagent, vortex, centrifuge
Sample volume: 10 μl of supernatant (+310 μl diluent)
Number of tests: 96
Controls - standards run in assay:
 Controls: Neg (1), Pos (1)
Incubation:
 30 min (37°C) + 30 min (37°C) + 30 min (RT)
Washes: 2 (+ preliminary plate wash)

CONTENTS

Antibodies, antigens, labelled components:
 Chlamydia Ag bound to well
 Anti-human IgM Ab HRP conjugated
Substrate: Not specified
Controls - standards supplied:
 Controls: Neg and Pos (human serum)
Additional reagents:
 None
Special equipment required:
 None

INTERPRETATION

Comments on interpretation:
 Equivocal: within cut-off ±0.03; retest using fresh
  specimen
No. of references: 27

NOTES

110594.0

*This kit also detects antibodies against C. psittaci, C.
 pneumoniae

Chlamydia trachomatis
ANTIBODY DETECTION

Manufacturer: bioMerieux
Cat. No./Trade name: 72071/Chlamydia-Spot IF-Kit

SUMMARY

[Slide-Ag]–**Ab**–[AHIg-FITC]–fluorescence

Assay type: Immunofluorescence assay (indirect)
Detection: Fluorescence microscopy
Format: Slide well, Ag coated
Sample type: Serum (not heat inactivated)
Sample pre-treatment:
 None
Sample volume: 20 μl of 1:16 and 1:64 dilutions (for
 screening)*
Number of tests: 200
Controls - standards run in assay:
 Controls: Neg (1), Pos (3)**
Incubation:
 30 min (37°C) + 30 min (37°C)
Washes: 2

CONTENTS

Antibodies, antigens, labelled components:
 C. trachomatis bound to slide
 Anti-human Ig Ab (g) fluorescein conjugated
Substrate:
Controls - standards supplied:
 Controls: Pos (human serum with assigned titre,
  prediluted 1:16)
Additional reagents:
 None
Special equipment required:
 None

INTERPRETATION

Comments on interpretation:
 Positive: fluorescent green spots on slightly red
  background; titre ⩾64 (women) or ⩾16 (men)
No. of references: 5

NOTES

110482.0

*Two-fold dilutions for quantitative determination
**two-fold dilutions (1:16, 1:32, 1:64, etc.)

© *KLUWER ACADEMIC PUBLISHERS 1994, ISSN 1381-5067*

Chlamydia trachomatis
ANTIBODY DETECTION

Manufacturer: Incstar
Cat. No./Trade name: 1680/Fluoro Kit® Chlamydia

SUMMARY

[Slide-Ag]–**Ab**–[AHIg-FITC]–fluorescence

Assay type: Immunofluorescence assay (indirect)
Detection: Fluorescence microscopy
Format: Slide well, Ag coated
Sample type: Serum
Sample pre-treatment:
   None
Sample volume: 20 µl of dilutions 1:8 to 1:1024
Number of tests: 60
Controls - standards run in assay:
   Controls: Neg (1), Pos (1)
Incubation:
   30 min (37°C) + 30 min (37°C)
Washes: 2

CONTENTS

Antibodies, antigens, labelled components:
   C. trachomas infected and uninfected tissue culture cells
      fixed to slide
   Anti-human immunoglobulins FITC conjugated
Substrate:
Controls - standards supplied:
   Controls: Pos and Neg (human serum)
Additional reagents:
   None
Special equipment required:
   None

INTERPRETATION

Comments on interpretation:
   Positive: (+1) fluorescence of Chlamydia particles
      within inclusions in the cytoplasm and/or perinuclear
      region of infected cells
   A method is available for the comparison of acute and
      convalescent sera
No. of references: 5

NOTES

110255.0

Chlamydia trachomatis
ANTIBODY DETECTION (IgG)

Manufacturer: Amico Laboratories Inc
Cat. No./Trade name: 5400FG/IFA Chlamydia IgG
Antibody Test

SUMMARY

[Slide-Ag]–**Ab**–[AHIgG-FITC]–fluorescence

Assay type: Immunofluorescence assay (indirect)
Detection: Fluorescence microscopy
Format: Slide well, Ag coated
Sample type: Serum
Sample pre-treatment:
   Dilute patient serum: 100 µl (+900 µl diluent)
Sample volume: 1 drop of diluted sample
Number of tests: 100
Controls - standards run in assay:
   Controls: Neg (1), Pos (1)
Incubation:
   25 min (RT) + 25 min (RT)
Washes: 1

CONTENTS

Antibodies, antigens, labelled components:
   C. trachomatis Ag bound to slide well
   Anti-human IgG Ab FITC conjugated
Substrate:
Controls - standards supplied:
   Controls: Neg and Pos (slides)
Additional reagents:
   None
Special equipment required:
   None

INTERPRETATION

Comments on interpretation:
   At test dilution of 1:10:
   Negative: red counterstained cells and no fluorescence
   Equivocal: colour intensity of apple green fluorescence
      (+/-)
   Positive: colour intensity of apple green fluorescence
      (+1) to (+4)
   Semiquantitative procedure is available using serial
      dilutions of samples
No. of references: 15

NOTES

110574.0

© *KLUWER ACADEMIC PUBLISHERS 1994, ISSN 1381-5067*

Chlamydia trachomatis
ANTIBODY DETECTION (IgG)

Manufacturer: Schiapparelli Biosystems Inc
Cat. No./Trade name: 3000/VIRGO C. trach IgG IFA

SUMMARY

[Slide-Ag]–**Ab**–[AHIgG-FITC]–fluorescence

Assay type: Immunofluorescence assay (indirect)
Detection: Fluorescence microscopy
Format: Slide well, Ag coated
Sample type: Serum
Sample pre-treatment:
    None
Sample volume: 20 µl 1:8 dilution
Number of tests: 96
Controls - standards run in assay:
    Controls: Neg (1), Pos (1)
Incubation:
    30 min (37°C) + 30 min (37°C)
Washes: 2

CONTENTS

Antibodies, antigens, labelled components:
    C. trachomatis infected and uninfected tissue culture
        cells bound to slide well
    Anti-human IgG Ab (g) FITC conjugated
Substrate:
Controls - standards supplied:
    Controls: Neg and Pos (human serum)
Additional reagents:
    None
Special equipment required:
    None

INTERPRETATION

Comments on interpretation:
    Positive: ≥(1+) specific apple green fluorescence at
        1:8 or greater
    Serial dilutions for quantitative assay
No. of references: 18

NOTES

110414.0

Chlamydia trachomatis
ANTIBODY DETECTION (IgM)

Manufacturer: Amico Laboratories Inc
Cat. No./Trade name: 5400FM/IFA Chlamydia IgM Antibody Test

SUMMARY

[Slide-Ag]–**Ab**–[AHIgM-FITC]–fluorescence

Assay type: Immunofluorescence assay (indirect)
Detection: Fluorescence microscopy
Format: Slide well, Ag coated
Sample type: Serum
Sample pre-treatment:
    Dilute patient serum: 100 µl (+900 µl diluent)
Sample volume: 1 drop of diluted sample
Number of tests: 100
Controls - standards run in assay:
    Controls: Neg (1), Pos (1)
Incubation:
    25 min (RT) + 25 min (RT)
Washes: 1

CONTENTS

Antibodies, antigens, labelled components:
    C. trachomatis Ag bound to slide well
    Anti-human IgM Ab FITC conjugated
Substrate:
Controls - standards supplied:
    Controls: Neg and Pos (slides)
Additional reagents:
    None
Special equipment required:
    None

INTERPRETATION

Comments on interpretation:
    At test dilution of 1:10:
    Negative: red counterstained cells and no fluorescence
    Equivocal: colour intensity of apple green fluorescence
        (+/-)
    Positive: colour intensity of apple green fluorescence
        (+1) to (+4)
    Semiquantitative procedure is available using serial
        dilutions of samples
No. of references: 15

NOTES

110573.0

© KLUWER ACADEMIC PUBLISHERS 1994, ISSN 1381-5067

Cytomegalovirus (CMV) (Cytomegalic inclusion body disease)

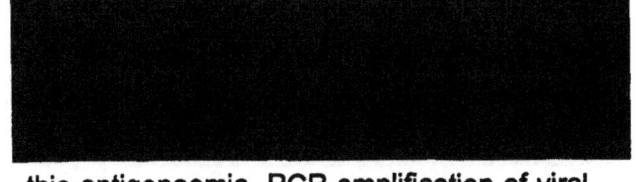

Natural history

Cytomegalovirus is a member of the herpes-virus family, and an important pathogen in immunocompromised hosts, although most infections in the immunocompetent are asymptomatic. CMV is one of the commonest of viral infections acquired *in utero*, but only 5% of congenitally infected neonates present with severe disease (jaundice, hepatosplenomegaly and purpura) in which infected cells show cytomegaly with characteristic inclusion bodies. Postnatal infection comes from intimate contact with infected cells in breast milk, saliva, genital secretions (thus sexually transmitted), or from seropositive blood or organ donors. In developing countries and overcrowded situations infection is acquired by early childhood, whilst in the industrialised regions 60% of young adults may remain susceptible. (However male homosexuals have a very high prevalence of CMV infection.) Adults with primary CMV infection may exhibit a mononucleosis-like syndrome but it is in those with cellular immune deficiency states that CMV disease is most evident. Pneumonitis after bone marrow transplant, retinitis in advanced AIDS, hepatitis and colitis post organ transplant are life and sight-threatening, and graft rejection results in many instances. Primary, recurrent and re-infections are all involved. Screening for antibody permits matching of seronegative donors and recipients in some situations. Prophylactic antiviral cover to delay disease and early treatment of systemic infection has been moderately successful in the transplant recipients.

Diagnosis and markers

Isolation of CMV in cell culture is highly sensitive but may take two to three weeks. Detection of early antigen fluorescent foci (DEAFF), in centrifugation-enhanced cultures (shell vials), provides a rapid diagnosis of CMV particularly in urine and respiratory samples. Monoclonal antibodies to the major immediate early non-structural 72 kD protein (encoded by the IE1 gene) are used 16–48 hours post-inoculation. CMV viraemia is increasingly demonstrated by the detection of CMV antigen in peripheral blood polymorphonuclear leuco-cytes. Monoclonal antibodies to the lower matrix phosphoprotein pp65 are used to detect this antigenaemia. PCR amplification of viral DNA or of mRNA (reverse transcribed) offers a significant advance in virus detection. Immunoassays for antibody continue to play an important part in the screening of donors and recipients. Assays incorporating recombinant/synthetic antigen (pp150 and pp65) promise improved sensitivity and specificity over those based on infected cell lysate or viral particle antigens. The performance of the rapid (latex agglutination) tests for antibody merits careful monitoring. IgM antibody to CMV is found in most but not all congenitally-infected neonates, and in primary infection except in severely compromised hosts, who will produce IgM after recurrent/reinfection but may fail to do so in a primary infection.

Comment

Detection of CMV indicates infection but not necessarily the cause of disease, for reactivated virus is shed asymptomatically in body fluids. Viraemia is associated with development of significant CMV disease in immunocompromised hosts, other than some patients with AIDS who have persisting viraemia. All seropositive individuals have latent CMV and may transmit infection through donated blood, organs, or semen.

Reference

Landini MP. New approaches and perspectives in cytomegalovirus diagnosis. Melnick JL (ed). Progress in Medical Virology. Basel, Karger. 1993;40:157–177.

Cytomegalovirus
ANTIGEN DETECTION

Manufacturer: Baxter Diagnostics Inc (Bartels Division)
Cat. No./Trade name: B1029-91/CMV IEA IFA Kit

SUMMARY

[Monolayer]–**Ag**–[MAb]–[AMIg-FITC]–fluorescence

Assay type: Immunofluorescence assay (indirect)
Detection: Fluorescence microscopy
Format: Vial with fixed cell monolayer
Sample type: Centrifuge-enhanced innoculated cell cultures*
Sample pre-treatment:
Rinse vial cultures with PBS, fix in acetone, air dry
Sample volume: One vial monolayer
Number of tests: 75
Controls - standards run in assay:
Controls: Neg (1), Pos (1)
Incubation:
30 min (37°C) + 30 min (37°C)
Washes: 2

CONTENTS

Antibodies, antigens, labelled components:
Anti-CMV MAb (m)
Anti-murine Ig Ab FITC conjugated
Substrate:
Controls - standards supplied:
Controls: Neg and Pos (antigen control slides with Neg and Pos wells)
Additional reagents:
None
Special equipment required:
None

INTERPRETATION

Comments on interpretation:
Negative: uninfected cells stained dull red and no fluorescence
Positive: specific green fluorescent nuclear staining
No. of references: 3

NOTES

110569.0

*Clinical samples are urine, throat swab, bronchoalveolar lavage, biopsy tissue and buffy coat cells, all in transport medium (vortexed and centrifuged prior to innoculation into tissue culture vials)

Cytomegalovirus
ANTIGEN DETECTION

Manufacturer: Baxter Diagnostics Inc (Bartels Division)
Cat. No./Trade name: B1029-81/CMV Monoclonal FA Kit

SUMMARY

[Slide]–**Ag**–[MAb-FITC]–fluorescence

Assay type: Immunofluorescence assay (indirect)
Detection: Fluorescence microscopy
Format: Slide well or vial/tube with fixed cell monolayer
Sample type: Clinical specimen in transport medium, tissue culture
Sample pre-treatment:
Clinical specimen: centrifuge, suspend pellet in PBS, apply one drop to slide, air dry, fix in acetone
Tissue culture: fix monolayer in acetone
Sample volume: 1 drop of clinical specimen suspension, one tube or vial monolayer
Number of tests: 75-100
Controls - standards run in assay:
Controls: Neg (1), Pos (1)
Incubation:
30 min (37°C)
Washes: 1

CONTENTS

Antibodies, antigens, labelled components:
Anti-CMV MAb (m) FITC conjugated
Substrate:
Controls - standards supplied:
Controls: Neg and Pos (antigen control slides with Neg and Pos wells)
Additional reagents:
None
Special equipment required:
None

INTERPRETATION

Comments on interpretation:
Negative: uninfected cells stained dull red and no fluorescence
Positive: bright apple-green fluorescence of inclusion bodies and/or fluorescence of cytoplasm
No. of references: 0

NOTES

110570.0

Cytomegalovirus
ANTIGEN DETECTION

Manufacturer: Sanofi Diagnostics Pasteur
Cat. No./Trade name: 52206/MONOFLUO® KIT CMV

SUMMARY

[Slide]–**Ag**–[MAb]–[AMIgG-FITC]–fluorescence

Assay type: Immunofluorescence assay (indirect)
Detection: Fluorescence microscopy
Format: Slide well, specimen coated
Sample type: Urinary, nasal, tracheo-bronchial cells; tissue
    culture cells inoculated with specimen 24 hr earlier
Sample pre-treatment:
    Washing (nasal or tracheo-bronchial cells only)
    Acetone fixation
Sample volume: 20 µl
Number of tests: 45
Controls - standards run in assay:
    Pos and Neg CMV cell cultures
Incubation:
    30 min (37°C) + 30 min (37°C)
Washes: 2

CONTENTS °

Antibodies, antigens, labelled components:
    Anti-CMV MAbs (m)
    Anti-murine IgG Ab (sh) FITC conjugated
Substrate:
Controls - standards supplied:
    Controls: Neg (tissue culture supernatant)
Additional reagents:
    Pos CMV cell culture
Special equipment required:
    None

INTERPRETATION

Comments on interpretation:
    Positive: granular greenish-yellow fluorescence in MAb
    treated well but absent in Neg control well
No. of references: 4

NOTES

110259.0

*Each specimen is tested in parallel with specific MAb and
    with control tissue culture supernatant

Cytomegalovirus
ANTIGEN DETECTION

Manufacturer: Syva Company
Cat. No./Trade name: 8H419/MicroTrak® CMV culture
identification test

SUMMARY

[Slide]–**Ag**–[MAb]–[AMIgG-FITC]–fluorescence

Assay type: Immunofluorescence assay (indirect)
Detection: Fluorescence microscopy
Format: Slide well, specimen coated
Sample type: Infected tissue culture cell*
Sample pre-treatment:
    Acetone fix air-dried smear or washed coverslip (10 min)
Sample volume:
Number of tests: 60-300**
Controls - standards run in assay:
    Controls: Neg (1), Pos (1)
Incubation:
    30 min (37°C) + 30 min (37°C)
Washes: 2

CONTENTS

Antibodies, antigens, labelled components:
    Anti-CMV MAbs (2) (m)
    Anti-murine IgG PAb (g) FITC conjugated
Substrate:
Controls - standards supplied:
    None
Additional reagents:
    Pos and Neg controls
Special equipment required:
    None

INTERPRETATION

Comments on interpretation:
    Negative: no fluorescent staining of at least 100 cells;
    confirm by repeating isolation procedure if necessary
    Positive: fluorescent staining of nucleus in at least one
    cell
No. of references: 8

NOTES

110525.0

*Test can be done on conventional cell culture and shell-vial
    cultures (MRC-5 cells)
**depending on sample format (smear or coverslip)

Cytomegalovirus
ANTIBODY DETECTION

Manufacturer: Centocor Inc
Cat. No./Trade name: M440/CAPTIA® CMV - TA

SUMMARY

$$[\text{Well-Ag}] \Big\langle {{}^{\text{Ab}} \atop {[\text{MAb-POD}]}} - [\text{TMB}] - A_{450}$$

Assay type: EIA (competitive)
Detection: Colorimetric A_{450}
Format: Microtitre well, Ag coated
Sample type: Serum
Sample pre-treatment:
  None
Sample volume: 50 µl
Number of tests: 96
Controls - standards run in assay:
  Controls: Neg (2), low Pos (3); high Pos (1)
Incubation:
  1 hr 30 min (37°C) + 30 min (RT)
Washes: 1

CONTENTS

Antibodies, antigens, labelled components:
  CMV Ag bound to well
  Anti-CMV MAb POD conjugated
Substrate: TMB, H_2O_2
Controls - standards supplied:
  Controls: Neg, low Pos, high Pos (human serum)
Additional reagents:
  H_2SO_4
Special equipment required:
  None

INTERPRETATION

Comments on interpretation:
  Equivocal: within cut-off ±10%; retest to confirm
  Repeatably equivocal: retest a fresh sample
No. of references: 8

NOTES

110013.0

Cytomegalovirus
ANTIBODY DETECTION

Manufacturer: Diesse
Cat. No./Trade name: 91013/CMV SCREEN

SUMMARY

$$[\text{Solid phase-Ag}] \Big\langle {{}^{\text{Ab}} \atop {[\text{MAb-POD}]}} - [\text{TMB}] - A_{450}$$

Assay type: EIA (competitive)
Detection: Colorimetric A_{450}
Format: Solid phase, Ag coated
Sample type: Serum, plasma
Sample pre-treatment:
  None
Sample volume: 20 µl
Number of tests: 96
Controls - standards run in assay:
  Not specified
Incubation:
  1 hr (37°C) + 15 min (RT)
Washes: 1

CONTENTS

Antibodies, antigens, labelled components:
  CMV Ag bound to solid phase (not specified)
  Anti-CMV MAb POD conjugated
Substrate: TMB, H_2O_2
Controls - standards supplied:
  Calibrator (bovine serum)
Additional reagents:
  None
Special equipment required:
  None

INTERPRETATION

Comments on interpretation:
  Classification of sample is according to cut-off; no further
    testing
No. of references: 0

NOTES

110597.0

© *KLUWER ACADEMIC PUBLISHERS 1994, ISSN 1381-5067*

Cytomegalovirus
ANTIBODY DETECTION

Manufacturer: Sanofi Diagnostics Pasteur
Cat. No./Trade name: 72275/PLATELIA® CMV

SUMMARY

$$[\text{Well-Ag}]\binom{\text{Ab}}{[\text{MAb-POD}]}-[\text{OPD}]-A_{492/620}$$

Assay type: EIA (competitive)
Detection: Colorimetric $A_{492/620}$
Format: Microtitre well, Ag coated
Sample type: Serum, plasma
Sample pre-treatment:
  None
Sample volume: 50 µl
Number of tests: 192
Controls - standards run in assay:
  Controls: Neg (3), Pos (2)
Incubation:
  2 hr (40°C) + 30 min (RT)
Washes: 1

CONTENTS

Antibodies, antigens, labelled components:
  CMV Ag antigen bound to well
  Anti-CMV MAb POD conjugated
Substrate: OPD
Controls - standards supplied:
  Controls: Neg and Pos (human serum)
Additional reagents:
  None
Special equipment required:
  None

INTERPRETATION

Comments on interpretation:
  Classification of samples is according to cut-off; no
    further testing
  Positive samples can be titrated to end-point
No. of references: 3

NOTES

110260.0

Cytomegalovirus
ANTIBODY DETECTION

Manufacturer: Behringwerke AG
Cat. No./Trade name: /OPUS® Anti-CMV

SUMMARY

[Glass fibre-A/G]–**Ab**–[Ag-AP]–[4-MP]–fluorescence

Assay type: EIA (non-competitive)
Detection: Fluorometric
Format: Test module, protein A/G coated glass fibre
Sample type: Serum, plasma
Sample pre-treatment:
  None
Sample volume: 10 µl (min fill level 100 µl)
Number of tests: 50
Controls - standards run in assay:
  Calibrators: Neg (2), Pos (2)
Incubation:
  Automated (23 min for first sample)
Washes: Automated

CONTENTS

Antibodies, antigens, labelled components:
  rec protein A/G bound to glass fibre
  rec CMV protein AP conjugated
Substrate: 4-MP
Controls - standards supplied:
  Controls: Neg and Pos (rabbit Ab in human serum)
Additional reagents:
  None
Special equipment required:
  OPUS® analyser
  OPUS® pipette tips and sample cups

INTERPRETATION

Comments on interpretation:
  Sample reactivity is calculated automatically and
    classified according to cut-off
  Equivocal: retest to confirm
No. of references: 8

NOTES

110139.0

Cytomegalovirus
ANTIBODY DETECTION (IgA)

Manufacturer: Savyon Diagnostics Ltd
Cat. No./Trade name: 018-01-096/IPAzyme® (CMV IgA)

SUMMARY

[Slide-Ag]–**Ab**–[AHIgA-HRP]–[substrate]–
dark blue precipitate

Assay type: EIA (non-competitive)
Detection: Light microscopy
Format: Slide well, Ag coated
Sample type: Serum
Sample pre-treatment:
None
Sample volume: 20 µl (+300 µl diluent)
Number of tests: 96
Controls - standards run in assay:
Controls: Neg (1), Pos (2)
Incubation:
1 hr (37°C) + 45 min (37°C) + 10 min (RT)
Washes: 3

CONTENTS

Antibodies, antigens, labelled components:
CMV Ag bound to slide well
Anti-human IgA Ab HRP conjugated
Substrate: Not specified
Controls - standards supplied:
Controls: Neg and Pos (human serum)
Additional reagents:
None
Special equipment required:
None

INTERPRETATION

Comments on interpretation:
Negative: (-) no dark blue precipitate in any cells. If (±)
precipitate in some cells; retest a fresh sample
Positive: (+) presence of dark blue precipitate in approx
20% of cells on slide
Invalid: dark blue precipitate in all cells
No. of references: 35

NOTES

110590.0

Cytomegalovirus
ANTIBODY DETECTION (IgG)

Manufacturer: Amico Laboratories Inc
Cat. No./Trade name: 5300G/AMIZYME® CMV IgG

SUMMARY

[Well-Ag]–**Ab**–[AHIgG-HRP]–[ABTS]–A_{405}

Assay type: EIA (non-competitive)
Detection: Colorimetric A_{405}
Format: Microtitre well, Ag coated
Sample type: Serum
Sample pre-treatment:
None
Sample volume: 5 µl (+245 µl diluent)
Number of tests: 96
Controls - standards run in assay:
Controls: Neg (1), Pos (1)
Calibrator: (1)
Incubation:
25 min (RT) + 25 min (RT) + 25 min (RT)
Washes: 2

CONTENTS

Antibodies, antigens, labelled components:
CMV Ag bound to well
Anti-human IgG Ab HRP conjugated
Substrate: ABTS
Controls - standards supplied:
Controls: Neg and Pos
Calibrator
Additional reagents:
None
Special equipment required:
None

INTERPRETATION

Comments on interpretation:
Equivocal: 19-24 U/ml; retest
Repeatably equivocal: repeat with fresh sample
No. of references: 4

NOTES

110290.0

© **KLUWER ACADEMIC PUBLISHERS** 1994, ISSN 1381-5067

Cytomegalovirus
ANTIBODY DETECTION (IgG)

Manufacturer: Baxter Diagnostics Inc (Bartels Division)
Cat. No./Trade name: B1029-330/Cytomegalovirus IgG EIA

SUMMARY

[Well-Ag]–**Ab**–[AHIgG-Enzyme]–[PNP]–A_{405}

Assay type: EIA (non-competitive)
Detection: Colorimetric A_{405}
Format: Microtitre well, Ag coated
Sample type: Serum
Sample pre-treatment:
  None
Sample volume: 100 µl of 1:21 dilution*
Number of tests: 96
Controls - standards run in assay:
  Controls: not specified
Incubation:
  30 min (37°C) + 30 min (37°C) + 30 min (37°C)
Washes: 2

CONTENTS

Antibodies, antigens, labelled components:
  CMV Ag bound to well
  Anti-human IgG Ab enzyme conjugated**
Substrate: PNP
Controls - standards supplied:
  Controls: Neg, Pos and reference serum
Additional reagents:
  None
Special equipment required:
  None

INTERPRETATION

Comments on interpretation:
  Classification of samples according to cut-off; further details not specified
No. of references: 7

NOTES

110628.0

*Diluent contains an absorbant to remove IgG and prevent IgG/rheumatoid factor complexes interfering with assay
**Enzyme label not specified

Cytomegalovirus
ANTIBODY DETECTION (IgG)

Manufacturer: Behringwerke AG
Cat. No./Trade name: OWBA/Enzygnost® Anti-CMV/IgG

SUMMARY

[Well-Ag]–**Ab**–[AHIgG-POD]–[TMB]–A_{450}

Assay type: EIA (non-competitive)
Detection: Colorimetric A_{450}
Format: Microtitre well, Ag coated
Sample type: Serum, plasma, Ig preparations
Sample pre-treatment:
  None
Sample volume: 20 µl of 1:21 dilution (+ 200 µl diluent) x 2* (final dilution 1:231)
Number of tests: 48
Controls - standards run in assay:
  Controls: Pos (2) per plate
Incubation:
  1 hr (37°C) + 1 hr (37°C) + 30 min (RT)
Washes: 2

CONTENTS

Antibodies, antigens, labelled components:
  CMV Ag or control tissue culture Ag bound to well
  Anti-human IgG (r) Fab' POD conjugated
Substrate: TMB, H_2O_2
Controls - standards supplied:
  Controls: Pos (human Ig)
Additional reagents:
  Substrate and H_2SO_4
Special equipment required:
  Behring ELISA processor (optional) or calculator with exponential and logarithmic functions for quantitative evaluating

INTERPRETATION

Comments on interpretation:
  Equivocal: within range of cut-off value and retest limit; retest to confirm. Interpretation of repeatably equivocal result depends on patient group
  Quantitative procedure available
No. of references: 17

NOTES

110108.0

*Samples are tested in parallel with Ag and control coated wells

© KLUWER ACADEMIC PUBLISHERS 1994, ISSN 1381-5067

Cytomegalovirus
ANTIBODY DETECTION (IgG)

Manufacturer: Bio-Stat Diagnostics
Cat. No./Trade name: 851203/ELISA - IgG Antibody Test

SUMMARY

$$[\text{Well-Ag}]\!-\!\mathbf{Ab}\!-\![\text{AHIgG-HRP}]\!-\![\text{TMB}]\!-\!A_{450}$$

Assay type: EIA (non-competitive)
Detection: Colorimetric A_{450}
Format: Microtitre well, Ag coated
Sample type: Serum
Sample pre-treatment:
   None
Sample volume: 10 µl (+ 1 ml diluent)
Number of tests: 96
Controls - standards run in assay:
   Controls: Neg (2), Pos (2)
Incubation:
   30 min (RT) + 30 min (RT) + 15 min (RT)
Washes: 2

CONTENTS

Antibodies, antigens, labelled components:
   CMV Ag bound to well
   Anti-human IgG Ab (r) HRP conjugated
Substrate: TMB, H_2O_2
Controls - standards supplied:
   Controls: Neg and Pos
Additional reagents:
   None
Special equipment required:
   None

INTERPRETATION

Comments on interpretation:
   Classification of samples is according to cut-off; no
     further testing
   Visual interpretation is possible
No. of references: 5

NOTES

110094.0

Cytomegalovirus
ANTIBODY DETECTION (IgG)

Manufacturer: Biologische Analysensystem GmbH
Cat. No./Trade name: 5220/BAG-CMV-EIA-G

SUMMARY

$$[\text{Well-Ag}]\!-\!\mathbf{Ab}\!-\![\text{AHIgG-HRP}]\!-\![\text{TMB}]\!-\!A_{450}$$

Assay type: EIA (non-competitive)
Detection: Colorimetric A_{450}
Format: Microtitre well, Ag coated
Sample type: Serum
Sample pre-treatment:
   None
Sample volume: 10 µl (+ 1 ml diluent)
Number of tests: 96
Controls - standards run in assay:
   Controls: Neg (1), Cut-off (2), Pos (1)
Incubation:
   30 min (RT) + 30 min (RT) + 10 min (RT)
Washes: 2

CONTENTS

Antibodies, antigens, labelled components:
   CMV Ag bound to well
   Anti-human IgG Ab (sh) HRP conjugated
Substrate: TMB
Controls - standards supplied:
   Controls: Neg, Pos and cut-off
Additional reagents:
   None
Special equipment required:
   None

INTERPRETATION

Comments on interpretation:
   Equivocal: within cut-off $\pm$ 20%; retest to confirm
No. of references: 0

NOTES

110282.0

Cytomegalovirus
ANTIBODY DETECTION (IgG)

Manufacturer: bioMerieux
Cat. No./Trade name: 30 204/VIDAS CMV IgG (CMVG)

SUMMARY

[Solid phase-Ag]–**Ab**–[AHIgG-AP]–[4-MP]–fluorescence

Assay type: EIA (non-competitive)
Detection: Fluorometric
Format: Solid phase receptacle (SPR), Ag coated and reagent strip
Sample type: Serum (not heat inactivated)
Sample pre-treatment:
  None
Sample volume: 100 µl
Number of tests: 60
Controls - standards run in assay:
  Controls: Neg (1), Pos (1)
  Calibrator: (1)
Incubation:
  Automated - total time 40 minutes
Washes: Automated

CONTENTS

Antibodies, antigens, labelled components:
  CMV Ag bound to solid phase
  Anti-human IgG MAb (m) AP conjugated
Substrate: 4-MP
Controls - standards supplied:
  Controls: Neg and Pos (human serum)
  Calibrator: Pos (human serum)
Additional reagents:
  None
Special equipment required:
  Vitek Immunodiagnostic assay system (VIDAS)

INTERPRETATION

Comments on Interpretation:
  Sample reactivity is calculated automatically and classification is according to cut-off
  Equivocal: retest to confirm value
  Quantitative assay
No. of references: 0

NOTES

110477.0

Cytomegalovirus
ANTIBODY DETECTION (IgG)

Manufacturer: Biotest Diagnostics
Cat. No./Trade name: /BIOTEST Anti-CMV IgG ELISA

SUMMARY

[Well-Ag]–**Ab**–[AHIgG-POD]–[OPD]–A_{492}

Assay type: EIA (non-competitive)
Detection: Colorimetric A_{492}
Format: Microtitre well, Ag coated
Sample type: Serum, plasma
Sample pre-treatment:
  None
Sample volume: a)25 µl (+100 µl diluent) x 2*
  b)20 µl (+200 µl diluent) x 2*
Number of tests: 96
Controls - standards run in assay:
  Controls: Neg (2), Pos (2)
Incubation:
  a) 30 min (40°C) + 30 min (40°C) + 10 min (RT)
  b) 1 hr (37°C) + 1 hr (37°C) + 30 min (RT)
Washes: 2

CONTENTS

Antibodies, antigens, labelled components:
  CMV Ag bound to well
  Control Ag (non-infected lysated cells) bound to well
  Anti-human IgG MAb POD conjugated
Substrate: OPD
Controls - standards supplied:
  Controls: Neg and Pos (human plasma)
Additional reagents:
  H_2SO_4
Special equipment required:
  None

INTERPRETATION

Comments on Interpretation:
  Procedure a: classification of sample is according to cut-off; no further testing
  Procedure b: grey zone samples with OD between 0.10 and 0.199; retest second sample to confirm
No. of references: 19

NOTES

110178.0

*Assay performed in parallel with antigen and control coated well

Cytomegalovirus
ANTIBODY DETECTION (IgG)

Manufacturer: Biowhittaker
Cat. No./Trade name: 30-627 U/CYTOMEGELISA II

SUMMARY

[Well-Ag]–**Ab**–[AHIgG-AP]–[PMP]–A_{550}

Assay type: EIA (non-competitive)
Detection: Colorimetric A_{550}
Format: Microtitre well, Ag coated
Sample type: Serum
Sample pre-treatment:
    None
Sample volume: 10 µl (+ 200 µl diluent)
Number of tests: 96
Controls - standards run in assay:
    Controls: Neg (1), Pos (1)
    Calibrators: (3)
Incubation:
    45 min (RT) + 45 min (RT) + 45 min (RT)
Washes: 2 (+ preliminary plate wash)

CONTENTS

Antibodies, antigens, labelled components:
    CMV Ag bound to plate
    Anti-human IgG Ab AP conjugated
Substrate: PMP
Controls - standards supplied:
    Controls: Neg and Pos (human serum)
    Calibrators: Neg, mid-Pos, high Pos (human serum) with
        assigned CYTOMEGELISA values
Additional reagents:
    None
Special equipment required:
    Biowhittaker automated system and software (optional)

INTERPRETATION

Comments on interpretation:
    Equivocal: Cytomegelisa value 0.23-0.24. Retest to
        confirm
    Repeatably equivocal: retest with an alternative method
        or repeat with a fresh sample
    A method is available for the comparison of acute and
        convalescent sera
No. of references: 6

NOTES

110183.0

Cytomegalovirus
ANTIBODY DETECTION (IgG)

Manufacturer: Biowhittaker
Cat. No./Trade name: 30-335 U/CMV STAT

SUMMARY

[Well-Ag]–**Ab**–[AHIgG]–[PMP]–A_{550}

Assay type: EIA (non-competitive)
Detection: Colorimetric A_{550}
Format: Microtitre well, Ag coated
Sample type: Serum
Sample pre-treatment:
    None
Sample volume: 10 µl (+ 200 µl diluent)
Number of tests: 192
Controls - standards run in assay:
    Controls: Neg (1), Pos (1)
    Calibrators: Neg (1), low Pos (3), high Pos (1)
Incubation:
    15 min (RT) + 15 min (RT) + 15 min (RT)
Washes: 2 (+1 preliminary plate wash)

CONTENTS

Antibodies, antigens, labelled components:
    CMV Ag bound to well
    Anti-human IgG Ab AP conjugated
Substrate: PMP
Controls - standards supplied:
    Controls: Neg and Pos (human)
    Calibrators: Neg, low Pos and high Pos (human) with
        assigned index value
Additional reagents:
    None
Special equipment required:
    Wellwash 4 automated plate washer (optional)
    Biowhittaker automated system and software (optional)

INTERPRETATION

Comments on interpretation:
    Equivocal: Predicted Index Value (PIV) 0.80-0.99.
        Retest to confirm
    Repeatably equivocal: retest with an alternative method
        or repeat with a fresh sample
    A method is available for the comparison of acute and
        convalescent sera
No. of references: 6

NOTES

110184.0

© KLUWER ACADEMIC PUBLISHERS 1994, ISSN 1381-5067

Cytomegalovirus
ANTIBODY DETECTION (IgG)

Manufacturer: Bouty Diagnostici
Cat. No./Trade name: 21465/BEIA CMV IgG Quant

SUMMARY

$$[\text{Well-Ag}]\text{–}\textbf{Ab}\text{–}[\text{AHIgG-HRP}]\text{–}[\text{OPD}]\text{–}A_{492/620}$$

Assay type: EIA (non-competitive)
Detection: Colorimetric $A_{492/620}$
Format: Microtitre well, Ag coated
Sample type: Serum
Sample pre-treatment:
  None
Sample volume: 10 µl (+800 µl diluent)*
Number of tests: 96, 192
Controls - standards run in assay:
  Controls: Neg (2)
  Calibrators: (8)
Incubation:
  30 min (RT) + 30 min (RT) + 15 min (RT)
Washes: 2

CONTENTS

Antibodies, antigens, labelled components:
  CMV Ag bound to well
  Anti-human IgG PAb (g) HRP conjugated
Substrate: OPD, H_2O_2
Controls - standards supplied:
  Controls: Neg (human serum)
  Calibrators: (4) (human serum with assigned values; 10-
  120 U Beia/ml)
Additional reagents:
  None
Special equipment required:
  None

INTERPRETATION

Comments on Interpretation:
  Negative: <10 U Beia/ml
  Low positive: 10-20 U Beia/ml
  Reactive: ≥20 U Beia/ml
No. of references: None

NOTES

110307.0

*Samples and controls run in duplicate

Cytomegalovirus
ANTIBODY DETECTION (IgG)

Manufacturer: Chimica Diagnostica
Cat. No./Trade name: 41500/CYTOMEGALOVIRUS IgG

SUMMARY

$$[\text{Well-Ag}]\text{–}\textbf{Ab}\text{–}[\text{AHIgG-POD}]\text{–}[\text{TMB}]\text{–}A_{450}$$

Assay type: EIA (non-competitive)
Detection: Colorimetric A_{450}
Format: Microtitre well, Ag coated
Sample type: Serum
Sample pre-treatment:
  None
Sample volume: 10 µl (+1 ml diluent) x 2
Number of tests: 96
Controls - standards run in assay:
  Controls: Neg (2), Pos (2)
Incubation:
  30 min (RT) + 30 min (RT) + 15 min (RT)
Washes: 2

CONTENTS

Antibodies, antigens, labelled components:
  CMV Ag bound to wells
  Anti-human IgG Ab (g) POD conjugated
Substrate: TMB, H_2O_2
Controls - standards supplied:
  Controls: Neg and Pos
Additional reagents:
  None
Special equipment required:
  None

INTERPRETATION

Comments on Interpretation:
  Classification of results is according to cut-off; no further
  testing
  Visual interpretation is possible if required
No. of references: 2

NOTES

110124.0

Cytomegalovirus
ANTIBODY DETECTION (IgG)

Manufacturer: Diagast Laboratories
Cat. No./Trade name: /Cytomegalovirus ELISA

SUMMARY

[Well-Ag]–**Ab**–[AHIgG-POD]–[TMB]–A_{450}

Assay type: EIA (non-competitive)
Detection: Colorimetric A_{450}
Format: Microtitre well, Ag coated
Sample type: Serum
Sample pre-treatment:
   None
Sample volume: 10 µl (+200 µl diluent)
Number of tests: 192
Controls - standards run in assay:
   Quantitative: Standards (6)
   Screening: Standards (3)
Incubation:
   30 min (37°C) + 30 min (37°C) + 30 min (37°C)
Washes: 4

CONTENTS

Antibodies, antigens, labelled components:
   CMV Ag bound to wells
   Anti-human IgG (g) POD conjugated
Substrate: TMB
Controls - standards supplied:
   Standards: 4 (human plasma, range in U/ml)
Additional reagents:
   None
Special equipment required:
   None

INTERPRETATION

Comments on interpretation:
   Equivocal: within 10% of cut-off; retest
   Quantitative procedures available
No. of references: 0

NOTES

110119.0

Cytomegalovirus
ANTIBODY DETECTION (IgG)

Manufacturer: Diamedix Corporation
Cat. No./Trade name: 783-320/CMV Microassay

SUMMARY

[Well-Ag]–**Ab**–[AHIgG-AP]–[PNP]–A_{405}

Assay type: EIA (non-competitive)
Detection: Colorimetric A_{405}
Format: Microtitre well, Ag coated
Sample type: Serum (do not heat inactivate)
Sample pre-treatment:
   None
Sample volume: 100 µl of 1:41 dilution
Number of tests: 96
Controls - standards run in assay:
   Controls: Neg (1), Pos (1)
   Calibrator: (1)
Incubation:
   20 min (RT) + 20 min (RT) + 20 min (RT)
Washes: 2

CONTENTS

Antibodies, antigens, labelled components:
   CMV Ag bound to well
   Anti-human IgG Ab AP conjugated
Substrate: PNP
Controls - standards supplied:
   Controls: Neg and Pos (human serum)
   Calibrators: (1) (human serum)
Additional reagents:
   None
Special equipment required:
   None

INTERPRETATION

Comments on interpretation:
   Equivocal: within range ≥18% and <23% of calibrator;
      retest to confirm
No. of references: 7

NOTES

110492.0

© *KLUWER ACADEMIC PUBLISHERS 1994, ISSN 1381-5067*

Cytomegalovirus
ANTIBODY DETECTION (IgG)

Manufacturer: E. Merck
Cat. No./Trade name: 14450/Cytomegalovirus IgG

SUMMARY

[Well-Ag]–**Ab**–[AHIgG-HRP]–[TMB]–A$_{450}$

Assay type: EIA (non-competitive)
Detection: Colorimetric A$_{450}$
Format: Microtitre well, Ag coated
Sample type: Serum
Sample pre-treatment:
　None
Sample volume: 10 µl (+1 ml diluent)
Number of tests: 96
Controls - standards run in assay:
　Controls: Neg (2), Pos (2)
Incubation:
　30 min (RT) + 30 min (RT) + 15 min (RT)
Washes: 2

CONTENTS

Antibodies, antigens, labelled components:
　CMV Ag bound to well
　Anti-human IgG PAb (r) HRP conjugated
Substrate: TMB
Controls - standards supplied:
　Controls: Neg and Pos
Additional reagents:
　None
Special equipment required:
　None

INTERPRETATION

Comments on interpretation:
　Classification of samples is according to cut-off; no
　further testing
No. of references: 5

NOTES
110318.0

Cytomegalovirus
ANTIBODY DETECTION (IgG)

Manufacturer: Eurogenetics
Cat. No./Trade name: /Eurogenetics CMV IgG ELISA

SUMMARY

[Well-Ag]–**Ab**–[AHIgG-POD]–[TMB]–A$_{450}$

Assay type: EIA (non-competitive)
Detection: Colorimetric A$_{450}$
Format: Microtitre well, Ag coated
Sample type: Serum, plasma
Sample pre-treatment:
　None
Sample volume: 10 µl (+1 ml diluent) x 2
Number of tests: 96
Controls - standards run in assay:
　Standards: (6) x 2
Incubation:
　1 hr (37°C) + 1 hr (37°C) + 15 min (RT)
Washes: 2

CONTENTS

Antibodies, antigens, labelled components:
　CMV Ag bound to wells
　Anti-human IgG Ab POD conjugated
Substrate: TMB, H$_2$O$_2$
Controls - standards supplied:
　Standards: 6 (human serum, 0-20 U/ml range of anti-
　CMV IgG Ab)
Additional reagents:
　None
Special equipment required:
　Eurogenetics microtitre plate reader (or similar)

INTERPRETATION

Comments on interpretation:
　Antibody concentration determined from calibration curve
　Equivocal:　0.7-1.2 U/ml; repeat on fresh sample
No. of references: 10

NOTES
110007.0

Eurogenetics ELISA AID computer programme can be used
　to calculate results

Cytomegalovirus
ANTIBODY DETECTION (IgG)

Manufacturer: Gamma SA
Cat. No./Trade name: /ELISA CMV IgG Test (quantitative)

SUMMARY

[Well-Ag]–**Ab**–[AHIgG-AP]–[PNP]–A_{405}

Assay type: EIA (non-competitive)
Detection: Colorimetric A_{405}
Format: Microtitre well, Ag coated
Sample type: Serum
Sample pre-treatment:
  None
Sample volume: 10 µl (+1 ml diluent)*
Number of tests: 192
Controls - standards run in assay:
  Controls: Neg (2), Pos a (2), Pos b (2), Pos c (2)
Incubation:
  1 hr (37°C) + 1 hr (37°C) + 30 min (37°C)
Washes: 2 (+preliminary plate wash)

CONTENTS

Antibodies, antigens, labelled components:
  CMV Ag bound to well
  Anti-human IgG Ab (r) AP conjugated
Substrate: PNP
Controls - standards supplied:
  Controls: Neg and 3 Pos (assigned values of 5, 10 and 20 units)
Additional reagents:
  None
Special equipment required:
  None

INTERPRETATION

Comments on interpretation:
  Quantitative assay: titre calculated using test parameters
No. of references: 0

NOTES

110368.0

*Samples assayed in duplicate

Cytomegalovirus
ANTIBODY DETECTION (IgG)

Manufacturer: Gamma SA
Cat. No./Trade name: /CYTOMEGALY-VIRUS IgG ELISA

SUMMARY

[Well-Ag]–**Ab**–[AHIgG-HRP]–[TMB]–A_{450}

Assay type: EIA (non-competitive)
Detection: Colorimetric A_{450}
Format: Microtitre well, Ag coated
Sample type: Serum
Sample pre-treatment:
  Predilution: 10 µl (+ 1 ml diluent)
Sample volume: 100 µl of diluted sample
Number of tests: 96
Controls - standards run in assay:
  Controls: Neg (2), Pos (2)
Incubation:
  30 min (RT) + 30 min (RT) + 15 min (RT)
Washes: 2

CONTENTS

Antibodies, antigens, labelled components:
  CMV Ag bound to well
  Anti-human IgG Ab (r) HRP conjugated
Substrate: TMB
Controls - standards supplied:
  Controls: Neg and Pos
Additional reagents:
  None
Special equipment required:
  None

INTERPRETATION

Comments on interpretation:
  Classification of sample is according to cut-off: no further testing
  Results may be expressed in GAMMA units
  Visual interpretation is possible
No. of references: 0

NOTES

110616.0

Cytomegalovirus
ANTIBODY DETECTION (IgG)

Manufacturer: Gull Laboratories
Cat. No./Trade name: CME 100/CMV IgG ELISA Test

SUMMARY

[Well-Ag]–**Ab**–[AHIgG-AP]–[PNP]–A_{405}

Assay type: EIA (non-competitive)
Detection: Colorimetric A_{405}
Format: Microtitre well, Ag coated
Sample type: Serum
Sample pre-treatment:
  None
Sample volume: 15 µl (+300 µl diluent)
Number of tests: 96
Controls - standards run in assay:
  Controls: Neg (1), Pos (1)
  Reference serum (3)
Incubation:
  30 min (37°C) + 30 min (37°C) + 30 min (37°C)
Washes: 2

CONTENTS

Antibodies, antigens, labelled components:
  CMV Ag bound to well
  Anti-human IgG Ab (g) AP conjugated
Substrate: PNP
Controls - standards supplied:
  Controls: Neg and Pos (human serum)
  Reference serum (human)
Additional reagents:
  None
Special equipment required:
  None

INTERPRETATION

Comments on interpretation:
  Equivocal: within cut-off and cut-off x 0.9; retest
  Repeatably equivocal: retest with alternative method
  (GULL product CM100 is recommended)
No. of references: 16

NOTES

110121.0

Cytomegalovirus
ANTIBODY DETECTION (IgG)

Manufacturer: Human GmbH
Cat. No./Trade name: 51 203/CYTOMEGALOVIRUS-IgG-ELISA

SUMMARY

[Well-Ag]–**Ab**–[AHIgG-HRP]–[TMB]–A_{450}

Assay type: EIA (non-competitive)
Detection: Colorimetric A_{450}
Format: Microtitre well, Ag coated
Sample type: Serum
Sample pre-treatment:
  None
Sample volume: 100 µl of 1:101 dilution
Number of tests: 96
Controls - standards run in assay:
  Controls: Neg (2), Pos (2)
Incubation:
  30 min (RT) + 30 min (RT) + 15 min (RT)
Washes: 2

CONTENTS

Antibodies, antigens, labelled components:
  CMV Ag bound to well
  Anti-human IgG Ab (r) HRP conjugated
Substrate: TMB, H_2O_2
Controls - standards supplied:
  Controls: Neg, Pos (human serum)
Additional reagents:
  None
Special equipment required:
  None

INTERPRETATION

Comments on interpretation:
  Equivocal: within cut-off ±15%; retest in parallel with
    sample taken 7-14 days later
No. of references: 5

NOTES

110511.0

Approved by Paul Ehrlich Institute, Germany

Cytomegalovirus
ANTIBODY DETECTION (IgG)

Manufacturer: IFCI Clone Systems
Cat. No./Trade name: 08.1004/EIAgen CMV IgG

SUMMARY

[Well-Ag]–**Ab**–[AHIgG-POD]–[TMB]–A_{450}

Assay type: EIA (non-competitive)
Detection: Colorimetric A_{450}
Format: Microtitre well, Ag coated
Sample type: Serum
Sample pre-treatment:
   None
Sample volume: 10 µl (+1 ml diluent)*
Number of tests: 96
Controls - standards run in assay:
   Controls: Neg (2), Pos (2), cut-off control (3)
Incubation:
   45 min (37°C) + 45 min (37°C) + 15 min (RT)
Washes: 2

CONTENTS

Antibodies, antigens, labelled components:
   CMV Ag bound to well
   Anti-human IgG MAb POD conjugated
Substrate: TMB, H_2O_2
Controls - standards supplied:
   Controls: Neg, Pos and cut-off control (serum)
Additional reagents:
   None
Special equipment required:
   None

INTERPRETATION

Comments on interpretation:
   Equivocal: within cut-off ±10%; retest to confirm
   Repeatably equivocal: retest fresh specimen
No. of references: 0

NOTES

110099.0

*Duplicate testing of sample is recommended

Cytomegalovirus
ANTIBODY DETECTION (IgG)

Manufacturer: Incstar
Cat. No./Trade name: 4535/Clin-ELISA CMV IgG

SUMMARY

[Well-Ag]–**Ab**–[AHIgG-AP]–[PNP]–A_{405}

Assay type: EIA (non-competitive)
Detection: Colorimetric A_{405}
Format: Microtitre well, Ag coated
Sample type: Serum
Sample pre-treatment:
   None
Sample volume: 10 µl (+500 µl diluent)
Number of tests: 96
Controls - standards run in assay:
   Controls: low Pos (1), high Pos (1)
   Calibrators: Neg (2), low Pos (2), high Pos (2)
Incubation:
   30 min (RT) + 30 min (RT) + 45 min (RT)
Washes: 2

CONTENTS

Antibodies, antigens, labelled components:
   CMV Ag (AD 169) bound to well
   Anti-human IgG Ab (g or sh) AP conjugated
Substrate: PNP
Controls - standards supplied:
   Controls: Low Pos, high Pos, human serum
   Calibrators: 3 (human) with assigned ELISA values
Additional reagents:
   None
Special equipment required:
   Clin-ELISA reader (optional)

INTERPRETATION

Comments on interpretation:
   Equivocal: ELISA value 26-34; retest to confirm and/or
   retest a fresh sample in 2-3 weeks
No. of references: 18

NOTES

110251.0

© KLUWER ACADEMIC PUBLISHERS 1994, ISSN 1381-5067

Cytomegalovirus
ANTIBODY DETECTION (IgG)

Manufacturer: International Immunodiagnostics
Cat. No./Trade name: 108 163/CMV-IgG

SUMMARY

[Well-Ag]–**Ab**–[AHIgG-HRP]–[TMB]–A$_{450}$

Assay type: EIA (non-competitive)
Detection: Colorimetric A$_{450}$
Format: Microtitre well, Ag coated
Sample type: Serum
Sample pre-treatment:
　None
Sample volume: 10 μl (+ 1 ml diluent)*
Number of tests: 96
Controls - standards run in assay:
　Controls: Neg (2), Pos (2)
Incubation:
　30 min (RT) + 30 min (RT) + 15 min (RT) (first two
　　incubations on plate shaker)
Washes: 2

CONTENTS

Antibodies, antigens, labelled components:
　CMV Ag bound to well
　Anti-human IgG Ab HRP conjugated
Substrate: TMB, H$_2$O$_2$
Controls - standards supplied:
　Controls: Neg and Pos (human serum)
Additional reagents:
　None
Special equipment required:
　None

INTERPRETATION

Comments on interpretation:
　Classification of results is according to cut-off; no further
　　testing
　Quantitative interpretation also available
No. of references: 0

NOTES

110332.0

*Samples assayed in duplicate

Cytomegalovirus
ANTIBODY DETECTION (IgG)

Manufacturer: Laboratoire Eurobio
Cat. No./Trade name: 900284/CYTOMEGALOVIRUS IgG ELIT®

SUMMARY

[Well-Ag]–**Ab**–[AHIgG-POD]–[OPD]–A$_{492/630}$

Assay type: EIA (non-competitive)
Detection: Colorimetric A$_{492/630}$
Format: Microtitre well, Ag coated
Sample type: Serum, plasma
Sample pre-treatment:
　None
Sample volume: 10 μl of 1:101 dilution
Number of tests: 96
Controls - standards run in assay:
　Standards: I (1), II (2), III (1), IV (1)
Incubation:
　1 hr (RT) + 1 hr (RT) + 30 min (RT)
Washes: 2

CONTENTS

Antibodies, antigens, labelled components:
　CMV Ag bound to well
　Anti-human IgG PAb (g) POD conjugated
Substrate: OPD, H$_2$O$_2$
Controls - standards supplied:
　Standards: 4 (human serum with defined EIA values)
Additional reagents:
　None
Special equipment required:
　None

INTERPRETATION

Comments on interpretation:
　Negative: ratio of sample: standard II absorbance < 0.5;
　　retest a fresh sample 1-2 weeks later
　Indeterminate: ratio of sample: standard absorbance
　　> 0.5 and < 1.0
　Positive: ratio of sample: standard absorbance > 1.0
　A quantitative assay can also be performed
No. of references: None

NOTES

110526.0

© *KLUWER ACADEMIC PUBLISHERS 1994, ISSN 1381-5067*

Cytomegalovirus
ANTIBODY DETECTION (IgG)

Manufacturer: Labsystems Oy
Cat. No./Trade name: 61 03 201/CYTOMEGALOVIRUS IgG EIA KIT

SUMMARY

[Well-Ag]–**Ab**–[AHIgG-AP]–[PNP]–A_{405}

Assay type: EIA (non-competitive)
Detection: Colorimetric A_{405}
Format: Microtitre well, Ag coated
Sample type: Serum*
Sample pre-treatment:
   None
Sample volume: 100 µl (of 1:100 dilution) x 2
Number of tests: 96
Controls - standards run in assay:
   Controls: Neg (2), Pos (2)
Incubation:
   1 hr (37°C) + 1 hr (37°C) + 30 min (37°C)
Washes: 2

CONTENTS

Antibodies, antigens, labelled components:
   CMV Ag bound to well
   Anti-human IgG PAb (sh) AP conjugated
Substrate: PNP
Controls - standards supplied:
   Controls: Neg and Pos (human serum)
Additional reagents:
   NaOH
Special equipment required:
   Auto-EIA II Analyzer (optional)
   MICROSTRIP® Reader (optional)

INTERPRETATION

Comments on Interpretation:
   This is a quantitative assay
No. of references: 22

NOTES

110537.0

*Heat treatment (30 min 56°C) may slightly change assay results

Cytomegalovirus
ANTIBODY DETECTION (IgG)

Manufacturer: Medac Diagnostika
Cat. No./Trade name: 115/12/CMV-IgG-ELA test medac

SUMMARY

[Well-RF]–**Ab**–[Ag-POD]–[OPD]–$A_{490-495}$

Assay type: EIA (non-competitive)
Detection: Colorimetric $A_{490-495}$
Format: Microtitre well, RF coated
Sample type: Serum, plasma
Sample pre-treatment:
   1:100 dilution
Sample volume: 50 µl
Number of tests: 96
Controls - standards run in assay:
   Controls: Neg (2), low Pos (2), Pos (2)
   Standards: (6)
Incubation:
   2 hr (RT) + 30 min (RT)
Washes: 2

CONTENTS

Antibodies, antigens, labelled components:
   Rheumatoid factor bound to well
   CMV Ag POD conjugated
Substrate: OPD
Controls - standards supplied:
   Controls: Neg, Borderline and Pos
   Standards: 0.5-20 U/ml
Additional reagents:
   H_2SO_4
   117 D CMV-IgG-ELA Standard Kit Medac
Special equipment required:
   None

INTERPRETATION

Comments on Interpretation:
   Equivocal: within cut-off ±30%; retest fresh specimen in 14 days
No. of references: 12

NOTES

110010.0

Cytomegalovirus
ANTIBODY DETECTION (IgG)

Manufacturer: Melotec S.A.
Cat. No./Trade name: MCMG/MELOTEST CMV IgG

SUMMARY

[Well-Ag]–**Ab**–[AHIgG-HRP]–[TMB]–A_{450}

Assay type: EIA (non-competitive)
Detection: Colorimetric A_{450}
Format: Microtitre well, Ag coated
Sample type: Serum, plasma
Sample pre-treatment:
  None
Sample volume: 10 µl (+190 µl diluent)
Number of tests: 96
Controls - standards run in assay:
  Controls: Neg (1), low Pos (2), high Pos (1)
Incubation:
  20 min (RT) + 20 min (RT) + 10 min (RT)
Washes: 2

CONTENTS

Antibodies, antigens, labelled components:
  CMV Ag bound to well
  Anti-human IgG Ab HRP conjugated
Substrate: TMB, H_2O_2
Controls - standards supplied:
  Controls: Neg, low Pos, high Pos (human serum)
Additional reagents:
  None
Special equipment required:
  None

INTERPRETATION

Comments on Interpretation:
  Equivocal: ratio of OD of sample to low Pos control is
    within the range 0.9 to 1.1; retest fresh sample
  Repeatably equivocal: retest fresh sample in 4-6 weeks
No. of references: 8

NOTES

110056.0

Cytomegalovirus
ANTIBODY DETECTION (IgG)

Manufacturer: Menarini Diagnostics
Cat. No./Trade name: M6158/HF CYTOMEGALOVIRUS IgG

SUMMARY

[Well-Ag]–**Ab**–[AHIgG-POD]–[TMB]–A_{405}

Assay type: EIA (non-competitive)
Detection: Colorimetric A_{405}
Format: Microtitre well, Ag coated
Sample type: Serum
Sample pre-treatment:
  None
Sample volume: 100 µl (of a 1:101 dilution)
Number of tests: 96
Controls - standards run in assay:
  Controls: Neg (1), Pos (1), cut-off (1)
Incubation:
  45 min (37°C) + 45 min (37°C) + 15 min (RT)
Washes: 2

CONTENTS

Antibodies, antigens, labelled components:
  CMV Ag bound to well
  Anti-human IgG Ab POD conjugated
Substrate: TMB, H_2O_2
Controls - standards supplied:
  Controls: Neg and Pos, and cut-off (serum)
Additional reagents:
  None
Special equipment required:
  Not specified

INTERPRETATION

Comments on Interpretation:
  Not specified
No. of references: 0

NOTES

110350.0

Cytomegalovirus
ANTIBODY DETECTION (IgG)

Manufacturer: Murex Diagnostics Limited
Cat. No./Trade name: MD02/04/05/Wellcozyme anti-CMV IgG

SUMMARY

[Well-IgM-RF]–**Ab**–[Ag-HRP]–[OPD]–A$_{490}$

Assay type: EIA (non-competitive)
Detection: Colorimetric A$_{490}$
Format: Microtitre well, Ab coated
Sample type: Serum, plasma
Sample pre-treatment:
  None
Sample volume: Screening: 10 µl (undiluted)
  Titration: 50 µl (of 1:100 and 1:1000 dilution)*
Number of tests: 48, 96, 384
Controls - standards run in assay:
  Controls: Neg (2), Borderline (2), Pos (2)
Incubation:
  Screening: 2 hr (RT) + 10 min (RT)
  Titration: 5 hr (RT) + 10 min (RT)
Washes: 1 (+ preliminary plate wash)

CONTENTS

Antibodies, antigens, labelled components:
  Human IgM-rheumatoid factor bound to well
  CMV Ag HRP conjugated
Substrate: OPD
Controls - standards supplied:
  Controls: Neg, Borderline, Pos (human serum)
Additional reagents:
  H$_2$SO$_4$
Special equipment required:
  Wellcozyme microwell plate washing system (optional)
  Wellcozyme microwell plate reader system (optional)

INTERPRETATION

Comments on interpretation:
  Equivocal: borderline control value ± 30%; retest now
    and repeat in 14 days if necessary
No. of references: 8

NOTES

110610.0

*If large numbers of samples are to be titrated, dilutions may
  be made directly in uncoated microtitre plates prior to
  transfer to test wells

Cytomegalovirus
ANTIBODY DETECTION (IgG)

Manufacturer: Radim
Cat. No./Trade name: K3CG/CYTOMEGALOVIRUS IgG EIA WELL

SUMMARY

[Well-Ag]–**Ab**–[AHIgG-HRP]–[TMB]–A$_{450}$

Assay type: EIA (non-competitive)
Detection: Colorimetric A$_{450}$
Format: Microtitre well, Ag coated
Sample type: Serum or plasma
Sample pre-treatment:
  None
Sample volume: 100 µl of 1:300 dilution x 2
Number of tests: 96, 192
Controls - standards run in assay:
  Controls: Neg (2)
  Standards: Neg (2), Pos (10)
Incubation:
  1 hr (37°C) + 30 min (37°C) + 10 min (37°C) or 15 min
  (RT)
Washes: 2

CONTENTS

Antibodies, antigens, labelled components:
  CMV Ag bound to well
  Anti-human IgG (g) HRP conjugate
Substrate: TMB, H$_2$O$_2$
Controls - standards supplied:
  Controls: Neg (serum)
  Standards: 5 with assigned values (0-240 RU/mL)
Additional reagents:
  None
Special equipment required:
  None

INTERPRETATION

Comments on interpretation:
  This is a quantitative assay
  Grey zone: within lowest standard ±10%; retest to
    confirm
No. of references: 5

NOTES

110445.0

© KLUWER ACADEMIC PUBLISHERS 1994, ISSN 1381-5067

Cytomegalovirus
ANTIBODY DETECTION (IgG)

Manufacturer: Roche Diagnostic Systems
Cat. No./Trade name: 07 3494 2/COBAS CORE CMV IgG EIA

SUMMARY

[Bead-Ag]–**Ab**–[AHIgG-HRP]–[TMB]–A_{450}

Assay type: EIA (non-competitive)
Detection: Colorimetric A_{450}
Format: Tube, Ag coated bead
Sample type: Serum or plasma (not heat inactivated)
Sample pre-treatment:
   None
Sample volume: 10 µl (+500 µl diluent)
Number of tests: 100
Controls - standards run in assay:
   Controls: Pos (2)
   Standards: Neg (2), Pos (10)
Incubation:
   15 min (37°C) + 30 min (37°C) + 15 min (37°C) all with
      shaking
Washes: 2

CONTENTS

Antibodies, antigens, labelled components:
   CMV Ag bound to beads
   Anti-human IgG (g) HRP conjugated
Substrate: TMB, H_2O_2
Controls - standards supplied:
   Controls: Pos (human serum)
   Standards: 6 with assigned values (human serum; 0-20
      U/ml)
Additional reagents:
   Substrate (supplied as separate kit)
Special equipment required:
   Cobas® EIA shaking incubator, tube washer and
      photometer (optional)
   Cobas® Core automated analyser (optional)

INTERPRETATION

Comments on Interpretation:
   This is a quantitative assay
No. of references: 5

NOTES

110411.0

Cytomegalovirus
ANTIBODY DETECTION (IgG)

Manufacturer: Schiapparelli Biosystems Inc
Cat. No./Trade name: 5772914/CYTOMEGALOVIRUS IgG ELISA SYSTEM

SUMMARY

[Well-Ag]–**Ab**–[AHIgG-HRP]–[OPD]–A_{492}

Assay type: EIA (non-competitive)
Detection: Colorimetric A_{492}
Format: Microtitre well, Ag coated
Sample type: Serum (do not heat inactivate)
Sample pre-treatment:
   None
Sample volume: 100 µl of 1:300 dilution x 2
Number of tests: 96
Controls - standards run in assay:
   Controls: Neg (2), Pos (2)
Incubation:
   1 hr (37°C) + 30 min (37°C) + 10 min (37°C)
Washes: 3

CONTENTS

Antibodies, antigens, labelled components:
   CMV specific Ag bound to well
   Anti-human IgG Ab (g) HRP conjugated
Substrate: OPD, H_2O_2
Controls - standards supplied:
   Controls: Neg and Pos (human serum)
Additional reagents:
   None
Special equipment required:
   None

INTERPRETATION

Comments on Interpretation:
   Doubtful range: within cut-off value and cut-off +0.100;
      retest to confirm
No. of references: 12

NOTES

110423.0

© *KLUWER ACADEMIC PUBLISHERS 1994, ISSN 1381-5067*

Cytomegalovirus
ANTIBODY DETECTION (IgG)

Manufacturer: Sigma Diagnostics
Cat. No./Trade name: SIA 405-A/SIA CMV IgG kit

SUMMARY

[Well-Ag]–**Ab**–[AHIgG-AP]–[PMP]–A_{550}

Assay type: EIA (non-competitive)
Detection: Colorimetric A_{550}
Format: Microtitre well, Ag coated
Sample type: Serum (do not heat inactivate)
Sample pre-treatment:
    None
Sample volume: 10 µl (+200 µl diluent)
Number of tests: 96
Controls - standards run in assay:
    Controls: Neg (1), Pos (1)
    Calibrator (3)
Incubation:
    45 min (RT) + 45 min (RT) + 45 min (RT)
Washes: 2 (+ preliminary plate wash)

CONTENTS

Antibodies, antigens, labelled components:
    CMV Ag bound to well
    Anti-human IgG PAb (g) AP conjugated
Substrate: PMP
Controls - standards supplied:
    Controls: Neg and Pos, human serum
    Calibrator (3) with assigned value
Additional reagents:
    None
Special equipment required:
    Sigma EIA microwell plate or strip reader (optional)

INTERPRETATION

Comments on interpretation:
    Results expressed as S.I.A. CMV IgG values
    Equivocal: 0.23-0.24; retest to confirm
No. of references: 6

NOTES

110118.0

Cytomegalovirus
ANTIBODY DETECTION (IgG)

Manufacturer: Sorin Biomedica
Cat. No./Trade name: 2860/ETI-CYTOK-G

SUMMARY

[Well-Ag]–**Ab**–[AHIgG-HRP]–[TMB]–A_{450}

Assay type: EIA (non-competitive)
Detection: Colorimetric A_{450}
Format: Microtitre well, Ag coated
Sample type: Serum, plasma
Sample pre-treatment:
    None
Sample volume: 10 µl (+ 1 ml diluent)
Number of tests: 192
Controls - standards run in assay:
    Controls: Neg (1)
    Calibrators: (4)
Incubation:
    1 hr (37°C) + 1 hr (37°C) + 30 min (RT)
Washes: 2

CONTENTS

Antibodies, antigens, labelled components:
    CMV Ag (AD 169 strain) bound to well
    Anti-human IgG IgG Ab (g) HRP conjugated
Substrate: TMB, H_2O_2
Controls - standards supplied:
    Controls: Neg (human serum)
    Calibrators: (4) 5-100 AU/ml
Additional reagents:
    None
Special equipment required:
    ETI-system reader and washer (optional)

INTERPRETATION

Comments on interpretation:
    Equivocal: Within cut-off ± 10%; retest to confirm
    Quantitative assay
No. of references: 7

NOTES

110245.0

© *KLUWER ACADEMIC PUBLISHERS 1994, ISSN 1381-5067*

Cytomegalovirus
ANTIBODY DETECTION (IgG)

Manufacturer: United Biotech Inc
Cat. No./Trade name: IA-201/MAGIWEL® CMV IgG

SUMMARY

$[Well-Ag]-Ab-[AHIgG-HRP]-[TMB]-A_{450}$

Assay type: EIA (non-competitive)
Detection: Colorimetric A_{450}
Format: Microtitre well, Ag coated
Sample type: Serum
Sample pre-treatment:
   None
Sample volume: 100 μl of 1:101 dilution
Number of tests: 96
Controls - standards run in assay:
   Reference standard set: Neg (1), Pos (1), calibrator (1)
Incubation:
   30 min (RT) + 30 min (RT) + 15 min (RT)
Washes: 2

CONTENTS

Antibodies, antigens, labelled components:
   CMV Ag bound to well
   Anti-human IgG Ab (g) HRP conjugated
Substrate: TMB, H_2O_2
Controls - standards supplied:
   Reference standard set: Neg, Pos and calibrator (100
      EU/ml)
Additional reagents:
   H_2SO_4
Special equipment required:
   None

INTERPRETATION

Comments on interpretation:
   Positive: $\geqslant 15$ EU/ml
No. of references: 16

NOTES

110498.0

Cytomegalovirus
ANTIBODY DETECTION (IgG)

Manufacturer: Zeus Scientific Inc
Cat. No./Trade name: 9500G series/CMV ELISA

SUMMARY

$[Well-Ag]-Ab-[AHIgG-HRP]-[OPD]-A_{490}$

Assay type: EIA (non-competitive)
Detection: Colorimetric A_{490}
Format: Microtitre well, Ag coated
Sample type: Serum
Sample pre-treatment:
   None
Sample volume: 10 μl (+200 μl diluent)
Number of tests: 96
Controls - standards run in assay:
   Controls: Neg (1), low Pos (3), high Pos (1)
Incubation:
   20 min (RT) + 20 min (RT) + 10 min (RT)
Washes: 2

CONTENTS

Antibodies, antigens, labelled components:
   CMV Ag (strain AD169) bound to well
   Anti-human IgG Ab HRP conjugated
Substrate: OPD
Controls - standards supplied:
   Controls: Neg, low Pos and high Pos (serum)
Additional reagents:
   None
Special equipment required:
   None

INTERPRETATION

Comments on interpretation:
   Equivocal: OD ratio of sample: cut-off between 0.91-
      1.09; retest using an alternative method
No. of references: 25

NOTES

110299.0

© *KLUWER ACADEMIC PUBLISHERS 1994, ISSN 1381-5067*

Cytomegalovirus
ANTIBODY DETECTION (IgG AND/OR IgM)

Manufacturer: Behringwerke AG
Cat. No./Trade name: OWGM/Enzygnost® Anti-CMV/ IgG + IgM

SUMMARY

[Well-Ag]–**Ab**–[AHIgG/IgM-POD]–[TMB]–A_{450}

Assay type: EIA (non-competitive)
Detection: Colorimetric A_{450}
Format: Microtitre well, Ag coated
Sample type: Serum, plasma (not heat inactivated)
Sample pre-treatment:
  None
Sample volume: 10 µl (+ 200 µl diluent)
Number of tests: 96
Controls - standards run in assay:
  Controls: Neg (4), Pos (2)
Incubation:
  30 min (37°C) + 30 min (37°C) + 30 min (RT)
Washes: 2

CONTENTS

Antibodies, antigens, labelled components:
  CMV Ag from cell culture bound to well
  Anti-human IgG (r) POD conjugated
  Anti-human IgM (g) POD conjugated
Substrate: TMB, H_2O_2
Controls - standards supplied:
  Controls: Neg and Pos (human serum)
Additional reagents:
  None
Special equipment required:
  Behring ELISA processor (optional)

INTERPRETATION

Comments on interpretation:
  Equivocal: within cut-off ±20%; retest to confirm.
    Interpretation of repeatably equivocal result depends
      on patient group
No. of references: 0

NOTES

110457.0

Cytomegalovirus
ANTIBODY DETECTION (IgG AND/OR IgM)

Manufacturer: Gamma SA
Cat. No./Trade name: /ELISA CMV Test IgG/IgM

SUMMARY

[Well-Ag]–**Ab**–[AHIgG/IgM-AP]–[PNP]–A_{405}

Assay type: EIA (non-competitive)
Detection: Colorimetric A_{405}
Format: Microtitre well, Ag coated
Sample type: Serum, plasma
Sample pre-treatment:
  For IgM assay: removal of RF with anti-RF reagent
Sample volume: 10 µl (+ 1 ml diluent)*
Number of tests: 192
Controls - standards run in assay:
  Controls: Neg (2), Pos a (2), Pos b (2), Pos c (2)
Incubation:
  1 hr (37°C) + 1 hr (37°C) + 30 min (37°C)
Washes: 2

CONTENTS

Antibodies, antigens, labelled components:
  CMV Ag bound to well
  Anti-human IgG Ab (r) AP conjugated
  Anti-human IgM Ab (r) AP conjugated
Substrate: PNP
Controls - standards supplied:
  Controls: Neg and Pos (serum assigned value 10 units)
Additional reagents:
  None
Special equipment required:
  None

INTERPRETATION

Comments on interpretation:
  Titre calculated using test parameters
No. of references: 0

NOTES

110369.0

Kit may be used to measure IgG and IgM both together and
  separately
*Samples assayed in duplicate

Cytomegalovirus
ANTIBODY DETECTION (IgM)

Manufacturer: Amico Laboratories Inc
Cat. No./Trade name: 5300M/AMIZYME® CMV IgM

SUMMARY

[Well-Ag]–**Ab**–[AHIgM-HRP]–[ABTS]–A_{405}

Assay type: EIA (non-competitive)
Detection: Colorimetric A_{405}
Format: Microtitre well, Ag coated
Sample type: Serum
Sample pre-treatment:
　None
Sample volume: 10 µl (+490 µl diluent)
Number of tests: 96
Controls - standards run in assay:
　Controls: Neg (1), Pos (1)
　Calibrator: (1)
Incubation:
　25 min (RT) + 25 min (RT) + 25 min (RT)
Washes: 2

CONTENTS

Antibodies, antigens, labelled components:
　CMV Ag bound to well
　Anti-human IgM Ab HRP conjugated
Substrate: ABTS
Controls - standards supplied:
　Controls: Neg and Pos
　Calibrator
Additional reagents:
　None
Special equipment required:
　None

INTERPRETATION

Comments on interpretation:
　Equivocal: 31-39 U/ml; retest to confirm or use a fresh
　sample
No. of references: 19

NOTES

110291.0

Cytomegalovirus
ANTIBODY DETECTION (IgM)

**Manufacturer: Baxter Diagnostics Inc
(Bartels Division)**
Cat. No./Trade name: B1029-335/Cytomegalovirus IgM
EIA

SUMMARY

[Well-Ag]–**Ab**–[AHIgM-Enzyme]–[PNP]–A_{405}

Assay type: EIA (non-competitive)
Detection: Colorimetric A_{405}
Format: Microtitre well, Ag coated
Sample type: Serum
Sample pre-treatment:
　None
Sample volume: 100 µl of 1:11 dilution*
Number of tests: 96
Controls - standards run in assay:
　Controls: not specified
Incubation:
　30 min (37°C) + 30 min (37°C) + 30 min (37°C)
Washes: 2

CONTENTS

Antibodies, antigens, labelled components:
　CMV Ag bound to well
　Anti-human IgM Ab enzyme conjugated**
Substrate:
Controls - standards supplied:
　Controls: Neg, Pos and reference serum
Additional reagents:
　None
Special equipment required:
　None

INTERPRETATION

Comments on interpretation:
　Classification of samples according to cut-off; further
　details not specified
No. of references: 7

NOTES

110629.0

*Diluent contains an absorbant to remove IgG and prevent
　IgG/rheumatoid factor complexes interfering with assay
**Enzyme label not specified

Cytomegalovirus
ANTIBODY DETECTION (IgM)

Manufacturer: Behringwerke AG
Cat. No./Trade name: OWBK/Enzygnost® Anti-CMV/IgM

SUMMARY

[Well-Ag]–**Ab**–[AHIgM-POD]–[TMB]–A$_{450}$

Assay type: EIA (non-competitive)
Detection: Colorimetric A$_{450}$
Format: Microtitre well, Ag coated
Sample type: Serum, plasma
Sample pre-treatment:
Incubate 1:21 prediluted sample with RF absorbent 15 min (RT) or overnight (4°C)
Sample volume: 150 μl of a 1:42 dilution*
Number of tests: 48
Controls - standards run in assay:
Controls: Neg (1) and Pos (2) per plate
Incubation:
1 hr (37°C) + 1 hr (37°C) + 30 min (RT)
Washes: 2

CONTENTS

Antibodies, antigens, labelled components:
CMV Ag or control tissue culture Ag bound to well
Anti-human IgM (g) POD conjugated
Substrate: TMB, H$_2$O$_2$
Controls - standards supplied:
Controls: Neg and Pos (human Ig)
Additional reagents:
Substrate and H$_2$SO$_4$
Special equipment required:
Behring ELISA processor (optional)

INTERPRETATION

Comments on interpretation:
Equivocal: within range of cut-off value and retest limit; retest to confirm
Quantitative procedure available
No. of references: 21

NOTES

110107.0

*Samples are tested in parallel in Ag and control-Ag coated wells

---

Cytomegalovirus
ANTIBODY DETECTION (IgM)

Manufacturer: Bio-Stat Diagnostics
Cat. No./Trade name: 851103/ELISA IgM Antibody Test

SUMMARY

[Well-Ag]–**Ab**–[AHIgM-HRP]–[TMB]–A$_{450}$

Assay type: EIA (non-competitive)
Detection: Colorimetric A$_{450}$
Format: Microtitre well, Ag coated
Sample type: Serum
Sample pre-treatment:
None
Sample volume: 10 μl (+1 ml diluent)
Number of tests: 96
Controls - standards run in assay:
Controls: Neg (2), Pos (2)
Incubation:
30 min (RT) + 30 min (RT) + 15 min (RT)
Washes: 2

CONTENTS

Antibodies, antigens, labelled components:
CMV Ag bound to wells
Anti-human IgM Ab (r) HRP conjugated
Substrate: TMB, H$_2$O$_2$
Controls - standards supplied:
Controls: Neg and Pos
Additional reagents:
None
Special equipment required:
None

INTERPRETATION

Comments on interpretation:
Classification of samples is according to cut-off; no further testing
Visual interpretation is possible
No. of references: 5

NOTES

110093.0

© KLUWER ACADEMIC PUBLISHERS 1994, ISSN 1381-5067

Cytomegalovirus
ANTIBODY DETECTION (IgM)

Manufacturer: Biologische Analysensytem GmbH
Cat. No./Trade name: 5222/BAG-CMV-EIA-M

SUMMARY

[Well-Ag]–**Ab**–[AHIgM-HRP]–[TMB]–A_{450}

Assay type: EIA (non-competitive)
Detection: Colorimetric A_{450}
Format: Microtitre well, Ag coated
Sample type: Serum
Sample pre-treatment:
    None
Sample volume: 10 µl (+ 1 ml diluent)*
Number of tests: 96
Controls - standards run in assay:
    Controls: Neg (1), Cut-off (2), Pos (1)
Incubation:
    30 min (RT) + 30 min (RT) + 10 min (RT)
Washes: 2

CONTENTS

Antibodies, antigens, labelled components:
    CMV Ag bound to well
    Anti-human IgM Ab (sh) HRP conjugated
Substrate: TMB
Controls - standards supplied:
    Controls: Neg, Pos and Cut-off
Additional reagents:
    None
Special equipment required:
    None

INTERPRETATION

Comments on interpretation:
    Equivocal: within cut-off ± 20%; retest to confirm
No. of references: 0

NOTES

110642.0

Cytomegalovirus
ANTIBODY DETECTION (IgM)

Manufacturer: bioMerieux
Cat. No./Trade name: 30205/VIDAS CMV IgM (CMVM)

SUMMARY

[Solid phase-Ag]–**Ab**–[AHIgM-AP]–[4-MP]–fluorescence

Assay type: EIA (non-competitive)
Detection: Fluorometric
Format: Solid phase receptacle (SPR), Ag coated and reagent strip
Sample type: Serum (not heat inactivated)
Sample pre-treatment:
    Automated: IgG and RF adsorption
Sample volume: 100 µl
Number of tests: 30
Controls - standards run in assay:
    Controls: Neg (1), Pos (1)
    Standard: (1)
Incubation:
    Automated - total time 1 hr
Washes: Automated

CONTENTS

Antibodies, antigens, labelled components:
    CMV Ag bound to solid phase
    Anti-human IgM MAb (m) AP conjugated
Substrate: 4-MP
Controls - standards supplied:
    Controls: Neg and Pos (human serum)
    Standard: Pos (human serum)
Additional reagents:
    None
Special equipment required:
    Vitek Immunodiagnostic assay system (VIDAS)

INTERPRETATION

Comments on interpretation:
    Sample reactivity is calculated automatically and
        classification is according to cut-off
    Equivocal: retest to confirm; if repeatably equivocal
        collect fresh sample 10-15 days later
No. of references: 0

NOTES

110476.0

© KLUWER ACADEMIC PUBLISHERS 1994, ISSN 1381-5067

Cytomegalovirus
ANTIBODY DETECTION (IgM)

Manufacturer: Bouty Diagnostici
Cat. No./Trade name: 21467/BEIA CMV-IgM capture

SUMMARY

[Well-AHIgM]–**Ab**–[Ag-biotin]–[strept-HRP]–[TMB]–
$A_{450/620}$

Assay type: EIA (non-competitive)
Detection: Colorimetric $A_{450/620}$
Format: Microtitre well, Ab coated
Sample type: Serum, plasma
Sample pre-treatment:
    None
Sample volume: 10 µl (+800 µl diluent)
Number of tests: 96
Controls - standards run in assay:
    Controls: Neg (1), Pos (1), cut-off (1)
Incubation:
    1 hr (RT) + 1 hr (RT) + 30 min (RT)
Washes: 2

CONTENTS

Antibodies, antigens, labelled components:
    Anti-human IgM Ab (IgG)
    CMV Ag biotinylated
    Streptavidin HRP conjugated
Substrate: TMB, H_2O_2
Controls - standards supplied:
    Controls: Neg, Pos and cut-off (human serum)
Additional reagents:
    None
Special equipment required:
    None

INTERPRETATION

Comments on interpretation:
    Equivocal: sample OD within 5% of the cut-off control;
    repeat
    Repeatably equivocal: retest a fresh sample
No. of references: None

NOTES

110306.0

Cytomegalovirus
ANTIBODY DETECTION (IgM)

Manufacturer: Centocor Inc
Cat. No./Trade name: M445/CAPTIA® CMV-M

SUMMARY

[Well-AHIgM]–**Ab**–[Ag-HRP]–[TMB]–A_{450}

Assay type: EIA (non-competitive)
Detection: Colorimetric A_{450}
Format: Microtitre well, Ab coated
Sample type: Serum
Sample pre-treatment:
    None
Sample volume: 10 µl (+1 ml diluent)
Number of tests: 96
Controls - standards run in assay:
    Controls: Neg (1), low Pos (2), Pos (1)
Incubation:
    1 hr (37°C) + 1 hr (37°C) + 30 min (RT)
Washes: 2

CONTENTS

Antibodies, antigens, labelled components:
    Anti-human IgM Ab bound to well
    CMV Ag HRP conjugated
Substrate: TMB, H_2O_2
Controls - standards supplied:
    Controls: Neg, low Pos, high Pos (human serum)
Additional reagents:
    H_2SO_4
Special equipment required:
    None

INTERPRETATION

Comments on interpretation:
    Equivocal: within cut-off ±10%; retest to confirm
    Repeatably equivocal: retest a fresh sample
No. of references: 10

NOTES

110012.0

© KLUWER ACADEMIC PUBLISHERS 1994, ISSN 1381-5067

Cytomegalovirus
ANTIBODY DETECTION (IgM)

Manufacturer: Chimica Diagnostica
Cat. No./Trade name: 41550/CYTOMEGALOVIRUS IgM

SUMMARY

[Well-Ag]–**Ab**–[AHIgM-POD]–[TMB]–A_{450}

Assay type: EIA (non-competitive)
Detection: Colorimetric A_{450}
Format: Microtitre well, Ag coated
Sample type: Serum
Sample pre-treatment:
    None
Sample volume: 10 µl (+ 1 ml diluent) x 2*
Number of tests: 96
Controls - standards run in assay:
    Controls: Neg (1), Cut-off (1), Pos (1)
Incubation:
    30 min (RT) + 30 min (RT) + 15 min (RT)
Washes: 2

CONTENTS

Antibodies, antigens, labelled components:
    CMV Ag bound to wells
    Anti-human IgM Ab (g) POD conjugated
Substrate: TMB, H_2O_2
Controls - standards supplied:
    Controls: Neg, Cut-off and Pos
Additional reagents:
    None
Special equipment required:
    None

INTERPRETATION

Comments on interpretation:
    Classification of results is according to cut-off; no further
        testing
    Visual interpretation is possible
No. of references: 2

NOTES

110125.0

*Dilution buffer contains anti-human IgG to prevent
    interference from RF or specific IgG

Cytomegalovirus
ANTIBODY DETECTION (IgM)

Manufacturer: Diamedix Corporation
Cat. No./Trade name: 783-330/CMV IgM Microassay

SUMMARY

[Well-Ag]–**Ab**–[AHIgM-AP]–[PNP]–A_{405}

Assay type: EIA (non-competitive)
Detection: Colorimetric A_{405}
Format: Microtitre well, Ag coated
Sample type: Serum (do not heat inactivate)
Sample pre-treatment:
    None
Sample volume: 100 µl of 1:21 dilution
Number of tests: 96
Controls - standards run in assay:
    Controls: Neg (1), Pos (1)
    Calibrators: (1)
Incubation:
    30 min (RT) + 30 min (RT) + 30 min (RT)
Washes: 2

CONTENTS

Antibodies, antigens, labelled components:
    CMV Ag bound to well
    Anti-human IgM Ab AP conjugated
Substrate: PNP
Controls - standards supplied:
    Controls: Neg and Pos (human serum)
    Calibrators: (1) (human serum)
Additional reagents:
    None
Special equipment required:
    None

INTERPRETATION

Comments on interpretation:
    Positive: > 30% of calibrator
No. of references: 5

NOTES

110491.0

© KLUWER ACADEMIC PUBLISHERS 1994, ISSN 1381-5067

Cytomegalovirus
ANTIBODY DETECTION (IgM)

Manufacturer: E. Merck
Cat. No./Trade name: 14451/Cytomegalovirus IgM

SUMMARY

[Well-Ag]–**Ab**–[AHIgM-HRP]–[TMB]–A_{450}

Assay type: EIA (non-competitive)
Detection: Colorimetric A_{450}
Format: Microtitre well, Ag coated
Sample type: Serum
Sample pre-treatment:
   None
Sample volume: 10 µl (+1 ml diluent)*
Number of tests: 96
Controls - standards run in assay:
   Controls: Neg (2), Pos (2)
Incubation:
   30 min (RT) + 30 min (RT) + 15 min (RT)
Washes: 2

CONTENTS

Antibodies, antigens, labelled components:
   CMV Ag bound to well
   Anti-human IgM PAb (r) HRP conjugated
Substrate: TMB
Controls - standards supplied:
   Controls: Neg and Pos
Additional reagents:
   None
Special equipment required:
   None

INTERPRETATION

Comments on interpretation:
   Classification of samples is according to cut-off; no
   further testing
No. of references: 5

NOTES

110317.0

*Dilution buffer contains anti-human IgG to prevent
   interference of rheumatoid factors or specific IgG

Cytomegalovirus
ANTIBODY DETECTION (IgM)

Manufacturer: Eurogenetics
Cat. No./Trade name: /Eurogenetics CMV IgM ELISA

SUMMARY

[Well-AHIgM]–**Ab**–[Ag]–[MAb-biotin]–[strept-HRP]–
[TMB]–A_{450}

Assay type: EIA (non-competitive)
Detection: Colorimetric A_{450}
Format: Microtitre well, Ab coated
Sample type: Serum, plasma
Sample pre-treatment:
   None
Sample volume: 10 µl (+1 ml diluent) x 2
Number of tests: 96
Controls - standards run in assay:
   Controls: (4) x 2
Incubation:
   1 hr (37°C) + 1 hr (37°C) + 30 min (37°C)
Washes: 2

CONTENTS

Antibodies, antigens, labelled components:
   Anti-human IgM (r) bound to wells
   CMV Ag
   Anti-CMV MAb biotinylated
   Streptavidin HRP conjugated
Substrate: TMB, H_2O_2
Controls - standards supplied:
   Controls: 4 (human serum, range 0-400 M-units/ml of
      anti-CMV IgM Ab)
Additional reagents:
   None
Special equipment required:
   Eurogenetics microtitre plate reader (or similar)

INTERPRETATION

Comments on interpretation:
   Antibody concentration determined from calibration curve
      calculated from OD of controls
   Equivocal: 100-150 M-units/ml; retest fresh sample
No. of references: 14

NOTES

110008.0

Eurogenetics ELISA AID computer programme can be used
   to calculate results

© KLUWER ACADEMIC PUBLISHERS 1994, ISSN 1381-5067

Cytomegalovirus
ANTIBODY DETECTION (IgM)

Manufacturer: Gamma SA
Cat. No./Trade name: /CYTOMEGALY-VIRUS IgM ELISA

SUMMARY

[Well-Ag]–**Ab**–[AHIgM-HRP]–[TMB]–A_{450}

Assay type: EIA (non-competitive)
Detection: Colorimetric A_{450}
Format: Microtitre well, Ag coated
Sample type: Serum
Sample pre-treatment:
　　Dilute sera 1:100 with dilution buffer and incubate at least 10 min prior to use
Sample volume: 100 µl of diluted sample
Number of tests: 96
Controls - standards run in assay:
　　Controls: Neg (2), Pos (2)
Incubation:
　　30 min (RT) + 30 min (RT) + 15 min (RT)
Washes: 2

CONTENTS

Antibodies, antigens, labelled components:
　　CMV Ag bound to well
　　Anti-human IgM Ab (r) HRP conjugated
Substrate: TMB
Controls - standards supplied:
　　Controls: Neg and Pos (titre 1:100 ± 10%)
Additional reagents:
　　None
Special equipment required:
　　None

INTERPRETATION

Comments on interpretation:
　　Equivocal: within cut-off ± 10%; retest duplicate samples in parallel with duplicates of fresh sample taken 7-14 days later
　　Visual interpretation is possible
No. of references: 0

NOTES

110589.0

Cytomegalovirus
ANTIBODY DETECTION (IgM)

Manufacturer: Gull Laboratories
Cat. No./Trade name: CME 150/CMV IgM ELISA Test

SUMMARY

[Well-Ag]–**Ab**–[AHIgM-AP]–[PNP]–A_{405}

Assay type: EIA (non-competitive)
Detection: Colorimetric A_{405}
Format: Microtitre well, Ag coated
Sample type: Serum
Sample pre-treatment:
　　None
Sample volume: 15 µl (+ 150 µl diluent)*
Number of tests: 96
Controls - standards run in assay:
　　Controls: Neg (1), Pos (1)
　　Reference serum: (3)
Incubation:
　　30 min (37°C) + 30 min (37°C) + 30 min (37°C)
Washes: 2

CONTENTS

Antibodies, antigens, labelled components:
　　CMV Ag bound to well
　　Anti-human IgM Ab (g) AP conjugated
Substrate: PNP
Controls - standards supplied:
　　Controls: Neg and Pos (human serum)
　　Reference serum (human)
Additional reagents:
　　None
Special equipment required:
　　None

INTERPRETATION

Comments on interpretation:
　　Equivocal: within cut-off and cut-off x 0.9; retest
　　Repeatably equivocal: retest with alternative method (GULL Product CM150 is recommended)
No. of references: 10

NOTES

110120.0

*Sample diluent contains an absorbent to remove IgG and RF

Cytomegalovirus
ANTIBODY DETECTION (IgM)

Manufacturer: Human GmbH
Cat. No./Trade name: 51 103/CYTOMEGALY-VIRUS-IgM-ELISA

SUMMARY

[Well-Ag]–**Ab**–[AHIgM-HRP]–[TMB]–A_{450}

Assay type: EIA (non-competitive)
Detection: Colorimetric A_{450}
Format: Microtitre well, Ag coated
Sample type: Serum
Sample pre-treatment:
   Removal of IgG - 5 min incubation with sample diluent
Sample volume: 100 µl of 1:101 dilution
Number of tests: 96
Controls - standards run in assay:
   Controls: Neg (2), Pos (2)
Incubation:
   30 min (RT) + 30 min (RT) + 15 min (RT)
Washes: 2

CONTENTS

Antibodies, antigens, labelled components:
   CMV Ag bound to well
   Anti-human IgM Ab (r) HRP conjugated
Substrate: TMB, H_2O_2
Controls - standards supplied:
   Controls: Neg, Pos (human serum)
Additional reagents:
   None
Special equipment required:
   None

INTERPRETATION

Comments on interpretation:
   Equivocal: within cut-off ± 15%; retest in parallel with
      sample taken 7-14 days later
No. of references: 5

NOTES

110512.0

Approved by Paul Ehrlich Institute, Germany

Cytomegalovirus
ANTIBODY DETECTION (IgM)

Manufacturer: IFCI Clone Systems
Cat. No./Trade name: 08.1005/ElAgen CMV IgM

SUMMARY

[Well-AHIgM]–**Ab**–[Ag]–[MAb-POD]–[TMB]–A_{450}

Assay type: EIA (non-competitive)
Detection: Colorimetric A_{450}
Format: Microtitre well, Ab coated
Sample type: Serum
Sample pre-treatment:
   None
Sample volume: 10 µl (+1 ml diluent)*
Number of tests: 96
Controls - standards run in assay:
   Controls: Neg (2), Pos (2), cut-off control (3)
Incubation:
   45 min (37°C) + 45 min (37°C) + 15 min (RT)
Washes: 2

CONTENTS

Antibodies, antigens, labelled components:
   Anti-human IgM MAb bound to well
   CMV Ag
   Anti-CMV MAb POD conjugated
Substrate: TMB, H_2O_2
Controls - standards supplied:
   Controls: Neg, Pos and cut-off control (serum)
Additional reagents:
   None
Special equipment required:
   None

INTERPRETATION

Comments on interpretation:
   Equivocal: within cut-off ± 10% retest
   Repeatably equivocal: retest fresh specimen
No. of references: 0

NOTES

110098.0

*Duplicate testing of samples is recommended

© KLUWER ACADEMIC PUBLISHERS 1994, ISSN 1381-5067

Cytomegalovirus
ANTIBODY DETECTION (IgM)

Manufacturer: Incstar
Cat. No./Trade name: 5530/Clin-ELISA CMV IgM

SUMMARY

[Well-Ag]–**Ab**–[AHIgM-AP]–[PNP]-A$_{405}$

Assay type: EIA (non-competitive)
Detection: Colorimetric A$_{405}$
Format: Microtitre well, Ag coated
Sample type: Serum
Sample pre-treatment:
Removal of IgG immunoglobulins (30 min incubation)
Sample volume: 10 µl (+500 µl pretreatment solution)
Number of tests: 96
Controls - standards run in assay:
Controls: Neg (1), Pos (1)
Calibrations: Neg (2), low Pos (2), high Pos (2)
Incubation:
30 min (RT) + 30 min (RT) + 45 min (RT)
Washes: 2

CONTENTS

Antibodies, antigens, labelled components:
CMV (AD 169) bound to well
Anti-human IgM Ab (g or sh) AP conjugated
Substrate: PNP
Controls - standards supplied:
Controls: Neg and Pos (human serum)
Calibrators: 3 (human) with assigned ELISA values
Additional reagents:
None
Special equipment required:
Clin-ELISA reader (optional)

INTERPRETATION

Comments on interpretation:
Equivocal: ELISA value 70-89; retest to confirm and/or test a fresh sample in 7 days
No. of references: 22

NOTES

110250.0

Cytomegalovirus
ANTIBODY DETECTION (IgM)

Manufacturer: International Immunodiagnostics
Cat. No./Trade name: 108 164/CMV-IgM

SUMMARY

[Well-Ag]–**Ab**–[AHIgM-HRP]–[TMB]–A$_{450}$

Assay type: EIA (non-competitive)
Detection: Colorimetric A$_{450}$
Format: Microtitre well, Ag coated
Sample type: Serum
Sample pre-treatment:
None
Sample volume: 10 µl (+ 1 ml diluent)*
Number of tests: 96
Controls - standards run in assay:
Controls: Neg (2), Pos (2)
Incubation:
30 min (RT) + 30 min (RT) + 15 min (RT) (first two incubations on plate shaker)
Washes: 2

CONTENTS

Antibodies, antigens, labelled components:
CMV Ag bound to well
Anti-human IgM Ab HRP conjugated
Substrate: TMB, H$_2$O$_2$
Controls - standards supplied:
Controls: Neg and Pos (human serum)
Additional reagents:
None
Special equipment required:
None

INTERPRETATION

Comments on interpretation:
Classification of results is according to cut-off; no further testing
Quantitative interpretation also available
No. of references: 0

NOTES

110333.0

*Samples assayed in duplicate

© KLUWER ACADEMIC PUBLISHERS 1994, ISSN 1381-5067

Cytomegalovirus
ANTIBODY DETECTION (IgM)

Manufacturer: Laboratoire Eurobio
Cat. No./Trade name: 900285/CYTOMEGALOVIRUS IgM ELIT®

SUMMARY

[Well-AHIgM]–**Ab**–[Ag]–[Ab-POD]–[OPD]–$A_{492/630}$

Assay type: EIA (non-competitive)
Detection: Colorimetric $A_{492/630}$
Format: Microtitre well, Ab coated
Sample type: Serum, plasma
Sample pre-treatment:
  None
Sample volume: 50 µl of 1:101 dilution
Number of tests: 96
Controls - standards run in assay:
  Standards: I (1), II (2), III (1)
Incubation:
  1 hr (RT) + 1 hr (RT) + 1 hr (RT) + 30 min (RT)
Washes: 3

CONTENTS

Antibodies, antigens, labelled components:
  Anti-human IgM MAb bound to well
  CMV Ag
  Anti-CMV PAb (h) POD conjugated
Substrate: OPD, H_2O_2
Controls - standards supplied:
  Standards: 3 (human serum with assigned values)
Additional reagents:
  None
Special equipment required:
  None

INTERPRETATION

Comments on interpretation:
  Negative: ratio of sample: standard II absorbance < 0.8
  Indeterminate: ratio of sample: standard absorbance
    between 0.8 and 1.2; retest a fresh sample 1-2 weeks
    later
  Positive: ratio of sample: standard absorbance > 1.2
No. of references: None

NOTES

110527.0

Cytomegalovirus
ANTIBODY DETECTION (IgM)

Manufacturer: Labsystems Oy
Cat. No./Trade name: 61 04 201/CYTOMEGALOVIRUS IgM EIA KIT

SUMMARY

[Well-Ag]–**Ab**–[AHIgM-AP]–[PNP]–A_{405}

Assay type: EIA (non-competitive)
Detection: Colorimetric A_{405}
Format: Microtitre well, Ag coated
Sample type: Serum
Sample pre-treatment:
  None
Sample volume: 100 µl (of 1:100 dilution) x 2
Number of tests: 96
Controls - standards run in assay:
  Controls: Neg (2), Pos (2)
Incubation:
  1 hr (37°C) + 1 hr (37°C) + 30 min (37°C)
Washes: 2

CONTENTS

Antibodies, antigens, labelled components:
  CMV Ag bound to well
  Anti-human IgM PAb (sh) AP conjugated
Substrate: PNP
Controls - standards supplied:
  Controls: Neg and Pos (human serum)
Additional reagents:
  NaOH
Special equipment required:
  Auto-EIA II Analyzer (optional)
  MICROSTRIP® Reader (optional)

INTERPRETATION

Comments on interpretation:
  This is a quantitative assay. All positive sera should be
    retested after pretreatment with LABSYSTEMS IgG
    blocking reagent (6106.020) to eliminate false
    positives caused by RF
No. of references: 20

NOTES

110538.0

© *KLUWER ACADEMIC PUBLISHERS 1994, ISSN 1381-5067*

Cytomegalovirus
ANTIBODY DETECTION (IgM)

Manufacturer: Medac Diagnostika
Cat. No./Trade name: 110/12/CMV-IgM-ELA test medac

SUMMARY

[Well-AHIgM]–**Ab**–[Ag-POD]–[OPD]–$A_{490-495}$

Assay type: EIA (non-competitive)
Detection: Colorimetric $A_{490-495}$
Format: Microtitre well, Ab coated
Sample type: Serum
Sample pre-treatment:
  None
Sample volume: 50 µl of 1:100 and 1:1000 dilution*
Number of tests: 96
Controls - standards run in assay:
  Controls: Neg (2), low Pos (2), Pos (2)
Incubation:
  1 hr (37°C) + 1 hr (37°C) + 30 min (RT)
Washes: 2 (+preliminary plate wash)

CONTENTS

Antibodies, antigens, labelled components:
  Anti-human IgM Ab bound to well
  CMV Ag POD labelled
Substrate: OPD
Controls - standards supplied:
  Controls: Neg, Borderline and Pos
Additional reagents:
  H_2SO_4
Special equipment required:
  None

INTERPRETATION

Comments on Interpretation:
  Equivocal: within cut-off ±30%; retest fresh specimen in
  14 days
No. of references: 19

NOTES

110009.0
*Samples assayed in duplicate (one of 1:100, one of 1:1000)

Cytomegalovirus
ANTIBODY DETECTION (IgM)

Manufacturer: Melotec S.A.
Cat. No./Trade name: MCMM/MELOTEST CMV IgM

SUMMARY

[Well-Ag]–**Ab**–[AHIgM-HRP]–[TMB]–A_{450}

Assay type: EIA (non-competitive)
Detection: Colorimetric A_{450}
Format: Microtitre well, Ag coated*
Sample type: Serum, plasma
Sample pre-treatment:
  Incubation with absorbant 20 min (RT) to remove IgG
Sample volume: 5 µl (+195 µl diluent)**
Number of tests: 96
Controls - standards run in assay:
  Controls: Neg (1), low Pos (2), high Pos (1)
Incubation:
  20 min (RT) + 20 min (RT) + 10 min (RT)
Washes: 2

CONTENTS

Antibodies, antigens, labelled components:
  CMV Ag bound to well
  Control coated well
  Anti-human IgM Ab HRP conjugated
Substrate: TMB, H_2O_2
Controls - standards supplied:
  Controls: Neg, low Pos, high Pos (human serum)
Additional reagents:
  None
Special equipment required:
  None

INTERPRETATION

Comments on interpretation:
  Equivocal: ratio of OD sample to low Pos control is within
    the range 0.9 to 1.1; retest fresh sample
  Repeatably equivocal: retest fresh sample in 1 week
No. of references: 8

NOTES

110055.0
*Samples and controls assayed simultaneously in antigen
  and control coated wells (control wells eliminate any antinuclear antibody interference not neutralised by the
  absorbant)

Cytomegalovirus
ANTIBODY DETECTION (IgM)

Manufacturer: Menarini Diagnostics
Cat. No./Trade name: M6159/CYTOMEGAOLVIRUS IgM

SUMMARY

[Well-AHIgM]–**Ab**–[Ag + MAb-POD]–[TMB]–A_{450}

Assay type: EIA (non-competitive)
Detection: Colorimetric A_{405}
Format: Microtitre well, Ab coated
Sample type: Serum
Sample pre-treatment:
  None
Sample volume: 100 µl (of a 1:100 dilution)
Number of tests: 96
Controls - standards run in assay:
  Controls: Neg (1), Pos (1), cut-off (1)
Incubation:
  45 min (37°C) + 45 min (37°C) + 15 min (RT)
Washes: 2

CONTENTS

Antibodies, antigens, labelled components:
  Anti-human IgM MAb bound to well
  MV Ag
  Anti-CMV MAb POD conjugated
Substrate: PNP
Controls - standards supplied:
  Controls: Neg and Pos (serum)
Additional reagents:
  None
Special equipment required:
  Not specified

INTERPRETATION

Comments on interpretation:
  Not specified
No. of references: 0

NOTES

110349.0

Cytomegalovirus
ANTIBODY DETECTION (IgM)

Manufacturer: Murex Diagnostics Limited
Cat. No./Trade name: MD01/03/Wellcozyme anti-CMV IgM

SUMMARY

[Well-AHIgM]–**Ab**–[Ag-HRP]–[OPD]–A_{490}

Assay type: EIA (non-competitive)
Detection: Colorimetric A_{490}
Format: Microtitre well, Ab coated
Sample type: Serum, plasma
Sample pre-treatment:
  None
Sample volume: Screening: 50 µl (of 1:100 dilution)
  Titration: 50 µl (of 1:100 and 1:1000 dilution)*
Number of tests: 48, 96
Controls - standards run in assay:
  Controls: Neg (2), Borderline (2), Pos (2)
Incubation:
  Screening: 2 hr (RT) + 2 hr (RT) + 30 min (RT)
  Titration: 1 hr (37°C) + 1 hr (37°C) + 30 min (RT)
Washes: 2 (+ preliminary plate wash)

CONTENTS

Antibodies, antigens, labelled components:
  Anti-human IgM Ab (g) bound to well
  CMV Ag HRP conjugated
Substrate: OPD
Controls - standards supplied:
  Controls: Neg, Borderline, Pos (human serum)
Additional reagents:
  H_2SO_4
Special equipment required:
  Wellcozyme microwell plate washing system (optional)
  Wellcozyme microwell plate reader system (optional)

INTERPRETATION

Comments on interpretation:
  Equivocal: borderline control value $\pm$ 30%; retest now
    and repeat in 14 days if necessary
No. of references: 11

NOTES

110611.0

*If large numbers of samples are to be titrated, dilutions may
be made directly in uncoated microtitre plates prior to
transfer to test wells

Cytomegalovirus
ANTIBODY DETECTION (IgM)

Manufacturer: Organon Teknika NV
Cat. No./Trade name: 80345/Vironostika® anti-CMV IgM II

SUMMARY

[Well-AHIgM]–**Ab**–[Ag]–[Ab-HRP]–[TMB]–A_{450}

Assay type: EIA (non-competitive)
Detection: Colorimetric A_{450}
Format: Microtitre well, Ab coated
Sample type: Serum, plasma (do not heat inactivate)
Sample pre-treatment:
  None
Sample volume: 10 µl (of 1:101 dilution)*
Number of tests: 96, 192
Controls - standards run in assay:
  Controls:
  Neg (1), Pos (1), strong Pos (1) (one strip)
  Neg (2), Pos (2), strong Pos (2) (two or more strips)
Incubation:
  1 hr (37°C) + 1 hr (37°C) + 30 min (RT)
Washes: 2

CONTENTS

Antibodies, antigens, labelled components:
  Anti-human IgM Ab (sh) bound to well
  CMV Ag
  Anti-CMV Ab (sh) HRP conjugated
Substrate: TMB
Controls - standards supplied:
  Controls: Neg, Pos and strong Pos (human serum)
Additional reagents:
  H_2SO_4
Special equipment required:
  None

INTERPRETATION

Comments on interpretation:
  Positive: ≥ cut-off and confirmed by viral isolation from
    urine, saliva or other secretions
  Semi-quantitative procedure is available
No. of references: 9

NOTES

110562.0

*Dilute samples from newborns 1:20

Cytomegalovirus
ANTIBODY DETECTION (IgM)

Manufacturer: Radim
Cat. No./Trade name: K3CM/CYTOMEGALOVIRUS IgM EIA WELL

SUMMARY

[Well-Ag]–**Ab**–[AHIgM-HRP]–[TMB]–A_{450}

Assay type: EIA (non-competitive)
Detection: Colorimetric A_{450}
Format: Microtitre well, Ag coated
Sample type: Serum or plasma
Sample pre-treatment:
  None
Sample volume: 100 µl of 1:300 dilution x 2
Number of tests: 96
Controls - standards run in assay:
  Controls: Neg (2), Pos (2), Cut-off (2)
Incubation:
  1 hr (37°C) + 30 min (37°C) + 10 min (37°C) or 15 min
    (RT)
Washes: 2

CONTENTS

Antibodies, antigens, labelled components:
  CMV Ag bound to well
  Anti-human IgM (g) HRP conjugated
Substrate: TMB, H_2O_2
Controls - standards supplied:
  Controls: Neg, Pos and Cut-off (serum)
Additional reagents:
  None
Special equipment required:
  None

INTERPRETATION

Comments on interpretation:
  Grey area: within cut-off value ± 10%
  Positive: > cut-off value; retest after treatment with
    protein A
No. of references: 4

NOTES

110446.0

Cytomegalovirus
ANTIBODY DETECTION (IgM)

Manufacturer: Roche Diagnostic Systems
Cat. No./Trade name: 07 3495 0/COBAS CORE CMV IgM EIA

SUMMARY

[Bead-AHIgM]–**Ab**–[Ag + Ab-HRP]–[TMB]–A_{450}

Assay type: EIA (non-competitive)
Detection: Colorimetric A_{450}
Format: Tube, Ab coated bead
Sample type: Serum or plasma (not heat inactivated)
Sample pre-treatment:
    None
Sample volume: 10 µl (+500 µl diluent) x 2
Number of tests: 50
Controls - standards run in assay:
    Controls: Neg (2), Pos (3)
Incubation:
    15 min (37°C) + 1 hr (37°C) + 15 min (37°C) all with shaking
Washes: 2

CONTENTS

Antibodies, antigens, labelled components:
    Anti-human IgM MAb (m) bound to beads
    CMV Ag
    Anti-CMV MAb (m) F(Ab')$_2$ HRP conjugated
Substrate: TMB, H_2O_2
Controls - standards supplied:
    Controls: Neg and Pos (human serum)
Additional reagents:
    Substrate (supplied as separate kit)
Special equipment required:
    Cobas® EIA shaking incubator, tube washer and photometer (optional)
    Cobas® Core automated analyser (optional)

INTERPRETATION

Comments on interpretation:
    Grey zone: within cut-off ±20%; retest using a later specimen
    Positive: >cut-off + 20: confirmed by supplemental tests
No. of references: 5

NOTES

110410.0

Cytomegalovirus
ANTIBODY DETECTION (IgM)

Manufacturer: Savyon Diagnostics Ltd
Cat. No./Trade name: 017-01-096/IPAzyme® CMV TRUEIgM®

SUMMARY

[Slide-Ag]–**Ab**–[AHIgM-HRP]–[substrate]– dark blue precipitate

Assay type: EIA (non-competitive)
Detection: Light microscopy
Format: Slide well, Ag coated
Sample type: Serum
Sample pre-treatment:
    IgG/RF strip treatment on samples and controls: add stripping solution, vortex, incubate 30 min (0-4°C), add strip/stop reagent, vortex, centrifuge
Sample volume: 50 µl supernatant (+350 µl diluent)
Number of tests: 96
Controls - standards run in assay:
    Controls: Neg (1), Pos (2)
Incubation:
    2 hr (37°C) + 45 min (37°C) + 10 min (RT)
Washes: 3

CONTENTS

Antibodies, antigens, labelled components:
    CMV Ag bound to slide well
    Anti-human IgM Ab HRP conjugated
Substrate: Not specified
Controls - standards supplied:
    Controls: Neg and Pos (human serum)
Additional reagents:
    None
Special equipment required:
    None

INTERPRETATION

Comments on interpretation:
    Negative: (-) no dark blue precipitate in any cells. If (±) precipitate in some cells; retest a fresh sample
    Positive: (+) presence of dark blue precipitate in approx 20% of cells on slide
    Invalid: dark blue precipitate in all cells
No. of references: 20

NOTES

110591.0

Cytomegalovirus
ANTIBODY DETECTION (IgM)

Manufacturer: Schiapparelli Biosystems Inc
Cat. No./Trade name: 5772915/CYTOMEGALOVIRUS IgM ELISA SYSTEM CAPTURE METHOD

SUMMARY

[Well-AHIgM]–**Ab**–[Ag:MAb + AMIgG-HRP]–[OPD]–A_{492}

Assay type: EIA (non-competitive)
Detection: Colorimetric A_{492}
Format: Microtitre well, Ag coated
Sample type: Serum (do not heat inactivate)
Sample pre-treatment:
    None
Sample volume: 100 µl of 1:100 dilution x 2
Number of tests: 96
Controls - standards run in assay:
    Controls: Neg (2), Pos (2)
Incubation:
    1 hr (37°C) + 1 hr (37°C) + 10 min (37°C)
Washes: 3

CONTENTS

Antibodies, antigens, labelled components:
    Anti-human IgM Ab bound to well
    Ag: MAb (m) complex
    Anti-murine Ig Ab (g) HRP conjugated
Substrate: OPD, H_2O_2
Controls - standards supplied:
    Controls: Neg and Pos (human serum)
Additional reagents:
    None
Special equipment required:
    None

INTERPRETATION

Comments on interpretation:
    Doubtful range: within cut-off value and cut-off + 0.100; retest to confirm
No. of references: 14

NOTES

110424.0

Cytomegalovirus
ANTIBODY DETECTION (IgM)

Manufacturer: Sigma Diagnostics
Cat. No./Trade name: SIA 410/SIA® CMV IgM

SUMMARY

[Well-Ag]–**Ab**–[AHIgM-AP]–[PMP]–A_{550}

Assay type: EIA (non-competitive)
Detection: Colorimetric A_{550}
Format: Microtitre well, Ag coated
Sample type: Serum (do not heat inactivate)
Sample pre-treatment:
    Pretreatment required but not specified
Sample volume: 50 µl (+ 200 µl diluent)
Number of tests: 96
Controls - standards run in assay:
    Controls: Neg (1), Pos (1)
    Calibrator: Pos (3)
Incubation:
    30 min (RT) + 30 min (RT) + 30 min (RT) on plate shaker
Washes: 2 (+ preliminary plate wash)

CONTENTS

Antibodies, antigens, labelled components:
    CMV Ag bound to well
    Anti-human IgM Ab (g) AP conjugated
Substrate: PMP
Controls - standards supplied:
    Controls: Neg and Pos (human serum)
    Calibrator: 1 with assigned EIA value (human serum)
Additional reagents:
    None
Special equipment required:
    Sigma EIA microwell or strip reader (optional)

INTERPRETATION

Comments on interpretation:
    Results expressed as S.I.A. CMV IgM values
No. of references: 26

NOTES

110400.0

To be used as an aid to diagnosis only

© *KLUWER ACADEMIC PUBLISHERS 1994, ISSN 1381-5067*

Cytomegalovirus
ANTIBODY DETECTION (IgM)

Manufacturer: Sigma Diagnostics
Cat. No./Trade name: SIA 301/SIA® CMV IgM (CAPTURE)

SUMMARY

[Well-AHIgM]–**Ab**–[Ag-HRP]–[TMB]–A_{450}

Assay type: EIA (non-competitive)
Detection: Colorimetric A_{450}
Format: Microtitre well, Ab coated
Sample type: Serum
Sample pre-treatment:
    None
Sample volume: 10 ml (+1 ml diluent)
Number of tests: 96
Controls - standards run in assay:
    Controls: Neg (1), Pos (2)
Incubation:
    1 hr (37°C) + 1 hr (37°C) + 30 min (RT)
Washes: 2

CONTENTS

Antibodies, antigens, labelled components:
    Anti-human IgM MAb bound to well
    CMV Ag HRP conjugated
Substrate: TMB, H_2O_2
Controls - standards supplied:
    Controls: Neg and Pos (human serum)
Additional reagents:
    None
Special equipment required:
    None

INTERPRETATION

Comments on interpretation:
    Equivocal: within cut-off ±10%; retest to confirm
No. of references: 10

NOTES

110401.0

To be used as an aid to diagnosis only

Cytomegalovirus
ANTIBODY DETECTION (IgM)

Manufacturer: Sorin Biomedica
Cat. No./Trade name: 3238/ETI-CYTOK-M reverse

SUMMARY

[Well-AHIgM]–**Ab**–[Ag]–[MAb-HRP]–[TMB]–A_{450}

Assay type: EIA (non-competitive)
Detection: Colorimetric A_{450}
Format: Microtitre well, Ab coated
Sample type: Serum, plasma
Sample pre-treatment:
    None
Sample volume: 10 µl (+1 ml diluent)
Number of tests: 96
Controls - standards run in assay:
    Controls: Neg (2), Pos (2), cut-off (4)
Incubation:
    1 hr (37°C) + 1 hr (37°C) + 30 min (RT)
Washes: 2

CONTENTS

Antibodies, antigens, labelled components:
    Anti-human IgM IgG MAb (m) bound to well
    CMV Ag
    Anti-CMV IgG MAb (m) HRP conjugated
Substrate: TMB, H_2O
Controls - standards supplied:
    Controls: Neg, cut-off and Pos (human serum)
Additional reagents:
    None
Special equipment required:
    ETI-system reader and washer (optional)

INTERPRETATION

Comments on interpretation:
    Equivocal: Within cut-off ± 10%; retest to confirm
No. of references: 15

NOTES

110246.0

Cytomegalovirus
ANTIBODY DETECTION (IgM)

Manufacturer: United Biotech Inc
Cat. No./Trade name: IA-202/MAGIWEL® CMV IgM

SUMMARY

[Well-Ag]–**Ab**–[AHIgM-HRP]–[TMB]–A_{450}

Assay type: EIA (non-competitive)
Detection: Colorimetric A_{450}
Format: Microtitre well, Ag coated
Sample type: Serum
Sample pre-treatment:
　None
Sample volume: 100 µl of 1:101 dilution
Number of tests: 96
Controls - standards run in assay:
　Controls: Neg (1)
　Calibrator: (1)
Incubation:
　30 min (RT) + 30 min (RT) + 15 min (RT)
Washes: 2

CONTENTS

Antibodies, antigens, labelled components:
　CMV Ag bound to well
　Anti-human IgM Ab (g) HRP conjugated
Substrate: TMB, H_2O_2
Controls - standards supplied:
　Controls: Neg
　Calibrator: IgM Pos (100 EU/ml)
Additional reagents:
　H_2SO_4
Special equipment required:
　None

INTERPRETATION

Comments on interpretation:
　Positive: ≥100 EU/ml
No. of references: 9

NOTES

110497.0

Cytomegalovirus
ANTIBODY DETECTION (IgM)

Manufacturer: Zeus Scientific Inc
Cat. No./Trade name: 9500M series/CMV IgM ELISA

SUMMARY

[Well-Ag]–**Ab**–[AHIgM-HRP]–[TMB]–A_{450}

Assay type: EIA (non-competitive)
Detection: Colorimetric A_{450}
Format: Microtitre well, Ag coated
Sample type: Serum
Sample pre-treatment:
　Incubation with absorbent to remove IgG (20 min RT)
Sample volume: 10 µl (+200 µl diluent)
Number of tests: 96
Controls - standards run in assay:
　Controls: Neg (1), low Pos (3), high Pos (1)
Incubation:
　20 min (RT) + 20 min (RT) + 10 min (RT)
Washes: 2

CONTENTS

Antibodies, antigens, labelled components:
　CMV Ag (strain AD169) bound to well
　Anti-human IgM Ab HRP conjugated
Substrate: TMB, H_2O_2
Controls - standards supplied:
　Controls: Neg, low Pos and high Pos serum
Additional reagents:
　None
Special equipment required:
　None

INTERPRETATION

Comments on interpretation:
　Equivocal: OD ratio of sample: cut-off between 0.91-
　1.09; retest using a fresh sample or an alternative
　method
No. of references: 35

NOTES

110300.0

Cytomegalovirus
ANTIBODY DETECTION (IgG)

Manufacturer: Gen Bio
Cat. No./Trade name: 4110/ImmunoDOT® TORCH TEST*

SUMMARY

[Membrane-Ag]–**Ab**–[AHIgG-AP]–[BCIP]–violet dot

Assay type: Immunoblot assay
Detection: Visual
Format: Reaction vessel, membrane strip, Ag coated
Sample type: Serum, whole blood
Sample pre-treatment:
  None
Sample volume: 10 µl (serum), 20 µl (whole blood)
Number of tests: 10, 50, 100
Controls - standards run in assay:
  Controls: Neg integral (1), Pos integral (1), Pos (1)
Incubation:
  5 x 4 min standing time in controlled temperature
    workstation
Washes: 4

CONTENTS

Antibodies, antigens, labelled components:
  CMV Ag bound as a discrete dot on membrane strip (one
    of 4 separate antigen dots)*
  Anti-human IgG Ab (g) AP conjugated
Substrate: BCIP
Controls - standards supplied:
  Controls: Integral Neg, Integral Pos
Additional reagents:
  Pos control serum (for all antigens) (no. 2215)
Special equipment required:
  Gen Bio workstation (Cat. no. 4001 or 4990)

INTERPRETATION

Comments on Interpretation:
  Negative: no dot or indistinct dot in CMV Ag window
  Positive: distinct blue-violet dot in CMV Ag window
No. of references: 17

NOTES

110378.0

*Simultaneous testing for T. gondii, Rubella virus, CMV and
  HSV with the ImmunoDOT® TORCH test system.
  Designed for preconception/postnatal screening

Cytomegalovirus
ANTIBODY DETECTION (IgG)

Manufacturer: Gen Bio
Cat. No./Trade name: 2210/ImmunoDOT® T.E.C.H. TEST*

SUMMARY

[Membrane-Ag]–**Ab**–[AHIgG-AP]–[BCIP]–violet dot

Assay type: Immunoblot assay
Detection: Visual
Format: Reaction vessel, membrane strip, Ag coated
Sample type: Serum, whole blood
Sample pre-treatment:
  None
Sample volume: 10 µl (serum), 20 µl (whole blood)
Number of tests: 10, 50, 100
Controls - standards run in assay:
  Controls: Neg integral (1), Pos integral (1), Pos (1)
Incubation:
  5 x 4 min standing time in controlled temperature
    workstation
Washes: 4

CONTENTS

Antibodies, antigens, labelled components:
  CMV Ag bound as a discrete dot on membrane strip (one
    of 4 separate antigen dots)*
  Anti-human IgG Ab (g) AP conjugated
Substrate: BCIP
Controls - standards supplied:
  Controls: Integral Neg, Integral Pos
Additional reagents:
  Pos control serum (for all antigens) (no. 2215)
Special equipment required:
  Gen Bio workstation (Cat. no. 4001 or 4990)

INTERPRETATION

Comments on Interpretation:
  Negative: no dot or indistinct dot in CMV Ag window
  Positive: distinct blue-violet dot in CMV Ag window
No. of references: 17

NOTES

110380.0

*Simultaneous testing for T. gondii, EBV, CMV and HSV with
  the ImmunoDOT® TECH Test system

© KLUWER ACADEMIC PUBLISHERS 1994, ISSN 1381-5067

Cytomegalovirus
ANTIBODY DETECTION

Manufacturer: Gull Laboratories
Cat. No./Trade name: CM 100/CMV Test

SUMMARY

[Slide well-Ag]–**Ab**–[AHIg-FITC]–fluorescence

Assay type: Immunofluorescence assay (indirect)
Detection: Fluorescence microscopy
Format: Slide well, Ag coated
Sample type: Serum*
Sample pre-treatment:
   None
Sample volume: 15 µl of a 1:10 dilution*
Number of tests: 100
Controls - standards run in assay:
   Controls: Neg (1), Pos (1)
Incubation:
   30 min (37°C) + 30 min (37°C)
Washes: 2

CONTENTS

Antibodies, antigens, labelled components:
   CMV Ag infected and uninfected cells: bound to slide well
   Anti-human Ig Ab (g) FITC conjugated
Substrate:
Controls - standards supplied:
   Controls: Neg and Pos (human serum - titre stated on label)
Additional reagents:
   None
Special equipment required:
   None

INTERPRETATION

Comments on interpretation:
   Negative: cells show red counterstain and no fluorescence
   Positive: fluorescence in ≥10% of infected cells per field at 1:10 or greater dilution
   A method is available for the comparison of acute and convalescent sera
No. of references: 12

NOTES

110123.0

*Sera found Pos at 1:10 can be titrated using serial two fold dilutions

---

Cytomegalovirus
ANTIBODY DETECTION

Manufacturer: Incstar
Cat. No./Trade name: 1706/CMV-Fluoro Kit®

SUMMARY

[Slide-Ag]–**Ab**–[AHIg-FITC]–fluorescence

Assay type: Immunofluorescence assay (indirect)
Detection: Fluorescence microscopy
Format: Slide well, Ag coated
Sample type: Serum, plasma
Sample pre-treatment:
   None
Sample volume: 20 µl of 1:16 dilution
Number of tests: 60, 120
Controls - standards run in assay:
   Controls: Neg (1), Pos (1)
Incubation:
   30 min (RT) + 30 min (RT)
Washes: 2

CONTENTS

Antibodies, antigens, labelled components:
   CMV infected and non-infected tissue culture cells bound to slide. At least 25% infected with CMV (D169)
   Anti-human Ig Ab FITC conjugated
Substrate:
Controls - standards supplied:
   Controls: Pos and Neg (human serum)
Additional reagents:
   None
Special equipment required:
   None

INTERPRETATION

Comments on interpretation:
   Positive: ≥(1+) specific apple-green fluorescence of the nucleus and/or cytoplasm of at least 10% to 75% of the cells
No. of references: 14

NOTES

110254.0

*Previously screened positive sera should be titred to end-point

Cytomegalovirus
ANTIBODY DETECTION (IgG)

Manufacturer: Amico Laboratories Inc
Cat. No./Trade name: 5300FG/IFA CMV IgG Antibody Test

SUMMARY

[Slide-Ag]–**Ab**–[AHIgG-FITC]–fluorescence

Assay type: Immunofluorescence assay (indirect)
Detection: Fluorescence microscopy
Format: Slide well, Ag coated
Sample type: Serum
Sample pre-treatment:
   Dilute patient serum: 100 μl (+900 μl diluent)
Sample volume: 1 drop of diluted sample
Number of tests: 100
Controls - standards run in assay:
   Controls: Neg (1), Pos (1)
Incubation:
   25 min (RT) + 25 min (RT)
Washes: 1

CONTENTS

Antibodies, antigens, labelled components:
   CMV Ag bound to slide well
   Anti-human IgG Ab FITC conjugated
Substrate:
Controls - standards supplied:
   Controls: Neg and Pos (slides)
Additional reagents:
   None
Special equipment required:
   None

INTERPRETATION

Comments on interpretation:
   At test dilution of 1:10:
   Negative: red counterstained cells and no fluorescence
   Equivocal: colour intensity of apple green fluorescence (+/-)
   Positive: colour intensity of apple green fluorescence (+1) to (+4)
   Semiquantitative procedure is available using serial dilutions of samples
No. of references: 15

NOTES

110576.0

Cytomegalovirus
ANTIBODY DETECTION (IgG)

Manufacturer: Bion Enterprises Ltd
Cat. No./Trade name: CMG-60/Cytomegalovirus IgG

SUMMARY

[Well-Ag]–**Ab**–[AHIgG-FITC]–fluorescence

Assay type: Immunofluorescence assay (indirect)
Detection: Fluorescence microscopy
Format: Slide/well, Ag coated
Sample type: Serum
Sample pre-treatment:
   None
Sample volume: 50 μl (+450 μl diluent)
Number of tests: 60, 120
Controls - standards run in assay:
   Controls: Neg (1), Pos (1)
Incubation:
   30 min (RT) + 30 min (RT)
Washes: 2

CONTENTS

Antibodies, antigens, labelled components:
   CMV infected and uninfected human diploid fibroblasts fixed to slide well
   Anti-human IgG Ab (g) FITC conjugated
Substrate:
Controls - standards supplied:
   Controls: Pos and Neg (human serum)
Additional reagents:
   None
Special equipment required:
   None

INTERPRETATION

Comments on interpretation:
   Positive: >(1+) grade fluorescence of well defined nuclear inclusuion body in ≥5 cells per x200 field at serum dilution ≥1:10
   For a quantitative assay, serial dilutions of sample (1:10-1:2560) are tested
No. of references: 20

NOTES

110207.0

© KLUWER ACADEMIC PUBLISHERS 1994, ISSN 1381-5067

Cytomegalovirus
ANTIBODY DETECTION (IgG)

Manufacturer: Biowhittaker
Cat. No./Trade name: 1232/FIAX®

SUMMARY

[Solid phase Ag]–**Ab**–[AHIgG-FITC]–fluorescence

Assay type: Immunofluorescence assay (indirect)
Detection: Fluorometric
Format: FIAX sampler, Ag coated
Sample type: Serum, plasma
Sample pre-treatment:
   None
Sample volume: 5 µl (+500 µl diluent)
Number of tests: 60, 240
Controls - standards run in assay:
   Controls: Neg (1), low Pos (1), high Pos (1)
   Standards: (4)
Incubation:
   1 hr (RT) + 30 min (RT)
Washes: 2 (each wash involves a 5 min incubation)

CONTENTS

Antibodies, antigens, labelled components:
   CMV Ag bound to side 1 of FIAX sampler (Side 2
      contains no antigen and serves as a blank)
   Anti-human IgG Ab (g) FITC conjugated
Substrate:
Controls - standards supplied:
   Controls: Neg, low Pos, high Pos (human serum)
   Calibrators: 4 (human serum) with assigned titre values
Additional reagents:
   None
Special equipment required:
   FIAX fluorometer, shaker, diluter

INTERPRETATION

Comments on interpretation:
   Equivocal: FIAX titre 20-30. Retest to confirm
   Repeatably equivocal: Retest with a fresh sample or
      using an alternative method
No. of references: 31

NOTES

110182.0

Cytomegalovirus
ANTIBODY DETECTION (IgG)

Manufacturer: Gen Bio
Cat. No./Trade name: 1800/The CMV IgG Test

SUMMARY

[Slide-Ag]–**Ab**–[AHIgG-FITC]–fluorescence

Assay type: Immunofluorescence assay (indirect)
Detection: Fluorescence microscopy
Format: Slide well, Ag coated
Sample type: Serum
Sample pre-treatment:
   None
Sample volume: 30 µl of 1:16 and 1:128 dilutions for
   screening
Number of tests: 100
Controls - standards run in assay:
   Controls: Neg (1), Pos (6) (serial dilutions 1:16 to 1:512)
Incubation:
   30 min (37°C) + 30 min (37°C)
Washes: 2

CONTENTS

Antibodies, antigens, labelled components:
   CMV infected and uninfected cells bound to slide well
   Anti-human IgG Ab (g) FITC conjugated
Substrate:
Controls - standards supplied:
   Controls: Neg and Pos (human serum)
Additional reagents:
   None
Special equipment required:
   None

INTERPRETATION

Comments on interpretation:
   Negative: no nuclear inclusions visible at 1:16 dilution
   Positive: nuclear inclusions visible at 1:16 dilution or
      greater at intensity (2+) to (4+) fluorescence
   Antibody titre of samples may be obtained by testing
      further serial sample dilutions
   Non-specific reaction: fluorescence in infected and
      uninfected cells usually due to antinuclear antibody in
      test serum
No. of references: 14

NOTES

110372.0

© KLUWER ACADEMIC PUBLISHERS 1994, ISSN 1381-5067

Cytomegalovirus
ANTIBODY DETECTION (IgG)

Manufacturer: Schiapparelli Biosystems Inc
Cat. No./Trade name: 2111/VIRGO CMV IFA

SUMMARY

[Slide-Ag]–**Ab**–[AHIgG-FITC]–fluorescence

Assay type: Immunofluorescence assay (indirect)
Detection: Fluorescence microscopy
Format: Slide well, Ag coated
Sample type: Serum
Sample pre-treatment:
    None
Sample volume: 20 μl of 1:16 dilution
Number of tests: 96, 200
Controls - standards run in assay:
    Controls: Neg (1), Pos (1)
Incubation:
    30 min (RT) + 30 min (RT)
Washes: 2

CONTENTS

Antibodies, antigens, labelled components:
    CMV infected and uninfected tissue culture cells bound to slide well
    Anti-human IgG Ab (g) FITC conjugated
Substrate:
Controls - standards supplied:
    Controls: Neg and Pos (human serum)
Additional reagents:
    None
Special equipment required:
    None

INTERPRETATION

Comments on interpretation:
    Positive: ⩾(1+) specific apple green fluorescence at 1:16 dilution or greater
    Serial dilutions for quantitative assay
No. of references: 27

NOTES

110415.0

Cytomegalovirus
ANTIBODY DETECTION (IgG)

Manufacturer: Stellar Bio Systems Inc
Cat. No./Trade name: /IFA for human CMV antibody

SUMMARY

[Slide-Ag]–**Ab**–[AHIgG-FITC]–fluorescence

Assay type: Immunofluorescence assay (indirect)
Detection: Fluorescence microscopy
Format: Slide well, Ag coated
Sample type: Serum
Sample pre-treatment:
    None
Sample volume: 200 μl of 1:16 dilution
Number of tests: 40, 120
Controls - standards run in assay:
    Controls: Neg (1), Pos (1)
Incubation:
    30 min (37°C) + 30 min (37°C)
Washes: 2

CONTENTS

Antibodies, antigens, labelled components:
    CMV infected tissue culture cells bound to slide
    Anti-human IgG PAb (g) FITC conjugated
Substrate:
Controls - standards supplied:
    Controls: Neg and Pos (human)
Additional reagents:
    None
Special equipment required:
    None

INTERPRETATION

Comments on interpretation:
    Negative: no fluorescent inclusions in the nucleii of infected cells at 1:16 dilution
    Positive: (1+) to (4+) fluorescent in inclusions in the nucleii of infected cells at a dilution of 1:16 or higher
    A quantitative assay may be performed testing serial dilutions
No. of references: 9

NOTES

110544.0

Cytomegalovirus
ANTIBODY DETECTION (IgG)

Manufacturer: Zeus Scientific Inc
Cat. No./Trade name: 9001

SUMMARY

[Slide-Ag]–**Ab**–[AHIgG-FITC]–fluorescence

Assay type: Immunofluorescence assay (indirect)
Detection: Fluorescence microscopy
Format: Slide well, Ag coated
Sample type: Serum
Sample pre-treatment:
   None
Sample volume: 20 µl of 1:8 and 1:16 dilutions (screening)*
Number of tests: 100
Controls - standards run in assay:
   Controls: Neg (1), Pos (1)
Incubation:
   30 min (RT) + 30 min (RT)
Washes: 2

CONTENTS

Antibodies, antigens, labelled components:
   CMV infected substrate cells fixed to slide well
   Anti-human IgG FITC conjugated**
Substrate:
Controls - standards supplied:
   Controls: Pos and Neg (human serum)
Additional reagents:
   None
Special equipment required:
   None

INTERPRETATION

Comments on interpretation:
   Positive: Bright applegreen fluorescence of inclusion
      bodies within the nucleus of infected cells
No. of references: 22

NOTES

110296.0

*Positive sera are titred to end-point
**Anti-human IgM Ab-FITC conjugated is also available

Cytomegalovirus
ANTIBODY DETECTION (IgM)

Manufacturer: Amico Laboratories Inc
Cat. No./Trade name: 5300FM/IFA CMV IgM Antibody
Test

SUMMARY

[Slide-Ag]–**Ab**–[AHIgM-FITC]–fluorescence

Assay type: Immunofluorescence assay (indirect)
Detection: Fluorescence microscopy
Format: Slide well, Ag coated
Sample type: Serum
Sample pre-treatment:
   Dilute patient serum: 100 µl (+900 µl diluent)
Sample volume: 1 drop of diluted sample
Number of tests: 100
Controls - standards run in assay:
   Controls: Neg (1), Pos (1)
Incubation:
   25 min (RT) + 25 min (RT)
Washes: 1

CONTENTS

Antibodies, antigens, labelled components:
   CMV Ag bound to slide well
   Anti-human IgM Ab FITC conjugated
Substrate:
Controls - standards supplied:
   Controls: Neg and Pos (slides)
Additional reagents:
   None
Special equipment required:
   None

INTERPRETATION

Comments on interpretation:
   At test dilution of 1:10:
   Negative: red counterstained cells and no fluorescence
   Equivocal: colour intensity of apple green fluorescence
      (+/-)
   Positive: colour intensity of apple green fluorescence
      (+1) to (+4)
   Semiquantitative procedure is available using serial
      dilutions of samples
No. of references: 15

NOTES

110575.0

Cytomegalovirus
ANTIBODY DETECTION (IgM)

Manufacturer: Gen Bio
Cat. No./Trade name: 1900/CMV IgM Test

SUMMARY

[Slide-Ag]–Ab–[AHIgM-FITC]–fluorescence

Assay type: Immunofluorescence assay (indirect)
Detection: Fluorescence microscopy
Format: Slide well, Ag coated
Sample type: Serum
Sample pre-treatment:
    None
Sample volume: 30 µl of serial dilutions 1:8 to 1:512
Number of tests: 100
Controls - standards run in assay:
    Controls: Neg (1), Pos (6) (serial dilutions 1:8 to 1:256)
Incubation:
    1 hr (37°C) + 30 min (37°C)
Washes: 2

CONTENTS

Antibodies, antigens, labelled components:
    CMV infected and uninfected cells bound to slide well
    Anti-human IgM Ab (g) FITC conjugated
Substrate:
Controls - standards supplied:
    Controls: Neg and Pos (human serum)
Additional reagents:
    None
Special equipment required:
    None

INTERPRETATION

Comments on interpretation:
    Negative: no nuclear inclusions visible at 1:8 dilution
    Positive: nuclear inclusions visible at 1:8 dilution or
        greater
    Antibody titre of samples may be obtained by testing
        further serial sample dilutions
    Non-specific reaction: fluorescence in infected and
        uninfected cells usually due to antinuclear antibody in
        test serum
No. of references: 40

NOTES

110373.0

*It is recommended that CMV IgG antibody testing be
    performed simultaneously with CMV-IgM antibody testing

Cytomegalovirus
ANTIBODY DETECTION (IgM)

Manufacturer: Gull Laboratories
Cat. No./Trade name: CM 150E/CMV IgM Test

SUMMARY

[Slide-Ag]–Ab–[AHIgM-FITC]–fluorescence

Assay type: Immunofluorescence assay (indirect)
Detection: Fluorescence microscopy
Format: Slide well, Ag coated
Sample type: Serum
Sample pre-treatment:
    Optional treatment with GULLSORB Reagent to remove
    IgG and RF
Sample volume: 15 µl of 1:10 and 1:40 dilution*
Number of tests: 50, 100
Controls - standards run in assay:
    Controls: Neg (1), Pos (1)
Incubation:
    1 hr 30 min (37°C) + 30 min (37°C)
Washes: 2

CONTENTS

Antibodies, antigens, labelled components:
    CMV Ag infected and uninfected cells bound to slide well
    Anti-human IgM Ab FITC conjugated
Substrate:
Controls - standards supplied:
    Controls: Neg and Pos (human serum - titre stated on
        label)
Additional reagents:
    None
Special equipment required:
    None

INTERPRETATION

Comments on interpretation:
    Negative: cells show red counterstain but no
        fluorescence
    Positive: fluorescence in 15% of infected cells per field at
        1:10 or greater dilution
No. of references: 8

NOTES

110122.0

*If treated with GULLSORB reagent only 1:10 dilution
    required in assay

© *KLUWER ACADEMIC PUBLISHERS 1994*, ISSN 1381-5067

Cytomegalovirus
ANTIBODY DETECTION (IgM)

Manufacturer: Schiapparelli Biosystems Inc
Cat. No./Trade name: 2112/VIRGO CMV IFA

SUMMARY

[Slide-Ag]–**Ab**–[AHIgM-FITC]–fluorescence

Assay type: Immunofluorescence assay (indirect)
Detection: Fluorescence microscopy
Format: Slide well, Ag coated
Sample type: Serum
Sample pre-treatment:
 Removal of rheumatoid factor
Sample volume: 20 µl of 1:8 dilution (exact dilution depends on pretreatment)
Number of tests: 96, 200
Controls - standards run in assay:
 Controls: Neg (1), Pos (1)
Incubation:
 1 hr (RT) + 30 min (RT)
Washes: 2

CONTENTS

Antibodies, antigens, labelled components:
 CMV infected and uninfected tissue culture cells bound to slide well
 Anti-human IgM Ag (g) FITC conjugated
Substrate:
Controls - standards supplied:
 Controls: Neg and Pos (human serum)
Additional reagents:
 None
Special equipment required:
 None

INTERPRETATION

Comments on Interpretation:
 Positive: ≥(1+) specific apple green fluorescence at 1:8 or greater
 Serial dilutions for quantitative assay
No. of references: 27

NOTES

110416.0

Cytomegalovirus
ANTIBODY DETECTION

Manufacturer: Becton Dickinson
Cat. No./Trade name: 8551-26/CMVScan®

SUMMARY

[Latex-Ag]–**Ab**–agglutination

Assay type: Particle agglutination assay
Detection: Visual
Format: Test card, Ag coated latex
Sample type: Serum, plasma
Sample pre-treatment:
 None
Sample volume: 25 µl
Number of tests: 30, 100, 500
Controls - standards run in assay:
 Controls: High Pos (1), Neg (1)
Incubation:
 8 min (RT) with rotation
Washes: None

CONTENTS

Antibodies, antigens, labelled components:
 CMV Ag bound to latex
Substrate:
Controls - standards supplied:
 Controls: High reactive, low reactive and negative (human serum)
Additional reagents:
 None
Special equipment required:
 None

INTERPRETATION

Comments on Interpretation:
 Positive: agglutination of CMVScan latex antigen
 Results may be assessed quantitatively by testing serial dilutions of the high Pos and low Pos controls and the samples
No. of references: 8

NOTES

110367.0

*The low reactive control is only used in the quantitative assay

Hepatitis A virus (HAV)

Natural history

Hepatitis A virus is classified as a distinct genus, hepatovirus, in the enterovirus family. Infection with hepatitis A virus occurs world-wide, spread principally by the faecal-oral route (including oral-anal sexual contact), with contaminated food or drink causing common-source outbreaks. HAV is acquired much less often by blood transfusion/blood contact from a viraemic case. Outbreaks have been noted in drug users and recently in haemophiliacs. The incubation period between clinical cases is around four weeks, but virus is shed in faeces prior to symptoms appearing. Poor sanitation and overcrowding account for a high rate of infection in early childhood in endemic areas; improved conditions lead to more cases in school children and adolescents, whilst in developed countries infection of the increasing number of susceptible adults results from exposure during travel or in other risk situations. Infection in childhood is asymptomatic or mild, the severity of systemic symptoms of a protracted influenza-like illness and hepatitis increasing with age. HAV is not a cytopathic virus; damage is considered to be immunopathological, and recovery within a few weeks is the rule. Compromised hosts (including neonates) can shed virus for weeks, and there are other prolonged cases with disease lasting for a few months, but no chronic persisting infection. Normal human immuno-globulin containing HAV antibody (immune serum globulin) is protective in the short-term pre-exposure and modifies disease if given after contact. Inactivated cell-culture grown HAV vaccines are now available and attenu-ated vaccines are being developed.

Diagnosis and markers

Immunoassays based on viral particle prep-arations as antigen have been widely used to detect antibody to the structural capsid proteins (from the P1 region of the genome), produced following infection or immunisation. IgM anti-body to HAV is usually detectable at disease presentation, lasting 3–6 months or occasion-ally one year. A low level IgM response is seen after vaccination. Total or IgG antibody assays are used to measure past infection/immunity. Radio-immunoprecipitation assays using recombinant-derived proteins have indicated that antibody to non-structural proteins (from P2 region especially) appear after infection, but are not seen post-vaccine. Isolation in cell culture is not attempted for routine diagnosis, and enzyme immunoassay for viral capsid antigen is largely a research tool. Amplification by PCR of cDNA obtained from reverse-transcription of viral RNA is coming into wider use for enterovirus diagnosis generally, including investigation of HAV.

Comment

Sensitive newer assays or modifications of existing protocols for diagnostic post-infection testing may be necessary when there is a need to demonstrate an antibody response to immunisation. Recently available Hepatitis A vaccines are being used to protect selected at-risk groups including non-immune travellers to endemic areas, certain health care personnel, haemophiliacs and homosexuals.

Reference

Flehmig B, Heinricy U, Pfisterer M. Prospects for a Hepatitis A virus vaccine. Melnick JI, ed. Progress in Medical Virology. Basel: Karger. 1990;37:56-71.

© KLUWER ACADEMIC PUBLISHERS 1994, ISSN 1381-5067

Hepatitis A virus
ANTIGEN DETECTION

Manufacturer: Organon Teknika NV
Cat. No./Trade name: 70071/Hepanostika® HAV
Microelisa system

SUMMARY

$$[Well-Ab]-Ag-[Ab-HRP]-[OPD]-A_{492}$$

Assay type: EIA (non-competitive)
Detection: Colorimetric A_{492}
Format: Microtitre well, Ab coated
Sample type: Faeces
Sample pre-treatment:
   Suspend 0.5 g of specimen in buffer add 1 ml chloroform,
      centrifuge, use aqueous upper layer
Sample volume: 100 µl of extract
Number of tests: 192
Controls - standards run in assay:
   Controls: Neg (1), Pos (1)
Incubation:
   16-20 hr (RT) + 2 hr (37°C) + 45 min (RT)
Washes: 2

CONTENTS

Antibodies, antigens, labelled components:
   Anti-HAV Ab (h) bound to well
   Anti-HAV Ab (h) HRP conjugated
Substrate: OPD, H_2O_2
Controls - standards supplied:
   Controls: Neg and Pos (extract of human faeces)
Additional reagents:
   H_2SO_4
Special equipment required:
   None

INTERPRETATION

Comments on interpretation:
   Positive: ≥cut-off and confirmed by confirmatory test
      using reagents provided with this kit
   Visual interpretation is possible
No. of references: None

NOTES

110553.0

This kit will be discontinued in 1995

Hepatitis A virus
ANTIBODY DETECTION

Manufacturer: Abbott Laboratories
Cat. No./Trade name: 2226-66/IMx® HAVAB®

SUMMARY

$$[Particle-Ag]\begin{cases} Ab \\ [Ab-AP] \end{cases}-[4-MP]-fluorescence$$

Assay type: EIA (competitive)
Detection: Fluorometric
Format: Reaction well, Ag coated microparticle
Sample type: Serum, plasma (do not heat inactivate)
Sample pre-treatment:
   None
Sample volume: 150 µl
Number of tests: 100
Controls - standards run in assay:
   Calibration assay: calibrators (1) x 2; Controls: Neg (1),
      Pos (1)
   Mode 1 assay: calibrators (1); Controls: Pos (1)*
Incubation:
   Automated
Washes: Automated

CONTENTS

Antibodies, antigens, labelled components:
   HAV Ag bound to microparticle
   Anti-HAV Ab (h) AP conjugated
Substrate: 4-MP
Controls - standards supplied:
   Calibrators: mode 1 calibrator (human plasma)
Additional reagents:
   IMx® HAVAB controls, IMx® MEIA diluent buffer
   IMx® probe cleaning solution
Special equipment required:
   IMx system

INTERPRETATION

Comments on interpretation:
   Sample reactivity is calculated automatically
   Classification of sample is according to cut-off; no further
      testing
No. of references: 11

NOTES

110061.0

*Minimum control requirement for mode 1 assay one positive
   control assayed once per 8 hr shift

© *KLUWER ACADEMIC PUBLISHERS 1994, ISSN 1381-5067*

Hepatitis A virus
ANTIBODY DETECTION

Manufacturer: ADI Diagnostics
Cat. No./Trade name: /Heprofile® Anti-HAV

SUMMARY

$$[\text{Well-Ag}] \left\langle \begin{array}{l} \text{Ab} \\ [\text{Ab-POD}] \end{array} \right. -[\text{TMB}] - A_{450}$$

Assay type: EIA (competitive)
Detection: Colorimetric A_{450}
Format: Microtitre well, Ag coated
Sample type: Serum, plasma (do not heat inactivate)
Sample pre-treatment:
   None
Sample volume: 10 μl
Number of tests: 96
Controls - standards run in assay:
   Controls: Neg (3), Pos (2)
Incubation:
   a) 12-20 hr (RT) + 30 min (RT)
   b) 3 hr (37°C) + 30 min (RT)
Washes: 1

CONTENTS

Antibodies, antigens, labelled components:
   HAV Ag bound to well
   Anti-HAV PAb (h) POD conjugated
Substrate: TMB, H_2O_2
Controls - standards supplied:
   Controls: Neg and Pos (human plasma)
Additional reagents:
   None
Special equipment required:
   None

INTERPRETATION

Comments on interpretation:
   Equivocal: Within cut-off ± 10%. Retest to confirm
   Positive: ≤ cut-off repeatably
   A quantitative assay may be performed using serial
      dilutions
No. of references: 0

NOTES

110194.0

Hepatitis A virus
ANTIBODY DETECTION

Manufacturer: Boehringer Mannheim
Cat. No./Trade name: 1354 639/Enzymun-Test® Anti-HAV

SUMMARY

$$[\text{Tube-strept}] - [\text{biotin-MAb}] - [\text{Ag}] \left\langle \begin{array}{l} \text{Ab} \\ [\text{MAb-POD}] \end{array} \right. -[\text{ABTS}] - A_{420}$$

Assay type: EIA (competitive)
Detection: Colorimetric A_{420}
Format: Tube, streptavidin coated
Sample type: Serum, plasma
Sample pre-treatment:
   None
Sample volume: 100 μl x 2
Number of tests: 145
Controls - standards run in assay:
   Controls: Neg (2), Pos (2)
Incubation:
   1 hr (RT) + 2 hr (RT) + 1 hr (RT)
Washes: 1

CONTENTS

Antibodies, antigens, labelled components:
   HAV Ag from cell culture
   Anti-HAV MAb (m) biotinylated
   Anti-HAV MAb (m) POD conjugated
Substrate: ABTS, H_2O_2
Controls - standards supplied:
   Controls: Neg and Pos (human serum with assigned EIA
      value)
Additional reagents:
   Substrate and streptavidin-coated tubes
Special equipment required:
   Automated Enzymun-Test Systems (optional)

INTERPRETATION

Comments on interpretation:
   Borderline: within cut-off ±10%; retest to confirm
   Quantitative procedure available
No. of references: 0

NOTES

110468.0

Hepatitis A virus
ANTIBODY DETECTION

Manufacturer: Laboratoire Eurobio
Cat. No./Trade name: 900271/HAV ELIT®

SUMMARY

$$[\text{Well-Ab}] \overset{\textbf{Ab}}{\Big)} [Ag]-[Ab\text{-POD}]-[OPD]-A_{492}$$

Assay type: EIA (competitive)
Detection: Colorimetric A_{492}
Format: Microtitre well, Ab coated
Sample type: Serum
Sample pre-treatment:
  None
Sample volume: 10 µl
Number of tests: 96
Controls - standards run in assay:
  Controls: Neg (2), Pos (2)
Incubation:
  1 hr (RT) + 1 hr (RT) + 30 min (RT)
Washes: 2

CONTENTS

Antibodies, antigens, labelled components:
  Anti-HAV PAb bound to well
  HAV Ag
  Anti-HAV PAb POD conjugated
Substrate: OPD, H_2O_2
Controls - standards supplied:
  Controls: Neg and Pos (serum)
Additional reagents:
  None
Special equipment required:
  None

INTERPRETATION

Comments on interpretation:
  Negative: % inhibition of enzyme activity < 30%
  Indeterminate: % inhibition of enzyme activity is within
    30-70%; retest using this assay or an alternative
    assay
  Positive: % inhibition of enzyme activity > 70%
No. of references: 5

NOTES

110530.0

Hepatitis A virus
ANTIBODY DETECTION

Manufacturer: Murex Diagnostics Limited
Cat. No./Trade name: VK37/Murex anti-HAV

SUMMARY

$$[\text{Well-MAb}]-[Ag] \Big(\overset{\textbf{Ab}}{\underset{[\text{MAb-HRP}]}{}} -[TMB]-A_{450}$$

Assay type: EIA (competitive)
Detection: Colorimetric A_{450}
Format: Microtitre well, Ab coated
Sample type: Serum, plasma
Sample pre-treatment:
  None
Sample volume: 10 µl
Number of tests: 96
Controls - standards run in assay:
  Controls: Neg (3), Pos (2)
Incubation:
  1 hr (37°C) + 1 hr (37°C) + 30 min (RT)
Washes: 2

CONTENTS

Antibodies, antigens, labelled components:
  Anti-HAV MAb bound to well
  HAV Ag
  Anti-HAV MAb (m) HRP conjugated
Substrate: TMB, H_2O_2
Controls - standards supplied:
  Controls: Neg and Pos (human serum)
Additional reagents:
  H_2SO_4
Special equipment required:
  Wellcozyme microwell plate washing system (optional)
  Wellcozyme microwell plate reader (optional)

INTERPRETATION

Comments on interpretation:
  Classification of samples is according to cut-off; no
    further testing
No. of references: 0

NOTES

110666.0

© *KLUWER ACADEMIC PUBLISHERS 1994, ISSN 1381-5067*

Hepatitis A virus
ANTIBODY DETECTION

Manufacturer: Organon Teknika NV
Cat. No./Trade name: 80224/Hepanostika® HAV Antibody

SUMMARY

$$\begin{array}{c} \text{Ab} \\ \text{[Well-Ab]} \end{array} \Big\rangle [Ag]-[Ab\text{-}HRP]-[TMB]-A_{450}$$

Assay type: EIA (competitive)
Detection: Colorimetric A_{450}
Format: Microtitre well, Ab coated
Sample type: Serum, plasma
Sample pre-treatment:
   None
Sample volume: 100 µl
Number of tests: 192
Controls - standards run in assay:
   Controls:
   Neg (1), Pos (1) (for one strip)
   Neg (2), Pos (2) (for two strips)
   Neg (3), Pos (3) (for three or more strips)
Incubation:
   2 hr (37°C) + 2 hr (37°C) + 30 min (RT)*
Washes: 2

CONTENTS

Antibodies, antigens, labelled components:
   Anti-HAV Ab (h) bound to well
   HAV Ag
   Anti-HAV Ab (h) HRP conjugated
Substrate: TMB, H_2O_2
Controls - standards supplied:
   Controls: Neg and Pos (human)
Additional reagents:
   H_2SO_4
Special equipment required:
   None

INTERPRETATION

Comments on interpretation:
   Positive: ⩽ cut-off repeatably
No. of references: 3

NOTES

110552.0

*1st incubation may be 16-24 hr (RT)

Hepatitis A virus
ANTIBODY DETECTION

Manufacturer: Roche Diagnostic Systems
Cat. No./Trade name: 07 3536 1/COBAS® CORE Anti-HAV EIA

SUMMARY

$$[\text{Bead-MAb:Ag}] \Big\langle \begin{array}{c} \text{Ab} \\ \text{[Ab-HRP]} \end{array} -[TMB]-A_{450}$$

Assay type: EIA (competitive)
Detection: Colorimetric A_{450}
Format: Tube, Ag-Ab complex coated bead
Sample type: Serum or plasma
Sample pre-treatment:
   None
Sample volume: 50 µl (+200 µl diluent)
Number of tests: 50
Controls - standards run in assay:
   Controls: Neg (3), Pos (2)
Incubation:
   1 hr (37°C) + 15 min (37°C) both with shaking
Washes: 1

CONTENTS

Antibodies, antigens, labelled components:
   Anti-HAV MAb complexed with
   HAV Ag bound to bead
   Anti-HAV Fab' (h) HRP conjugated
Substrate: TMB, H_2O_2
Controls - standards supplied:
   Controls: Neg and Pos (human serum)
Additional reagents:
   Substrate (supplied as separate kit)
Special equipment required:
   Cobas® EIA shaking incubator, tube washer and
      photometer (optional)
   Cobas® Core automated analyser (optional)

INTERPRETATION

Comments on interpretation:
   Grey zone: within cut-off ±10%; retest to confirm
   Positive: < cut-off - 10% repeatably
No. of references: 6

NOTES

110402.0

Hepatitis A virus
ANTIBODY DETECTION

Manufacturer: Schiapparelli Biosystems Inc
Cat. No./Trade name: 5853550/ELISA HAVAb MAB

SUMMARY

$$[\text{Well-MAb}] \rangle^{\mathbf{Ab}} [Ag]-[MAb\text{-}POD]-[TMB]-A_{450}$$

Assay type: EIA (competitive)
Detection: Colorimetric A_{450}
Format: Microtitre well, Ab coated
Sample type: Serum or plasma (do not heat inactivate)
Sample pre-treatment:
  None
Sample volume: 10 µl (x 2 optional)
Number of tests: 96
Controls - standards run in assay:
  Controls: Neg (3), Pos (2)
Incubation:
  a) 1 hr (37°C) + 1 hr (37°C) + 30 min (RT)
  b) 16-20 hr (RT) + 1 hr (37°C) + 30 min (RT)
Washes: 2

CONTENTS

Antibodies, antigens, labelled components:
  Anti-HAV MAb bound to well
  HAV Ag
  Anti-HAV MAb POD conjugated
Substrate: TMB, H_2O_2
Controls - standards supplied:
  Controls: Neg and Pos (human serum)
Additional reagents:
  None
Special equipment required:
  None

INTERPRETATION

Comments on interpretation:
  Equivocal: within cut-off value ±10%; retest to confirm
No. of references: 12

NOTES

110431.0

Hepatitis A virus
ANTIBODY DETECTION

Manufacturer: Sorin Biomedica
Cat. No./Trade name: 2885/ETI-AB-HAVK-2

SUMMARY

$$[\text{Well-Ag}] \langle \begin{matrix} \mathbf{Ab} \\ [Ab\text{-}HRP] \end{matrix} -[TMB]-A_{450}$$

Assay type: EIA (competitive)
Detection: Colorimetric A_{450}
Format: Microtitre well, Ag coated
Sample type: Serum, plasma
Sample pre-treatment:
  None
Sample volume: 10 µl
Number of tests: 96
Controls - standards run in assay:
  Controls: Neg (3), Pos (2)
Incubation:
  3 hr (37°C) + 30 min (RT)
Washes: 1

CONTENTS

Antibodies, antigens, labelled components:
  HAV Ag (h) bound to well
  Anti-HAV IgG Ab (h) HRP conjugated
Substrate: TMB, H_2O_2
Controls - standards supplied:
  Controls: Neg and Pos (human serum)
Additional reagents:
  None
Special equipment required:
  ETI-system reader and software (optional)
  ETI-system washer (optional)

INTERPRETATION

Comments on interpretation:
  Equivocal: Within cut-off ± 10%; retest to confirm
  A quantitative assay may be performed using serial
    sample dilutions 1:100 to 1:6400
No. of references: 5

NOTES

110233.0

© *KLUWER ACADEMIC PUBLISHERS 1994, ISSN 1381-5067*

Hepatitis A virus
ANTIBODY DETECTION

Manufacturer: Syva Company
Cat. No./Trade name: 8HG29UL/MicroTrak® II Total Anti-HAV EIA

SUMMARY

$$[\text{Well-Ag}]\left\langle\begin{array}{l}\textbf{Ab}\\{}[\text{Ab-HRP}]\end{array}\right.-[\text{TMB}]-A_{450/630}$$

Assay type: EIA (competitive)
Detection: Colorimetric $A_{450/630}$
Format: Microtitre well, Ag coated
Sample type: Serum, plasma
Sample pre-treatment:
  None
Sample volume: 10 µl
Number of tests: 96
Controls - standards run in assay:
  Controls: Neg (3), Pos (2)
Incubation:
  3 hr (37°C) + 30 min (37°C)
Washes: 1

CONTENTS

Antibodies, antigens, labelled components:
  HAV bound to well
  Anti-HAV IgG Ab (h) HRP conjugated
Substrate: TMB, H_2O_2
Controls - standards supplied:
  Controls: Neg and Pos (human serum)
Additional reagents:
  MicroTrak® II EIA universal reagents (8K209UL)
Special equipment required:
  Syva MicroTrak® EIA autowasher and autoreader

INTERPRETATION

Comments on interpretation:
  Grey zone: within cut-off ±25%; retest to confirm
No. of references: 9

NOTES

110062.0

Hepatitis A virus
ANTIBODY DETECTION (IgG)

Manufacturer: Amico Laboratories Inc
Cat. No./Trade name: 1300G/AMIZYME® Hepatitis A IgG

SUMMARY

$$[\text{Well-Ag}]-\textbf{Ab}-[\text{AHIgG-HRP}]-[\text{ATBS}]-A_{450}$$

Assay type: EIA (non-competitive)
Detection: Colorimetric A_{405}
Format: Microtitre well, Ag coated
Sample type: Serum
Sample pre-treatment:
  None
Sample volume: 5 µl (+245 µl diluent)
Number of tests: 96
Controls - standards run in assay:
  Controls: Neg (1), Pos (1)
  Calibrator: (1)
Incubation:
  25 min (RT) + 25 min (RT) + 25 min (RT)
Washes: 2

CONTENTS

Antibodies, antigens, labelled components:
  HAV Ag bound to well
  Anti-human IgG Ab (g) HRP conjugated
Substrate: ABTS
Controls - standards supplied:
  Controls: Neg and Pos
  Calibrator
Additional reagents:
  None
Special equipment required:
  None

INTERPRETATION

Comments on interpretation:
  Equivocal area: retest
  Repeatably equivocal: retest a fresh specimen
No. of references: 18

NOTES

110572.0

Hepatitis A virus
ANTIBODY DETECTION (IgM)

Manufacturer: Abbott Laboratories
Cat. No./Trade name: 2263-66/IMx® HAVAB® - M

SUMMARY

[Particle-AHIgM]–**Ab**–[Ag]–[MAb-AP]–[4-MP]–
fluorescence

Assay type: EIA (non-competitive)
Detection: Fluorometric
Format: Reaction well, Ab coated microparticle
Sample type: Serum, plasma (do not heat inactivate)
Sample pre-treatment:
  None
Sample volume: 150 µl
Number of tests: 100
Controls - standards run in assay:
  Calibration assay: calibrators (1) x 2; Controls: Neg (1),
  Pos (1)
  Mode 1 assay: calibrators (1); Controls: Pos (1)*
Incubation:
  Automated
Washes: Automated

CONTENTS

Antibodies, antigens, labelled components:
  Anti-human IgM Ab (g) bound to microparticle
  HAV Ag (h)
  Anti-HAV MAb (m) AP conjugated
Substrate: 4-MP
Controls - standards supplied:
  Calibrators: mode 1 calibrator (human plasma)
Additional reagents:
  IMx® HAVAB®-M controls, IMx® MEIA diluent buffer,
  IMx® probe cleaning solution
Special equipment required:
  IMx system

INTERPRETATION

Comments on interpretation:
  Sample reactivity is calculated automatically
  Grey zone: sample with values between 0.8 and 1.2;
  report as borderline and advise patient follow-up
No. of references: 14

NOTES

110060.0

Hepatitis A virus
ANTIBODY DETECTION (IgM)

Manufacturer: ADI Diagnostics
Cat. No./Trade name: /Heprofile® Anti-HAV IgM

SUMMARY

[Well-AHIgM]–**Ab**–[Ag]–[Ab-POD]–[TMB]–A_{450}

Assay type: EIA (non-competitive)
Detection: Colorimetric A_{450}
Format: Microtitre well, Ab coated
Sample type: Serum, plasma
Sample pre-treatment:
  None
Sample volume: 10 µl (+2 ml diluent)
Number of tests: 96
Controls - standards run in assay:
  Controls: Neg (3), Pos (2)
Incubation:
  2 hr (37°C) + 18 hr (RT) + 30 min (RT)
Washes: 2

CONTENTS

Antibodies, antigens, labelled components:
  Anti-human IgM MAb (m) bound to well
  HAV Ag (h)
  Anti-HAV Ab POD conjugated
Substrate: TMB, H_2O_2
Controls - standards supplied:
  Controls: Neg and Pos (human plasma)
Additional reagents:
  None
Special equipment required:
  None

INTERPRETATION

Comments on interpretation:
  Positive: ≥cut-off repeatably
No. of references: 19

NOTES

110014.0

Hepatitis A virus
ANTIBODY DETECTION (IgM)

Manufacturer: Amico Laboratories Inc
Cat. No./Trade name: 1300M/AMIZYME® Hepatitis A IgM

SUMMARY

[Well-Ag]–Ab–[AHIgM-HRP]–[ATBS]–A_{450}

Assay type: EIA (non-competitive)
Detection: Colorimetric A_{405}
Format: Microtitre well, Ag coated
Sample type: Serum
Sample pre-treatment:
  None
Sample volume: 5 µl (+245 µl diluent)
Number of tests: 96
Controls - standards run in assay:
  Controls: Neg (1), Pos (1)
  Calibrator: (1)
Incubation:
  25 min (RT) + 25 min (RT) + 25 min (RT)
Washes: 2

CONTENTS

Antibodies, antigens, labelled components:
  HAV Ag bound to well
  Anti-human IgM Ab (g) HRP conjugated
Substrate: ABTS
Controls - standards supplied:
  Controls: Neg and Pos
  Calibrator
Additional reagents:
  None
Special equipment required:
  None

INTERPRETATION

Comments on Interpretation:
  Equivocal area: retest
  Repeatably equivocal: retest a fresh specimen
No. of references: 18

NOTES

110571.0

Hepatitis A virus
ANTIBODY DETECTION (IgM)

Manufacturer: bioMerieux
Cat. No./Trade name: 30307/VIDAS HAV IgM (HAVM)

SUMMARY

[Solid phase-AHIgM]–Ab–[Ag:MAb-AP]–[4-MP]– fluorescence

Assay type: EIA (non-competitive)
Detection: Fluorometric
Format: Solid phase receptacle (SPR), Ab coated reagent strip
Sample type: Serum, plasma
Sample pre-treatment:
  None
Sample volume: 100 µl
Number of tests: 30
Controls - standards run in assay:
  Controls: Neg (1), Pos (1)
  Standard: (1)*
Incubation:
  Automated - total time 1 hr
Washes: Automated

CONTENTS

Antibodies, antigens, labelled components:
  Anti-human IgM (g) bound to solid phase
  HAV Ag
  Anti-HAV Ag MAb (m) AP conjugated
Substrate: 4-MP
Controls - standards supplied:
  Controls: Neg and Pos (human serum)
  Standard: Pos (human serum)
Additional reagents:
  None
Special equipment required:
  Vitek Immunodiagnostic assay system (VIDAS)

INTERPRETATION

Comments on Interpretation:
  Sample reactivity is calculated automatically and classification is according to cut-off
  Equivocal: retest with fresh sample
No. of references: 6

NOTES

110475.0

*Recalibrate with each new lot of reagents and every 14 days

© KLUWER ACADEMIC PUBLISHERS 1994, ISSN 1381-5067

Hepatitis A virus
ANTIBODY DETECTION (IgM)

Manufacturer: Boehringer Mannheim
Cat. No./Trade name: 1352 474/Enzymun-Test® Anti-HAV IgM

SUMMARY

[Tube-strept]–[AHIgM-biotin]–**Ab**–[Ag:MAb-POD]–[ABTS]–A_{420}

Assay type: EIA (non-competitive)
Detection: Colorimetric A_{420}
Format: Tube, streptavidin coated
Sample type: Serum, plasma
Sample pre-treatment:
    None
Sample volume: 20 µl
Number of tests: 140
Controls - standards run in assay:
    Controls: Neg (2), Pos (2)
Incubation:
    1 hr 30 min (RT) + 1 hr 30 min (RT) + 1 hr (RT)
Washes: 2

CONTENTS

Antibodies, antigens, labelled components:
    HAV Ag
    Anti-human IgM MAb (m) biotinylated
    Anti-HAV MAb (m) POD conjugated
Substrate: ABTS, H_2O_2
Controls - standards supplied:
    Controls: Neg and Pos (human serum)
Additional reagents:
    Substrate and streptavidin-coated tubes
Special equipment required:
    Automated Enzymun-Test Systems (optional)

INTERPRETATION

Comments on interpretation:
    Borderline: within cut-off ±10%; retest to confirm
No. of references: 0

NOTES

110469.0

Hepatitis A virus
ANTIBODY DETECTION (IgM)

Manufacturer: Laboratoire Eurobio
Cat. No./Trade name: 900272/HAV-M ELIT®

SUMMARY

[Well-AMIgG]–[AHIgM(MAb)-**Ab**]–[Ag]–[Ab-POD]–[OPD]–A_{492}

Assay type: EIA (non-competitive)
Detection: Colorimetric A_{492}
Format: Microtitre well, Ab coated
Sample type: Serum
Sample pre-treatment:
    None
Sample volume: 100 µl of 1:201 dilution
Number of tests: 96
Controls - standards run in assay:
    Controls: Neg (2), Pos (2)
Incubation:
    1 hr (RT) + 1 hr (RT) + 1 hr (RT) + 30 min (RT)
Washes: 3

CONTENTS

Antibodies, antigens, labelled components:
    Anti-murine IgG PAb bound to well
    Anti-human IgM MAb (IgG) (m)
    HAV antigen
    Anti-HAV PAb POD conjugated
Substrate: OPD, H_2O_2
Controls - standards supplied:
    Controls: Neg, Pos
Additional reagents:
    None
Special equipment required:
    None

INTERPRETATION

Comments on interpretation:
    Classification of sample is according to cut-off; no further testing
No. of references: 5

NOTES

110531.0

© *KLUWER ACADEMIC PUBLISHERS 1994, ISSN 1381-5067*

Hepatitis A virus
ANTIBODY DETECTION (IgM)

Manufacturer: Murex Diagnostics Limited
Cat. No./Trade name: VK36/Murex anti-HAV IgM

SUMMARY

[Well-AHIgM]–**Ab**–[Ag:MAb-HRP]–[TMB]–A_{450}

Assay type: EIA (non-competitive)
Detection: Colorimetric A_{450}
Format: Microtitre well, Ab coated
Sample type: Serum, plasma
Sample pre-treatment:
  None
Sample volume: 10 μl (+1.99 ml diluent)
Number of tests: 96
Controls - standards run in assay:
  Controls: Neg (2), Pos (3)
Incubation:
  1 hr (37°C) + 1 hr (37°C) + 30 min (RT)
Washes: 2

CONTENTS

Antibodies, antigens, labelled components:
  Anti-human IgM MAb bound to well
  HAV Ag
  Anti-HAV MAb HRP conjugated
Substrate: TMB, H_2O_2
Controls - standards supplied:
  Controls: Neg and Pos (human serum)
Additional reagents:
  H_2SO_4
Special equipment required:
  Wellcozyme microwell plate washing system (optional)
  Wellcozyme microwell plate reader (optional)

INTERPRETATION

Comments on interpretation:
  Equivocal: within cut-off ± 10%; retest to confirm
No. of references: 0

NOTES

110665.0

Hepatitis A virus
ANTIBODY DETECTION (IgM)

Manufacturer: Organon Teknika NV
Cat. No./Trade name: 80223/Hepanostika® HAV IgM

SUMMARY

[Well-AHIgM]–**Ab**–[Ag]–[Ab-HRP]–[TMB]–A_{450}

Assay type: EIA (non-competitive)
Detection: Colorimetric A_{450}
Format: Microtitre well, Ab coated
Sample type: Serum, plasma
Sample pre-treatment:
  None
Sample volume: 100 μl
Number of tests: 192
Controls - standards run in assay:
  Controls:
  Neg (1), Pos (1) (for one strip)
  Neg (2), Pos (2) (for two strips)
  Neg (3), Pos (3) (for three or more strips)
Incubation:
  2 hr (37°C) + 2 hr (37°C) + 30 min (RT)*
Washes: 2

CONTENTS

Antibodies, antigens, labelled components:
  Anti-human IgM Ab (ovine) bound to well
  HAV Ag (monkey)
  Anti-HAV Fab Ab (h) HRP conjugated
Substrate: TMB, H_2O_2
Controls - standards supplied:
  Controls: Neg and Pos (human)
Additional reagents:
  H_2SO_4
Special equipment required:
  None

INTERPRETATION

Comments on interpretation:
  Positive: ≥ cut-off repeatably
No. of references: 5

NOTES

110551.0

*1st incubation may be 16-24 hr (RT)

© KLUWER ACADEMIC PUBLISHERS 1994, ISSN 1381-5067

Hepatitis A virus
ANTIBODY DETECTION (IgM)

Manufacturer: Roche Diagnostic Systems
Cat. No./Trade name: 07 3443 8/COBAS CORE Anti-HAV IgM EIA

SUMMARY

[Bead-AHIgM]–**Ab**–[Ag:MAb-HRP]–[TMB]–A_{450}

Assay type: EIA (non-competitive)
Detection: Colorimetric A_{450}
Format: Tube, Ab coated bead
Sample type: Serum or plasma
Sample pre-treatment:
    None
Sample volume: 10 µl (+1 ml diluent)
Number of tests: 50
Controls - standards run in assay:
    Controls: Neg (2); Pos (3)
Incubation:
    15 min (37°C) + 30 min (37°C) + 15 min (37°C) all with
        shaking
Washes: 2

CONTENTS

Antibodies, antigens, labelled components:
    Anti-human IgM MAb (m) bound to beads
    HAV Ag complexed with
    Anti-HAV F(ab')$_2$ MAb (m) HRP conjugated
Substrate: TMB, H_2O_2
Controls - standards supplied:
    Controls: Neg and Pos (human serum)
Additional reagents:
    Substrate (supplied as separate kit)
Special equipment required:
    Cobas® EIA shaking incubator, tube washer and
        photometer (optional)
    Cobas® Core automated analyser (optional)

INTERPRETATION

Comments on interpretation:
    Grey zone: within cut-off ±10%; retest to confirm
    Positive: > cut-off +10% or repeatably within grey
        zone range
No. of references: 10

NOTES

110403.0

Hepatitis A virus
ANTIBODY DETECTION (IgM)

Manufacturer: Schiapparelli Biosystems Inc
Cat. No./Trade name: 5853700/ELISA HAVAb IgM MAB

SUMMARY

[Well-AHIgM]–**Ab**–[Ag:MAb-POD]–[TMB]–A_{450}

Assay type: EIA (non-competitive)
Detection: Colorimetric A_{450}
Format: Microtitre well, Ab coated
Sample type: Serum or plasma (do not heat inactivate)
Sample pre-treatment:
    None
Sample volume: a)100 µl of 1:10 or 1:100 dilution
    b)100 µl of 1:200 or 1:2000 dilution
Number of tests: 96
Controls - standards run in assay:
    Controls: Neg (2), Pos (3)
Incubation:
    a) 1 hr (37°C) + 1 hr (37°C) + 30 min (RT)
    b) 16-20 hr (RT) + 1 hr (37°C) + 30 min (RT)
Washes: 2

CONTENTS

Antibodies, antigens, labelled components:
    Anti-human IgM MAb bound to well
    HAV Ag
    Anti-HAV MAb POD conjugated
Substrate: TMB, H_2O_2
Controls - standards supplied:
    Controls: Neg and Pos (human serum)
Additional reagents:
    None
Special equipment required:
    None

INTERPRETATION

Comments on interpretation:
    Equivocal: within cut-off value ±10%; retest to confirm
No. of references: 12

NOTES

110432.0

© *KLUWER ACADEMIC PUBLISHERS 1994, ISSN 1381-5067*

Hepatitis A virus
ANTIBODY DETECTION (IgM)

Manufacturer: Sorin Biomedica
Cat. No./Trade name: 2034/ETI-HA-IGMK-2

SUMMARY

[Well-AHIgM]–**Ab**–[Ag]–[Ab-HRP]–[TMB]–A$_{450}$

Assay type: EIA (non-competitive)
Detection: Colorimetric A$_{450}$
Format: Microtitre well, Ab coated
Sample type: Serum, plasma
Sample pre-treatment:
  None
Sample volume: 10 µl (+1.0 ml diluent)
Number of tests: 96
Controls - standards run in assay:
  Controls: Neg (3), Pos (3)
Incubation:
  1 hr (37°C) + 1 hr (37°C) + 30 min (RT)
Washes: 3

CONTENTS

Antibodies, antigens, labelled components:
  Anti-human IgM IgG Ab (r) bound to well
  HAV Ag (h)
  Anti-HAV IgG Ab (h) HRP conjugated
Substrate: TMB, H$_2$O$_2$
Controls - standards supplied:
  Controls: Neg and Pos (human serum)
Additional reagents:
  None
Special equipment required:
  ETI system reader and washer (optional)

INTERPRETATION

Comments on interpretation:
  Equivocal: Within cut-off ± 10%; retest to confirm
No. of references: 6

NOTES

110234.0

Hepatitis A virus
ANTIBODY DETECTION (IgM)

Manufacturer: Syva Company
Cat. No./Trade name: 8K629UL/MicroTrak® II IgM Anti-HAV EIA

SUMMARY

[Well-strept]–[biotin-AHIgM]–**Ab**–[Ag]–[MAb-HRP]–[TMB]–A$_{450/630}$

Assay type: EIA (non-competitive)
Detection: Colorimetric A$_{450/630}$
Format: Microtitre well, streptavidin coated
Sample type: Serum, plasma
Sample pre-treatment:
  None
Sample volume: 5 µl (diluted 1:441 with Ab-biotin solution)
Number of tests: 96
Controls - standards run in assay:
  Controls: Neg (2), Pos (3)
Incubation:
  1 hr (37°C) + 1 hr (37°C) + 1 hr (37°C) + 30 min (37°C)
Washes: 3

CONTENTS

Antibodies, antigens, labelled components:
  HAV
  Anti-human IgM Ab (g) biotinylated
  Anti-HAV MAb (m) HRP conjugated
  Streptavidin coated well
Substrate: TMB, H$_2$O$_2$
Controls - standards supplied:
  Controls: Neg and Pos (human plasma)
Additional reagents:
  MicroTrak® II EIA universal reagents (8K209UL)
Special equipment required:
  Syva MicroTrak® EIA autowasher and autoreader

INTERPRETATION

Comments on interpretation:
  Equivocal: sample absorbance within ±25% of the cut-off; retest to confirm
No. of references: 10

NOTES

110059.0

Not available until 1995

Hepatitis A virus
ANTIBODY DETECTION (IgM)

Manufacturer: Kodak Clinical Diagnostics
Cat. No./Trade name: LAN.6206/KODAK Amerlite anti-HAV IgM assay

SUMMARY

[Well-AHIgM]–**Ab**–[Ag]–[MAb-HRP]–[signal reagent]–luminescence

Assay type: Luminometric immunoassay (non-competitive)
Detection: Luminometric
Format: Microtitre well, Ab coated
Sample type: Serum, plasma
Sample pre-treatment:
    None
Sample volume: 10 µl of 1:201 dilution
Number of tests: 48
Controls - standards run in assay:
    Controls: Neg (1), Pos (3)
Incubation:
    1 hr (37°C) + 1 hr (37°C) both with shaking + 2-20 min (RT)
Washes: 2

CONTENTS

Antibodies, antigens, labelled components:
    Anti-human IgM MAb (m) bound to well
    HAV Ag
    Anti-HAV MAb (m) HRP conjugated
Substrate: Amerlite signal reagent
Controls - standards supplied:
    Controls: Neg and Pos (human serum)
Additional reagents:
    Amerlite signal reagent and serology wash reagent
Special equipment required:
    Amerlite Kodak immunoassay system

INTERPRETATION

Comments on interpretation:
    Sample reactivity is calculated automatically and classification is according to cut-off
    Equivocal samples are marked 'retest'; retest to confirm
No. of references: 7

NOTES

110484.0

Hepatitis A virus
ANTIBODY DETECTION

Manufacturer: Abbott Laboratories
Cat. No./Trade name: 5786-24/HAVAB®

SUMMARY

$$[\text{Bead-Ag}] \begin{cases} \textbf{Ab} \\ [\text{Ab-}^{125}\text{I}] \end{cases} - \text{radioactivity}$$

Assay type: RIA (competitive)
Detection: Radioisotopic
Format: Reaction well, Ag coated bead
Sample type: Serum, plasma
Sample pre-treatment:
    None
Sample volume: 10 µl
Number of tests: 100
Controls - standards run in assay:
    Controls: Neg (3), Pos (2)
Incubation:
    a) 4 hr (45°C)
    b) 18-24 hr (RT)
Washes: 1

CONTENTS

Antibodies, antigens, labelled components:
    HAV Ag (h) bound to beads
    Anti-HAV Ab (h) ^{125}I labelled
Substrate:
Controls - standards supplied:
    Controls: Neg and Pos (human plasma)
Additional reagents:
    None
Special equipment required:
    None

INTERPRETATION

Comments on interpretation:
    Positive: ≤ cut-off repeatably
    Quantitative procedure also available
No. of references: 10

NOTES

110015.0

© *KLUWER ACADEMIC PUBLISHERS 1994, ISSN 1381-5067*

Hepatitis A virus
ANTIBODY DETECTION

Manufacturer: Sorin Biomedica
Cat. No./Trade name: 2405/Ab-HAVK

SUMMARY

$$[\text{Bead-Ag}]\begin{cases} \text{Ab} \\ [\text{Ab-}^{125}\text{I}] \end{cases} - \text{radioactivity}$$

Assay type: RIA (competitive)
Detection: Radioisotopic
Format: Tray/Tube, Ag coated bead
Sample type: Serum, plasma
Sample pre-treatment:
　None
Sample volume: 10 µl
Number of tests: 100
Controls - standards run in assay:
　Controls: Neg (3), Pos (2)
Incubation:
　a) 18-22 hr (RT)
　b) 3 hr (45°C)
Washes: 1

CONTENTS

Antibodies, antigens, labelled components:
　HAV Ag (h) bound to bead
　Anti-HAV IgG Ab (h) ^{125}I labelled
Substrate:
Controls - standards supplied:
　Controls: Neg and Pos (human serum)
Additional reagents:
　None
Special equipment required:
　Automatic rinsing device, PLA-2 (optional)
　Bead dispenser, MEDI-578 (optional)

INTERPRETATION

Comments on interpretation:
　Equivocal:　Within cut-off ± 10%; retest to confirm
　Sample dilutions 1:100 to 1:3200 are used for the
　　quantitative assay
No. of references: 5

NOTES

110278.0

Hepatitis A virus
ANTIBODY DETECTION (IgM)

Manufacturer: Abbott Laboratories
Cat. No./Trade name: 7180-22/HAVAB® - M

SUMMARY

$$[\text{Bead-AHIgM}]-\textbf{Ab}-[\text{Ag}]-[\text{Ab-}^{125}\text{I}]-\text{radioactivity}$$

Assay type: RIA (non-competitive)
Detection: Radioisotopic
Format: Reaction well, Ab coated bead
Sample type: Serum, plasma
Sample pre-treatment:
　None
Sample volume: 10 µl (+2 ml diluent)
Number of tests: 50
Controls - standards run in assay:
　Controls: Neg (2), Pos (3)
Incubation:
　2 hr (RT) + 18-22 hr (RT) + 4 hr (45°C)
Washes: 3

CONTENTS

Antibodies, antigens, labelled components:
　Anti-human IgM Ab (g) bound to bead
　HAV Ag (h)
　Anti-HAV PAb (h) ^{125}I labelled
Substrate:
Controls - standards supplied:
　Controls: Neg and Pos (human plasma)
Additional reagents:
　None
Special equipment required:
　None

INTERPRETATION

Comments on interpretation:
　Equivocal: within cut-off ±10%; retest to confirm
　Positive: ≥cut-off repeatably
No. of references: 17

NOTES

110016.0

Hepatitis A virus
ANTIBODY DETECTION (IgM)

Manufacturer: Sorin Biomedica
Cat. No./Trade name: 2440/HA-IGMK

SUMMARY

[Bead-AHIgM]–**Ab**–[Ag]–[Ab-^{125}I]–radioactivity

Assay type: RIA (non-competitive)
Detection: Radioisotopic
Format: Tray/Tube, Ab coated bead
Sample type: Serum, plasma
Sample pre-treatment:
None
Sample volume: 10 µl (+2 ml diluent)
Number of tests: 50
Controls - standards run in assay:
Controls: Neg (3), Pos (3)
Incubation:
2 hr (RT) + overnight (RT) + 3 hr (45°C)
Washes: 2

CONTENTS

Antibodies, antigens, labelled components:
Anti-human IgM Ab (g) bound to bead
HAV Ag
Anti-HAV IgG Ab ^{125}I labelled
Substrate:
Controls - standards supplied:
Controls: Neg and Pos (human serum)
Additional reagents:
None
Special equipment required:
Automatic rinser, PLA-2 (optional)
Bead dispenser, MEDI-578 (optional)

INTERPRETATION

Comments on interpretation:
Equivocal: Within cut-off ± 10%; retest to confirm
Positive: ≥ cut-off repeatably
No. of references: 6

NOTES

110221.0

© KLUWER ACADEMIC PUBLISHERS 1994, ISSN 1381-5067

Hepatitis B virus (HBV)

Natural history

Hepatitis B is endemic in areas such as eastern Asia and sub-Saharan Africa where infection is acquired perinatally from carrier mothers or early in childhood. Most of these infections are sub-clinical and in a high proportion (70–90% of infected neonates, 20–50% of those infected as children) a persistent carrier state is established. HBV infection in the West occurs mostly in adults, transmitted sexually, or by percutaneous exposure or mucosal contamination. Half the adults present with a clinical illness, including immune complex related rash or arthritis preceding hepatitis, but persistent infection occurs in less than 10% of adults. The HBV carrier may remain asymptomatic over many years, later developing an active hepatitis during spontaneous immune clearance of the infection, or have a mild persistent hepatitis, or there may be more significant chronic active hepatitis followed by cirrhosis. Hepatocellular carcinoma is associated with long term carriage of hepatitis B and cirrhosis. Carriers may have a high titre of infectious virus in blood, or predominantly non-infectious particles composed of virion surface antigen. HB immunoglobulin and HBV surface-antigen vaccines are available and are used to prevent infection in neonates, sexual contacts, health care workers and others at risk from exposure. Universal childhood immunisation is now offered in N. America and some major European countries. The goal of universal neonatal immunisation in high prevalence countries is to eliminate the carrier stage and its long term sequelae. Screening antenatal women for HBV carriage permits selective immunisation of neonates in areas of low prevalence. Interferon therapy has been successful in reducing viral replication in some 50% of chronic cases, and new antiviral regimes are on trial.

Diagnosis and markers

HBV, a member of the hepadnovirus family, cannot be isolated in cell culture. Acute infection and persistent carriage are detected by immunoassays for the virion surface (envelope) antigen, HBsAg, which bears the common group (a) as well as subtype specific (d,y,w,r) epitopes. HBsAg may be found in serum weeks before the icteric stage in the long incubation of this disease (6 weeks to 6 months). Persistence of HBsAg beyond 6 months marks the carrier state. Antibodies to the internal core protein (anti-HBc) are found soon after HBsAg appears; IgM anti-HBc indicates recent infection, while IgG anti-HBc persists throughout life as a marker of past HBV infection, even in those who have cleared infection. A soluble HBeAg found in serum during active viral replication is a marker of acute infection and of the highly infectious viraemic carriers. Clearance of HBeAg and sero-conversion to anti-HBe indicates a change to lower infectivity. HBV DNA detection by PCR is a more sensitive and direct method of determining infectivity than HBeAg detection. PCR can also be used to study viral replication in special cases, including mutant HBV variants such as the pre-core mutants which do not express HBeAg, and vaccine-induced escape mutants not neutralised by anti-HBs. Antibody to HBsAg resulting from natural infection or immunisation neutralises HBV and is protective. It is recommended that the level of antibody is maintained above 100 mIU/ml in health care workers.

Comment

Immunoassays for HBs antigen capable of detecting a minimum of 0.5 IU/ml are recommended for quality assurance in screening. HBV DNA detection should be undertaken when serological results are not consistent with the clinical presentation.

Reference

Koff RS. Hepatitis B today: clinical and diagnostic overview. Pediatric Infectious Diseases Journal. 1993;12:428–432.

Hepatitis B virus (core antigen)
ANTIBODY DETECTION

Manufacturer: Abbott Laboratories
Cat. No./Trade name: 9977/CORZYME

SUMMARY

$$[\text{Bead-Ag}] \Big\langle {}^{\text{Ab}}_{[\text{Ab-HRP}]} -[\text{OPD}]-A_{492}$$

Assay type: EIA (competitive)
Detection: Colorimetric A_{492}
Format: Reaction well, Ag coated bead
Sample type: Serum, plasma
Sample pre-treatment:
    None
Sample volume: 100 µl
Number of tests: 100, 500
Controls - standards run in assay:
    Controls: Neg (3), Pos (2)
Incubation:
    a) 2 hr (40°C) + 30 min (RT)
    b) 12-20 hr (RT) + 30 min (RT)
Washes:

CONTENTS

Antibodies, antigens, labelled components:
    rec HBcAg bound to beads
    Anti-HBc Ab (h) HRP conjugated
Substrate: OPD
Controls - standards supplied:
    Controls: Neg and Pos (human plasma)
Additional reagents:
    H_2SO_4
Special equipment required:
    None

INTERPRETATION

Comments on interpretation:
    Negative: > cut-off but where absorbance value is
        greater than 2.0; retest to confirm negative
    Equivocal: within cut-off ±10%; retest to confirm
    Semi-quantitative procedure available
No. of references: 13

NOTES

110026.0

Hepatitis B virus (core antigen)
ANTIBODY DETECTION

Manufacturer: Abbott Laboratories
Cat. No./Trade name: 2259-20/IMx® CORE®

SUMMARY

$$[\text{Particle-Ag}] \Big\langle {}^{\text{Ab}}_{[\text{Ab-AP}]} -[\text{4-MP}]-\text{fluorescence}$$

Assay type: EIA (competitive)
Detection: Fluorometric
Format: Reaction well, Ag coated microparticle
Sample type: Serum, plasma (do not heat inactivate)
Sample pre-treatment:
    None
Sample volume: 150 µl
Number of tests: 100
Controls - standards run in assay:
    Calibration assay: calibrators (1) x 2; Controls: Neg (1),
        Pos (1)
    Mode 1 assay: calibrators (1); Controls: Pos (1)*
Incubation:
    Automated
Washes: Automated

CONTENTS

Antibodies, antigens, labelled components:
    rec HBcAg bound to microparticle
    Anti-HBc Ab (h) AP conjugated
Substrate: 4-MP
Controls - standards supplied:
    Calibrator: mode 1 calibrator (human plasma)
Additional reagents:
    IMx® CORE® controls, IMx® MEIA diluent buffer, IMx®
        probe cleaning solution
Special equipment required:
    IMx system

INTERPRETATION

Comments on interpretation:
    Sample reactivity is calculated automatically
    Positive: ≤ cut-off repeatably
No. of references: 12

NOTES

110075.0

*Minimum control requirement for mode 1 assay: one
    positive control assayed once per 8 hr shift

© *KLUWER ACADEMIC PUBLISHERS 1994, ISSN 1381-5067*

Hepatitis B virus (core antigen)
ANTIBODY DETECTION

Manufacturer: ADI Diagnostics
Cat. No./Trade name: /Heprofile® Anti-HBc

SUMMARY

$$[\text{Well-Ag}]\Big\langle{}^{\textbf{Ab}}_{[\text{Ab-POD}]}-[\text{TMB}]-A_{450}$$

Assay type: EIA (competitive)
Detection: Colorimetric A_{450}
Format: Microtitre well, Ag coated
Sample type: Serum, plasma
Sample pre-treatment:
　None
Sample volume: 50 µl
Number of tests: 96
Controls - standards run in assay:
　Controls: Neg (3), Pos (2)
Incubation:
　a) 12-20 hr (RT) + 30 min (RT)
　b) 2 hr (37°C) + 30 min (RT)
Washes: 1

CONTENTS

Antibodies, antigens, labelled components:
　rec HBcAg bound to microtitre well
　Anti-HBc Ab (h) POD conjugated
Substrate: TMB, H_2O_2
Controls - standards supplied:
　Controls: Neg and Pos (human plasma)
Additional reagents:
　None
Special equipment required:
　None

INTERPRETATION

Comments on interpretation:
　Equivocal: Within cut-off ± 10%. Retest to confirm
　Positive: < cut-off - 10% repeatably
No. of references: 10

NOTES

110031.0

Hepatitis B virus (core antigen)
ANTIBODY DETECTION

Manufacturer: Behringwerke AG
Cat. No./Trade name: OUWE/Enzygnost® Anti-HBc monoclonal

SUMMARY

$$[\text{Well-Ag}]\Big\langle{}^{\textbf{Ab}}_{[\text{MAb-POD}]}-[\text{TMB}]-A_{450}$$

Assay type: EIA (competitive)
Detection: Colorimetric A_{450}
Format: Microtitre well, Ag coated
Sample type: Serum, plasma
Sample pre-treatment:
　None
Sample volume: 25 µl
Number of tests: 96
Controls - standards run in assay:
　Controls: Neg (4), Pos (2)
Incubation:
　1 hr (37°C) + 30 min (RT)
Washes: 1

CONTENTS

Antibodies, antigens, labelled components:
　rec HBcAg bound to well
　Anti-HBc MAb POD conjugated
Substrate: TMB, H_2O_2
Controls - standards supplied:
　Controls: Neg and Pos (human serum)
Additional reagents:
　None
Special equipment required:
　Behring ELISA processor (optional)

INTERPRETATION

Comments on interpretation:
　Equivocal: within cut-off ±10%; retest to confirm
No. of references: 5

NOTES

110454.0

Hepatitis B virus (core antigen)
ANTIBODY DETECTION

Manufacturer: bioMerieux
Cat. No./Trade name: 30302/VIDAS anti-HBc Total (HBCT)

SUMMARY

$$[\text{Solid phase-Ag}] \Big\langle {{\text{Ab}} \atop {[\text{MAb-AP}]}} - [\text{4-MP}] - \text{fluorescence}$$

Assay type: EIA (competitive)
Detection: Fluorometric
Format: Solid phase receptacle (SPR), Ag coated reagent strip
Sample type: Serum, plasma
Sample pre-treatment:
  None
Sample volume: 200 µl
Number of tests: 60
Controls - standards run in assay:
  Controls: Neg (1), Pos (1)
  Standard: (1)*
Incubation:
  Automated - total time 1 hr 30 minutes
Washes: Automated

CONTENTS

Antibodies, antigens, labelled components:
  rec HBcAg bound to solid phase
  Anti-HBc MAb (m) AP conjugated
Substrate: 4-MP
Controls - standards supplied:
  Controls: Neg and Pos (human serum)
  Standard: Pos (human serum)
Additional reagents:
  None
Special equipment required:
  Vitek Immunodiagnostic assay system (VIDAS)

INTERPRETATION

Comments on interpretation:
  Sample reactivity is calculated automatically and
    classification is according to cut-off
  Equivocal sample should be retested
No. of references: 4

NOTES

110474.0

*Recalibrate with each new lot of reagents and every 14
  days

Hepatitis B virus (core antigen)
ANTIBODY DETECTION

Manufacturer: Boehringer Mannheim
Cat. No./Trade name: 1123 882/Enzymun-Test® Anti-HBc

SUMMARY

$$[\text{Tube-strept}] - [\text{biotin-Ag}] \Big\langle {{\text{Ab}} \atop {[\text{MAb-POD}]}} - [\text{ABTS}] - A_{420}$$

Assay type: EIA (competitive)
Detection: Colorimetric A_{420}
Format: Tube, streptavidin coated
Sample type: Serum, plasma
Sample pre-treatment:
  None
Sample volume: 200 µl
Number of tests: 125
Controls - standards run in assay:
  Controls: Neg (2), Pos (2)
Incubation:
  1 hr (RT) + 1 hr (RT) + 1 hr (RT)
Washes: 2 (+ preliminary tube pre-wash)

CONTENTS

Antibodies, antigens, labelled components:
  rec HBcAg biotinylated
  Anti-HBc MAb (m) POD conjugated
Substrate: ABTS, H_2O_2
Controls - standards supplied:
  Controls: Neg and Pos (human serum)
Additional reagents:
  Streptavidin-coated tubes
  Substrate
Special equipment required:
  Automated Enzymun-Test Systems (optional)

INTERPRETATION

Comments on interpretation:
  Borderline: within cut-off ±10%; retest to confirm
No. of references: 0

NOTES

110465.0

Hepatitis B virus (core antigen)
ANTIBODY DETECTION

Manufacturer: IFCI Clone Systems
Cat. No./Trade name: 07.1002/EIAgen Anti-CORE IgG Kit

SUMMARY

$$[\text{Well-Ag}]\Big\langle\begin{matrix}\textbf{Ab}\\ [\text{Ab-POD}]\end{matrix}-[\text{TMB}]-A_{450}$$

Assay type: EIA (competitive)
Detection: Colorimetric A_{450}
Format: Microtitre well, Ag coated
Sample type: Serum, plasma
Sample pre-treatment:
    None
Sample volume: 50 µl
Number of tests: 96
Controls - standards run in assay:
    Controls: Neg (3), Pos (2)
Incubation:
    a) 16 hr (RT) + 30 min (RT)
    b) 2 hr (37°C) + 30 min (RT)
Washes: 1

CONTENTS

Antibodies, antigens, labelled components:
    rec HBcAg bound to well
    Anti-HBc Ab (h) POD conjugated
Substrate: TMB, H_2O_2
Controls - standards supplied:
    Controls: Neg and Pos (human plasma)
Additional reagents:
    None
Special equipment required:
    None

INTERPRETATION

Comments on interpretation:
    Equivocal: within cut-off ± 10%; retest in duplicate. If duplicate values do not agree result is inconclusive and retest fresh sample
    Positive: ≤ cut-off - 10% repeatably
No. of references: 0

NOTES

110089.0

Hepatitis B virus (core antigen)
ANTIBODY DETECTION

Manufacturer: Labsystems Oy
Cat. No./Trade name: 61 10 370/Anti-HBc EIA

SUMMARY

$$[\text{Well-Ag}]\Big\langle\begin{matrix}\textbf{Ab}\\ [\text{MAb-HRP}]\end{matrix}-[\text{TMB}]-A_{450}$$

Assay type: EIA (competitive)
Detection: Colorimetric A_{450}
Format: Microtitre well, Ag coated
Sample type: Serum, plasma
Sample pre-treatment:
    None
Sample volume: 50 µl
Number of tests: 96
Controls - standards run in assay:
    Controls: Neg (3), Pos (2)
Incubation:
    a) 2 hr (37°C) + 30 min (RT)
    b) 16-22 hr (RT) + 30 min (RT)
Washes: 1

CONTENTS

Antibodies, antigens, labelled components:
    rec HBcAg bound to well
    Anti-HBc MAb (m) HRP conjugated
Substrate: TMB, H_2O_2
Controls - standards supplied:
    Controls: Neg (human serum), Pos (murine MAb)
Additional reagents:
    H_2SO_4
Special equipment required:
    Auto-EIA II Analyzer (optional)

INTERPRETATION

Comments on interpretation:
    Grey zone: within range ≥ 0.5 x cut-off and ≤ 1.1 x cut-off; retest to confirm; repeatable reaction in this zone should be confirmed by testing for anti-HBs (e.g. LABSYSTEMS anti-HBs EIA)
    Positive: ≤ cut-off repeatably
No. of references: 14

NOTES

110532.0

© KLUWER ACADEMIC PUBLISHERS 1994, ISSN 1381-5067

Hepatitis B virus (core antigen)
ANTIBODY DETECTION

Manufacturer: Melotec S.A.
Cat. No./Trade name: /MELOTEST Anti-HBc

SUMMARY

$$[\text{Well-Ag}]\genfrac{}{}{0pt}{}{\text{Ab}}{[\text{Ab-HRP}]}-[\text{TMB}]-A_{450}$$

Assay type: EIA (competitive)
Detection: Colorimetric A_{450}
Format: Microtitre well
Sample type: Serum, plasma
Sample pre-treatment:
  None
Sample volume: 50 µl
Number of tests: 96
Controls - standards run in assay:
  Controls: Neg (2), Pos (2)
Incubation:
  Overnight: 16 ± 4 hr (RT) + 30 min (RT)
  Rapid: 2 hr (37°C) + 30 min (RT)
Washes: 1

CONTENTS

Antibodies, antigens, labelled components:
  HBcAg bound to well
  Anti-HBc Ab HRP conjugated
Substrate: TMB, H_2O_2
Controls - standards supplied:
  Controls: Neg and Pos
Additional reagents:
  None
Special equipment required:
  None

INTERPRETATION

Comments on interpretation:
  Equivocal: cut-off ± 10%; retest to confirm
  Repeatably equivocal: retest a fresh sample in 1–2
    weeks
  Positive: ≤cut-off–10% repeatably and confirmed by
    supplemental tests
No. of references: 0

NOTES

110638.0

Hepatitis B virus (core antigen)
ANTIBODY DETECTION

Manufacturer: Murex Diagnostics Limited
Cat. No./Trade name: VK26/28/Wellcozyme anti-HBc

SUMMARY

$$[\text{Well-Ag}]\genfrac{}{}{0pt}{}{\text{Ab}}{[\text{Ab-HRP}]}-[\text{TMB}]-A_{450}$$

Assay type: EIA (competitive)
Detection: Colorimetric A_{450}
Format: Microtitre well, Ag coated
Sample type: Serum
Sample pre-treatment:
  None
Sample volume: 200 µl
Number of tests: 96, 480
Controls - standards run in assay:
  Controls: Neg (3), Pos (2)
Incubation:
  Serum: 1 hr 30 min (45-50°C) + 30 min (45-50°C) + 30
    min (RT)
  Plasma: 2 hr (37°C) + 1 hr (37°C) + 30 min (RT)
Washes: 2

CONTENTS

Antibodies, antigens, labelled components:
  rec HBcAg bound to well
  Anti-HBc Ab (h) HRP conjugated
Substrate: TMB, H_2O_2
Controls - standards supplied:
  Controls: Neg and Pos (human serum)
Additional reagents:
  H_2SO_4
Special equipment required:
  Wellcozyme microwell plate washing system (optional)
  Wellcozyme microwell plate reader system (optional)

INTERPRETATION

Comments on interpretation:
  Classification of samples is according to cut-off; no
    further testing
  Visual interpretation is possible but sensitivity will be
    reduced
No. of references: 5

NOTES

110157.0

Hepatitis B virus (core antigen)
ANTIBODY DETECTION

Manufacturer: Organon Teknika NV
Cat. No./Trade name: 72811/Hepanostika® anti-HBc Uni-Form

SUMMARY

$$[\text{Well-Ag}]\left\langle\begin{array}{l}\textbf{Ab}\\ [\text{Ab-HRP}]\end{array}\right.-[\text{OPD}]-A_{450}$$

Assay type: EIA (competitive)
Detection: Colorimetric A_{450}
Format: Microtitre well, Ag coated
Sample type: Serum, plasma
Sample pre-treatment:
 None
Sample volume: 100 µl
Number of tests: 576
Controls - standards run in assay:
 Controls: Neg (3), Pos (3) per plate
Incubation:
 1 hr 30 min (37°C) + 30 min (RT)
Washes: 1

CONTENTS

Antibodies, antigens, labelled components:
 rec HBcAg bound to well
 Anti-HBc Ab (h) HRP conjugated
Substrate: OPD, H_2O_2
Controls - standards supplied:
 Controls: Neg and Pos (human serum)
Additional reagents:
 H_2SO_4
Special equipment required:
 None

INTERPRETATION

Comments on interpretation:
 Positive: $\leq$ cut-off repeatably
No. of references: 0

NOTES

110550.0

Hepatitis B virus (core antigen)
ANTIBODY DETECTION

Manufacturer: Organon Teknika NV
Cat. No./Trade name: 72148/Hepanostika® anti-HBc Microelisa system

SUMMARY

$$[\text{Well-Ag}]\left\langle\begin{array}{l}\textbf{Ab}\\ [\text{Ab-HRP}]\end{array}\right.-[\text{TMB}]-A_{450}$$

Assay type: EIA (competitive)
Detection: Colorimetric A_{450}
Format: Microtitre well, Ag coated
Sample type: Serum, plasma
Sample pre-treatment:
 None
Sample volume: 100 µl
Number of tests: 192, 576
Controls - standards run in assay:
 Controls:
 Neg (1), Pos (1) (for one strip)
 Neg (2), Pos (2) (for two or more strips)
Incubation:
 a) 1 hr (37°C) + 1 hr (37°C) + 30 min (RT)
 b) 30 min (50°C) + 30 min (50°C) + 30 min (RT)
 c) 16-24 hr (RT) + 1 hr (37°C) + 30 min (RT)*
Washes: 2

CONTENTS

Antibodies, antigens, labelled components:
 rec HBc Ag bound to well
 Anti-HBc Ab (h) HRP conjugated
Substrate: TMB
Controls - standards supplied:
 Controls: Neg and Pos (human serum)
Additional reagents:
 H_2SO_4
Special equipment required:
 None

INTERPRETATION

Comments on interpretation:
 Positive: $\leq$ cut-off repeatably
 Semi-quantitative procedure available
 Visual interpretation is possible
No. of references: 1

NOTES

110559.0

*Procedure 3 is more sensitive than procedures 1 or 2

© *KLUWER ACADEMIC PUBLISHERS 1994, ISSN 1381-5067*

Hepatitis B virus (core antigen)
ANTIBODY DETECTION

Manufacturer: Radim
Cat. No./Trade name: KHB2EW/ANTI-HBc EIA WELL

SUMMARY

$$[\text{Well-Ag}] \Big\langle {}^{\textstyle\textbf{Ab}}_{\textstyle[\text{MAb-HRP}]} - [\text{TMB}] - A_{450}$$

Assay type: EIA (competitive)
Detection: Colorimetric A_{450}
Format: Microtitre well, Ag coated
Sample type: Serum or plasma
Sample pre-treatment:
  None
Sample volume: 50 µl
Number of tests: 96, 192
Controls - standards run in assay:
  Controls: Neg (4), Pos (2)
Incubation:
  1 hr 30 min (37°C) + 20 min (37°C)
Washes: 1

CONTENTS

Antibodies, antigens, labelled components:
  rec HBcAg bound to well
  Anti-HBc MAb HRP conjugated
Substrate: TMB, H_2O_2
Controls - standards supplied:
  Controls: Neg and Pos (serum)
Additional reagents:
  None
Special equipment required:
  None

INTERPRETATION

Comments on interpretation:
  Grey area: within cut-off value ± 10%; retest to confirm
  Positive: < cut-off value repeatably
No. of references: 7

NOTES

110433.0

Hepatitis B virus (core antigen)
ANTIBODY DETECTION

Manufacturer: Randox Laboratories Ltd
Cat. No./Trade name: HT 1486/Anti-HBc

SUMMARY

$$[\text{Well-Ag}] \Big\langle {}^{\textstyle\textbf{Ab}}_{\textstyle[\text{Ab-POD}]} - [\text{OPD}] - A_{492}$$

Assay type: EIA (competitive)
Detection: Colorimetric A_{492}
Format: Microtitre well, Ag coated
Sample type: Serum, plasma
Sample pre-treatment:
  None
Sample volume: 50 µl
Number of tests: 96
Controls - standards run in assay:
  Controls: Neg (3), Pos (2)
Incubation:
  a) 20 hr (RT) + 30 min (RT)
  b) 3 hr (40°C) + 30 min (RT)
Washes: 1

CONTENTS

Antibodies, antigens, labelled components:
  HBcAg bound to well
  Anti-HBc Ab POD conjugated
Substrate: OPD, H_2O_2
Controls - standards supplied:
  Controls: Neg and Pos
Additional reagents:
  None
Special equipment required:
  None

INTERPRETATION

Comments on interpretation:
  Retest range: within cut-off ± 10%; retest to confirm
  Positive: ≤ cut-off repeatably and confirmed by
    supplemental tests
No. of references: 3

NOTES

110507.0

© *KLUWER ACADEMIC PUBLISHERS 1994, ISSN 1381-5067*

Hepatitis B virus (core antigen)
ANTIBODY DETECTION

Manufacturer: Roche Diagnostic Systems
Cat. No./Trade name: 07 3444 6/COBAS CORE Anti-HBc EIA

SUMMARY

$$[\text{Bead-Ag}] \Big\langle \begin{array}{c} \textbf{Ab} \\ [\text{Ab-HRP}] \end{array} - [\text{TMB}] - A_{450}$$

Assay type: EIA (competitive)
Detection: Colorimetric A_{450}
Format: Tube, Ag coated bead
Sample type: Serum or plasma
Sample pre-treatment:
 None
Sample volume: 50 µl
Number of tests: 100, 500
Controls - standards run in assay:
 Controls: Neg (3), Pos (1)
Incubation:
 1 hr (37°C) + 15 min (37°C) both with shaking
Washes: 1

CONTENTS

Antibodies, antigens, labelled components:
 rec HBcAg bound to beads
 Anti-HBc F(Ab')$_2$ (h) HRP conjugated
Substrate: TMB, H_2O_2
Controls - standards supplied:
 Controls: Neg and Pos (human serum
Additional reagents:
 Substrate (supplied as separate kit)
Special equipment required:
 Cobas® EIA shaking incubator, tube washer and
  photometer (optional)
 Cobas® Core automated analyser (optional)

INTERPRETATION

Comments on interpretation:
 Grey zone: within cut-off ± 10%; repeat to confirm
 Positive: < cut-off -10% repeatably
No. of references: 10

NOTES

110407.0

Hepatitis B virus (core antigen)
ANTIBODY DETECTION

Manufacturer: Sanofi Diagnostics Pasteur
Cat. No./Trade name: 72209/MONOLISA® ANTI HBc

SUMMARY

$$[\text{Well-Ag}] \Big\langle \begin{array}{c} \textbf{Ab} \\ [\text{Ab-POD}] \end{array} - [\text{OPD}] - A_{492/620}$$

Assay type: EIA (competitive)
Detection: Colorimetric $A_{492/620}$
Format: Microtitre well, Ag coated
Sample type: Serum
Sample pre-treatment:
 None
Sample volume: 50 µl
Number of tests: 192
Controls - standards run in assay:
 Controls: Neg (3), Pos (2)
Incubation:
 1 hr 30 min (40°C) + 30 min (RT)
Washes: 1 (+ preliminary plate prewash)

CONTENTS

Antibodies, antigens, labelled components:
 HBcAg bound to well
 Anti-HBc PAb (h) POD conjugated
Substrate: OPD, H_2O_2
Controls - standards supplied:
 Controls: Neg and Pos (human serum)
Additional reagents:
 None
Special equipment required:
 None

INTERPRETATION

Comments on interpretation:
 Equivocal: inhibition of absorbance in the range 54-66%;
  retest to confirm
 Positive: inhibition of absorbance > 60% repeatably
No. of references: 0

NOTES

110265.0

© KLUWER ACADEMIC PUBLISHERS 1994, ISSN 1381-5067

Hepatitis B virus (core antigen)
ANTIBODY DETECTION

Manufacturer: Schiapparelli Biosystems Inc
Cat. No./Trade name: 5770328/HEPATITIS B - HBcAb ELISA SYSTEM

SUMMARY

$$[\text{Well-Ag}]\left\langle\begin{array}{l}\textbf{Ab}\\ [\text{MAb-HRP}]\end{array}\right.-[\text{TMB}]-A_{450}$$

Assay type: EIA (competitive)
Detection: Colorimetric A_{450}
Format: Microtitre well, Ag coated
Sample type: Serum (do not heat inactivate)
Sample pre-treatment:
  None
Sample volume: 100 µl x 2
Number of tests: 96
Controls - standards run in assay:
  Controls: Neg (2), Pos (3)
Incubation:
  1 hr (40°C) + 1 hr (40°C) + 20 min (RT)
Washes: 2

CONTENTS

Antibodies, antigens, labelled components:
  rec HBcAg bound to well
  Anti-HBc MAb HRP conjugated
Substrate: TMB, H_2O_2
Controls - standards supplied:
  Controls: Neg and Pos (human serum)
Additional reagents:
  None
Special equipment required:
  None

INTERPRETATION

Comments on interpretation:
  Classification of sample is according to cut-off; no further testing
No. of references: 6

NOTES

110425.0

Hepatitis B virus (core antigen)
ANTIBODY DETECTION

Manufacturer: Sorin Biomedica
Cat. No./Trade name: 2862/ETI-AB-COREK-2

SUMMARY

$$[\text{Well-Ag}]\left\langle\begin{array}{l}\textbf{Ab}\\ [\text{Ab-HRP}]\end{array}\right.-[\text{TMB}]-A_{450}$$

Assay type: EIA (competitive)
Detection: Colorimetric A_{450}
Format: Microtitre well, Ag coated
Sample type: Serum, plasma
Sample pre-treatment:
  None
Sample volume: 50 µl
Number of tests: 96
Controls - standards run in assay:
  Controls: Neg (3), Pos (2)
Incubation:
  2 hr (37°C) + 30 min (RT)
Washes: 1

CONTENTS

Antibodies, antigens, labelled components:
  rec HBcAg bound to well
  Anti-HBc IgG Ab (h) HRP conjugated
Substrate: TMB, H_2O_2
Controls - standards supplied:
  Controls: Neg (human serum) and Pos (human plasma)
Additional reagents:
  None
Special equipment required:
  ETI system reader and washer (optional)

INTERPRETATION

Comments on interpretation:
  Equivocal: Within cut-off ± 10%; retest to confirm
No. of references: 6

NOTES

110225.0

Hepatitis B virus (core antigen)
ANTIBODY DETECTION

Manufacturer: Sorin Biomedica
Cat. No./Trade name: 2082/AB-COREK eia

SUMMARY

$$[\text{Bead-Ag}]\binom{\text{Ab}}{[\text{Ab-HRP}]}-[\text{OPD}]-A_{492}$$

Assay type: EIA (competitive)
Detection: Colorimetric A_{492}
Format: Tray/Tube, Ag coated bead
Sample type: Serum, plasma
Sample pre-treatment:
　None
Sample volume: 100 µl
Number of tests: 100
Controls - standards run in assay:
　Controls: Neg (3), Pos (2)
Incubation:
　a) 2 hr (45°C) + 30 min (RT)
　b) Overnight (RT) + 30 min (RT)
Washes: 1

CONTENTS

Antibodies, antigens, labelled components:
　rec HBcAg bound to bead
　Anti-HBc IgG Ab (h) HRP conjugated
Substrate: OPD; H_2O_2
Controls - standards supplied:
　Controls: Neg and Pos (human serum)
Additional reagents:
　None
Special equipment required:
　Automated rinser, PLA-2 (optional)
　Bead dispenser, MEDI-578 (optional)

INTERPRETATION

Comments on interpretation:
　Equivocal:　Within cut-off ± 10%; retest to confirm
No. of references: 6

NOTES

110235.0

This kit will be discontinued in December 1994

Hepatitis B virus (core antigen)
ANTIBODY DETECTION

Manufacturer: Syva Company
Cat. No./Trade name: 8HD29UL/MicroTrak® II Total Anti-HBcore EIA

SUMMARY

$$[\text{Well-Ag}]\binom{\text{Ab}}{[\text{Ab-HRP}]}-[\text{TMB}]-A_{450/630}$$

Assay type: EIA (competitive)
Detection: Colorimetric $A_{450/630}$
Format: Microtitre well, Ag coated
Sample type: Serum, plasma
Sample pre-treatment:
　None
Sample volume: 50 µl
Number of tests: 96
Controls - standards run in assay:
　Controls: Neg (3), Pos (2)
Incubation:
　2 hr (37°C) + 30 min (37°C)
Washes: 1

CONTENTS

Antibodies, antigens, labelled components:
　rec HBcAg bound to well
　Anti-HBc IgG Ab (h) HRP conjugated
Substrate: TMB, H_2O_2
Controls - standards supplied:
　Controls: Neg (human serum), Pos (human plasma)
Additional reagents:
　MicroTrak® II EIA universal reagents (8K209UL)
Special equipment required:
　Syva MicroTrak® EIA autowasher and autoreader

INTERPRETATION

Comments on interpretation:
　Positive: ≤ cut-off repeatably
No. of references: 11

NOTES

110066.0

Hepatitis B virus (core antigen)
ANTIBODY DETECTION

Manufacturer: VEDA-LAB
Cat. No./Trade name: 1551/HBc Ab EIA

SUMMARY

$$[\text{Well-Ab}]\text{--}[\text{Ag}]\begin{cases}\textbf{Ab}\\ [\text{Ab-HRP}]\end{cases}\text{--}[\text{TMB}]\text{--}A_{450}$$

Assay type: EIA (competitive)
Detection: Colorimetric A_{450}
Format: Microtitre well, Ab coated
Sample type: Serum, plasma
Sample pre-treatment:
    None
Sample volume: 10 µl (+500 µl diluent)
Number of tests: 96
Controls - standards run in assay:
    Controls: Neg (1), Pos (1)
Incubation:
    1 hr (37°C) + 15 min (RT)
Washes: 1

CONTENTS

Antibodies, antigens, labelled components:
    Anti-HBc PAb bound to well
    HBcAg (neutralizing reagent)
    Anti-HBc Ab HRP conjugated
Substrate: TMB, H_2O_2
Controls - standards supplied:
    Controls: Neg and Pos
Additional reagents:
    None
Special equipment required:
    None

INTERPRETATION

Comments on interpretation:
    Equivocal: within cut-off ±10%; retest to confirm
No. of references: 5

NOTES

110393.0

Hepatitis B virus (core antigen)
ANTIBODY DETECTION (IgM)

Manufacturer: Abbott Laboratories
Cat. No./Trade name: 2260-66/IMx® CORE® - M

SUMMARY

$$[\text{Particle-AHIgM}]\text{--}\textbf{Ab}\text{--}[\text{Ag}]\text{--}[\text{Ab-AP}]\text{--}[\text{4-MP}]\text{--}\text{fluorescence}$$

Assay type: EIA (non-competitive)
Detection: Fluorometric
Format: Reaction well, Ab coated microparticle
Sample type: Serum, plasma (do not heat inactivate)
Sample pre-treatment:
    None
Sample volume: 150 µl
Number of tests: 100
Controls - standards run in assay:
    Calibration assay: calibrators (1) x 2; controls: Neg (1);
        Pos (1)
    Mode 1 Assay: calibrators (1); controls: Pos (1)*
Incubation:
    Automated
Washes: Automated

CONTENTS

Antibodies, antigens, labelled components:
    Anti-human IgM Ab (g) bound to microparticle
    rec HBCAg
    Anti-HBc Ab (h) AP conjugated
Substrate: 4-MP
Controls - standards supplied:
    Calibrators: Mode 1 calibrator (human plasma)
Additional reagents:
    IMx® CORE® controls; IMx® MEIA diluent buffer; IMx®
        probe cleaning solution
Special equipment required:
    IMx system

INTERPRETATION

Comments on interpretation:
    Sample reactivity is calculated automatically
    Grey zone: samples with values between 0.8 and 1.2:
        report as borderline and advise patient follow-up
No. of references: 15

NOTES

110023.0

*Minimum control requirement for Mode 1 assay: one control
    (Pos or Neg) assayed once per 8 hr shift

Hepatitis B virus (core antigen)
ANTIBODY DETECTION (IgM)

Manufacturer: Abbott Laboratories
Cat. No./Trade name: 1236/CORZYME-M (rDNA) test

SUMMARY

[Bead-AHIgM]–**Ab**–[Ag]–[Ab-HRP]–[OPD]–A$_{492}$

Assay type: EIA (non-competitive)
Detection: Colorimetric A$_{492}$
Format: Reaction well, Ab coated bead
Sample type: Serum, plasma (do not heat inactivate)
Sample pre-treatment:
    None
Sample volume: 10 µl (+500 µl diluent)
Number of tests: 100
Controls - standards run in assay:
    Controls: Neg (2), Pos (3)
Incubation:
    a) 1 hr (40°C) + 3 hr (40°C) + 30 min (RT)
    b) 1 hr (40°C) + 18-22 hr (RT) + 30 min (RT)
Washes: 2

CONTENTS

Antibodies, antigens, labelled components:
    Anti-human IgM Ab (g) bound to beads
    rec HBcAg
    Anti-HBc Ab (h) HRP conjugated
Substrate: OPD, H$_2$O$_2$
Controls - standards supplied:
    Controls: Neg and Pos (human plasma)
Additional reagents:
    H$_2$SO$_4$
Special equipment required:
    None

INTERPRETATION

Comments on interpretation:
    Equivocal: within cut-off ±10%; retest to confirm and if
        sample is consistently within cut-off ±10%; report
        borderline nature of result and advise patient follow-
        up
    Positive: ≥cut-off repeatably
No. of references: 19

NOTES

110074.0

Hepatitis B virus (core antigen)
ANTIBODY DETECTION (IgM)

Manufacturer: ADI Diagnostics
Cat. No./Trade name: /Heprofile® Anti-HBc IgM

SUMMARY

[Well-AHIgM]–**Ab**–[Ag]–[Ab-POD]–[TMB]–A$_{450}$

Assay type: EIA (non-competitive)
Detection: Colorimetric A$_{450}$
Format: Microtitre well, Ab coated
Sample type: Serum, plasma
Sample pre-treatment:
    None
Sample volume: 10 µl (+1 ml diluent)
Number of tests: 96
Controls - standards run in assay:
    Controls: Neg (3), Pos (2)
Incubation:
    2 hr (37°C) + 20 hr (RT) + 30 min (RT)
Washes: 2

CONTENTS

Antibodies, antigens, labelled components:
    Anti-human IgM MAb (m) bound to well
    HBcAg
    Anti-HBc Ab POD conjugated
Substrate: TMB, H$_2$O$_2$
Controls - standards supplied:
    Controls: Neg and Pos (human plasma)
Additional reagents:
    None
Special equipment required:
    None

INTERPRETATION

Comments on interpretation:
    Positive: ≥cut-off repeatably
No. of references: 20

NOTES

110196.0

© KLUWER ACADEMIC PUBLISHERS 1994, ISSN 1381-5067

Hepatitis B virus (core antigen)
ANTIBODY DETECTION (IgM)

Manufacturer: Behringwerke AG
Cat. No./Trade name: OWSE/Enzygnost® Anti-HBc/IgM

SUMMARY

[Well-AHIgM]–**Ab**–[Ag-POD]–[TMB]–A$_{450}$

Assay type: EIA (non-competitive)
Detection: Colorimetric A$_{450}$
Format: Microtitre well, Ab coated
Sample type: Serum, plasma
Sample pre-treatment:
 None
Sample volume: 10 µl of 1:101 dilution
Number of tests: 96
Controls - standards run in assay:
 Controls: Neg (4), Pos (2)
Incubation:
 15-30 min (RT) + 1 hr (37°C) + 30 min (RT)
Washes: 1

CONTENTS

Antibodies, antigens, labelled components:
 Anti-human IgM MAb bound to well
 rec HBcAg, POD conjugated
Substrate: TMB, H$_2$O$_2$
Controls - standards supplied:
 Controls: Neg and Pos (human serum)
Additional reagents:
 None
Special equipment required:
 Behring ELISA processor (optional)
 Dual wavelength spectrophotometer (optional)

INTERPRETATION

Comments on interpretation:
 Equivocal: within cut-off ±10%; retest to confirm
No. of references: 0

NOTES

110453.0

Hepatitis B virus (core antigen)
ANTIBODY DETECTION (IgM)

Manufacturer: bioMerieux
Cat. No./Trade name: 30303/VIDAS HBc IgM (HBCM)

SUMMARY

[Solid phase-AHIgM]–**Ab**–[Ag:MAb-AP]–[4-MP]–
fluorescence

Assay type: EIA (non-competitive)
Detection: Fluorometric
Format: Solid phase receptacle (SPR), Ab coated reagent strip
Sample type: Serum, plasma (do not heat inactivate)
Sample pre-treatment:
 None
Sample volume: 100 µl
Number of tests: 60
Controls - standards run in assay:
 Controls: Neg (1), Pos (1)
 Calibrator: (1)*
Incubation:
 Automated - total time under 55 minutes
Washes: Automated

CONTENTS

Antibodies, antigens, labelled components:
 Anti-human IgM (g) bound to solid phase
 rec HBcAg
 Anti-HBc MAb (m) AP conjugated
Substrate: 4-MP
Controls - standards supplied:
 Controls: Neg and Pos (human serum)
 Calibrator: Pos (human serum)
Additional reagents:
 None
Special equipment required:
 Vitek Immunodiagnostic assay system (VIDAS)

INTERPRETATION

Comments on interpretation:
 Sample reactivity is calculated automatically and
 classification is according to cut-off
 Equivocal sample should be retested
No. of references: 9

NOTES

110473.0

*Recalibrate with each new lot of reagents and every 14
 days

© KLUWER ACADEMIC PUBLISHERS 1994, ISSN 1381-5067

Hepatitis B virus (core antigen)
ANTIBODY DETECTION (IgM)

Manufacturer: Boehringer Mannheim
Cat. No./Trade name: 1141 538/Enzymun-Test® Anti-HBc-IgM

SUMMARY

[Tube-strept]–[AHIgM-biotin]–**Ab**–[Ag:MAb-POD]–[ABTS]–A_{420}

Assay type: EIA (non-competitive)
Detection: Colorimetric A_{420}
Format: Tube, streptavidin coated
Sample type: Serum, plasma
Sample pre-treatment:
    None
Sample volume: 10 µl
Number of tests: 145
Controls - standards run in assay:
    Controls: Neg (2), Pos (2)
Incubation:
    1 hr (RT) + 1 hr (RT) + 1 hr (RT)
Washes: 2

CONTENTS

Antibodies, antigens, labelled components:
    Anti-human IgM MAb biotinylated
    rec HBcAg
    Anti-HBc MAb POD conjugated
Substrate: ABTS, H_2O_2
Controls - standards supplied:
    Controls: Neg and Pos (human serum)
Additional reagents:
    Substrate and streptavidin-coated tubes
Special equipment required:
    Automated Enzymun-Test Systems (optional)

INTERPRETATION

Comments on interpretation:
    Borderline: within cut-off ±10%; retest to confirm
No. of references: 0

NOTES

110464.0

Hepatitis B virus (core antigen)
ANTIBODY DETECTION (IgM)

Manufacturer: IFCI Clone Systems
Cat. No./Trade name: 07.1003/EIAgen Anti-CORE IgM Kit

SUMMARY

[Well-AHIgM]–**Ab**–[Ag]–[Ab-POD]–[TMB]–A_{450}

Assay type: EIA (non-competitive)
Detection: Colorimetric A_{450}
Format: Microtitre well, Ab coated
Sample type: Serum, plasma
Sample pre-treatment:
    None
Sample volume: 10 µl (+ 1 ml diluent)
Number of tests: 96
Controls - standards run in assay:
    Controls: Neg (3), Pos (2)
Incubation:
    2 hr (37°C) + 20 hr (RT) + 30 min (RT)
Washes: 2

CONTENTS

Antibodies, antigens, labelled components:
    Anti-human IgM MAb (m) bound to well
    HBcAg
    Anti-HBc Ab POD conjugated
Substrate: TMB, H_2O_2
Controls - standards supplied:
    Controls: Neg and Pos (human plasma)
Additional reagents:
    None
Special equipment required:
    None

INTERPRETATION

Comments on interpretation:
    Positive: ≥ cut-off repeatably
No. of references: 18

NOTES

110066.0

© *KLUWER ACADEMIC PUBLISHERS 1994, ISSN 1381-5067*

Hepatitis B virus (core antigen)
ANTIBODY DETECTION (IgM)

Manufacturer: Labsystems Oy
Cat. No./Trade name: 61 10 380/Anti-HBc IgM EIA

SUMMARY

[Well-AHIgM]–**Ab**–[Ag:MAb-HRP]–[TMB]–A_{450}

Assay type: EIA (non-competitive)
Detection: Colorimetric A_{450}
Format: Microtitre well, Ab coated
Sample type: Serum, plasma
Sample pre-treatment:
   None
Sample volume: 25 µl of 1:200 dilution (+200 µl diluent)
Number of tests: 96
Controls - standards run in assay:
   Controls: Neg (3), Pos (2)
Incubation:
   1 hr (37°C) + 1 hr (37°C) + 30 min (RT)
Washes: 2

CONTENTS

Antibodies, antigens, labelled components:
   Anti-human IgM PAb (sh) bound to well
   rec HBcAg
   Anti-HBc MAb (m) HRP conjugated
Substrate: TMB, H_2O_2
Controls - standards supplied:
   Controls: Neg and Pos (human serum)
Additional reagents:
   H_2SO_4
Special equipment required:
   Auto-EIA II Analyzer (optional)

INTERPRETATION

Comments on interpretation:
   Positive: ⩾cut-off repeatably
No. of references: 10

NOTES

110533.0

Hepatitis B virus (core antigen)
ANTIBODY DETECTION (IgM)

Manufacturer: Murex Diagnostics Limited
Cat. No./Trade name: VK27/Wellcozyme anti-HBc IgM

SUMMARY

[Well-AHIgM]–**Ab**–[Ag-HRP]–[TMB]–A_{450}

Assay type: EIA (non-competitive)
Detection: Colorimetric A_{450}
Format: Microtitre well, Ab coated
Sample type: Serum, plasma (do not heat inactivate)
Sample pre-treatment:
   None
Sample volume: 10 µl (+1 ml diluent)
Number of tests: 96, 480
Controls - standards run in assay:
   Controls: Neg (2), Pos (3)
Incubation:
   a) 30 min (37°C) + 30 min (37°C) + 30 min (RT)
   b) 1 hr (RT) + 45 min (RT) + 30 min (RT)
Washes: 2

CONTENTS

Antibodies, antigens, labelled components:
   Anti-human IgM MAb (m) bound to wells
   rec HBcAg HRP conjugated
Substrate: TMB, H_2O_2
Controls - standards supplied:
   Controls: Neg and Pos (human serum)
Additional reagents:
   H_2SO_4
Special equipment required:
   Wellcozyme microwell plate washing system (optional)
   Wellcozyme microwell plate reader (optional)

INTERPRETATION

Comments on interpretation:
   Borderline: within cut-off ±10%; retest a fresh sample
No. of references: 11

NOTES

110158.0

© KLUWER ACADEMIC PUBLISHERS 1994, ISSN 1381-5067

Hepatitis B virus (core antigen)
ANTIBODY DETECTION (IgM)

Manufacturer: Organon Teknika NV
Cat. No./Trade name: 70333/Hepanostika® anti-HBc IgM Microelisa system

SUMMARY

[Well-AHIgM]–**Ab**–[Ag]–[Ab-HRP]–[TMB]–A$_{450}$

Assay type: EIA (non-competitive)
Detection: Colorimetric A$_{450}$
Format: Microtitre well, Ab coated
Sample type: Serum, plasma
Sample pre-treatment:
    None
Sample volume: 100 μl
Number of tests: 192
Controls - standards run in assay:
    Controls:
    Neg (1), Pos (1) (for one strip)
    Neg (2), Pos (2) (for two or more strips)
    Optional: strong Pos control (1)
Incubation:
    2 hr (37°C) + 16-24 hr (37°C) + 1 hr (37°C) + 30 min (RT)
Washes: 3

CONTENTS

Antibodies, antigens, labelled components:
    Anti-human IgM Ab (sh) bound to well
    rec HBc Ag
    Anti-HBc Ab (h) HRP conjugated
Substrate: TMB
Controls - standards supplied:
    Controls: Neg and Pos (human serum)
Additional reagents:
    H$_2$SO$_4$
Special equipment required:
    None

INTERPRETATION

Comments on interpretation:
    Positive: ⩾cut-off repeatably
    Semi-quantitative procedure available
No. of references: 1

NOTES

110558.0

Hepatitis B virus (core antigen)
ANTIBODY DETECTION (IgM)

Manufacturer: Radim
Cat. No./Trade name: KHB2IM/ANTI-HBc IgM IEMA WELL

SUMMARY

[Well-AHIgM]–**Ab**–Ag]–[MAb-HRP]–[TMB]–A$_{450}$

Assay type: EIA (non-competitive)
Detection: Colorimetric A$_{450}$
Format: Microtitre well, Ab coated
Sample type: Serum or plasma
Sample pre-treatment:
    None
Sample volume: 10 μl of 1:51 dilution (+200 μl diluent)
Number of tests: 96
Controls - standards run in assay:
    Controls: Neg (4), Pos (2)
Incubation:
    1 hr (37°C) + 1 hr (37°C) + 20 min (37°C)
Washes: 2

CONTENTS

Antibodies, antigens, labelled components:
    Anti-human IgM MAb bound to well
    rec HBcAg
    Anti-HBc MAb HRP conjugated
Substrate: TMB, H$_2$O$_2$
Controls - standards supplied:
    Controls: Neg and Pos (serum)
Additional reagents:
    None
Special equipment required:
    None

INTERPRETATION

Comments on interpretation:
    Grey area: within cut-off value ± 10%; retest to confirm
    Positive: > cut-off value repeatably
    A set of standards is available to make this a quantitative assay
No. of references: 7

NOTES

110434.0

© KLUWER ACADEMIC PUBLISHERS 1994, ISSN 1381-5067

Hepatitis B virus (core antigen)
ANTIBODY DETECTION (IgM)

Manufacturer: Randox Laboratories Ltd
Cat. No./Trade name: HT 1487/Anti-HBc IgM

SUMMARY

[Well-AHIgM]–**Ab**–[Ag + Ab-POD]–[OPD]–A_{492}

Assay type: EIA (non-competitive)
Detection: Colorimetric A_{492}
Format: Microtitre well, Ab coated
Sample type: Serum, plasma
Sample pre-treatment:
Predilute sample 5 µl (+500 µl diluent)
Sample volume: 5 µl of prediluted sample (+100 µl diluent)
Number of tests: 96
Controls - standards run in assay:
Controls: Neg (3), Pos (2)
Incubation:
1 hr (40°C) + 20 hr (RT) + 30 min (RT)
Washes: 2

CONTENTS

Antibodies, antigens, labelled components:
Anti-human IgM Ab bound to well
HBcAg
Anti-HBc Ab POD conjugated
Substrate: OPD, H_2O_2
Controls - standards supplied:
Controls: Neg, Pos
Additional reagents:
H_2SO_4
Special equipment required:
None

INTERPRETATION

Comments on interpretation:
Retest range: within cut-off ±10%; retest to confirm
Positive: ⩾cut-off repeatably
No. of references: 4

NOTES

110508.0

Hepatitis B virus (core antigen)
ANTIBODY DETECTION (IgM)

Manufacturer: Roche Diagnostic Systems
Cat. No./Trade name: 07 3441 1/COBAS CORE Anti-HBc IgM EIA

SUMMARY

[Bead-AHIgM]–**Ab**–[Ag + Ab-HRP]–[TMB]–A_{450}

Assay type: EIA (non-competitive)
Detection: Colorimetric A_{450}
Format: Tube, Ab coated bead
Sample type: Serum or plasma
Sample pre-treatment:
None
Sample volume: 10 µl (+1 ml diluent)
Number of tests: 50
Controls - standards run in assay:
Controls: Neg (1), Pos (3)
Incubation:
30 min (37°C) + 1 hr (37°C) + 15 min (37°C) all with
shaking
Washes: 2

CONTENTS

Antibodies, antigens, labelled components:
Anti-human IgM MAb (m) bound to beads
rec HBcAg
Anti-HBc F(Ab')$_2$ HRP conjugate
Substrate: TMB, H_2O_2
Controls - standards supplied:
Controls: Neg and Pos (human serum)
Additional reagents:
Substrate (supplied as separate kit)
Special equipment required:
Cobas® EIA shaking incubator, tube washer and
photometer (optional)
Cobas® Core automated analyser (optional)

INTERPRETATION

Comments on interpretation:
Grey zone: within cut-off ±10%; retest to confirm
No. of references: 10

NOTES

110408.0

© *KLUWER ACADEMIC PUBLISHERS 1994, ISSN 1381-5067*

Hepatitis B virus (core antigen)
ANTIBODY DETECTION (IgM)

Manufacturer: Sanofi Diagnostics Pasteur
Cat. No./Trade name: 72211/MONOLISA® HBc IgM

SUMMARY

[Well-AHIgM]–**Ab**–[Ag-POD]–[OPD]–$A_{492/620}$

Assay type: EIA (non-competitive)
Detection: Colorimetric $A_{492/620}$
Format: Microtitre well, Ab coated
Sample type: Serum, plasma
Sample pre-treatment:
    None
Sample volume: 100 µl of 1:101 dilution
Number of tests: 96
Controls - standards run in assay:
    Controls: Neg (3), Pos (3)
Incubation:
    30 min (40°C) + 1 hr (40°C) + 30 min (RT)
Washes: 2 (+ preliminary plate prewash)

CONTENTS

Antibodies, antigens, labelled components:
    Anti-human IgM Ab (g) bound to well
    rec HBcAg POD conjugated
Substrate: OPD, H_2O_2
Controls - standards supplied:
    Controls: Neg and Pos (human serum)
Additional reagents:
    None
Special equipment required:
    None

INTERPRETATION

Comments on interpretation:
    Equivocal: within cut-off value ± 10%; retest to confirm
No. of references: 7

NOTES

110266.0

Hepatitis B virus (core antigen)
ANTIBODY DETECTION (IgM)

Manufacturer: Schiapparelli Biosystems Inc
Cat. No./Trade name: 5770330/HEPATITIS B - HBc IgM ELISA SYSTEM

SUMMARY

[Well-AHIgM]–**Ab**–[Ag:MAb-HRP]–[TMB]–A_{450}

Assay type: EIA (non-competitive)
Detection: Colorimetric A_{450}
Format: Microtitre well, Ab coated
Sample type: Serum (do not heat inactivate)
Sample pre-treatment:
    None
Sample volume: 10 µl (+ 190 µl diluent) x 2
Number of tests: 96
Controls - standards run in assay:
    Controls: Neg (3), Pos (2)
Incubation:
    1 hr (RT) + 1 hr (RT) + 10 min (RT)
Washes: 2

CONTENTS

Antibodies, antigens, labelled components:
    Anti-human IgM MAb bound to well
    rec HBcAg
    Anti-HBc MAb HRP conjugated
Substrate: TMB, H_2O_2
Controls - standards supplied:
    Controls: Neg and Pos (human serum)
Additional reagents:
    None
Special equipment required:
    None

INTERPRETATION

Comments on interpretation:
    Classification of sample is according to cut-off; no further testing
No. of references: 7

NOTES

110426.0

© KLUWER ACADEMIC PUBLISHERS 1994, ISSN 1381-5067

Hepatitis B virus (core antigen)
ANTIBODY DETECTION (IgM)

Manufacturer: Sorin Biomedica
Cat. No./Trade name: 2876/ETI-CORE-IGMK-2

SUMMARY

[Well-AHIgM]–**Ab**–[Ag]–[Ab-HRP]–[TMB]–A_{450}

Assay type: EIA (non-competitive)
Detection: Colorimetric A_{450}
Format: Microtitre well, Ab coated
Sample type: Serum, plasma
Sample pre-treatment:
　None
Sample volume: 10 µl (+0.4 ml diluent)
Number of tests: 96
Controls - standards run in assay:
　Controls: Neg (3), Pos (2)
Incubation:
　1 hr (37°C) + 1 hr (37°C) + 30 min (RT)
Washes: 2

CONTENTS

Antibodies, antigens, labelled components:
　Anti-human IgM IgG Ab (r) bound to well
　rec HBcAg
　Anti-HBc IgG Ab (h) HRP conjugated
Substrate: TMB, H_2O_2
Controls - standards supplied:
　Controls: Neg and Pos (human serum)
Additional reagents:
　None
Special equipment required:
　ETI-system reader and software (optional)
　ETI-system washer (optional)

INTERPRETATION

Comments on interpretation:
　Classification of samples is according to cut-off; no
　　further testing
No. of references: 6

NOTES

110229.0

Hepatitis B virus (core antigen)
ANTIBODY DETECTION (IgM)

Manufacturer: Sorin Biomedica
Cat. No./Trade name: 2449/CORF-IGMK eia

SUMMARY

[Bead-AHIgM]–**Ab**–[Ag]–[Ab-HRP]–[OPD]–A_{492}

Assay type: EIA (non-competitive)
Detection: Colorimetric A_{492}
Format: Tray/Tube, Ab coated bead
Sample type: Serum, plasma
Sample pre-treatment:
　None
Sample volume: 10 µl (+2 ml diluent)
Number of tests: 50
Controls - standards run in assay:
　Controls: Neg (2), Pos (3)
Incubation:
　18-22 hr (RT) + 3 hr (45°C) + 30 min (RT)
Washes: 2

CONTENTS

Antibodies, antigens, labelled components:
　Anti-human IgM IgG Ab (r) bound to beads
　HBcAg rec
　Anti-HBc IgG Ab (h) HRP conjugated
Substrate: OPD; H_2O_2
Controls - standards supplied:
　Controls: Neg and Pos (human serum)
Additional reagents:
　None
Special equipment required:
　Automatic rinsing device PLA-2 (optional)
　Bead dispenser MEDI-578 (optional)

INTERPRETATION

Comments on interpretation:
　Equivocal:　Within cut-off ± 10%; retest to confirm
　Positive:　≥cut-off repeatably
No. of references: 6

NOTES

110240.0

This kit will be discontinued in December 1994

© *KLUWER ACADEMIC PUBLISHERS 1994, ISSN 1381-5067*

Hepatitis B virus (core antigen)
ANTIBODY DETECTION (IgM)

Manufacturer: Syva Company
Cat. No./Trade name: 8HC29UL/MicroTrak® II IgM Anti-HBcore EIA

SUMMARY

[Well-AHIgM]–**Ab**–[Ag]–[Ab-HRP]–[TMB]–$A_{450/630}$

Assay type: EIA (non-competitive)
Detection: Colorimetric $A_{450/630}$
Format: Microtitre well, Ab coated
Sample type: Serum, plasma
Sample pre-treatment:
   None
Sample volume: 10 µl of 1:4000 dilution
Number of tests: 96
Controls - standards run in assay:
   Controls: Neg (3), Pos (2)
Incubation:
   1 hr (37°C) + 1 hr (37°C) + 30 min (37°C)
Washes: 2

CONTENTS

Antibodies, antigens, labelled components:
   Anti-human IgM MAb (m) bound to well
   rec HBcAg
   Anti-HBc IgG Ab (h) HRP conjugated
Substrate: TMB, H_2O_2
Controls - standards supplied:
   Controls: Neg and Pos (human serum)
Additional reagents:
   MicroTrak® II EIA universal reagents (8K209UL)
Special equipment required:
   Syva MicroTrak® EIA autowasher and autoreader

INTERPRETATION

Comments on interpretation:
   Grey zone: within cut-off ±25%; retest to confirm
No. of references: 9

NOTES

110063.0

Hepatitis B virus (core antigen)
ANTIBODY DETECTION

Manufacturer: Kodak Clinical Diagnostics
Cat. No./Trade name: LAN.1204/KODAK Amerlite anti-HBc assay

SUMMARY

[Well-Ag] $\begin{cases} \textbf{Ab} \\ \text{[Ab-HRP]} \end{cases}$ –[signal reagent]–luminescence

Assay type: Luminometric immunoassay
   (competitive)
Detection: Luminometric
Format: Microtitre well, Ag coated
Sample type: Serum, plasma
Sample pre-treatment:
   None
Sample volume: 50 µl
Number of tests: 96
Controls - standards run in assay:
   Controls: Neg (3), Pos (1)
Incubation:
   1 hr (37°C) with shaking + 2-20 min (RT)
Washes: 1

CONTENTS

Antibodies, antigens, labelled components:
   HBcAg bound to well
   Anti-HBc PAb (human) HRP conjugated
Substrate: Amerlite signal reagent
Controls - standards supplied:
   Controls: Neg and Pos (human serum)
Additional reagents:
   Amerlite signal reagent and serology wash reagent
Special equipment required:
   Amerlite Kodak immunoassay system

INTERPRETATION

Comments on interpretation:
   Sample reactivity is calculated automatically and
      classification is according to cut-off
   Equivocal samples are marked 'retest'; retest to confirm
   Positive: retest to confirm
No. of references: 12

NOTES

110486.0

© *KLUWER ACADEMIC PUBLISHERS 1994, ISSN 1381-5067*

Hepatitis B virus (core antigen)
ANTIBODY DETECTION (IgM)

Manufacturer: Kodak Clinical Diagnostics
Cat. No./Trade name: LAN.6205/KODAK Amerlite anti-HBc IgM assay

SUMMARY

[Well-AHIgM]–**Ab**–[Ag-HRP]–[signal reagent]–
luminescence

Assay type: Luminometric immunoassay (non-competitive)
Detection: Luminometric
Format: Microtitre well, Ab coated
Sample type: Serum, plasma
Sample pre-treatment:
None
Sample volume: 10 µl of 1:201 dilution
Number of tests: 48
Controls - standards run in assay:
Controls: Neg (1), Pos (3)
Incubation:
30 min (37°C) + 30 min (37°C) both with shaking + 2-20 min (RT)
Washes: 2

CONTENTS

Antibodies, antigens, labelled components:
Anti-human IgM MAb (m) bound to well
HBcAg HRP conjugated
Substrate: Amerlite signal reagent
Controls - standards supplied:
Controls: Neg and Pos (human serum)
Additional reagents:
Amerlite signal reagent and serology wash reagent
Special equipment required:
Amerlite Kodak immunoassay system

INTERPRETATION

Comments on interpretation:
Sample reactivity is calculated automatically and classification is according to cut-off
Equivocal samples are marked 'retest'; retest to confirm
No. of references: 7

NOTES

110485.0

Hepatitis B virus (core antigen)
ANTIBODY DETECTION

Manufacturer: Abbott Laboratories
Cat. No./Trade name: IA16/CORAB®

SUMMARY

$$[\text{Bead-Ag}] \begin{cases} \textbf{Ab} \\ [\text{Ab-}^{125}\text{I}] \end{cases} \text{–radioactivity}$$

Assay type: RIA (competitive)
Detection: Radioisotopic
Format: Reaction well, Ag coated bead
Sample type: Serum, plasma (do not heat inactivate)
Sample pre-treatment:
None
Sample volume: 100 µl
Number of tests: 100
Controls - standards run in assay:
Controls: Neg (3), Pos (2)
Incubation:
20 hr (RT)
Washes: 1

CONTENTS

Antibodies, antigens, labelled components:
rec HBcAg bound to bead
Anti-HBc Ab (h) ^{125}I labelled
Substrate:
Controls - standards supplied:
Controls: Pos and Neg (human plasma)
Additional reagents:
None
Special equipment required:
None

INTERPRETATION

Comments on interpretation:
Positive: ≤ cut-off repeatably
Semi-quantitative procedure available
No. of references: 11

NOTES

110029.0

© *KLUWER ACADEMIC PUBLISHERS 1994, ISSN 1381-5067*

Hepatitis B virus (core antigen)
ANTIBODY DETECTION

Manufacturer: Radim
Cat. No./Trade name: KHB2CT/ANTI-HBc RIA CT

SUMMARY

$$[\text{Tube-Ag}]\binom{\text{Ab}}{[\text{MAb-}^{125}\text{I}]} -\text{radioactivity}$$

Assay type: RIA (competitive)
Detection: Radioisotopic
Format: Tube, Ag coated
Sample type: Serum or plasma
Sample pre-treatment:
   None
Sample volume: 50 µl
Number of tests: 100
Controls - standards run in assay:
   Controls: Neg (4), Pos (2)
Incubation:
   2 hr (RT) with shaking
Washes: 1

CONTENTS

Antibodies, antigens, labelled components:
   rec HBcAg bound to tube
   Anti-HBc MAb ^{125}I labelled
Substrate:
Controls - standards supplied:
   Controls: Neg and Pos (human serum)
Additional reagents:
   None
Special equipment required:
   None

INTERPRETATION

Comments on interpretation:
   Grey area: within cut-off value ± 10%; retest to confirm
   Positive: < cut-off value repeatably
No. of references: 7

NOTES

110435.0

Hepatitis B virus (core antigen)
ANTIBODY DETECTION

Manufacturer: Sorin Biomedica
Cat. No./Trade name: 2967/AB-COREK

SUMMARY

$$[\text{Ab-}^{125}\text{I}]\binom{\text{Ab}}{}[\text{Bead-Ag}]-\text{radioactivity}$$

Assay type: RIA (competitive)
Detection: Radioisotopic
Format: Tray/Tube, Ag coated bead
Sample type: Serum, plasma
Sample pre-treatment:
   None
Sample volume: 100 µl
Number of tests: 100
Controls - standards run in assay:
   Controls: Neg (3), Pos (3)
Incubation:
   Overnight (RT)
Washes: 1

CONTENTS

Antibodies, antigens, labelled components:
   rec HBcAg bound to bead
   Anti-HBc IgG Ab ^{125}I labelled
Substrate:
Controls - standards supplied:
   Controls: Neg (human serum) and Pos
Additional reagents:
   None
Special equipment required:
   Automatic rinser, PLA-2 (optional)
   Bead dispenser, MEDI-578 (optional)

INTERPRETATION

Comments on interpretation:
   Equivocal: Within cut-off ± 10%; retest to confirm
No. of references: 6

NOTES

110226.0

© *KLUWER ACADEMIC PUBLISHERS 1994, ISSN 1381-5067*

Hepatitis B virus (core antigen)
ANTIBODY DETECTION (IgM)

Manufacturer: Abbott Laboratories
Cat. No./Trade name: 1234-22/CORAB® - M

SUMMARY

[Bead-AHIgM]–**Ab**–[Ag]–[Ab-^{125}I]–radioactivity

Assay type: RIA (non-competitive)
Detection: Radioisotopic
Format: Reaction well, Ab coated bead
Sample type: Serum, plasma
Sample pre-treatment:
   None
Sample volume: 10 µl (+500 µl diluent)
Number of tests: 50
Controls - standards run in assay:
   Controls: Neg (2), Pos (3)
Incubation:
   1 hr (45°C) + 18-22 hr (RT) + 2 hr (45°C)
Washes: 3

CONTENTS

Antibodies, antigens, labelled components:
   Anti-human IgM Ab (g) bound to bead
   HBcAg (h)
   Anti-HBc Ab (h) ^{125}I labelled
Substrate:
Controls - standards supplied:
   Controls: Pos and Neg (human plasma)
Additional reagents:
   None
Special equipment required:
   None

INTERPRETATION

Comments on interpretation:
   Equivocal: within cut-off ±10%; retest to confirm. If
      sample is consistently within cut-off ±10%; report as
      such and advise patient follow-up
   Positive: ≥cut-off repeatably
No. of references: 14

NOTES

110028.0

Hepatitis B virus (core antigen)
ANTIBODY DETECTION (IgM)

Manufacturer: Radim
Cat. No./Trade name: KHB2CM/ANTI-HBc IgM IRMA CT

SUMMARY

[Tube-AHIgM]–**Ab**-[Ag]–[MAb-^{125}I]–radioactivity

Assay type: RIA (non-competitive)
Detection: Radioisotopic
Format: Tube, Ab coated
Sample type: Serum or plasma
Sample pre-treatment:
   None
Sample volume: 10 µl of 1:200 dilution (+200 µl diluent)
Number of tests: 100
Controls - standards run in assay:
   Controls: Neg (4), Pos (1)
Incubation:
   1 hr (RT) + 1 hr (RT) both with shaking
Washes: 2

CONTENTS

Antibodies, antigens, labelled components:
   Anti-human IgM MAb (r) bound to tube
   rec HBcAg
   Anti-HBc MAb ^{125}I labelled
Substrate:
Controls - standards supplied:
   Controls: Neg and Pos (human serum)
Additional reagents:
   None
Special equipment required:
   None

INTERPRETATION

Comments on interpretation:
   Grey area: within cut-off value ± 10%; retest to confirm
   Positive: > cut-off value repeatably
No. of references: 9

NOTES

110436.0

© KLUWER ACADEMIC PUBLISHERS 1994, ISSN 1381-5067

Hepatitis B virus (core antigen)
ANTIBODY DETECTION (IgM)

Manufacturer: Sorin Biomedica
Cat. No./Trade name: 2489/CORE-IGMK

SUMMARY

[Bead-AHIgM]–**Ab**–[Ag]–[Ab-^{125}I]–radioactivity

Assay type: RIA (non-competitive)
Detection: Radioisotopic
Format: Tray/Tube, Ab coated bead
Sample type: Serum, plasma
Sample pre-treatment:
 None
Sample volume: 10 µl (+ 2 ml diluent)
Number of tests: 50
Controls - standards run in assay:
 Controls: Neg (3), Pos (3)
Incubation:
 18-22 hr (RT) + 3 hr (45°C)
Washes: 2

CONTENTS

Antibodies, antigens, labelled components:
 Anti-human IgM Ab (r) bound to bead
 rec HBcAg
 Anti-HBc IgG Ab (h) ^{125}I labelled
Substrate:
Controls - standards supplied:
 Controls: Neg and Pos (human serum)
Additional reagents:
 None
Special equipment required:
 Automatic rinser, PLA-2 (optional)
 Bead dispenser, MEDI-578

INTERPRETATION

Comments on interpretation:
 Classification of samples is according to cut-off; no
 further testing
No. of references: 6

NOTES

110216.0

Hepatitis B virus (e antigen)
ANTIGEN DETECTION*

Manufacturer: Abbott Laboratories
Cat. No./Trade name: 1235/ABBOTT HBe (rDNA) EIA

SUMMARY

[Bead-Ab]–**Ag**–[Ab-HRP]–[OPD]–A_{492}

Assay type: EIA (non-competitive)
Detection: Colorimetric A_{492}
Format: Reaction well, Ab coated bead
Sample type: Serum, plasma (do not heat inactivate)
Sample pre-treatment:
 None
Sample volume: 200 µl
Number of tests: 100
Controls - standards run in assay:
 Controls: Neg (3), Pos (2)
Incubation:
 20 hr (RT) + 2 hr (40°C) + 30 min (RT)
Washes: 2

CONTENTS

Antibodies, antigens, labelled components:
 Anti-HBe Ab (h) bound to bead
 rec HBeAg (for Ab detection only)
 Anti-HBe Ab (h) HRP conjugated
Substrate: OPD, H_2O_2
Controls - standards supplied:
 Controls: Neg and Pos (human plasma)
Additional reagents:
 H_2SO_4
Special equipment required:
 None

INTERPRETATION

Comments on interpretation:
 Equivocal: within 10% of cut-off; retest to confirm
 Semi-quantitative procedure available
No. of references: 13

NOTES

110025.0

*This kit is used for the detection of both HBeAg and anti-
 HBe. Details of antibody detection are given in the
 appropriate section

Hepatitis B virus (e antigen)
ANTIGEN DETECTION

Manufacturer: Abbott Laboratories
Cat. No./Trade name: 2227-66/IMx® HBe Assay

SUMMARY

[Particle-PAb]–**Ag**–[MAb-AP]–[4-MP]–fluorescence

Assay type: EIA (non-competitive)
Detection: Fluorometric
Format: Reaction well, Ab coated microparticle
Sample type: Serum, plasma (do not heat inactivate)
Sample pre-treatment:
  None
Sample volume: 150 µl
Number of tests: 100
Controls - standards run in assay:
  Calibration assay: calibrators (1) x 2; Controls: Neg (1),
    Pos (1)
  Mode 1 assay: calibrators (1); Controls: Pos (1)*
Incubation:
  Automated
Washes: Automated

CONTENTS

Antibodies, antigens, labelled components:
  Anti-HBe PAb (h) bound to microparticle
  Anti-HBe MAb (m) AP conjugated
Substrate: 4-MP
Controls - standards supplied:
  Calibrators: mode 1 calibrator (human plasma)
Additional reagents:
  IMx ®HBe controls, IMx® MEIA diluent buffer, IMx®
    probe cleaning solution
Special equipment required:
  IMx system

INTERPRETATION

Comments on interpretation:
  Sample reactivity is calculated automatically
  Positive: ⩾cut-off repeatably
No. of references: 10

NOTES

110021.0

For research use only
*Minimum control requirement for mode 1 assay: one
  positive control assayed once per 8 hr shift

Hepatitis B virus (e antigen)
*ANTIGEN DETECTION**

Manufacturer: ADI Diagnostics
Cat. No./Trade name: /Heprofile® HBe/Anti-HBe

SUMMARY

[Well-MAb]–**Ag**–[MAb-POD]–[TMB]–A_{450}

Assay type: EIA (non-competitive)
Detection: Colorimetric A_{450}
Format: Microtitre well, Ab coated
Sample type: Serum, plasma (do not heat inactivate)
Sample pre-treatment:
  None
Sample volume: 200 µl
Number of tests: 96
Controls - standards run in assay:
  Controls: Neg (3), Pos (2)
Incubation:
  12-20 hr (RT) + 2 hr (37°C) + 30 min (RT)
Washes: 2

CONTENTS

Antibodies, antigens, labelled components:
  Anti-HBe MAb (m) bound to well
  HBeAg (h) (for use in Ab detection assay only)
  Anti-HBe MAb (m) POD conjugated
Substrate: TMB, H_2O_2
Controls - standards supplied:
  Controls: Neg and Pos (human plasma)
Additional reagents:
  None
Special equipment required:
  None

INTERPRETATION

Comments on interpretation:
  Positive: ⩾cut-off repeatably
No. of references: 19

NOTES

110019.0

*This kit is used for the detection of both HBeAg and anti-
  HBeAg. Details of the antibody detection are given in the
  appropriate section

© *KLUWER ACADEMIC PUBLISHERS 1994, ISSN 1381-5067*

Hepatitis B virus (e antigen)
ANTIGEN DETECTION*

Manufacturer: Behringwerke AG
Cat. No./Trade name: OUMG/Enzygnost® HBe

SUMMARY

[Well-Ab]–**Ag**–[Ab-POD]–[TMB]–A_{450}

Assay type: EIA (non-competitive)
Detection: Colorimetric A_{450}
Format: Microtitre well, Ab coated
Sample type: Serum, plasma
Sample pre-treatment:
   None
Sample volume: 100 µl
Number of tests: 96
Controls - standards run in assay:
   Controls: Neg (4), Pos (2)
Incubation:
   16-24 hr (RT) + 1 hr (37°C) + 30 min (RT)
Washes: 2

CONTENTS

Antibodies, antigens, labelled components:
   Anti-HBe (human) bound to well
   HBe Ag (for Ab assay)
   Anti-HBe (human) POD conjugated
Substrate: TMB, H_2O_2
Controls - standards supplied:
   Controls: Neg and Pos (human serum)
Additional reagents:
   None
Special equipment required:
   Behring ELISA processor (optional)

INTERPRETATION

Comments on interpretation:
   Classification of samples is according to cut-off; no
   further testing
No. of references: 11

NOTES

110455.0

*The kit is used for the detection of both HBe Ag and anti-
HBe. Details of antibody detection are given in the
appropriate section

Hepatitis B virus (e antigen)
ANTIGEN DETECTION*

Manufacturer: Boehringer Mannheim
Cat. No./Trade name: 1335 995/Enzymun-Test® HBeAg
+ Anti-HBe

SUMMARY

[Tube-strept]–[biotin-MAb]–**Ag**–[MAb-POD]–[ABTS]–
A_{420}

Assay type: EIA (non-competitive)
Detection: Colorimetric A_{420}
Format: Tube, streptavidin coated
Sample type: Serum, plasma
Sample pre-treatment:
   None
Sample volume: 100 µl
Number of tests: 145
Controls - standards run in assay:
   Controls: Neg (2), Pos (2)
Incubation:
   3 hr (RT) + 1 hr (RT)
Washes: 1

CONTENTS

Antibodies, antigens, labelled components:
   Anti-HBe MAb (m) biotinylated
   rec HBe Ag (for Ab assay)
   Anti-HBe MAb (m) POD conjugated
Substrate: ABTS, H_2O_2
Controls - standards supplied:
   Controls: Neg (human serum), Pos (Ag)
Additional reagents:
   Substrate and streptavidin-coated tubes
Special equipment required:
   Automated Enzymun-Test Systems (optional)

INTERPRETATION

Comments on interpretation:
   Borderline: within cut-off ±10%; retest to confirm
No. of references: 0

NOTES

110466.0

*This kit is used for the detection of both HBe Ag and Anti-
HBe. Details of the antibody detection are given in the
appropriate section

© **KLUWER ACADEMIC PUBLISHERS** 1994, ISSN 1381-5067

Hepatitis B virus (e antigen)
ANTIGEN DETECTION

Manufacturer: IFCI Clone Systems
Cat. No./Trade name: 07.1004/EIAgen HBeAg Kit

SUMMARY

[Well-MAb]–**Ag**–[Ab-HRP]–[TMB]–A_{450}

Assay type: EIA (non-competitive)
Detection: Colorimetric A_{450}
Format: Microtitre well, Ab coated
Sample type: Serum, plasma (do not heat inactivate)
Sample pre-treatment:
　None
Sample volume: 200 µl
Number of tests: 96
Controls - standards run in assay:
　Controls: Neg (3), Pos (2)
Incubation:
　2 hr (40°C) + 1 hr (40°C) + 20 min (RT)
Washes: 2

CONTENTS

Antibodies, antigens, labelled components:
　Anti-HBe IgG MAb bound to well
　Anti-HBe IgG Ab HRP conjugated
Substrate: TMB, H_2O_2
Controls - standards supplied:
　Controls: Neg and Pos (human serum)
Additional reagents:
　None
Special equipment required:
　None

INTERPRETATION

Comments on interpretation:
　Classification of sample is according to cut-off; no further
　testing
No. of references: 8

NOTES

110091.0

Hepatitis B virus (e antigen)
ANTIGEN DETECTION*

Manufacturer: Melotec S.A.
Cat. No./Trade name: /MELOTEST HBeAg/Anti-HBe

SUMMARY

[Well-MAb]–**Ag**–[Ab-HRP]–[TMB]–A_{450}

Assay type: EIA (non-competitive)
Detection: Colorimetric A_{450}
Format: Microtitre well, Ab coated
Sample type: Serum, plasma
Sample pre-treatment:
　None
Sample volume: 200 µl**
Number of tests: 96
Controls - standards run in assay:
　Controls: Neg (3), Pos (1)
Incubation:
　16 ± 4 h (RT) + 2 hr (37°C) + 30 min (RT)
Washes: 2

CONTENTS

Antibodies, antigens, labelled components:
　Anti-HBe MAb (m) bound to well
　HBeAg (for Ab detection only)
　Anti-HBe Ab HRP conjugated
Substrate: TMB, H_2O_2
Controls - standards supplied:
　Controls: Neg, Pos (anti-HBe) and Pos (HBeAg)
Additional reagents:
　None
Special equipment required:
　None

INTERPRETATION

Comments on interpretation:
　Equivocal: within cut-off and cut-off–10%; retest to
　confirm
　Repeatably equivocal: test a fresh sample after 1–2
　weeks
　Positive: ≥ cut-off repeatably and confirmed by
　supplemental tests
No. of references: 5

NOTES

110640.0

*This kit is used for the detection of both HBeAg and anti-
　HBe. Details of antibody detection are given in the
　appropriate section
**It is recommended to run duplicates of samples for greater
　precision

© *KLUWER ACADEMIC PUBLISHERS 1994, ISSN 1381-5067*

Hepatitis B virus (e antigen)
ANTIGEN DETECTION*

Manufacturer: Organon Teknika NV
Cat. No./Trade name: 70170/Hepanostika® HBe Ag/ anti-HBe Microelisa system

SUMMARY

[Well-Ab]–**Ag**–[Ab-HRP]–[TMB]–A_{450}

Assay type: EIA (non-competitive)
Detection: Colorimetric A_{450}
Format: Microtitre well, Ab coated
Sample type: Serum, plasma
Sample pre-treatment:
   None
Sample volume: 100 µl
Number of tests: 192
Controls - standards run in assay:
   Controls: Neg (3), Pos HBe Ag (1)
Incubation:
   2 hr (37°C) + 2 hr (37°C) + 30 min (RT)
Washes: 2

CONTENTS

Antibodies, antigens, labelled components:
   Anti-HBe Ab (h) bound to well
   HBeAg (Pos control used in anti-HBe screening test)
   Anti-HBe Ab (h) HRP conjugated
Substrate: TMB, H_2O_2
Controls - standards supplied:
   Controls: Neg, Pos (HBe Ag), Pos (anti-HBe) (human serum)
Additional reagents:
   H_2SO_4
Special equipment required:
   None

INTERPRETATION

Comments on Interpretation:
   Positive: ⩾ cut-off and confirmed by using this Hepanostika HBe Ag kit as a confirmatory neutralization test
   Semi-quantitative procedure available
No. of references: 0

NOTES

110556.0

*This kit is used for the detection of both HBe Ag and Ab. Details of the Ab detection are in the appropriate section

---

Hepatitis B virus (e antigen)
ANTIGEN DETECTION*

Manufacturer: Radim
Cat. No./Trade name: KHB4IW/HBe Ag/Ab IEMA WELL

SUMMARY

[Well-MAb]–**Ag**–[MAb-HRP]–[TMB]–A_{450}

Assay type: EIA (non-competitive)
Detection: Colorimetric A_{450}
Format: Microtitre well, Ab coated
Sample type: Serum or plasma
Sample pre-treatment:
   None
Sample volume: 100 µl
Number of tests: 96
Controls - standards run in assay:
   Controls: Neg (4), Pos (2)
Incubation:
   3 hr (37°C) + 20 min (37°C)
Washes: 1

CONTENTS

Antibodies, antigens, labelled components:
   Anti-HBe MAb bound to well
   rec HBeAg (for Ab assay)
   Anti-HBe MAb HRP conjugated
Substrate: TMB, H_2O_2
Controls - standards supplied:
   Controls: Neg and Pos (serum)
Additional reagents:
   None
Special equipment required:
   None

INTERPRETATION

Comments on Interpretation:
   Grey area: within cut-off value ± 10%; retest to confirm
   Positive: > cut-off value repeatably
No. of references: 5

NOTES

110437.0

*The kit is used for detection of both HBeAg and anti-HBe. Details of the antibody detection are given in the appropriate section

© *KLUWER ACADEMIC PUBLISHERS 1994, ISSN 1381-5067*

Hepatitis B virus (e antigen)
ANTIGEN DETECTION*

Manufacturer: Randox Laboratories Ltd
Cat. No./Trade name: HT 1488/HBe Ag/Anti-HBe Ag

SUMMARY

$$[Well-Ab]-Ag-[Ab-POD]-[OPD]-A_{492}$$

Assay type: EIA (non-competitive)
Detection: Colorimetric A_{492}
Format: Microtitre well, Ab coated
Sample type: Serum, plasma (do not heat inactivate)
Sample pre-treatment:
   None
Sample volume: 100 µl
Number of tests: 96
Controls - standards run in assay:
   Controls: Neg (3), Pos (2)
Incubation:
   a) 20 hr (RT) + 1 hr (40°C) + 30 min (RT)
   b) 2 hr (40°C) + 1 hr (40°C) + 30 min (RT)
Washes: 2

CONTENTS

Antibodies, antigens, labelled components:
   Anti-HBe Ab bound to well
   HBe Ag (for Ab assay)
   Anti-HBe Ab POD conjugated
Substrate: OPD, H_2O_2
Controls - standards supplied:
   Controls: Neg, Pos
Additional reagents:
   None
Special equipment required:
   None

INTERPRETATION

Comments on interpretation:
   Classification of samples is according to cut-off; no
   further testing
No. of references: 3

NOTES

110509.0

*This test is for the detection of both HBe Ag and anti-HBe.
   Details of the antibody detection are given in the
   appropriate section

Hepatitis B virus (e antigen)
ANTIGEN DETECTION

Manufacturer: Sanofi Diagnostics Pasteur
Cat. No./Trade name: 72212/MONOLISA® HBe

SUMMARY

$$[Well-Ab]-Ag-[MAb-POD]-[OPD]-A_{492/620}$$

Assay type: EIA (non-competitive)
Detection: Colorimetric $A_{492/620}$
Format: Microtitre well, Ab coated
Sample type: Serum, plasma
Sample pre-treatment:
   None
Sample volume: 100 µl
Number of tests: 96
Controls - standards run in assay:
   Controls: Neg (3), Pos (1)
Incubation:
   Overnight (RT) + 30 min (40°C) + 30 min (RT)
Washes: 2 (+ preliminary plate prewash)

CONTENTS

Antibodies, antigens, labelled components:
   Anti-HBe PAb (h) bound to well
   Anti-HBe MAb_1 and MAb_2 (m) POD conjugated
Substrate: OPD, H_2O_2
Controls - standards supplied:
   Controls: Neg (human serum) and Pos (human plasma)
Additional reagents:
   None
Special equipment required:
   None

INTERPRETATION

Comments on interpretation:
   Classification of samples is according to cut-off; no
   further testing
No. of references: 7

NOTES

110267.0

Hepatitis B virus (e antigen)
ANTIGEN DETECTION*

Manufacturer: Schiapparelli Biosystems Inc
Cat. No./Trade name: 5770333/HEPATITIS B - HBeAg/HBeAb ELISA SYSTEM

SUMMARY

[Well-MAb]–**Ag**–[MAb-HRP]–[TMB]–A_{450}

Assay type: EIA (non-competitive)
Detection: Colorimetric A_{450}
Format: Microtitre well, Ab coated
Sample type: Serum (do not heat inactivate)
Sample pre-treatment:
　None
Sample volume: 200 µl x 2
Number of tests: 96
Controls - standards run in assay:
　Controls: Neg (3), Pos (2)
Incubation:
　2 hr (40°C) + 1 hr (40°C) + 20 min (RT)
Washes: 2

CONTENTS

Antibodies, antigens, labelled components:
　Anti-HBe MAb bound to well
　rec HBeAg (for Ab assay)
　Anti-HBe MAb HRP conjugated
Substrate: TMB, H_2O_2
Controls - standards supplied:
　Controls: Neg (human serum) and Pos (rec Ag)
Additional reagents:
　None
Special equipment required:
　Biochromatic microplate spectrophotometer (optional)

INTERPRETATION

Comments on interpretation:
　Classification of sample is according to cut-off; no further testing
No. of references: 9

NOTES

110427.0

*The kit is used for the detection of both HBeAg and anti-HBe. Details of the antibody detection are given in the appropriate section

Hepatitis B virus (e antigen)
ANTIGEN DETECTION

Manufacturer: Sorin Biomedica
Cat. No./Trade name: 2877/ETI-EBK-2

SUMMARY

[Well-MAb]–**Ag**–[MAb-HRP]–[TMB]–A_{450}

Assay type: EIA (non-competitive)
Detection: Colorimetric A_{450}
Format: Microtitre well, Ab coated
Sample type: Serum, plasma
Sample pre-treatment:
　None
Sample volume: 100 µl
Number of tests: 96
Controls - standards run in assay:
　Controls: Neg (3), Pos (2)
Incubation:
　2 hr (37°C) + 1 hr (37°C) + 30 min (RT)
Washes: 2

CONTENTS

Antibodies, antigens, labelled components:
　Anti-HBe IgG MAb (m) bound to well
　Anti-HBe IgG MAb (m) HRP conjugated
Substrate: TMB, H_2O_2
Controls - standards supplied:
　Controls: Neg and Pos (human plasma)
Additional reagents:
　None
Special equipment required:
　None

INTERPRETATION

Comments on interpretation:
　Equivocal:　Within cut-off ± 10%; retest to confirm
No. of references: 11

NOTES

110228.0

Hepatitis B virus (e antigen)
ANTIGEN DETECTION*

Manufacturer: Sorin Biomedica
Cat. No./Trade name: 2439/EBK eia

SUMMARY

[Bead-MAb]–**Ag**-[MAb-HRP]–[OPD]–A$_{492}$

Assay type: EIA (non-competitive)
Detection: Colorimetric A$_{492}$
Format: Tray/Tube, Ab coated bead
Sample type: Serum, plasma
Sample pre-treatment:
  None
Sample volume: 200 µl
Number of tests: 100
Controls - standards run in assay:
  Controls: Neg (3), Pos (2)
Incubation:
  18-22 hr (RT) + 3 hr (RT) + 30 min (RT)
Washes: 2

CONTENTS

Antibodies, antigens, labelled components:
  Anti-HBe IgG MAb (m) bound to bead
  HBeAg (h) (for Ab detection assay)
  Anti-HBe IgG MAb (m) HRP conjugated
Substrate: OPD; H$_2$O$_2$
Controls - standards supplied:
  Controls: Neg and Pos for both HBeAg and anti-HBeAg
  (human)
Additional reagents:
  None
Special equipment required:
  Automatic rinsing device, PLA-2 (optional)
  Bead dispenser, MEDI-578 (optional)

INTERPRETATION

Comments on interpretation:
  Equivocal: Within cut-off ± 10%; retest to confirm
  Positive: ≥cut-off repeatably
No. of references: 11

NOTES

110242.0

*This kit measures both HBeAg and anti-HBe. Details of the
  assay for anti-HBe are given in the appropriate section
This kit will be discontinued in December 1994

Hepatitis B virus (e antigen)
ANTIGEN DETECTION

Manufacturer: Syva Company
Cat. No./Trade name: 8HE29UL/MicroTrak® II HBe Ag
EIA

SUMMARY

[Well-MAb]–**Ag**–[MAb-HRP]–[TMB]–A$_{450/630}$

Assay type: EIA (non-competitive)
Detection: Colorimetric A$_{450/630}$
Format: Microtitre well, Ab coated
Sample type: Serum, plasma
Sample pre-treatment:
  None
Sample volume:
Number of tests: 96
Controls - standards run in assay:
  Controls: Neg (3), Pos (2)
Incubation:
  2 hr (37°C) + 1 hr (37°C) + 30 min (37°C)
Washes: 2

CONTENTS

Antibodies, antigens, labelled components:
  Anti-HBe IgG MAb bound to well
  Anti-HBe IgG MAb HRP conjugated
Substrate: TMB, H$_2$O$_2$
Controls - standards supplied:
  Controls: Neg and Pos (human plasma)
Additional reagents:
  MicroTrak® II EIA universal reagents (8K209UL)
Special equipment required:
  Syva MicroTrak® EIA autowasher and autoreader

INTERPRETATION

Comments on interpretation:
  Equivocal: absorbance values within ±20% of the cut-
    off; retest to confirm
No. of references: 12

NOTES

110071.0

Hepatitis B virus (e antigen)
ANTIGEN DETECTION

Manufacturer: VEDA-LAB
Cat. No./Trade name: 1061/HBe Ag EIA

SUMMARY

[Well-MAb]–**Ag**–[Ab-HRP]–[TMB]–A$_{450}$

Assay type: EIA (non-competitive)
Detection: Colorimetric A$_{450}$
Format: Microtitre well, Ab coated
Sample type: Serum, plasma
Sample pre-treatment:
    None
Sample volume: 50 µl
Number of tests: 96
Controls - standards run in assay:
    Controls: Neg (1), Pos (1)
Incubation:
    1 hr (37°C) + 15 min (RT)
Washes: 1

CONTENTS

Antibodies, antigens, labelled components:
    Anti-HBe MAb bound to well
    Anti-HBe Ab HRP conjugated
Substrate: TMB, H$_2$O$_2$
Controls - standards supplied:
    Controls: Neg and Pos
Additional reagents:
    None
Special equipment required:
    None

INTERPRETATION

Comments on interpretation:
    Classification of sample is according to cut-off; no further
    testing
No. of references: 5

NOTES

110394.0

Hepatitis B virus (e antigen)
*ANTIGEN DETECTION**

Manufacturer: Radim
Cat. No./Trade name: KHB4CT/HBe Ag/Ab IRMA CT

SUMMARY

[Tube-MAb]–**Ag**–[MAb-^{125}I]–radioactivity

Assay type: RIA (non-competitive)
Detection: Radioisotopic
Format: Tube, Ab coated
Sample type: Serum or plasma
Sample pre-treatment:
    None
Sample volume: 200 µl
Number of tests: 100
Controls - standards run in assay:
    Controls: Neg (4), Pos (2)
Incubation:
    a) 1 hr (45°C) + 1 hr (45°C)
    b) 18-22 hr (RT) + 1 hr (45°C)
Washes: 2

CONTENTS

Antibodies, antigens, labelled components:
    Anti-HBe MAb (r) bound to tube
    rec HBeAg (for Ab assay)
    Anti-HBe MAb ^{125}I labelled
Substrate:
Controls - standards supplied:
    Controls: Neg and Pos (human serum)
Additional reagents:
    None
Special equipment required:
    None

INTERPRETATION

Comments on interpretation:
    Grey area: within cut-off value ± 10%; retest to confirm
    Positive: > cut-off value repeatably
No. of references: 7

NOTES

110439.0

*The kit is used for detection of both HBeAg and anti-HBe.
    Details of the antibody detection are given in the
    appropriate section

Hepatitis B virus (e antigen)
ANTIGEN DETECTION*

Manufacturer: Sorin Biomedica
Cat. No./Trade name: 2502/EBK

SUMMARY

[Bead-MAb]–**Ag**–[MAb-^{125}I]–radioactivity

Assay type: RIA (non-competitive)
Detection: Radioisotopic
Format: Tray/Tube, Ab coated bead
Sample type: Serum, plasma
Sample pre-treatment:
  None
Sample volume: 200 µl
Number of tests: 100
Controls - standards run in assay:
  Controls: Neg (3), Pos (3)
Incubation:
  18-22 hr (RT) + 3 hr (45°C)
Washes: 2

CONTENTS

Antibodies, antigens, labelled components:
  Anti-HBe IgG MAb (m) bound to beads
  rec HBeAg (for antibody assay only)
  Anti-HBe IgG MAb (m) ^{125}I labelled
Substrate:
Controls - standards supplied:
  Controls: Neg and Pos
Additional reagents:
  None
Special equipment required:
  Automated rinser, PLA-2 (optional)
  Bead dispenser, MEDI-578 (optional)

INTERPRETATION

Comments on interpretation:
  Positive: ≥ cut-off repeatably
  Due to the low radioactivity employed, initially reactive
    samples (> cut-off) whose net count rate is < 5 times
    the Neg control mean should be repeated
No. of references: 11

NOTES

110214.0

*The kit is used for the detection of both HBeAg and Anti-
  HBe. Details of the antibody detection are given in the
  appropriate section

Hepatitis B virus (e antigen)
ANTIGEN AND ANTIBODY DETECTION*

Manufacturer: Murex Diagnostics Limited
Cat. No./Trade name: VK30/HBeAg/anti-HBe

SUMMARY

[Well-MAb]–**Ag**–[MAb-HRP]–[TMB]–A$_{450}$

$$[\text{Well-MAb}]-[\text{Ag}]\left\langle\begin{array}{l}\textbf{Ab}\\ [\text{MAb-HRP}]\end{array}\right. -[\text{TMB}]-A_{450}$$

Assay type: EIA (non-competitive)
Detection: Colorimetric A$_{450}$
Format: Microtitre well, Ab coated
Sample type: Serum, plasma
Sample pre-treatment:
  None
Sample volume: 100 µl x 2*
Number of tests: 96
Controls - standards run in assay:
  Controls: Neg (4), HBeAg Pos (2), anti-HBe Pos (2)
Incubation:
  Serum: 1 hr (45°C) + 30 min (RT)
  Plasma: 1 hr 30 min (37°C) + 30 min (RT)
Washes: 1

CONTENTS

Antibodies, antigens, labelled components:
  Anti-HBe MAb (m) bound to well
  rec HBeAg (for anti-HBe assay only)
  Anti-HBe MAb (m) HRP conjugated
Substrate: TMB, H$_2$O$_2$
Controls - standards supplied:
  Controls: Neg and anti-HBe Pos (human serum); HBeAg
    Pos (rec)
Additional reagents:
  H$_2$SO$_4$
Special equipment required:
  Wellcozyme microwell plate washing system (optional)
  Wellcozyme microwell plate reader (optional)

INTERPRETATION

Comments on interpretation:
  Antibody and antigen: classification of sample is
    according to cut-off; no further testing
No. of references: None

NOTES

110159.0

*Test for HBe antigen and anti-HBe performed in parallel in
  adjacent microtitre wells for each sample

© KLUWER ACADEMIC PUBLISHERS 1994, ISSN 1381-5067

Hepatitis B virus (e antigen)
ANTIGEN AND ANTIBODY DETECTION*

Manufacturer: Kodak Clinical Diagnostics
Cat. No./Trade name: LAN.1209/KODAK Amerlite HBe/
anti-HBe

SUMMARY

$$[\text{Well-Ab}] \left\langle \begin{array}{l} \textbf{Ag--[Ab-HRP]--luminescence increase} \\ \textbf{Ab--[Ag-HRP]--luminescence decrease} \end{array} \right.$$

Assay type: Luminometric immunoassay (non-competitive)
Detection: Luminometric
Format: Microtitre well, Ab coated
Sample type: Serum, plasma
Sample pre-treatment:
   None
Sample volume: 50 µl
Number of tests: 96
Controls - standards run in assay:
   Controls: Neg (3), Ab Pos (2), Ag Pos (1)
Incubation:
   2 hr (37°C) with shaking + 2-20 min (RT)
Washes: 1

CONTENTS

Antibodies, antigens, labelled components:
   Anti-HBe MAb (m) bound to well
   Anti-HBe MAb (m) HRP conjugated complexed to rec
      HBeAg (MAb-HRP in excess)
Substrate: Amerlite signal reagent
Controls - standards supplied:
   Controls: Neg and Ab Pos (human plasma) and Ag Pos
      (rec Ag)
Additional reagents:
   Amerlite signal reagent and serology wash reagent
Special equipment required:
   Amerlite Kodak immunoassay system

INTERPRETATION

Comments on interpretation:
   Results are calculated automatically as a normalized
      signal relative to the cut-off
Anti-HBe positive: 0-0.45
HBe Ag positive: >1.3
Non-reactive: 0.45-1.3, meaning that neither HBe Ag nor
   anti-HBe are present OR that both Ag and Ab are in
   equivalence. Further tests for HBV infection and the
   overall clinical history of the patient should be
   considered
No. of references: 7

NOTES

110487.0

*This assay measures both Ag and Ab simultaneously

Hepatitis B virus (e antigen)
ANTIBODY DETECTION*

Manufacturer: Abbott Laboratories
Cat. No./Trade name: 1235/ABBOTT HBe (rDNA) EIA

SUMMARY

$$\begin{array}{l} \textbf{Ab} \\ [\text{Bead-Ab}] \end{array} \Big/ [\text{Ag}]\text{--}[\text{Ab-HRP}]\text{--}[\text{OPD}]\text{--}A_{492}$$

Assay type: EIA (competitive)
Detection: Colorimetric A_{492}
Format: Reaction well, Ab coated bead
Sample type: Serum, plasma (do not heat inactivate)
Sample pre-treatment:
   None
Sample volume: 50 µl
Number of tests: 100
Controls - standards run in assay:
   Controls: Neg (3), Pos (2)
Incubation:
   20 hr (RT) + 2 hr (40°C) + 30 min (RT)
Washes: 2

CONTENTS

Antibodies, antigens, labelled components:
   Anti-HBe Ab (h) bound to beads
   rec HBeAg
   Anti-HBe Ab (h) HRP conjugated
Substrate: OPD, H_2O_2
Controls - standards supplied:
   Controls: Neg and Pos (human plasma)
Additional reagents:
   H_2SO_4
Special equipment required:
   None

INTERPRETATION

Comments on interpretation:
   Equivocal within 10% of cut-off; retest to confirm
   Semi-quantitative procedure available
No. of references: 13

NOTES

110024.0

*This kit is used for the detection of both HBeAg and anti-
   HBe. Details of antigen detection are given in the
   appropriate section

Hepatitis B virus (e antigen)
ANTIBODY DETECTION

Manufacturer: Abbott Laboratories
Cat. No./Trade name: 2261-66/IMx® Anti-HBe Assay

SUMMARY

$$[\text{Particle-Ab}]-[\text{Ag}]\genfrac{}{}{0pt}{}{\text{Ab}}{[\text{MAb-AP}]}-[\text{4-MP}]-\text{fluorescence}$$

Assay type: EIA (competitive)
Detection: Fluorometric
Format: Reaction well, Ab coated microparticle
Sample type: Serum, plasma (do not heat inactivate)
Sample pre-treatment:
  None
Sample volume: 150 μl
Number of tests: 100
Controls - standards run in assay:
  Calibration assay: calibrators (1) x 2, Controls: Neg (1),
    Pos (1)
  Mode 1 assay: calibrators (1), Controls: Pos (1)*
Incubation:
  Automated
Washes: Automated

CONTENTS

Antibodies, antigens, labelled components:
  Anti-HBe PAb (h) bound to microparticle
  rec HBeAg
  Anti-HBe MAb (m) AP conjugated
Substrate: 4-MP
Controls - standards supplied:
  Calibrators: mode 1 calibrator (human plasma)
Additional reagents:
  IMx® Anti-HBe controls, IMx® MEIA diluent buffer, IMx®
    probe cleaning solution
Special equipment required:
  IMx system

INTERPRETATION

Comments on interpretation:
  Sample reactivity is calculated automatically
  Classification of samples is according to cut-off; no
    further testing
No. of references: 8

NOTES

110022.0

For research use only
Minimum control requirement for mode 1 assay: one positive
  control assayed once per 8 hr shift

Hepatitis B virus (e antigen)
ANTIBODY DETECTION*

Manufacturer: ADI Diagnostics
Cat. No./Trade name: /Heprofile® HBe/Anti-HBe

SUMMARY

$$\genfrac{}{}{0pt}{}{\text{Ab}}{[\text{Well-Ab}]}[\text{Ag}]-[\text{Ab-POD}]-[\text{TMB}]-A_{450}$$

Assay type: EIA (competitive)
Detection: Colorimetric A_{450}
Format: Microtitre well, Ab coated
Sample type: Serum, plasma (do not heat inactivate)
Sample pre-treatment:
  None
Sample volume: 100 μl (+100 μl neutralising reagent)
Number of tests: 96
Controls - standards run in assay:
  Controls: Neg (3), Pos (2)
Incubation:
  12-20 hr (RT) + 2 hr (37°C) + 30 min (RT)
Washes: 2

CONTENTS

Antibodies, antigens, labelled components:
  Anti-HBe MAb (m) bound to well
  HBeAg (h)
  Anti-HBe MAb (m) POD conjugated
Substrate: TMB, H_2O_2
Controls - standards supplied:
  Controls: Neg and Pos (human plasma)
Additional reagents:
  None
Special equipment required:
  None

INTERPRETATION

Comments on interpretation:
  Positive: ≤cut-off repeatably
  A quantitative assay may be performed using serial
    dilutions
No. of references: 19

NOTES

110017.0

*This kit is used for the detection of both HBeAg and anti-
  HBeAg. Details of the antigen detection are given in the
  appropriate section

© KLUWER ACADEMIC PUBLISHERS 1994, ISSN 1381-5067

Hepatitis B virus (e antigen)
ANTIBODY DETECTION*

Manufacturer: Behringwerke AG
Cat. No./Trade name: OUMG/Enzygnost® HBe

SUMMARY

$$\left.\begin{array}{c}\textbf{Ab} \\ \text{[Well-Ab]}\end{array}\right\rangle\text{[Ag]--[Ab-POD]--[TMB]--A}_{450}$$

Assay type: EIA (competitive)
Detection: Colorimetric A_{450}
Format: Microtitre well, Ab coated
Sample type: Serum, plasma
Sample pre-treatment:
    None
Sample volume: 100 µl (+50 µl neutralization reagent)
Number of tests: 96
Controls - standards run in assay:
    Controls: Neg (4), Pos (2)
Incubation:
    16-24 hr (RT) + 1 hr (37°C) + 30 min (RT)
Washes: 2

CONTENTS

Antibodies, antigens, labelled components:
    Anti-HBe Ab (h) bound to well
    HBeAg
    Anti-HBe Ab (h) POD conjugated
Substrate: TMB, H_2O_2
Controls - standards supplied:
    Controls: Neg and Pos (human serum)
Additional reagents:
    None
Special equipment required:
    Behring ELISA processor (optional)

INTERPRETATION

Comments on interpretation:
    Classification of samples is according to cut-off; no
    further testing
No. of references: 11

NOTES

110456.0

*The kit is used for the detection of both HBe Ag and anti-
    HBe. Details of antigen detection are given in the
    appropriate section

Hepatitis B virus (e antigen)
ANTIBODY DETECTION*

Manufacturer: Boehringer Mannheim
Cat. No./Trade name: 1335 995/Enzymun-Test® HBeAg
+ Anti-HBe

SUMMARY

$$\text{[Tube-strept]--[biotin-MAb]--[Ag]}\left(\begin{array}{c}\textbf{Ab} \\ \text{[MAb-POD]} \\ \text{[ABTS]--A}_{420}\end{array}\right. -$$

Assay type: EIA (competitive)
Detection: Colorimetric A_{420}
Format: Tube, streptavidin coated
Sample type: Serum, plasma
Sample pre-treatment:
    None
Sample volume: 100 µl
Number of tests: 145
Controls - standards run in assay:
    Controls: Neg (2), Pos (2)
Incubation:
    1 hr (RT) + 1 hr (RT) + 1 hr (RT)
Washes: 1

CONTENTS

Antibodies, antigens, labelled components:
    rec HBeAg
    Anti-HBe MAb (m) biotinylated
    Anti-HBe MAb (m) POD conjugated
Substrate: ABTS, H_2O_2
Controls - standards supplied:
    Controls: Neg (human serum), Pos (Ag)
Additional reagents:
    Substrate and streptavidin-coated tubes
Special equipment required:
    Automated Enzymun-Test Systems (optional)

INTERPRETATION

Comments on interpretation:
    Borderline: within cut-off ±10%; retest to confirm
No. of references: 0

NOTES

110467.0

*This kit is used for the detection of both HBe Ag and Anti-
    HBe. Details of the antigen detection are given in the
    appropriate section

© KLUWER ACADEMIC PUBLISHERS 1994, ISSN 1381-5067

Hepatitis B virus (e antigen)
ANTIBODY DETECTION

Manufacturer: IFCI Clone Systems
Cat. No./Trade name: 07.1005/EIAgen Anti-HBe Kit

SUMMARY

$$\left.\begin{array}{c}\textbf{Ab} \\ \text{[Well-MAb]}\end{array}\right\rangle\text{[Ag]--[Ab-HRP]--[TMB]--}A_{450}$$

Assay type: EIA (competitive)
Detection: Colorimetric A_{450}
Format: Microtitre well, Ab coated
Sample type: Serum, plasma (do not heat inactivate)
Sample pre-treatment:
　None
Sample volume: 100 µl
Number of tests: 96
Controls - standards run in assay:
　Controls: Neg (2), Pos (3)
Incubation:
　2 hr (40°C) + 1 hr (40°C) + 20 min (RT)
Washes: 2

CONTENTS

Antibodies, antigens, labelled components:
　Anti-HBe IgG MAb bound to well
　rec HBeAg
　Anti-HBe IgG Ab HRP conjugated
Substrate: TMB, H_2O_2
Controls - standards supplied:
　Controls: Neg and Pos (human serum)
Additional reagents:
　None
Special equipment required:
　None

INTERPRETATION

Comments on interpretation:
　Classification of sample is according to cut-off; no further
　　testing
No. of references: 8

NOTES

110090.0

Hepatitis B virus (e antigen)
ANTIBODY DETECTION*

Manufacturer: Melotec S.A.
Cat. No./Trade name: /MELOTEST HBeAg/Anti-HBe

SUMMARY

$$\left.\begin{array}{c}\textbf{Ab} \\ \text{[Well-MAb]}\end{array}\right\rangle\text{--[Ag]--[Ab-HRP]--[TMB]--}A_{450}$$

Assay type: EIA (competitive)
Detection: Colorimetric A_{450}
Format: Microtitre well, Ab coated
Sample type: Serum, plasma
Sample pre-treatment:
　None
Sample volume: 100 µl*
Number of tests: 96
Controls - standards run in assay:
　Controls: Neg (3), Pos (1)
Incubation:
　16 ± 4 h (RT) + 2 hr (37°C) + 30 min (RT)
Washes: 2

CONTENTS

Antibodies, antigens, labelled components:
　Anti-HBe MAb (m) bound to well
　HBeAg
　Anti-HBe Ab HRP conjugated
Substrate: TMB, H_2O_2
Controls - standards supplied:
　Controls: Neg, Pos (anti-HBe) and Pos (HBeAg)
Additional reagents:
　None
Special equipment required:
　None

INTERPRETATION

Comments on interpretation:
　Equivocal: within cut-off and cut-off + 10%; retest to
　　confirm
　Repeatably equivocal: test a fresh sample after 1–2
　　weeks
　Positive: ≤ cut-off repeatably and confirmed by
　　supplemental tests
No. of references: 5

NOTES

110641.0

*This kit is used for the detection of both HBeAg and anti-
　HBe. Details of antigen detection are given in the
　appropriate section
**It is recommended to run duplicates of samples for greater
　precision

© KLUWER ACADEMIC PUBLISHERS 1994, ISSN 1381-5067

Hepatitis B virus (e antigen)
ANTIBODY DETECTION*

Manufacturer: Organon Teknika NV
Cat. No./Trade name: 70170/Hepanostika® HBe Ag/ anti-HBe Microelisa system

SUMMARY

$$[\text{Well-Ab}] \Big\rangle^{\text{Ab}} [\text{Ag}]\text{—}[\text{Ab-HRP}]\text{—}[\text{TMB}]\text{—}A_{450}$$

Assay type: EIA (competitive)
Detection: Colorimetric A_{450}
Format: Microtitre well, Ab coated
Sample type: Serum, plasma
Sample pre-treatment:
None
Sample volume: 100 µl
Number of tests: 192
Controls - standards run in assay:
Controls: Neg (3), Pos anti-HBe (1)
Incubation:
16-20 hr (37°C) + 2 hr (37°C) + 2 hr (37°C) + 30 min (RT)
Washes: 2

CONTENTS

Antibodies, antigens, labelled components:
Anti-HBe Ab (h) bound to well
HBeAg (Pos control used in anti-HBe screening test)
Anti-HBe Ab (h) HRP conjugated
Substrate: TMB, H_2O_2
Controls - standards supplied:
Controls: Neg, Pos (HBe Ag), Pos (anti-HBe) (human serum)
Additional reagents:
H_2SO_4
Special equipment required:
None

INTERPRETATION

Comments on interpretation:
Positive: < cut-off
Possible positive for HBe Ag if value > 1.25; check with Hepanostika HBe Ag kit used as confirmatory test
Semi-quantitative procedure available
No. of references: None

NOTES

110557.0

*This kit is used for the detection of both HBe Ag and Ab.
Details of the Ag detection are in the appropriate section

Hepatitis B virus (e antigen)
ANTIBODY DETECTION*

Manufacturer: Radim
Cat. No./Trade name: KHB4IW/HBe Ag/Ab IEMA WELL

SUMMARY

$$[\text{Well-MAb}]\text{—}[\text{Ag}]\Big\langle^{\text{Ab}}_{[\text{MAb-HRP}]}\text{—}[\text{TMB}]\text{—}A_{450}$$

Assay type: EIA (competitive)
Detection: Colorimetric A_{450}
Format: Microtitre well, Ab coated
Sample type: Serum or plasma
Sample pre-treatment:
None
Sample volume: 50 µl
Number of tests: 96
Controls - standards run in assay:
Controls: Neg (4), Pos (2)
Incubation:
3 hr (37°C) + 20 min (37°C)
Washes: 1

CONTENTS

Antibodies, antigens, labelled components:
Anti-HBe MAb bound to well
rec HBeAg
Anti-HBe MAb HRP conjugated
Substrate: TMB, H_2O_2
Controls - standards supplied:
Controls: Neg and Pos (serum)
Additional reagents:
None
Special equipment required:
None

INTERPRETATION

Comments on interpretation:
Grey area: within cut-off value ± 10%; retest to confirm
Positive: < cut-off value repeatably
No. of references: 5

NOTES

110438.0

*The kit is used for detection of both HBeAg and anti-HBe.
Details of the antigen detection are given in the appropriate section

© KLUWER ACADEMIC PUBLISHERS 1994, ISSN 1381-5067

Hepatitis B virus (e antigen)
ANTIBODY DETECTION*

Manufacturer: Randox Laboratories Ltd
Cat. No./Trade name: HT 1488/HBe Ag/Anti-HBe Ag

SUMMARY

$$\left.{Ab \atop [Well\text{-}Ab]}\right\rangle [Ag]-[Ab\text{-}POD]-OPD-A_{492}$$

Assay type: EIA (competitive)
Detection: Colorimetric A_{492}
Format: Microtitre well, Ab coated
Sample type: Serum, plasma
Sample pre-treatment:
    None
Sample volume: 50 µl (+50 µl neutralizing solution)
Number of tests: 96
Controls - standards run in assay:
    Controls: Neg (3), Pos (2)
Incubation:
    20 hr (RT) + 1 hr (40°C) + 30 min (RT)
Washes: 2

CONTENTS

Antibodies, antigens, labelled components:
    Anti-HBe Ab bound to well
    HBeAg
    Anti-HBe Ab POD conjugated
Substrate: OPD, H_2O_2
Controls - standards supplied:
    Controls: Neg, Pos
Additional reagents:
    None
Special equipment required:
    None

INTERPRETATION

Comments on Interpretation:
    Classification of samples is according to cut-off; no
        further testing
No. of references: 3

NOTES

110510.0

*This test is for the detection of both HBe Ag and anti-HBe.
    Details of the antigen detection are given in the
    appropriate section

Hepatitis B virus (e antigen)
ANTIBODY DETECTION

Manufacturer: Roche Diagnostic Systems
Cat. No./Trade name: 07 3446 2/COBAS CORE Anti-HBe EIA

SUMMARY

$$[Bead\text{-}MAb]-[Ag]\left\langle{Ab \atop [Ab\text{-}HRP]}\right.-[TMB]-A_{450}$$

Assay type: EIA (competitive)
Detection: Colorimetric A_{450}
Format: Tube, Ab coated bead
Sample type: Serum (do not heat inactivate)
Sample pre-treatment:
    None
Sample volume: 50 µl
Number of tests: 50
Controls - standards run in assay:
    Controls: Neg (3), Pos (1)
Incubation:
    45 min (37°C) + 15 min (37°C) both with shaking
Washes: 1

CONTENTS

Antibodies, antigens, labelled components:
    Anti-HBe MAb (m) bound to beads
    rec HBeAg
    Anti-HBe F(Ab')₂ (h) HRP conjugated
Substrate: TMB, H_2O_2
Controls - standards supplied:
    Controls: Neg (human serum) and Pos (sheep anti-HBe
        in human serum)
Additional reagents:
    Substrate (supplied as separate kit)
Special equipment required:
    Cobas® EIA shaking incubator, tube washer and
        photometer (optional)
    Cobas® Core automated analyser (optional)

INTERPRETATION

Comments on Interpretation:
    Grey zone: within cut-off ±10%; retest unless this
        result expected from clinical course
    Positive: <cut-off -10% or <cut-off repeatably
No. of references: 4

NOTES

110406.0

Hepatitis B virus (e antigen)
ANTIBODY DETECTION

Manufacturer: Sanofi Diagnostics Pasteur
Cat. No./Trade name: 72212/MONOLISA® HBe

SUMMARY

$$\left.\begin{array}{c}\textbf{Ab}\\ \text{[Well-Ab]}\end{array}\right\rangle [Ag]\text{--}[MAb\text{-}POD]\text{--}[OPD]\text{--}A_{492/620}$$

Assay type: EIA (competitive)
Detection: Colorimetric $A_{492/620}$
Format: Microtitre well, Ab coated
Sample type: Serum, plasma
Sample pre-treatment:
  None
Sample volume: 100 µl (+50 µl neutralizing Ag)
Number of tests: 96
Controls - standards run in assay:
  Controls: Neg (3), Pos (1)
Incubation:
  Overnight (RT) + 30 min (40°C) + 30 min (RT)
Washes: 2 (+ preliminary plate wash)

CONTENTS

Antibodies, antigens, labelled components:
  Anti-HBe PAb (h) bound to well
  HBeAg
  Anti-HBe MAb_1 (m) and MAb_2 (m) POD conjugated
Substrate: OPD, H_2O_2
Controls - standards supplied:
  Controls: Neg (human serum) and Pos (human plasma)
Additional reagents:
  None
Special equipment required:
  None

INTERPRETATION

Comments on interpretation:
  Equivocal: inhibition of absorbance between 55 and 60%; retest to confirm
  Positive: inhibition >60%
No. of references: 7

NOTES

110496.0

Hepatitis B virus (e antigen)
ANTIBODY DETECTION*

Manufacturer: Schiapparelli Biosystems Inc
Cat. No./Trade name: 5770333/HEPATITIS B - HBeAg/HbeAb ELISA SYSTEM

SUMMARY

$$\left.\begin{array}{c}\textbf{Ab}\\ \text{[Well-MAb]}\end{array}\right\rangle [Ag]\text{--}[MAb\text{-}HRP]\text{--}[TMB]\text{--}A_{450}$$

Assay type: EIA (competitive)
Detection: Colorimetric A_{450}
Format: Microtitre well, Ab coated
Sample type: Serum (do not heat inactivate)
Sample pre-treatment:
  None
Sample volume: 100 µl x 2
Number of tests: 96
Controls - standards run in assay:
  Controls: Neg (2), Pos (3)
Incubation:
  2 hr (40°C) + 1 hr (40°C) + 20 min (RT)
Washes: 2

CONTENTS

Antibodies, antigens, labelled components:
  Anti-HBe MAb bound to well
  rec HBeAg
  Anti-HBe MAb HRP conjugated
Substrate: TMB, H_2O_2
Controls - standards supplied:
  Controls: Neg and Pos (human serum)
Additional reagents:
  None
Special equipment required:
  None

INTERPRETATION

Comments on interpretation:
  Classification of sample is according to cut-off; no further testing
No. of references: 9

NOTES

110428.0

*The kit is used for the detection of both HBeAg and anti-HBe. Details of the antigen detection are given in the appropriate section

© KLUWER ACADEMIC PUBLISHERS 1994, ISSN 1381-5067

Hepatitis B virus (e antigen)
ANTIBODY DETECTION

Manufacturer: Sorin Biomedica
Cat. No./Trade name: 2879/ETI-AB-EBK

SUMMARY

$$\left.\begin{array}{c}\text{Ab}\\ \text{[Well-MAb]}\end{array}\right\rangle \text{Ag--[MAb-HRP]--[TMB]--A}_{450}$$

Assay type: EIA (competitive)
Detection: Colorimetric A_{450}
Format: Microtitre well, Ab coated
Sample type: Serum, plasma
Sample pre-treatment:
    None
Sample volume: 10 µl (+ 150 µl neutralising solution)
Number of tests: 96
Controls - standards run in assay:
    Controls: Neg (3), Pos (2)
Incubation:
    2 hr (37°C) + 1 hr (37°C) + 30 min (RT)
Washes: 2

CONTENTS

Antibodies, antigens, labelled components:
    Anti-HBe IgG MAb (m) bound to well
    HBeAg
    Anti-HBe IgG MAb (m) HRP conjugated
Substrate: TMB, H_2O_2
Controls - standards supplied:
    Controls: Neg and Pos (human plasma)
Additional reagents:
    None
Special equipment required:
    None

INTERPRETATION

Comments on interpretation:
    Equivocal: Within cut-off ± 10%; retest to confirm
No. of references: 11

NOTES

110275.0

Hepatitis B virus (e antigen)
ANTIBODY DETECTION*

Manufacturer: Sorin Biomedica
Cat. No./Trade name: 2439/EBK eia

SUMMARY

$$\left.\begin{array}{c}\text{MAb}\\ \text{[Bead-MAb]}\end{array}\right\rangle \text{[Ag]--[Ab-HRP]--[OPD]--A}_{492}$$

Assay type: EIA (competitive)
Detection: Colorimetric A_{492}
Format: Tray/Tube, Ab coated bead
Sample type: Serum, plasma
Sample pre-treatment:
    None
Sample volume: 50 µl (+ 200 µl neutralising solution)
Number of tests: 100
Controls - standards run in assay:
    Controls: Neg (3), Pos (2)
Incubation:
    18-22 hr (RT) + 3 hr (RT) + 30 min (RT)
Washes: 2

CONTENTS

Antibodies, antigens, labelled components:
    Anti-HBe IgG MAb (m) bound to bead
    HBeAg (h)
    Anti-HBe IgG MAb (m) HRP conjugated
Substrate: OPD; H_2O_2
Controls - standards supplied:
    Controls: Neg and Pos for both HBeAg and anti-HBeAg
        (human)
Additional reagents:
    None
Special equipment required:
    Automatic rinsing device, PLA-2 (optional)
    Bead dispenser, MEDI-578 (optional)

INTERPRETATION

Comments on interpretation:
    Equivocal: Within cut-off ± 10%; retest to confirm
    Positive: ≤ cut-off repeatably
No. of references: 11

NOTES

110279.0

*This kit measures both HBeAg and anti-HBe. Details of the
    HBeAg detection are given in the appropriate section
This kit will be discontinued in December 1994

© KLUWER ACADEMIC PUBLISHERS 1994, ISSN 1381-5067

Hepatitis B virus (e antigen)
ANTIBODY DETECTION

Manufacturer: Syva Company
Cat. No./Trade name: 8HE39UL/MicroTrak® II Anti-HBe EIA

SUMMARY

$$[\text{Well-MAb}]\genfrac{}{}{0pt}{}{\text{Ab}}{}\Big)[\text{Ag}]-[\text{MAb-HRP}]-[\text{TMB}]-A_{450/630}$$

Assay type: EIA (competitive)
Detection: Colorimetric $A_{450/630}$
Format: Microtitre well, Ab coated
Sample type: Serum, plasma
Sample pre-treatment:
   None
Sample volume: 10 µl
Number of tests: 96
Controls - standards run in assay:
   Controls: Neg (3), Pos (2)
Incubation:
   2 hr (37°C) + 1 hr (37°C) + 30 min (37°C)
Washes: 2

CONTENTS

Antibodies, antigens, labelled components:
   Anti-HBe MAb (g) bound to well
   rec HBeAg
   Anti-HBe IgG MAb HRP conjugated
Substrate: TMB, H_2O_2
Controls - standards supplied:
   Controls: Neg and Pos (human plasma)
Additional reagents:
   MicroTrak® II EIA universal reagents (8K209UL)
Special equipment required:
   Syva MicroTrak® EIA autowasher and autoreader

INTERPRETATION

Comments on interpretation:
   Equivocal: absorbance values within 15% of the cut-off;
   retest to confirm
No. of references: 13

NOTES

110069.0

Hepatitis B virus (e antigen)
ANTIBODY DETECTION

Manufacturer: VEDA-LAB
Cat. No./Trade name: 1561/HBe Ab EIA

SUMMARY

$$[\text{Well-Ab}]-[\text{Ag}]\genfrac{}{}{0pt}{}{\text{Ab}}{[\text{Ab-HRP}]}-[\text{TMB}]-A_{450}$$

Assay type: EIA (competitive)
Detection: Colorimetric A_{450}
Format: Microtitre well, Ab coated
Sample type: Serum, plasma
Sample pre-treatment:
   None
Sample volume: 50 µl
Number of tests: 96
Controls - standards run in assay:
   Controls: Neg (1), Pos (1)
Incubation:
   1 hr (37°C) + 15 min (RT)
Washes: 1

CONTENTS

Antibodies, antigens, labelled components:
   Anti-HBe PAb bound to well
   HBeAg (neutralizing reagent)
   Anti-HBe Ab HRP conjugated
Substrate: TMB, H_2O_2
Controls - standards supplied:
   Controls: Neg and Pos
Additional reagents:
   None
Special equipment required:
   None

INTERPRETATION

Comments on interpretation:
   Equivocal: within cut-off $\pm$ 10%; retest to confirm
No. of references: 4

NOTES

110395.0

© *KLUWER ACADEMIC PUBLISHERS 1994, ISSN 1381-5067*

Hepatitis B virus (e antigen)
ANTIBODY DETECTION*

Manufacturer: Radim
Cat. No./Trade name: KHB4CT/HBe Ag/Ab IRMA CT

SUMMARY

$$[\text{Tube-MAb}]\text{--}[\text{Ag}]\Big\langle\begin{array}{l}\textbf{Ab}\\ [\text{MAb-}^{125}\text{I}]\end{array}\text{--radioactivity}$$

Assay type: RIA (competitive)
Detection: Radioisotopic
Format: Tube, Ab coated
Sample type: Serum or plasma
Sample pre-treatment:
   None
Sample volume: 100 µl
Number of tests: 100
Controls - standards run in assay:
   Controls: Neg (4), Pos (2)
Incubation:
   a) 2 hr (45°C)
   b) 18-22 hr (RT)
Washes: 1

CONTENTS

Antibodies, antigens, labelled components:
   Anti-HBe MAb (r) bound to tube
   rec HBeAg
   Anti-HBe MAb ^{125}I labelled
Substrate:
Controls - standards supplied:
   Controls: Neg and Pos (human serum)
Additional reagents:
   None
Special equipment required:
   None

INTERPRETATION

Comments on interpretation:
   Grey area: within cut-off value ± 10%; retest to confirm
   Positive: < cut-off value repeatably
No. of references: 7

NOTES

110440.0

*The kit is used for detection of both HBeAg and anti-HBe.
   Details of the antigen detection are given in the
   appropriate section

Hepatitis B virus (e antigen)
ANTIBODY DETECTION*

Manufacturer: Sorin Biomedica
Cat. No./Trade name: 2502/EBK

SUMMARY

$$\begin{array}{l}\textbf{Ab}\\ [\text{Bead-MAb}]\end{array}\Big\rangle[\text{Ag}]\text{--}[\text{MAb-}^{125}\text{I}]\text{--radioactivity}$$

Assay type: RIA (competitive)
Detection: Radioisotopic
Format: Tray/Tube, Ab coated bead
Sample type: Serum, plasma
Sample pre-treatment:
   None
Sample volume: 100 µl
Number of tests: 100
Controls - standards run in assay:
   Controls: Neg (3), Pos (3)
Incubation:
   18-22 hr (RT) + 3 hr (45°C)
Washes: 2

CONTENTS

Antibodies, antigens, labelled components:
   Anti-HBe IgG MAb (m) bound to beads
   rec HBeAg
   Anti-HBe IgG MAb (m) ^{125}I labelled
Substrate:
Controls - standards supplied:
   Controls: Neg and Pos
Additional reagents:
   None
Special equipment required:
   Automated rinser, PLA-2 (optional)
   Bead dispenser, MEDI-578 (optional)

INTERPRETATION

Comments on interpretation:
   Equivocal: Within cut-off ± 10%; retest to confirm
   Positive: ≤ cut-off repeatably
No. of references: 11

NOTES

110274.0

*The kit is used for the detection of both HBeAg and Anti-
   HBe. Details of the antigen detection are given in the
   appropriate section

Hepatitis B virus (surface antigen)
ANTIGEN DETECTION

Manufacturer: Abbott Laboratories
Cat. No./Trade name: 1980/AUSZYME®
MONOCLONAL

SUMMARY

[Bead-MAb]–**Ag**–[MAb-HRP]–[OPD]–A$_{492}$

Assay type: EIA (non-competitive)
Detection: Colorimetric A$_{492}$
Format: Reaction well, Ag coated bead
Sample type: Serum, plasma (do not heat inactivate)
Sample pre-treatment:
   None
Sample volume: 200 µl
Number of tests: 100, 1000
Controls - standards run in assay:
   Controls: Neg (3), Pos (2)
Incubation:
   a) 3 hr (40°C) + 30 min (RT)*
   b) 16 hr (RT) + 30 min (RT)
   c) 1 hr 15 min (40°C) + 30 min (RT)
Washes: 1*

CONTENTS

Antibodies, antigens, labelled components:
   Anti-HBs MAb (m) bound to beads
   Anti-HBs MAb (m) HRP conjugated
Substrate: OPD, H$_2$O$_2$
Controls - standards supplied:
   Controls: Neg and Pos (human plasma)
Additional reagents:
   H$_2$SO$_4$
Special equipment required:
   None

INTERPRETATION

Comments on interpretation:
   Positive: ⩾ cut-off repeatably and confirmed by
   neutralization test (eg. ABBOTT HBsAg Confirmatory
   Assay)
No. of references: 20

NOTES

110027.0

*Alternative procedure available for samples containing
   sodium azide

Hepatitis B virus (surface antigen)
ANTIGEN DETECTION

Manufacturer: Abbott Laboratories
Cat. No./Trade name: 2228-66/IMx® HBsAg

SUMMARY

[Particle-MAb]–**Ag**–[Ab-biotin + anti-biotin-AP]–
[4-MP]–fluorescence

Assay type: EIA (non-competitive)
Detection: Fluorometric
Format: Reaction well, Ab coated microparticle
Sample type: Serum, plasma
Sample pre-treatment:
   None
Sample volume: 150 µl
Number of tests: 100
Controls - standards run in assay:
   Calibration assay: calibrators (1) x 2, Controls: Neg (1),
   Pos (1)
   Mode 1 assay: calibrators (1), Controls: Pos (1)*
Incubation:
   Automated
Washes: Automated

CONTENTS

Antibodies, antigens, labelled components:
   Anti-HBs MAb (m) bound to microparticle
   Anti-HBs Ab (g) biotinylated
   Anti-biotin (r) AP conjugated
Substrate: 4-MP
Controls - standards supplied:
   Calibrators: mode 1 calibrator (human plasma)
Additional reagents:
   IMx® HBs Ag controls, IMx® MEIA diluent buffer, IMx®
   probe cleaning solution
Special equipment required:
   IMx system

INTERPRETATION

Comments on interpretation:
   Sample reactivity is calculated automatically
   Positive: ⩾ cut-off repeatably and confirmed by
   supplemental testing with IMx® HBs Ag Confirmatory
   Test
No. of references: 14

NOTES

110076.0

*Minimum control requirement for mode 1 assay: one
   positive control assayed once per 8 hr shift

Hepatitis B virus (surface antigen)
ANTIGEN DETECTION

Manufacturer: ADI Diagnostics
Cat. No./Trade name: Heprofile® HBsAg

SUMMARY

[Well-Ab]–**Ag**–[Ab-POD]–[TMB]–A$_{450}$

Assay type: EIA (non-competitive)
Detection: Colorimetric A$_{450}$
Format: Microtitre well, Ab coated
Sample type: Serum, plasma
Sample pre-treatment:
  None
Sample volume: 200 µl
Number of tests: 96
Controls - standards run in assay:
  Controls: Neg (3), Pos (2)
Incubation:
  a) 12-20 hr (RT) + 2 hr (RT) + 30 min (RT)
  b) 3 hr (37°C) + 1 hr (37°C) + 30 min (RT)
  c) 30 min (37°C) + 30 min (37°C) + 30 min (RT)
Washes: 2

CONTENTS

Antibodies, antigens, labelled components:
  Anti-HBs Ab bound to well
  Anti-HBs Ab (chimp) POD conjugated
Substrate: TMB, H$_2$O$_2$
Controls - standards supplied:
  Controls: Neg and Pos (human plasma)
Additional reagents:
  None
Special equipment required:
  None

INTERPRETATION

Comments on interpretation:
  Positive: ≥cut-off repeatably
No. of references: 6

NOTES

110669.0

Hepatitis B virus (surface antigen)
ANTIGEN DETECTION

Manufacturer: Behringwerke AG
Cat. No./Trade name: OWND/Enzygnost® HBs Ag monoclonal

SUMMARY

[Well-Ab]–**Ag**–[MAb-POD]–[TMB]–A$_{450}$

Assay type: EIA (non-competitive)
Detection: Colorimetric A$_{450}$
Format: Microtitre well, Ab coated
Sample type: Serum, plasma
Sample pre-treatment:
  None
Sample volume: 100 µl
Number of tests: 192, 960
Controls - standards run in assay:
  Controls: Neg (4), Pos (2)
Incubation:
  1 hr 30 min (37°C) + 30 min (RT)
Washes: 1

CONTENTS

Antibodies, antigens, labelled components:
  Anti-HBs PAb (sh) bound to well
  Anti-HBs MAb (m) POD conjugated
Substrate: TMB, H$_2$O$_2$
Controls - standards supplied:
  Controls: Neg and Pos (human serum)
Additional reagents:
  None
Special equipment required:
  Behring ELISA processor (optional)

INTERPRETATION

Comments on interpretation:
  Positive: ≥cut-off repeatably and confirmed by
    supplemental tests*
No. of references: 0

NOTES

110126.0

*Enzygnost HBs Ag confirmatory test available

Hepatitis B virus (surface antigen)
ANTIGEN DETECTION

Manufacturer: BIOKIT SA
Cat. No./Trade name: /Bioelisa HBs Ag

SUMMARY

[Well-Ab]–**Ag**–[Ab-POD]–[TMB]–$A_{450/620}$

Assay type: EIA (non-competitive)
Detection: Colorimetric $A_{450/620}$
Format: Microtitre well, Ab coated
Sample type: Serum, plasma
Sample pre-treatment:
    None
Sample volume: 100 μl
Number of tests: 96, 480
Controls - standards run in assay:
    Controls:
    Neg (3), Pos (1) (1-6 strips of wells)
    Neg (4), Pos (1) (7-9 strips of wells)
    Neg (5), Pos (1) (10-12 strips of wells)
Incubation:
    a) 1 hr (40°C) + 30 min (40°C) + 30 min (RT)
    b) 16-24 hr (RT) + 30 m in (40°C) + 30 min (RT)
    c) 20 min (40°C) + 20 min (40°C) + 10 min (RT)*
Washes: 2

CONTENTS

Antibodies, antigens, labelled components:
    Anti-HBs Ab (gp) bound to well
    Anti-HBs Ab (g) POD conjugated
Substrate: TMB
Controls - standards supplied:
    Controls: Neg and Pos (human serum)
Additional reagents:
    H_2SO_4 (for 5 plate kits)
Special equipment required:
    None

INTERPRETATION

Comments on interpretation:
    Positive: ≥cut-off repeatably and confirmed by a similar
    assay or by Bioelisa HBs Ag confirmatory assay (Cat.
    no. 3000-1090)
No. of references: 9

NOTES

110583.0

Method (a) is the standard incubation. Incubation at 37°C is
    also suitable

Hepatitis B virus (surface antigen)
ANTIGEN DETECTION

Manufacturer: bioMerieux
Cat. No./Trade name: 30300/VIDAS HBs Ag (HBS)

SUMMARY

[Solid phase-MAb]–**Ag**–[MAb-biotin]–[strept-AP]–
[4-MP]–fluorescence

Assay type: EIA (non-competitive)
Detection: Fluorometric
Format: Solid phase receptacle (SPR), Ab coated reagent
strip
Sample type: Serum, plasma
Sample pre-treatment:
    None
Sample volume: 150 μl
Number of tests: 60
Controls - standards run in assay:
    Controls: Neg (1), Pos (1)
    Standard: (1)*
Incubation:
    Automated - total time 1 hr
Washes: Automated

CONTENTS

Antibodies, antigens, labelled components:
    Anti-HBs MAb (m) bound to solid phase
    Anti-HBs MAb (m) biotinylated
    Streptavidin AP conjugated
Substrate: 4-MP
Controls - standards supplied:
    Controls: Neg and Pos
    Standard: Pos (human serum and rec Ag)
Additional reagents:
    None
Special equipment required:
    Vitek Immunodiagnostic assay system (VIDAS)

INTERPRETATION

Comments on interpretation:
    Sample reactivity is calculated automatically and
    classification is according to cut-off
    Positive: retest after centrifuging specimen and confirm
    in VIDAS HBs Ag Confirmation test
No. of references: 4

NOTES

110472.0

*Recalibrate with each new lot of reagents and every 14
days

Hepatitis B virus (surface antigen)
ANTIGEN DETECTION

Manufacturer: Biotest Diagnostics
Cat. No./Trade name: /BIOTEST HBs Ag ELISA

SUMMARY

[Well-MAb]–**Ag**–[Ab-HRP]–[TMB]–A$_{450}$

Assay type: EIA (non-competitive)
Detection: Colorimetric A$_{450}$
Format: Microtitre well, Ab coated
Sample type: Serum, plasma
Sample pre-treatment:
　None
Sample volume: 100 µl
Number of tests: 192
Controls - standards run in assay:
　Controls: Neg (2), low Pos (3), Pos (2)
Incubation:
　a) 1 hr (37°C) + 1 hr (37°C) + 30 min (RT)
　b) 18-22 hr (RT) + 1 hr (37°C) + 30 min (RT)
　c) 30 min (37°C) + 30 min (37°C) + 30 min (RT)
Washes: 2

CONTENTS

Antibodies, antigens, labelled components:
　Anti-HBs IgG MAb (m) bound to well
　Anti-HBs IgG Ab (sh) HRP conjugated
Substrate: TMB, H$_2$O$_2$
Controls - standards supplied:
　Controls: Neg, low Pos and Pos (human plasma)
Additional reagents:
　None
Special equipment required:
　None

INTERPRETATION

Comments on interpretation:
　Grey area: within cut-off ±12%; retest to confirm
　Confirm results obtained by procedure (c) with procedure
　　(a) or (b)
　Visual interpretation is possible
No. of references: 10

NOTES

110175.0

Hepatitis B virus (surface antigen)
ANTIGEN DETECTION

Manufacturer: Boehringer Mannheim
Cat. No./Trade name: 1288 989/Enzymun-Test® HBsAg

SUMMARY

[Tube-strept]–[MAb-biotin]–**Ag**–[MAb-POD]–[ABTS]–
A$_{420}$

Assay type: EIA (non-competitive)
Detection: Colorimetric A$_{420}$
Format: Tube, streptavidin coated
Sample type: Serum, plasma
Sample pre-treatment:
　None
Sample volume: 200 µl
Number of tests: 125
Controls - standards run in assay:
　Controls: Neg (2), Pos (2)
Incubation:
　5 hr (RT) + 1 hr (RT)*
Washes: 1 (+tube pre-wash)

CONTENTS

Antibodies, antigens, labelled components:
　Anti-HBs MAb (m) POD conjugated
　Anti-HBs MAb (m) biotinylated
Substrate: ABTS, H$_2$O$_2$
Controls - standards supplied:
　Controls: Neg (human serum), Pos (Ag in bovine serum)
Additional reagents:
　Streptavidin-coated tubes
　Substrate (for certain Enzymun-Test Systems)
Special equipment required:
　Automated Enzymun-Test Systems (optional)

INTERPRETATION

Comments on interpretation:
　Positive: ≥cut-off and confirmed by a supplemental test
　　(Enzymun-Test® HBsAg Confirmatory Test)
No. of references: 0

NOTES

110462.0

*Time and temperature of incubations varies with Test
　system used

Hepatitis B virus (surface antigen)
ANTIGEN DETECTION

Manufacturer: Genetic Systems Corporation/Sanofi Diagnostics Pasteur
Cat. No./Trade name: 0254-02/GENETIC SYSTEMS® HBsAg EIA

SUMMARY

[Well-MAb]–**Ag**–[MAb-HRP]–[TMB]–A_{450}

Assay type: EIA (non-competitive)
Detection: Colorimetric A_{450}
Format: Microtitre well, Ab coated
Sample type: Serum, plasma
Sample pre-treatment:
  None
Sample volume: 200 µl
Number of tests: 192, 960, 4800
Controls - standards run in assay:
  Controls: Neg (3), Pos (2)
Incubation:
  1 hr (37°C) + 1 hr (37°C) + 30 min (RT)
Washes: 2

CONTENTS

Antibodies, antigens, labelled components:
  Anti-HBs MAb (m) bound to wells
  Anti-HBs MAb (m) HRP conjugated
Substrate: TMB, H_2O_2
Controls - standards supplied:
  Controls: Neg and Pos (human serum)
Additional reagents:
  None
Special equipment required:
  None

INTERPRETATION

Comments on interpretation:
  Positive: ⩾ cut-off repeatably and confirmed by a
    neutralization test, e.g. Genetic Systems HBsAg
    Confirmatory Assay
No. of references: 9

NOTES

110018.0

Hepatitis B virus (surface antigen)
ANTIGEN DETECTION

Manufacturer: Human GmbH
Cat. No./Trade name: 51 048/HBsAg HUMAN ELISA Test

SUMMARY

[Well-MAb]–**Ag**–[Ab-HRP]–[TMB]–A_{450}

Assay type: EIA (non-competitive)
Detection: Colorimetric A_{450}
Format: Microtitre well, Ab coated
Sample type: Serum, plasma (do not heat inactivate)
Sample pre-treatment:
  None
Sample volume: 100 µl
Number of tests: 96
Controls - standards run in assay:
  Controls: Neg (3), Pos (2)
Incubation:
  1 hr (37°C) + 30 min (37°C) + 30 min (RT)
Washes: 2

CONTENTS

Antibodies, antigens, labelled components:
  Anti-HBs MAb bound to well
  Anti-HBs Ab HRP conjugated
Substrate: TMB
Controls - standards supplied:
  Controls: Neg and Pos (human serum)
Additional reagents:
  None
Special equipment required:
  None

INTERPRETATION

Comments on interpretation:
  Equivocal: within cut-off and cut-off x 0.9; retest to
    confirm
  Repeatably equivocal: retest using a confirmatory test
  Positive: ⩾ cut-off and confirmed by supplemental tests
No. of references: None

NOTES

110658.0

© **KLUWER ACADEMIC PUBLISHERS** 1994, ISSN 1381-5067

Hepatitis B virus (surface antigen)
ANTIGEN DETECTION

Manufacturer: Labsystems Oy
Cat. No./Trade name: 61 10 800/HBs Ag EIA Plus

SUMMARY

[Well-MAb]–**Ag**–[MAb-HRP]–[TMB]–A_{450}

Assay type: EIA (non-competitive)
Detection: Colorimetric A_{450}
Format: Microtitre well, Ab coated
Sample type: Serum, plasma (do not heat inactivate)
Sample pre-treatment:
　　None
Sample volume: 100 µl
Number of tests: 96, 480
Controls - standards run in assay:
　　Controls: Neg (3), Pos (2)
Incubation:
　　a) 2 hr (37°C) with shaking + 30 min (RT)
　　b) 16-22 hr (RT) + 30 min (RT)
Washes: 1

CONTENTS

Antibodies, antigens, labelled components:
　　Anti-HBs MAb (m) bound to well
　　Anti-HBs PAb (sh) and MAb (m) HRP conjugated
Substrate: TMB, H_2O_2
Controls - standards supplied:
　　Controls: Neg (foetal bovine serum), Pos (rec Ag)
Additional reagents:
　　H_2SO_4
Special equipment required:
　　Auto-EIA II Analyzer (optional)

INTERPRETATION

Comments on interpretation:
　　Positive: ≥ cut-off repeatably and must be confirmed by a
　　neutralization assay (e.g. LABSYSTEM HBs Ag
　　Confirmatory Test - Cat. no. 61 06 070)
No. of references: 7

NOTES

110534.0

Hepatitis B virus (surface antigen)
ANTIGEN DETECTION

Manufacturer: Melotec S.A.
Cat. No./Trade name: MHBS/MELOTEST HBsAg

SUMMARY

[Well-MAb]–**Ag**–[MAb-HRP]–[TMB]–A_{450}

Assay type: EIA (non-competitive)
Detection: Colorimetric A_{450}
Format: Microtitre well, Ab coated
Sample type: Serum, plasma
Sample pre-treatment:
　　None
Sample volume: 50 µl x 2*
Number of tests: 96
Controls - standards run in assay:
　　Controls: Neg (3), Pos (1)
Incubation:
　　a) 30 min (45°C) + 15 min (45°C) + 30 min (RT)
　　b) 40 min (37°C) + 20 min (37°C) + 30 min (RT)
Washes: 2

CONTENTS

Antibodies, antigens, labelled components:
　　Anti-HBs MAb bound to well
　　Anti-HBs MAb HRP conjugated
Substrate: TMB, H_2O_2
Controls - standards supplied:
　　Controls: Neg and Pos
Additional reagents:
　　None
Special equipment required:
　　None

INTERPRETATION

Comments on interpretation:
　　Equivocal: within cut-off and cut-off-10%; retest to
　　confirm
　　Repeatably equivocal: retest a fresh sample in 1-2 weeks
　　Positive: ≥ cut-off repeatably and confirmed by
　　supplemental neutralization tests
No. of references: 10

NOTES

110072.0

*It is recommended to run duplicate of sample for greater
　precision

Hepatitis B virus (surface antigen)
ANTIGEN DETECTION

Manufacturer: Melotec S.A.
Cat. No./Trade name: /MELOTEST HBsAg

SUMMARY

[Well-MAb]–**Ag**–[MAb-HRP]–[TMB]–A_{450}

Assay type: EIA (non-competitive)
Detection: Colorimetric A_{450}
Format: Microtitre well, Ab coated
Sample type: Serum, plasma
Sample pre-treatment:
  None
Sample volume: 50 µl
Number of tests: 96
Controls - standards run in assay:
  Controls: Neg (3), Pos (1)
Incubation:
  a) 30 min (45°C) + 15 min (45°C) + 30 min (RT)
  b) 40 min (37°C) + 20 min (37°C) + 30 min (RT)
Washes: 1

CONTENTS

Antibodies, antigens, labelled components:
  Anti-HBs MAb bound to well
  Anti-HBs MAb HRP conjugated
Substrate: TMB, H_2O_2
Controls - standards supplied:
  Controls: Neg and Pos
Additional reagents:
  None
Special equipment required:
  None

INTERPRETATION

Comments on interpretation:
  Equivocal: within cut-off and cut-off–10%; retest to
    confirm
  Repeatably equivocal: retest a fresh sample in 1–2
    weeks
  Positive: ≥cut-off repeatably and confirmed by a
    neutralization test
No. of references: 10

NOTES

110636.0

Hepatitis B virus (surface antigen)
ANTIGEN DETECTION

Manufacturer: Mitsui Pharmaceuticals Inc
Cat. No./Trade name: MP-5000/HBs Ag- MP MITSUI

SUMMARY

[Particle-PAb]–**Ag**–[PAb-HRP]–[TMB]–A_{450}

Assay type: EIA (non-competitive)
Detection: Colorimetric A_{450}
Format: Tube, Ab coated particle
Sample type: Serum
Sample pre-treatment:
  None
Sample volume: 80 µl
Number of tests: 100
Controls - standards run in assay:
  Controls: Neg (1), Pos (1), Calibrators (2)
Incubation:
  5 min (37°C) + 5 min (37°C) + 5 min (37°C)
Washes: 2

CONTENTS

Antibodies, antigens, labelled components:
  Anti-HBs PAb (r) bound to particles
  Anti-HBs PAb (r) HRP conjugated
Substrate: TMB
Controls - standards supplied:
  None
Additional reagents:
  Quality controls bought separately: H_2SO_4, cell
    detergent, concentrated buffer
Special equipment required:
  MITSUI QUARTUS Fully Automated EIAsystem

INTERPRETATION

Comments on interpretation:
  Not specified
No. of references: 4

NOTES

110600.0

© **KLUWER ACADEMIC PUBLISHERS 1994, ISSN 1381-5067**

Hepatitis B virus (surface antigen)
ANTIGEN DETECTION

Manufacturer: Murex Diagnostics Limited
Cat. No./Trade name: VK20/21/Wellcozyme HBsAg

SUMMARY

[Well-MAb]–**Ag**–[MAb-AP]–[NADP+ampl]–A_{492}

Assay type: EIA (non-competitive, amplified)
Detection: Colorimetric A_{492}
Format: Microtitre well, Ab coated
Sample type: Serum, plasma*
Sample pre-treatment:
　None
Sample volume: 150 μl
Number of tests: 96, 480
Controls - standards run in assay:
　Controls: Neg (4), Pos (2)
Incubation:
　4-20 hr** (RT) + 40 min (RT) + 10 min (RT)
Washes: 1

CONTENTS

Antibodies, antigens, labelled components:
　Anti-HBs MAb (m) bound to well
　Anti-HBs MAb (m) AP conjugated
Substrate: NADP + amplifier
Controls - standards supplied:
　Controls: Neg and Pos (human serum)
Additional reagents:
　H_2SO_4
Special equipment required:
　Wellcozyme microwell plate washing system (optional)
　Wellcozyme microwell plate reader system (optional)

INTERPRETATION

Comments on interpretation:
　Positive: ≥cut-off repeatably and confirmed using
　　Wellcozyme HBsAg confirmatory kit (VK25)
　Visual interpretation is possible
No. of references: 6

NOTES

110323.0

*Plasma samples collected in EDTA or sodium citrate may
　be tested
**Overnight incubation at RT leads to a more sensitive assay
Alternative incubation times and temperatures are available
　for serum and plasma

Hepatitis B virus (surface antigen)
ANTIGEN DETECTION

Manufacturer: Murex Diagnostics Limited
Cat. No./Trade name: GE14/15/16/Murex HBsAg

SUMMARY

[Well-Ab]–**Ag**–[MAb-HRP]–[TMB]–A_{450}

Assay type: EIA (non-competitive)
Detection: Colorimetric A_{450}
Format: Microtitre well, Ab coated
Sample type: Serum, plasma
Sample pre-treatment:
　None
Sample volume: 75 μl (+25 μl diluent)
Number of tests: 96, 480, 2400
Controls - standards run in assay:
　Controls: Neg (3), Pos (1)
Incubation:
　a)1 hr 30 min (37°C) + 30 min (37°C)
　b)10-18 hr (RT) + 60 min (37°C)
Washes: 1

CONTENTS

Antibodies, antigens, labelled components:
　Anti-HBs PAb (g) bound to well
　Anti-HBs MAb (m) HRP conjugated
Substrate: TMB, H_2O_2
Controls - standards supplied:
　Controls: Neg and Pos (human serum)
Additional reagents:
　H_2SO_4
Special equipment required:
　Wellcozyme microwell plate washing system (optional)
　Wellcozyme microwell plate reader (optional)

INTERPRETATION

Comments on interpretation:
　Positive: ≥cut-off repeatably and confirmed by Murex
　　HBsAg Confirmatory Kit (GE17)
No. of references: 2

NOTES

110664.0

Hepatitis B virus (surface antigen)
ANTIGEN DETECTION

Manufacturer: Omega Diagnostics Ltd
Cat. No./Trade name: OD 037/Hepatitis B Surface Antigen EIA

SUMMARY

[Well-MAb]–**Ag**–[MAb-HRP]–[TMB]–A$_{450}$

Assay type: EIA (non-competitive)
Detection: Colorimetric A$_{450}$
Format: Microtitre well, Ab coated
Sample type: Serum, plasma
Sample pre-treatment:
   None
Sample volume: 50 µl
Number of tests: 192
Controls - standards run in assay:
   Controls: Neg (3), Pos (1)
Incubation:
   Rapid assay: 40 min (37°C) + 20 min (37°C) + 30 min (37°C)*
   Slow assay: 2 hr 30 min (37°C) + 1 hr 30 min (37°C) + 30 min (37°C)
Washes: 2

CONTENTS

Antibodies, antigens, labelled components:
   Anti-HBs MAb bound to well
   Anti-HBs MAb HRP conjugated
Substrate: TMB
Controls - standards supplied:
   Controls: Neg and Pos
Additional reagents:
   None
Special equipment required:
   None

INTERPRETATION

Comments on interpretation:
   Positive: ⩾ cut-off repeatably and confirmed by further neutralisation test
   Equivocal: within cut-off – 10% and cut-off; retest and if consistently equivocal repeat with fresh sample in 1-2 weeks
No. of references: 10

NOTES

110617.0

*Rapid and slow assays offer different sensitivity. Use of different incubation temperature of 45°C reduces total test time but does not affect sensitivity

Hepatitis B virus (surface antigen)
ANTIGEN DETECTION

Manufacturer: Organon Teknika NV
Cat. No./Trade name: 80251/Hepanostika® HBs Ag Uni-Form II

SUMMARY

[Well-MAb]–**Ag**–[Ab-HRP]–[TMB]–A$_{450}$

Assay type: EIA (non-competitive)
Detection: Colorimetric A$_{450}$
Format: Microtitre well, Ab coated
Sample type: Serum, plasma
Sample pre-treatment:
   None
Sample volume: 100 µl
Number of tests: 192, 576
Controls - standards run in assay:
   Controls:
   Neg (2), Pos (1) (for one strip)
   Neg (3), Pos (1) (for two or more strips)
Incubation:
   1 hr (37°C) + 30 min (RT)
Washes: 1

CONTENTS

Antibodies, antigens, labelled components:
   Anti-HBs MAb (m) bound to well
   Anti-HBs Ab (sh) HRP conjugated
Substrate: TMB, H$_2$O$_2$
Controls - standards supplied:
   Controls: Neg and Pos (human serum)
Additional reagents:
   H$_2$SO$_4$
Special equipment required:
   None

INTERPRETATION

Comments on interpretation:
   Positive: ⩾ cut-off repeatably and confirmed by a neutralization test
No. of references: 5

NOTES

110549.0

Hepatitis B virus (surface antigen)
ANTIGEN DETECTION

Manufacturer: Organon Teknika NV
Cat. No./Trade name: 6029/Hepanostika® HBs Ag

SUMMARY

[Well-MAb]–**Ag**–[Ab-HRP]–[OPD]–A_{492}

Assay type: EIA (non-competitive)
Detection: Colorimetric A_{492}
Format: Microtitre well, Ab coated
Sample type: Serum, plasma
Sample pre-treatment:
  None
Sample volume:
Number of tests: 192, 576
Controls - standards run in assay:
  Controls:
  Neg (1), Pos (1) (one strip)
  Neg (2), Pos (2) (two or more strips)
Incubation:
  a) 1 hr (37°C) + 1 hr (37°C) + 30 min (RT)
  b) 30 min (50°C) + 30 min (50°C) + 30 min (RT)
Washes: 2

CONTENTS

Antibodies, antigens, labelled components:
  Anti-HBs MAb bound to well
  Anti-HBs Ab (sh) HRP conjugated
Substrate: OPD
Controls - standards supplied:
  Controls: Neg and Pos
Additional reagents:
  H_2SO_4
Special equipment required:
  None

INTERPRETATION

Comments on interpretation:
  Positive: ≥cut-off repeatably and confirmed by
    supplemental tests
  Visual interpretation is possible
No. of references: 0

NOTES

110561.0

This kit will be discontinued in 1995

Hepatitis B virus (surface antigen)
ANTIGEN DETECTION

Manufacturer: Radim
Cat. No./Trade name: KHB1IWT/HBsAg IEMA WELL

SUMMARY

[Well-MAb]–**Ag**–[MAb-HRP]–[TMB]–A_{450}

Assay type: EIA (non-competitive)
Detection: Colorimetric A_{450}
Format: Microtitre well, Ab coated
Sample type: Serum or plasma
Sample pre-treatment:
  None
Sample volume: 100 µl
Number of tests: 96, 192
Controls - standards run in assay:
  Controls: Neg (4), Pos (2)
Incubation:
  a)3 hr (37°C) or b) 1 hr 30 min (37°C) + 20 min (37°C)
Washes: 1

CONTENTS

Antibodies, antigens, labelled components:
  Anti-HBs MAb (r) bound to well
  Anti-HBs MAb HRP conjugated
Substrate: TMB, H_2O_2
Controls - standards supplied:
  Controls: Neg (serum, Pos (HBsAg)
Additional reagents:
  None
Special equipment required:
  None

INTERPRETATION

Comments on interpretation:
  Grey area: within cut-off value ±10%; retest to confirm
  Positive: >cut-off value repeatably
  A set of standards is available to make this a quantitative
    assay
No. of references: 9

NOTES

110443.0

Hepatitis B virus (surface antigen)
ANTIGEN DETECTION

Manufacturer: Randox Laboratories Ltd
Cat. No./Trade name: HT 1482/HBs Ag

SUMMARY

[Well-Ab]–**Ag**–[Ab-POD]–[OPD]–A_{492}

Assay type: EIA (non-competitive)
Detection: Colorimetric A_{492}
Format: Microtitre well, Ab coated
Sample type: Serum, plasma
Sample pre-treatment:
    None
Sample volume: 50 µl*
Number of tests: 96
Controls - standards run in assay:
    Controls: Neg (3), Pos (2)
Incubation:
    a) 3 hr (40°C) + 30 min RT
    b) 20 hr (RT) + 30 min (RT)
    c) 1 hr 20 min (40°C) + 30 min (RT)**
Washes: 1

CONTENTS

Antibodies, antigens, labelled components:
    Anti-HBs Ab bound to well
    Anti-HBs Ab POD conjugated
Substrate: OPD, H_2O_2
Controls - standards supplied:
    Controls: Neg and Pos
Additional reagents:
    None
Special equipment required:
    None

INTERPRETATION

Comments on interpretation:
    Positive: ≥ cut-off repeatably and confirmed by
        supplemental tests
No. of references: 4

NOTES

110505.0

*Sample and positive control can be diluted to perform a
    quantitative assay
**Method c for emergency rapid testing only

Hepatitis B virus (surface antigen)
ANTIGEN DETECTION

Manufacturer: Roche Diagnostic Systems
Cat. No./Trade name: 07.5350.5/COBAS® CORE
HBsAg II EIA

SUMMARY

[Bead-MAb]–**Ag**–[MAb-HRP]–[TMB]–A_{450}

Assay type: EIA (non-competitive)
Detection: Colorimetric A_{450}
Format: Tube, Ab coated bead
Sample type: Serum, plasma
Sample pre-treatment:
    None
Sample volume: 200 µl
Number of tests: 100, 500
Controls - standards run in assay:
    Controls: Neg (3), Pos (1)
Incubation:
    1 hr 30 min (37°C) + 15 min (37°C) with shaking
Washes: 1

CONTENTS

Antibodies, antigens, labelled components:
    Anti-HBs MAb (m) bound to beads
    Anti-HBs MAb (m) HRP conjugated
Substrate: Bought separately
Controls - standards supplied:
    Controls: Neg (human serum), Pos (rec DNA)
Additional reagents:
    TMB (automated method)
    TMB, H_2SO_4 (semi-automated method)
Special equipment required:
    Cobas® Core Immunoassay Analyzer (optional)

INTERPRETATION

Comments on interpretation:
    Positive: > cut-off repeatably and confirmed by Cobas®
        Core HBsAg II Confirmatory EIA or other similar test
    Semi-quantitative procedure available
No. of references: 6

NOTES

110631.0

Hepatitis B virus (surface antigen)
ANTIGEN DETECTION

Manufacturer: Sanofi Diagnostics Pasteur
Cat. No./Trade name: 72204/MONOLISA® Ag HBs

SUMMARY

[Well-MAb]–**Ag**–[MAb-POD]–[OPD]–$A_{492/620}$

Assay type: EIA (non-competitive)
Detection: Colorimetric $A_{492/620}$
Format: Microtitre well, Ab coated
Sample type: Serum, plasma
Sample pre-treatment:
    None
Sample volume: 100 µl
Number of tests: 96, 480
Controls - standards run in assay:
    Controls: Neg (4), Pos (2)
Incubation:
    a) 1 hr 30 min (40°C) + 30 min (RT)
    b) 45 min (40°C) + 30 min (RT)*
Washes: 1 (+ preliminary plate prewash)

CONTENTS

Antibodies, antigens, labelled components:
    Anti-HBs Ab MAb bound to well
    Anti-HBs MAbs (two) POD conjugated
Substrate: OPD, H_2O_2
Controls - standards supplied:
    Controls: Neg and Pos (human serum)
Additional reagents:
    None
Special equipment required:
    None

INTERPRETATION

Comments on interpretation:
    Classification of samples is according to cut-off; no
    further testing
No. of references: 12

NOTES

110264.0

*Method (a) is with or without shaking for incubation at 40°C
and method (b) is with shaking for incubation at 40°C

Hepatitis B virus (surface antigen)
ANTIGEN DETECTION

Manufacturer: Schiapparelli Biosystems Inc
Cat. No./Trade name: 5770347/ELISA SYSTEM HEPATITIS B - HBsAg

SUMMARY

[Well-MAb]–**Ag**–[MAb-HRP]–[TMB]–A_{450}

Assay type: EIA (non-competitive)
Detection: Colorimetric A_{450}
Format: Microtitre well, Ab coated
Sample type: Serum (do not heat inactivate)
Sample pre-treatment:
    None
Sample volume: 200 µl x 2
Number of tests: 192
Controls - standards run in assay:
    Controls: Neg (3), Pos (2)
Incubation:
    2 hr (40°C) + 1 hr (40°C) + 20 min (RT)
Washes: 2

CONTENTS

Antibodies, antigens, labelled components:
    Anti-HBs MAb bound to well
    Anti-HBs MAb HRP conjugated
Substrate: TMB, H_2O_2
Controls - standards supplied:
    Controls: Neg and Pos (human serum)
Additional reagents:
    None
Special equipment required:
    None

INTERPRETATION

Comments on interpretation:
    Classification of sample is according to cut-off; no further
    testing
No. of references: 7

NOTES

110429.0

Hepatitis B virus (surface antigen)
ANTIGEN DETECTION

Manufacturer: Sorin Biomedica
Cat. No./Trade name: 2075/AUK eiaS

SUMMARY

[Bead-MAb]–**Ag**–[MAb-HRP]–[OPD]–A_{492}

Assay type: EIA (non-competitive)
Detection: Colorimetric A_{492}
Format: Tray/Tube, Ab coated bead
Sample type: Serum, plasma
Sample pre-treatment:
  None
Sample volume: 200 µl
Number of tests: 100
Controls - standards run in assay:
  Controls: Neg (3), Pos (2)
Incubation:
  *a) 3 hr (40°C) + 30 min (RT)
  b) Overnight (RT) + 30 min (RT)
  c) 1 hr (45°C) + 30 min (RT)
Washes: 1

CONTENTS

Antibodies, antigens, labelled components:
  Anti-HBs IgG MAb (m) bound to bead
  Anti-HBs IgG MAb (m) HRP conjugated
Substrate: OPD
Controls - standards supplied:
  Controls: Neg and Pos (human serum)
Additional reagents:
  None
Special equipment required:
  Automatic rinser, PLA-2 (optional)
  Bead dispenser, MEDI-578 (optional)

INTERPRETATION

Comments on interpretation:
  Positive: ⩾ cut-off repeatably and also confirmed by a
    confirmatory test
No. of references: 10

NOTES

110237.0

Method (a) large scale routine sampling
Method (b) highest assay sensitivity
Method (c) rapid screening: results must be confirmed using
  method a or b
This kit will be discontinued in December 1994

Hepatitis B virus (surface antigen)
ANTIGEN DETECTION

Manufacturer: Sorin Biomedica
Cat. No./Trade name: 2448/AUK eia

SUMMARY

[Bead-MAb]–**Ag**–[Ab-HRP]–[OPD]–A_{492}

Assay type: EIA (non-competitive)
Detection: Colorimetric A_{492}
Format: Tray/Tube, Ab coated bead
Sample type: Serum, plasma, recalcified plasma*
Sample pre-treatment:
  None
Sample volume: 200 µl
Number of tests: 100
Controls - standards run in assay:
  Controls: Neg (3), Pos (2)
Incubation:
  *a) 2 hr (45°C) + 1 hr (45°C) + 30 min (RT)
  b) Overnight (RT) + 1 hr (45°C) + 30 min (RT)
  c) 30 min (45°C) + 30 min (45°C) + 30 min (RT)
Washes: 2

CONTENTS

Antibodies, antigens, labelled components:
  Anti-HBs IgG MAb (m) bound to bead
  Anti-HBs IgG Ab (sh) HRP conjugated
Substrate: OPD
Controls - standards supplied:
  Controls: Neg and Pos (human plasma)
Additional reagents:
  None
Special equipment required:
  None

INTERPRETATION

Comments on interpretation:
  Positive: ⩾ cut-off repeatably and confirmed by a
    confirmatory test
No. of references: 10

NOTES

110238.0

*Method (a) routine large scale screening: serum or
  recalcified plasma
Method (b) high sensitivity: serum or plasma
Method (c) rapid screening: serum or recalcified plasma
This kit will be discontinued in December 1994

Hepatitis B virus (surface antigen)
ANTIGEN DETECTION

Manufacturer: Sorin Biomedica
Cat. No./Trade name: 3142/ETI-MAK-3

SUMMARY

[Well-MAb]–**Ag**–[Ab-HRP]–[TMB]–A_{450}

Assay type: EIA (non-competitive)
Detection: Colorimetric A_{450}
Format: Microtitre well, Ab coated
Sample type: Serum, plasma
Sample pre-treatment:
  None
Sample volume: 100 µl
Number of tests: 192
Controls - standards run in assay:
  Controls: Neg (3), Pos (2)
Incubation:
  a) 30 min (37°C) + 30 min (37°C) + 30 min (RT)*
  b) 1 hr (37°C) + 1 hr (37°C) + 30 min (RT)
Washes: 2

CONTENTS

Antibodies, antigens, labelled components:
  Anti-HBs MAb (m), ad and ay subtype, bound to well
  Anti-HBs Ab (sh) HRP conjugated
Substrate: TMB, H_2O_2
Controls - standards supplied:
  Controls: Neg and Pos
Additional reagents:
  None
Special equipment required:
  ETI-system shaker/incubator and washer
  ETI-system reader

INTERPRETATION

Comments on interpretation:
  Positive: ⩾ cut-off repeatably and also confirmed by a confirmatory test (REAC 801)
No. of references: 10

NOTES

110222.0

*Procedure (a): first 2 incubations using a plate-shaker

Hepatitis B virus (surface antigen)
ANTIGEN DETECTION

Manufacturer: Syva Company
Cat. No./Trade name: 8HB29UL/MicroTrak® II HBs Ag EIA

SUMMARY

[Well-MAb]–**Ag**–[Ab-HRP]–[TMB]–$A_{450/630}$

Assay type: EIA (non-competitive)
Detection: Colorimetric $A_{450/630}$
Format: Microtitre well, Ab coated
Sample type: Serum, plasma (do not heat inactivate)
Sample pre-treatment:
  None
Sample volume: 100 µl
Number of tests: 192
Controls - standards run in assay:
  Controls: Neg (2), Pos (3)
Incubation:
  1 hr (37°C) + 30 min (37°C)
Washes: 2

CONTENTS

Antibodies, antigens, labelled components:
  Anti-HBs IgG MAb (m) bound to well
  Anti-HBs IgG PAb (sh) HRP conjugated
Substrate: TMB, H_2O_2
Controls - standards supplied:
  Controls: Neg and Pos (human plasma)
Additional reagents:
  MicroTrak® II EIA universal reagents (8K209UL)
Special equipment required:
  Syva MicroTrak® EIA autowasher and autoreader

INTERPRETATION

Comments on interpretation:
  Positive: ⩾ cut-off repeatably; confirm with neutralization test (MicroTrak® II HBs Ag confirmatory test)
No. of references: 10

NOTES

110073.0

EDTA as anticoagulant may cause false negative results

© *KLUWER ACADEMIC PUBLISHERS 1994, ISSN 1381-5067*

Hepatitis B virus (surface antigen)
ANTIGEN DETECTION

Manufacturer: United Biotech Inc
Cat. No./Trade name: IA-501/MAGIWEL® HBsAg

SUMMARY

[Well-Ab]–**Ag**–[Ab-HRP]–[TMB]–A_{450}

Assay type: EIA (non-competitive)
Detection: Colorimetric A_{450}
Format: Microtitre well, Ab coated
Sample type: Serum
Sample pre-treatment:
  None
Sample volume: 100 μl
Number of tests: 96
Controls - standards run in assay:
  Controls: Neg (1), Pos (1)
Incubation:
  2 hr (37°C) + 10 min (RT)
Washes: 1

CONTENTS

Antibodies, antigens, labelled components:
  Anti-HBs Ab bound to well
  Anti-HBs Ab HRP conjugated
Substrate: TMB, H_2O_2
Controls - standards supplied:
  Controls: Neg, Pos
Additional reagents:
  H_2SO_4
Special equipment required:
  None

INTERPRETATION

Comments on interpretation:
  Visual: positive samples develop blue colour greater than or equal to the Pos control (no addition of stop solution)
  Reading at A_{450}: classification of samples is according to cut-off; no further testing
No. of references: 0

NOTES

110503.0

Hepatitis B virus (surface antigen)
ANTIGEN DETECTION

Manufacturer: VEDA-LAB
Cat. No./Trade name: 1011/HBs Ag EIA

SUMMARY

[Well-MAb]–**Ag**–[Ab-HRP]–[TMB]–A_{450}

Assay type: EIA (non-competitive)
Detection: Colorimetric A_{450}
Format: Microtitre well, Ab coated
Sample type: Serum, plasma
Sample pre-treatment:
  None
Sample volume: 100 μl
Number of tests: 96
Controls - standards run in assay:
  Controls: Neg (1), Pos (1)
Incubation:
  1 hr (37°C) + 15 min (RT)
Washes: 1

CONTENTS

Antibodies, antigens, labelled components:
  Anti-HBs MAb bound to well
  Anti-HBs PAb HRP conjugated
Substrate: TMB, H_2O_2
Controls - standards supplied:
  Controls: Neg and Pos
Additional reagents:
  None
Special equipment required:
  None

INTERPRETATION

Comments on interpretation:
  Classification of sample is according to cut-off; no further testing
No. of references: 8

NOTES

110391.0

© KLUWER ACADEMIC PUBLISHERS 1994, ISSN 1381-5067

Hepatitis B virus (surface antigen)
ANTIGEN DETECTION

Manufacturer: Chembio Diagnostic Systems Inc
Cat. No./Trade name: HB101/Hepatitis B STAT-PAK

SUMMARY

[Membrane-Ab]–Ag–[MAb-gold]–rose band

Assay type: Immunochromatographic assay
Detection: Visual
Format: Testcard, Ab coated membrane
Sample type: Serum, plasma
Sample pre-treatment:
  None
Sample volume: 6 drops (= 200 μl)
Number of tests: 20, 50
Controls - standards run in assay:
  Controls: Pos (1)* bought separately
  Integral control (1)
Incubation:
  Read results 15-30 min after adding sample to sample window of test card
Washes:

CONTENTS

Antibodies, antigens, labelled components:
  Anti-HBs PAb bound to membrane (test well)
  Anti-HBs MAb (m) colloidal gold labelled (absorbent pad)
  Anti-murine Ab (g) (control well)
Substrate:
Controls - standards supplied:
  None
Additional reagents:
  Positive, quantitative Hepatitis B antigen commercial control
Special equipment required:
  None

INTERPRETATION

Comments on interpretation:
  Negative: rose coloured band in control well, and no rose coloured band in test well
  Positive: rose coloured band in control well and distinct rose coloured band in test well
  Inconclusive: no rose coloured band in control well. Test a fresh specimen or repeat if present specimen less than 1 hr old
  If test is negative and clinical symptoms persist follow-up using additional clinically available methods
No. of references: 8

NOTES

110602.0

*Positive control should be run at least once per day

Hepatitis B virus (surface antigen)
ANTIGEN DETECTION

Manufacturer: Savyon Diagnostics Ltd
Cat. No./Trade name: /HEPATITIS B MEMBRANE TEST

SUMMARY

[Membrane-Ab]–Ag–[MAb-gold]–pink line

Assay type: Immunochromatographic assay
Detection: Visual
Format: Test slide unit, Ab coated membrane
Sample type: Serum, plasma
Sample pre-treatment:
  None
Sample volume: 200 μl
Number of tests: 20
Controls - standards run in assay:
  Batch controls: Pos (1)
  Integral reagent control (1)
Incubation:
  Result read 10-20 min after addition of patient sample to slide unit
Washes: NA

CONTENTS

Antibodies, antigens, labelled components:
  Anti-HBs PAb bound to membrane (test window)
  Anti-murine Ig Ab (g) bound to membrane (reagent control window)
  Anti-HBs MAb colloidal gold labelled (in absorbent pad)
Substrate:
Controls - standards supplied:
  Controls: Pos
  Integral reagent control bound to membrane
Additional reagents:
  Positive control (HBsAg calibrated) bought separately
Special equipment required:
  None

INTERPRETATION

Comments on interpretation:
  Negative: pink line in control window, no line in test window
  Positive: pink line in control window and test window
  Inconclusive: no line in control window; repeat with fresh unit using same or fresh sample
No. of references: 8

NOTES

110359.0

Hepatitis B virus (surface antigen)
ANTIGEN DETECTION

Manufacturer: Kodak Clinical Diagnostics
Cat. No./Trade name: LAN.2212/KODAK Amerlite HBs Ag assay

SUMMARY

[Well–MAb]–**Ag**–[MAb–HRP]–[signal reagent]–
luminescence

Assay type: Luminometric immunoassay (non-competitive)
Detection: Luminometric
Format: Microtitre well, Ab coated
Sample type: Serum, plasma
Sample pre-treatment:
    None
Sample volume: 100 μl
Number of tests: 144*
Controls - standards run in assay:
    Controls: Neg (3), Pos (3)
Incubation:
    1 hr (37°C) with shaking + 2-20 min (RT)
Washes: 2

CONTENTS

Antibodies, antigens, labelled components:
    Anti-HBs MAb (m) bound to well
    Anti-HBs MAb (m) HRP conjugated
Substrate: Amerlite signal reagent
Controls - standards supplied:
    Controls: Neg (human serum), Pos (human serum)
Additional reagents:
    Amerlite signal reagent and serology wash reagent
Special equipment required:
    Amerlite Kodak immunoassay system

INTERPRETATION

Comments on interpretation:
    Sample reactivity is calculated automatically and classification is according to cut-off
    Positive: repeatably reactive and confirmed in Ab neutralization assay (Amerlite HBs Ag confirmatory assay)
No. of references: 4

NOTES

110490.0

*450 tests by special request

Hepatitis B virus (surface antigen)
ANTIGEN DETECTION

Manufacturer: Agen Biomedical Ltd
Cat. No./Trade name: BSRK1/SimpliRED® HBsAg Test

SUMMARY

[RBC]–[MAb$_1$–MAb$_2$]–**Ag**–agglutination

Assay type: Particle RBC agglutination assay*
Detection: Visual
Format: Agglutination tray, patient/donor RBC
Sample type: Whole blood, serum, plasma**
Sample pre-treatment:
    None
Sample volume: 10 μl x 2
Number of tests: 40
Controls - standards run in assay:
    Controls: Neg (1), Pos (1)
Incubation:
    Total time 4 minutes
Washes: 0

CONTENTS

Antibodies, antigens, labelled components:
    Anti-RBC MAb$_1$ - anti-HBs MAb$_2$ conjugate
Substrate:
Controls - standards supplied:
    Controls: Neg and Pos
Additional reagents:
    None
Special equipment required:
    None

INTERPRETATION

Comments on interpretation:
    Negative: no agglutination in test well but agglutination after addition of Pos control reagent
    Positive: agglutination in test well, and no agglutination in control well repeatably
No. of references: None

NOTES

110103.0

*In the assay, patient/donor RBC are coated with the MAb-MAb conjugate. This causes cross-linking and visible agglutination when HBsAg in the patient sample binds to the RBC + conjugate
**If using serum or plasma, whole blood from a donor must be added

© KLUWER ACADEMIC PUBLISHERS 1994, ISSN 1381-5067

Hepatitis B virus (surface antigen)
ANTIGEN DETECTION

Manufacturer: Human GmbH
Cat. No./Trade name: 40 048/HEPATITIS B QUICK TEST

SUMMARY

[Latex-Ab]–**Ag**–agglutination

Assay type: Particle agglutination assay
Detection: Visual
Format: Slide, Ab coated latex
Sample type: Serum, plasma (fresh if possible)
Sample pre-treatment:
   None
Sample volume: 50 µl undiluted and 1:41 dilution
Number of tests: 40, 100, 300
Controls - standards run in assay:
   Controls: Neg (1), Pos (1)
Incubation:
   5 min with rotation
Washes: None

CONTENTS

Antibodies, antigens, labelled components:
   Anti-HBs PAb bound to latex particle
Substrate:
Controls - standards supplied:
   Controls: Neg, Pos (human serum)
Additional reagents:
   None
Special equipment required:
   None

INTERPRETATION

Comments on Interpretation:
   Negative: no agglutination with diluted or undiluted sample
   Positive (low): agglutination only with undiluted sample
   Positive (med/high): agglutination with diluted and undiluted sample
   Positive (very high): agglutination only with diluted sample
No. of references: 1

NOTES

110517.0

Hepatitis B virus (surface antigen)
ANTIGEN DETECTION

Manufacturer: Omega Diagnostics Ltd
Cat. No./Trade name: OD018/VIROTECT - HBsAg

SUMMARY

[Latex-Ab]–**Ag**–agglutination

Assay type: Particle agglutination assay
Detection: Visual
Format: Slide, Ab coated latex
Sample type: Serum, plasma
Sample pre-treatment:
   None
Sample volume: 50 µl x 2 (diluted 1:40 and undiluted)*
Number of tests: 100
Controls - standards run in assay:
   Controls: Neg (1), Pos (1)**
Incubation:
   Read test 5 min after mixing reagents
Washes: 0

CONTENTS

Antibodies, antigens, labelled components:
   Anti-HBs Ab bound to latex particles
Substrate:
Controls - standards supplied:
   Controls: Neg and Pos
Additional reagents:
   None
Special equipment required:
   None

INTERPRETATION

Comments on interpretation:
   Positive (low level): agglutination only with undiluted sample
   Positive (medium/high level): agglutination with both dilutions
   Positive (very high level): agglutination only with diluted sample
No. of references: 0

NOTES

110020.0

*Sample assayed in duplicate on slide (diluted and undiluted)
**Pos and Neg controls to run in parallel with each batch

Hepatitis B virus (surface antigen)
ANTIGEN DETECTION

Manufacturer: VEDA-LAB
Cat. No./Trade name: /Hepatitis B DIRECT LATEX TEST for HBs Ag

SUMMARY

[Latex-Ab]–**Ag**–agglutination

Assay type: Particle agglutination assay
Detection: Visual
Format: Slide, latex particles, Ab coated
Sample type: Serum, plasma (serum preferred)
Sample pre-treatment:
 None
Sample volume: 50 µl (+2 ml saline)*
Number of tests: 50, 100, 200
Controls - standards run in assay:
 Conrols: Neg (1), Pos (1)
Incubation:
 Results read after 5 minutes
Washes: 0

CONTENTS

Antibodies, antigens, labelled components:
 Anti-HBs Ab bound to latex particles
Substrate:
Controls - standards supplied:
 Controls: Neg and Pos
Additional reagents:
 None
Special equipment required:
 None

INTERPRETATION

Comments on interpretation:
 Negative: no agglutination
 Low level Positive: agglutination only with undiluted
  sample
 Medium/high Positive: agglutination with both diluted and
  undiluted samples
 High level Positive: agglutination only with diluted sample
 Positives should be confirmed by supplemental tests
No. of references: None

NOTES

110399.0

*Assay run with diluted and undiluted sample in parallel

Hepatitis B virus (surface antigen)
ANTIGEN DETECTION

Manufacturer: Radim
Cat. No./Trade name: KHB1CT/HBsAg IRMA CT

SUMMARY

[Tube-MAb]–**Ag**–[MAb-^{125}I]–radioactivity

Assay type: RIA (non-competitive)
Detection: Radioisotopic
Format: Tube, Ab coated
Sample type: Serum or plasma
Sample pre-treatment:
 None
Sample volume: 200 µl
Number of tests: 100
Controls - standards run in assay:
 Controls: Neg (4), Pos (2)
Incubation:
 (a) 1 hr (45°C) + 1 hr (45°C)
 (b) 2 hr (45°C) + 1 hr (45°C)*
 (c) 18-22 hr (RT) + 1 hr (45°C)*
Washes: 2

CONTENTS

Antibodies, antigens, labelled components:
 Anti-HBs MAb (r) bound to tube
 Anti-HBs MAb ^{125}I labelled
Substrate:
Controls - standards supplied:
 Controls: Neg (serum) and Pos (HBsAg)
Additional reagents:
 None
Special equipment required:
 None

INTERPRETATION

Comments on interpretation:
 Grey zone: within cut-off ±10%; retest to confirm
 Positive: >cut-off value repeatably
 A set of standards is available to make this a quantitative
  assay
No. of references: 8

NOTES

110441.0

*Incubation formats (b) and (c) provide increased sensitivity

---

© **KLUWER ACADEMIC PUBLISHERS 1994, ISSN 1381-5067**

Hepatitis B virus (surface antigen)
ANTIGEN DETECTION

Manufacturer: Sorin Biomedica
Cat. No./Trade name: 2506/AUK-3

SUMMARY

[Bead-MAb]–**Ag**–[Ab-^{125}I]–radioactivity

Assay type: RIA (non-competitive)
Detection: Radioisotopic
Format: Tray/Tube, Ab coated bead
Sample type: Serum, plasma, recalcified plasma
Sample pre-treatment:
   None
Sample volume: 200 µl
Number of tests: 100, 500
Controls - standards run in assay:
   Controls: Neg (5), Pos (3)
Incubation:
   a) 2 hr (45°C) + 1 hr (45°C)*
   b) 18-22 hr (RT) + 1 hr (45°C)
   c) 30 min (50°C) + 15 min (50°C)
Washes: 2

CONTENTS

Antibodies, antigens, labelled components:
   Anti-HBs MAb (m) bound to bead
   Anti-HBs Ab (sh) ^{125}I labelled
Substrate:
Controls - standards supplied:
   Controls: Neg and Pos (human plasma)
Additional reagents:
   None
Special equipment required:
   Automatic rinser, PLA-2 (optional)
   Bead dispenser, MEDI-578 (optional)

INTERPRETATION

Comments on Interpretation:
   Positive: ≥ cut-off repeatably and confirmed by a
   confirmatory test [REAC-801]
No. of references: 8

NOTES

110217.0

*Method (a): Routine screening
Method (b): Highest sensitivity
Method (c): Rapid screening only: results require
   confirmation

Hepatitis B virus (surface antigen)
ANTIBODY DETECTION

Manufacturer: Abbott Laboratories
Cat. No./Trade name: 2262-66/IMx® AUSAB®

SUMMARY

[Particle-Ag]–**Ab**–[Ag-biotin + anti-biotin-AP]–
[4-MP]–fluorescence

Assay type: EIA (non-competitive)
Detection: Fluorometric
Format: Reaction well, Ag coated microparticle
Sample type: Serum, plasma (do not heat inactivate)
Sample pre-treatment:
   None
Sample volume: 150 µl
Number of tests: 100
Controls - standards run in assay:
   Calibration assay: calibrators (6) x 2; Controls: Neg (1),
      Pos (1)
   Mode 1 assay: calibrators (1); Controls: Pos (1)*
Incubation:
   Automated
Washes: Automated

CONTENTS

Antibodies, antigens, labelled components:
   rec HBsAg bound to microparticle
   rec HBsAg (ad, ay) biotinylated
   Anti-biotin (r) AP conjugated
Substrate: 4-MP
Controls - standards supplied:
   Calibrators: mode 1 calibrator (human plasma)
Additional reagents:
   IMx® AUSAB® calibrators (conc. range of Anti-HBs 0-
      1000 mIU/ml)
   IMx® AUSAB® controls
   IMx® AUSAB® specimen diluent
   IMx® probe cleaning solution
Special equipment required:
   IMx system

INTERPRETATION

Comments on Interpretation:
   Sample reactivity is calculated automatically
   Classification of samples is according to cut-off; no
      further retesting
   Quantitative procedure available
No. of references: 6

NOTES

110067.0

*Minimum control requirement for mode 1 assay: one
   positive control on each carousel

© *KLUWER ACADEMIC PUBLISHERS 1994, ISSN 1381-5067*

Hepatitis B virus (surface antigen)
ANTIBODY DETECTION

Manufacturer: ADI Diagnostics
Cat. No./Trade name: /Heprofile® Anti-HBs

SUMMARY

[Well-Ag]–**Ab**–[Ag-POD]–[TMB]–A_{450}

Assay type: EIA (non-competitive)
Detection: Colorimetric A_{450}
Format: Microtitre well, Ag coated
Sample type: Serum, plasma
Sample pre-treatment:
  None
Sample volume: 200 µl
Number of tests: 96
Controls - standards run in assay:
  Controls: Neg (3), Pos (2)
Incubation:
  a) 12-20 hr (RT) + 4 hr (RT) + 30 min (RT)
  b) 3 hr (37°C) + 1 hr (37°C) + 30 min (RT)
Washes: 2

CONTENTS

Antibodies, antigens, labelled components:
  HBsAg (h) bound to well
  HBsAg POD conjugated
Substrate: TMB, H_2O_2
Controls - standards supplied:
  Controls: Neg and Pos (human plasma)
Additional reagents:
  None
Special equipment required:
  None

INTERPRETATION

Comments on interpretation:
  Positive: ⩾ cut-off repeatably
No. of references: 6

NOTES

110030.0

Hepatitis B virus (surface antigen)
ANTIBODY DETECTION

Manufacturer: Behringwerke AG
Cat. No./Trade name: OWRT/Enzygnost® Anti-HBs micro

SUMMARY

[Well-Ag]–**Ab**–[Ag-POD]–[TMB]–A_{450}

Assay type: EIA (non-competitive)
Detection: Colorimetric A_{450}
Format: Microtitre well, Ag coated
Sample type: Serum, plasma
Sample pre-treatment:
  None
Sample volume: 100 µl*
Number of tests: 96
Controls - standards run in assay:
  Controls: Neg (4), Pos (2) (qualitative)
Incubation:
  1 hr (37°C) + 30 min (RT)
Washes: 1

CONTENTS

Antibodies, antigens, labelled components:
  HBsAg bound to well
  HBsAg POD conjugated
Substrate: TMB, H_2O_2
Controls - standards supplied:
  Controls: Neg (human serum), and Pos (human serum
    with defined value)
Additional reagents:
  None
Special equipment required:
  Behring ELISA processor (optional)

INTERPRETATION

Comments on interpretation:
  Classification of samples is according to cut-off; no
    further testing
No. of references: 0

NOTES

110452.0

*Samples must be diluted if Ab concentration is expected to
  be ⩾ 100 IU/L
Quantitative procedure available using dilutions of the HBs
  standard serum

© KLUWER ACADEMIC PUBLISHERS 1994, ISSN 1381-5067

Hepatitis B virus (surface antigen)
ANTIBODY DETECTION

Manufacturer: Boehringer Mannheim
Cat. No./Trade name: 1123 866/Enzymun-Test® Anti-HBs

SUMMARY

[Tube-strept]–[Ag-biotin]–**Ab**–[Ag-POD]–[ABTS]–A_{420}

Assay type: EIA (non-competitive)
Detection: Colorimetric A_{420}
Format: Tube, streptavidin coated
Sample type: Serum, plasma (not citrated)
Sample pre-treatment:
   None
Sample volume: 200 µl
Number of tests: 125
Controls - standards run in assay:
   Controls: Neg (2), Pos (2)
Incubation:
   3 hr (RT) + 1 hr (RT)
Washes: 1

CONTENTS

Antibodies, antigens, labelled components:
   HBsAg POD conjugated
   HBsAg biotinylated
Substrate: ABTS, H_2O_2
Controls - standards supplied:
   Controls: Neg and Pos (human serum with assigned EIA
   value)
Additional reagents:
   Streptavidin-coated tubes
   Substrate
Special equipment required:
   Automated Enzymun-Test Systems (optional)

INTERPRETATION

Comments on interpretation:
   Equivocal: within cut-off ±15%; retest to confirm
   Quantitative procedure available
No. of references: 0

NOTES

110463.0

Hepatitis B virus (surface antigen)
ANTIBODY DETECTION

Manufacturer: Melotec S.A.
Cat. No./Trade name: /MELOTEST Anti-HBs

SUMMARY

[Well-Ag]–**Ab**–[Ag-HRP]–[TMB]–A_{450}

Assay type: EIA (non-competitive)
Detection: Colorimetric A_{450}
Format: Microtitre well, Ag coated
Sample type: Serum, plasma
Sample pre-treatment:
   None
Sample volume: 200 µl
Number of tests: 96
Controls - standards run in assay:
   Controls: Neg (3), Pos (2)
Incubation:
   Overnight: 16 ± 4 hr (RT) + 4 hr (RT) + 30 min (RT)
   Rapid: 3 hr (37°C) + 1 hr (37°C) + 30 min (RT)
Washes: 2

CONTENTS

Antibodies, antigens, labelled components:
   HBsAg bound to well
   HBsAg HRP conjugated
Substrate: TMB, H_2O_2
Controls - standards supplied:
   Controls: Neg and Pos
Additional reagents:
   None
Special equipment required:
   None

INTERPRETATION

Comments on interpretation:
   Equivocal: within cut-off and cut-off–10%; retest to
   confirm
   Repeatably equivocal: retest a fresh sample in 1–2
   weeks
   Positive: ≥cut-off repeatably and confirmed by
   supplemental tests
No. of references: 5

NOTES

110639.0

© *KLUWER ACADEMIC PUBLISHERS 1994, ISSN 1381-5067*

Hepatitis B virus (surface antigen)
ANTIBODY DETECTION

Manufacturer: Mitsui Pharmaceuticals Inc
Cat. No./Trade name: MP-5100/HBsAb-MP MITSUI

SUMMARY

[Particle-Ag]–**Ab**–[Ag-HRP]–[TMB]–A_{450}

Assay type: EIA (non-competitive)
Detection: Colorimetric A_{450}
Format: Tube, Ag coated particles (magnetisable)
Sample type: Serum
Sample pre-treatment:
   None
Sample volume: 80 µl
Number of tests: 100
Controls - standards run in assay:
   Controls: Neg (1), Pos (1), Calibrators (2)
Incubation:
   5 min (37°C) + 5 m in (37°C) + 5 min (37°C)
Washes: 2

CONTENTS

Antibodies, antigens, labelled components:
   HBsAg bound to particles
   HBsAg HRP conjugated
Substrate: TMB
Controls - standards supplied:
   None
Additional reagents:
   Quality controls bought separately: H_2SO_4, Mitsui
     common reagent, concentrated buffer, cell detergent
Special equipment required:
   MITSUI QUARTUS Fully Automated EIAsystem

INTERPRETATION

Comments on interpretation:
   Not specified
No. of references: 4

NOTES

110599.0

Hepatitis B virus (surface antigen)
ANTIBODY DETECTION

Manufacturer: Murex Diagnostics Limited
Cat. No./Trade name: VK40/Wellcozyme anti-HBs

SUMMARY

[Well-Ag]–**Ab**–[Ag-AP]–[NADP + ampl]–A_{492}

Assay type: EIA (non-competitive, amplified)
Detection: Colorimetric $A_{492\text{-}496}$
Format: Microtitre well, Ag coated
Sample type: Serum, plasma*
Sample pre-treatment:
   None
Sample volume: 100 µl
Number of tests: 96
Controls - standards run in assay:
   Controls: Neg (4), Pos (2)
   If required: Pos reference (2)
Incubation:
   2 hr (37°C) + 1 hr (37°C) + 20 min (37°C) + 10 min
     (RT)
Washes: 2

CONTENTS

Antibodies, antigens, labelled components:
   HBsAg bound to well
   HBsAg AP conjugated
Substrate: NADP + amplifier
Controls - standards supplied:
   Controls: Neg and Pos (human serum)
   Positive reference (10 mIU/ml, anti-HBs)
Additional reagents:
   H_2SO_4
Special equipment required:
   Wellcozyme microwell plate washing system (optional)
   Wellcozyme microwell plate reader system (optional)

INTERPRETATION

Comments on interpretation:
   Positive: ⩾ cut-off repeatably; perform an anti-HBc assay
     for collaborative evidence of positivity
   Positive reference serum may be used to evaluate
     immune status of vaccinees
   Visual interpretation may be used but sensitivity may be
     reduced
No. of references: None

NOTES

110160.0

*Plasma samples may be collected in EDTA
Do not test plasma collected in sodium citrate

© *KLUWER ACADEMIC PUBLISHERS 1994, ISSN 1381-5067*

Hepatitis B virus (surface antigen)
ANTIBODY DETECTION

Manufacturer: Organon Teknika NV
Cat. No./Trade name: 72193/Hepanostika® anti-HBs

SUMMARY

[Well-Ag]–**Ab**–[Ag-HRP]–[TMB]–A_{450}

Assay type: EIA (non-competitive)
Detection: Colorimetric A_{450}
Format: Microtitre well, Ag coated
Sample type: Serum, plasma
Sample pre-treatment:
  None
Sample volume: 100 µl
Number of tests: 192
Controls - standards run in assay:
  Controls:
  Neg (1), low Pos (1), high Pos (1) (one strip)
  Neg (2), low Pos (2), high Pos (2) (two or more strips)
Incubation:
  a) 1 hr (37°C) + 1 hr (37°C) + 30 min (RT)
  b) 16-24 hr (RT) + 1 hr (37°C) + 30 min (RT)
Washes: 2

CONTENTS

Antibodies, antigens, labelled components:
  HBs (subtype ay) Ag bound to well
  HBs (subtype ad) Ag HRP conjugated
Substrate: TMB
Controls - standards supplied:
  Controls: Neg, low Pos, high Pos (human serum)
Additional reagents:
  H_2SO_4
Special equipment required:
  None

INTERPRETATION

Comments on interpretation:
  Positive: ⩾ cut-off repeatably
  A quantitative procedure available
No. of references: 0

NOTES

110560.0

Hepatitis B virus (surface antigen)
ANTIBODY DETECTION

Manufacturer: Randox Laboratories Ltd
Cat. No./Trade name: HT 1484/Anti-HBs

SUMMARY

[Well-Ag]–**Ab**–[Ag-POD]–[OPD]–A_{492}

Assay type: EIA (non-competitive)
Detection: Colorimetric A_{492}
Format: Microtitre well, Ag coated
Sample type: Serum, plasma
Sample pre-treatment:
  None
Sample volume: 50 µl*
Number of tests: 96
Controls - standards run in assay:
  Controls: Neg (3), Pos (2)
Incubation:
  a) 3 hr (RT) + 30 min
  b) 50 min (40°C)** + 30 min (RT)
  c) 20 ± 4 hr (RT) + 30 min (RT)
Washes: 1

CONTENTS

Antibodies, antigens, labelled components:
  HBsAg bound to well
  HBsAg POD conjugated
Substrate: OPD, H_2O_2
Controls - standards supplied:
  Controls: Neg and Pos
Additional reagents:
  None
Special equipment required:
  None

INTERPRETATION

Comments on interpretation:
  Retest range: within cut-off ± 10%; retest to confirm
  Positive: ⩾ cut-off repeatably
No. of references: 4

NOTES

110506.0

*Sample and positive control can be diluted to perform a
  quantitative assay
**Incubation (b) for emergency rapid testing only

© *KLUWER ACADEMIC PUBLISHERS 1994, ISSN 1381-5067*

Hepatitis B virus (surface antigen)
ANTIBODY DETECTION

Manufacturer: Roche Diagnostic Systems
Cat. No./Trade name: 07 3438 1/COBAS CORE Anti-HBs EIA

SUMMARY

[Bead-Ag]–**Ab**–[Ag-POD]–[TMB]–A_{450}

Assay type: EIA (non-competitive)
Detection: Colorimetric A_{450}
Format: Tube, Ag coated bead
Sample type: Serum or plasma (do not heat inactivate)
Sample pre-treatment:
　None
Sample volume: 200 µl (+50 µl diluent)
Number of tests: 100, 500
Controls - standards run in assay:
　Controls: Neg (3), Pos (1)
Incubation:
　1 hr (37°C) + 15 min (37°C) both with shaking
Washes: 1

CONTENTS

Antibodies, antigens, labelled components:
　HBsAg bound to beads
　HBsAg POD conjugated
Substrate: TMB, H_2O_2
Controls - standards supplied:
　Controls: Neg and Pos (human serum)
Additional reagents:
　Substrate (supplied as separate kit)
Special equipment required:
　Cobas® EIA shaking incubator, tube washer and
　　photometer (optional)
　Cobas® Core automated analyser (optional)

INTERPRETATION

Comments on interpretation:
　Grey zone:　within cut-off ±10%; retest to confirm
　Positive:　≥cut-off repeatably
　A kit for quantitative determination is also available
No. of references: 8

NOTES

110404.0

Hepatitis B virus (surface antigen)
ANTIBODY DETECTION

Manufacturer: Roche Diagnostic Systems
Cat. No./Trade name: 07 5111 1/COBAS CORE Anti-HBsAg Quant.EIA

SUMMARY

[Bead-Ag]–**Ab**–[Ag-POD]–[TMB]–A_{450}

Assay type: EIA (non-competitive)
Detection: Colorimetric A_{450}
Format: Tube, Ag coated bead
Sample type: Serum or plasma (do not heat inactivate)
Sample pre-treatment:
　None
Sample volume: 200 µl undiluted and diluted 1:11
Number of tests: 100, 500
Controls - standards run in assay:
　Controls: Pos (2)
　Calibrators: Neg (2), Pos (8)
Incubation:
　1 hr (37°C) + 15 min (37°C) both with shaking
Washes: 1

CONTENTS

Antibodies, antigens, labelled components:
　HBsAg bound to beads
　HBsAg POD conjugated
Substrate: TMB, H_2O_2
Controls - standards supplied:
　Controls: Pos (human serum)
　Calibrators: 5 with assigned EIA values (human serum;
　　0-150 mIU/ml)
Additional reagents:
　Substrate (supplied as separate kit)
Special equipment required:
　Cobas® EIA shaking incubator, tube washer and
　　photometer (optional)
　Cobas® Core automated analyser (optional)

INTERPRETATION

Comments on interpretation:
　This is a quantitative assay
No. of references: 9

NOTES

110405.0

© KLUWER ACADEMIC PUBLISHERS 1994, ISSN 1381-5067

Hepatitis B virus (surface antigen)
ANTIBODY DETECTION

Manufacturer: Sanofi Diagnostics Pasteur
Cat. No./Trade name: 72198/MONOLISA® Anti-HBs

SUMMARY

[Well-Ag]–**Ab**–[Ag-biotin]–[strept-POD]–[OPD]–
$A_{492/620}$

Assay type: EIA (non-competitive)
Detection: Colorimetric $A_{492/620}$
Format: Microtitre well, Ag coated
Sample type: Serum
Sample pre-treatment:
   None
Sample volume: 100 µl
Number of tests: 96
Controls - standards run in assay:
   Controls: Neg (3), Pos (2)
Incubation:
   1 hr (40°C) + 1 hr (40°C) + 30 min (RT)
Washes: 2 (+ preliminary plate prewash)

CONTENTS

Antibodies, antigens, labelled components:
   rec HBsAg bound to well
   rec HBsAg biotin conjugated
   Streptavidin-POD conjugated
Substrate: OPD, H_2O_2
Controls - standards supplied:
   Controls: Neg and Pos (human Ig)
Additional reagents:
   None
Special equipment required:
   None

INTERPRETATION

Comments on interpretation:
   In the screening assay, classification of samples is
      according to the threshold cut-off; no further testing
   Quantitative procedure available using standards from
      MONOLISA® Anti-HBs kit
No. of references: 8

NOTES

110263.0

Hepatitis B virus (surface antigen)
ANTIBODY DETECTION

Manufacturer: Schiapparelli Biosystems Inc
Cat. No./Trade name: 5770334/ELISA SYSTEM
HEPATITIS B - HBsAb 2nd Generation

SUMMARY

[Well-Ag]–**Ab**–[Ag-HRP]–[TMB]–$A_{450/405}$

Assay type: EIA (non-competitive)
Detection: Colorimetric $A_{450/405}$
Format: Microtitre well, Ag coated
Sample type: Serum (do not heat inactivate)
Sample pre-treatment:
   None
Sample volume: 200 µl x 2
Number of tests: 96
Controls - standards run in assay:
   Standards: Neg (2), Pos (8)
Incubation:
   2 hr (40°C) + 1 hr (40°C) + 20 min (RT)
Washes: 2

CONTENTS

Antibodies, antigens, labelled components:
   HBsAg bound to well
   HBsAg HRP conjugated
Substrate: TMB, H_2O_2
Controls - standards supplied:
   Standards: 5 with assigned EIA values (human serum; 0-
      750 mIU/ml)
Additional reagents:
   None
Special equipment required:
   None

INTERPRETATION

Comments on interpretation:
   This is a quantitative assay
   Non reactive: <10 mIU/ml
No. of references: 6

NOTES

110430.0

© *KLUWER ACADEMIC PUBLISHERS 1994, ISSN 1381-5067*

Hepatitis B virus (surface antigen)
ANTIBODY DETECTION

Manufacturer: Sorin Biomedica
Cat. No./Trade name: 2857/ETI-AB-AUK-2

SUMMARY

$$[Well\text{-}Ag]\text{--}\textbf{Ab}\text{--}[Ag\text{-}HRP]\text{--}[TMB]\text{--}A_{450}$$

Assay type: EIA (non-competitive)
Detection: Colorimetric A_{450}
Format: Microtitre well, Ag coated
Sample type: Serum, plasma
Sample pre-treatment:
  None
Sample volume: 100 µl
Number of tests: 96
Controls - standards run in assay:
  Controls: Neg (3), Pos (2)
Incubation:
  2 hr (37°C) + 1 hr (37°C) + 30 min (RT)
Washes: 2

CONTENTS

Antibodies, antigens, labelled components:
  HBsAg (h), subtypes ad and ay bound to well
  HBsAg (h) HRP conjugated
Substrate: TMB H_2O_2
Controls - standards supplied:
  Controls: Neg (human serum), Pos (human plasma)
Additional reagents:
  None
Special equipment required:
  ETI system reader and washer (optional)

INTERPRETATION

Comments on interpretation:
  Equivocal: Within cut-off ± 10%; retest to confirm
  Positive: ≥ cut-off repeatably
No. of references: 9

NOTES

110215.0

Hepatitis B virus (surface antigen)
ANTIBODY DETECTION

Manufacturer: Sorin Biomedica
Cat. No./Trade name: 3498/ETI-AB-AUK QUANT

SUMMARY

$$[Well\text{-}Ag]\text{--}\textbf{Ab}\text{--}[Ag\text{-}HRP]\text{--}[TMB]\text{--}A_{450}$$

Assay type: EIA (non-competitive)
Detection: Colorimetric A_{450}
Format: Microtitre well, Ag coated
Sample type: Serum
Sample pre-treatment:
  Samples with Ab levels > 1000 IU/ml should be diluted
    prior to assay
Sample volume: 100 µl
Number of tests: 96
Controls - standards run in assay:
  Calibrators (5) in duplicate
Incubation:
  2 hr (37°C) + 1 hr (37°C) + 30 min (RT)
Washes: 2

CONTENTS

Antibodies, antigens, labelled components:
  HBsAg (h) subtypes ad and ay bound to well
  HBsAg (h) HRP conjugated
Substrate: TMB, H_2O_2
Controls - standards supplied:
  Calibrators: human serum, WHO anti-hepatitis B
    immunoglobulin, 10-1000 mIU/ml
Additional reagents:
  None
Special equipment required:
  ETI-system reader and software (optional)
  ETI-system washer (optional)

INTERPRETATION

Comments on interpretation:
  Quantitative assay
No. of references: 2

NOTES

110232.0

© *KLUWER ACADEMIC PUBLISHERS 1994, ISSN 1381-5067*

Hepatitis B virus (surface antigen)
ANTIBODY DETECTION

Manufacturer: Sorin Biomedica
Cat. No./Trade name: 2447/AB-AUK-eia

SUMMARY

[Bead-Ag]–**Ab**–[Ag-HRP]–[OPD]–A_{492}

Assay type: EIA (non-competitive)
Detection: Colorimetric A_{492}
Format: Tray/Tube, Ag coated bead
Sample type: Serum, plasma
Sample pre-treatment:
None
Sample volume: 200 μl
Number of tests: 100
Controls - standards run in assay:
Controls: Neg (3), Pos (2)
Incubation:
Overnight (RT) + 4 hr (RT) + 30 min (RT)
Washes: 2

CONTENTS

Antibodies, antigens, labelled components:
HBsAg (h) subtypes ad and ay bound to bead
HBsAg HRP conjugated
Substrate: OPD
Controls - standards supplied:
Controls: Neg and Pos (human plasma)
Additional reagents:
None
Special equipment required:
Automatic rinser, PLA-2 (optional)
Bead dispenser, MEDI-578 (optional)

INTERPRETATION

Comments on interpretation:
Equivocal: Within cut-off ± 10%; retest to confirm
No. of references: 9

NOTES

110236.0

Quantitative assay version may be performed using the
ABAU-STD standards set
This kit will be discontinued in December 1994

Hepatitis B virus (surface antigen)
ANTIBODY DETECTION

Manufacturer: Syva Company
Cat. No./Trade name: 8HA29UL/MicroTrak® II Anti-HBsurface EIA

SUMMARY

[Well-Ag]–**Ab**–[Ag-HRP]–[TMB]–$A_{450/630}$

Assay type: EIA (non-competitive)
Detection: Colorimetric $A_{450/630}$
Format: Microtitre well, Ag coated
Sample type: Serum, plasma
Sample pre-treatment:
None
Sample volume: 100 μl
Number of tests: 96
Controls - standards run in assay:
Controls: Neg (3), Pos (2)
Incubation:
2 hr (37°C) + 1 hr (37°C) + 30 min (37°C)
Washes: 2

CONTENTS

Antibodies, antigens, labelled components:
HBsAg (h) bound to well
HBsAg (h) HRP conjugated
Substrate: TMB, H_2O_2
Controls - standards supplied:
Controls: Neg (human serum), Pos (human plasma)
Additional reagents:
MicroTrak® II EIA universal reagents (8K209UL)
Special equipment required:
Syva MicroTrak® EIA autowasher and autoreader

INTERPRETATION

Comments on interpretation:
Positive: ⩾ cut-off repeatably
No. of references: 10

NOTES

110070.0

Hepatitis B virus (surface antigen)
ANTIBODY DETECTION

Manufacturer: VEDA-LAB
Cat. No./Trade name: 1511/HBs Ab EIA

SUMMARY

[Well-Ag]–**Ab**–[Ag-HRP]–[TMB]–A_{450}

Assay type: EIA (non-competitive)
Detection: Colorimetric A_{450}
Format: Microtitre well, Ag coated
Sample type: Serum, plasma
Sample pre-treatment:
    None
Sample volume: 50 µl
Number of tests: 96
Controls - standards run in assay:
    Controls: Neg (1), Pos (1)
Incubation:
    1 hr (37°C) + 15 min (RT)
Washes: 1

CONTENTS

Antibodies, antigens, labelled components:
    HBsAg bound to well
    HBsAg HRP conjugated
Substrate: TMB, H_2O_2
Controls - standards supplied:
    Controls: Neg and Pos
Additional reagents:
    None
Special equipment required:
    None

INTERPRETATION

Comments on interpretation:
    Classification of sample is according to cut-off; no further testing
No. of references: 11

NOTES

110392.0

Hepatitis B virus (surface antigen)
ANTIBODY DETECTION

Manufacturer: Kodak Clinical Diagnostics
Cat. No./Trade name: LAN.1203/KODAK Amerlite anti-HBs (Antibody to Hepatitis B Surface Antigen) Assay

SUMMARY

[Well-Ag]–**Ab**–[Ag-HRP]–[signal reagent]–luminescence

Assay type: Luminometric immunoassay (non-competitive)
Detection: Luminometric
Format: Microtitre well, Ag coated
Sample type: Serum, plasma
Sample pre-treatment:
    None
Sample volume: 200 µl
Number of tests: 96
Controls - standards run in assay:
    Controls: Neg (2), low Pos (3), high Pos (1)
Incubation:
    2 hr (37°C) + 2 hr (37°C) both with shaking + 2-20 min (RT)
Washes: 2

CONTENTS

Antibodies, antigens, labelled components:
    HBsAg bound to well
    HBsAg HRP conjugated
Substrate: Amerlite signal reagent
Controls - standards supplied:
    Controls: Neg, low Pos, high Pos (human serum)
Additional reagents:
    Amerlite signal reagent and serology wash reagent
    Amerlite anti-HBs quantitation panel (for quantitative assay)
Special equipment required:
    Amerlite Kodak immunoassay system

INTERPRETATION

Comments on interpretation:
    Sample reactivity is calculated automatically and classification is according to cut-off
    Equivocal samples are marked 'retest'; retest to confirm
    Quantitative format available
No. of references: 7

NOTES

110489.0

© KLUWER ACADEMIC PUBLISHERS 1994, ISSN 1381-5067

Hepatitis B virus (surface antigen)
ANTIBODY DETECTION

Manufacturer: Radim
Cat. No./Trade name: KHB3CT/ANTI-HBs IRMA CT

SUMMARY

[Tube-Ag]–**Ab**–[Ag-^{125}I]–radioactivity

Assay type: RIA (non-competitive)
Detection: Radioisotopic
Format: Tube, Ag coated
Sample type: Serum or plasma
Sample pre-treatment:
  None
Sample volume: 200 µl
Number of tests: 100
Controls - standards run in assay:
  Controls: Neg (4), Pos (2)
Incubation:
  2 hr (45°C)
Washes: 1

CONTENTS

Antibodies, antigens, labelled components:
  HBsAg bound to tube
  HBsAg ^{125}I labelled
Substrate:
Controls - standards supplied:
  Controls: Neg and Pos (human serum)
Additional reagents:
  None
Special equipment required:
  None

INTERPRETATION

Comments on interpretation:
  Grey zone: within cut-off ±10%; retest to confirm
  Positive: > cut-off value repeatably
  A set of standards is available to make this a quantitative
    assay
No. of references: 5

NOTES

110442.0

Hepatitis B virus (surface antigen)
ANTIBODY DETECTION

Manufacturer: Sorin Biomedica
Cat. No./Trade name: 2521/AB-AUK-3

SUMMARY

[Bead-Ag]–**Ab**–[Ag-^{125}I]–radioactivity

Assay type: RIA (non-competitive)
Detection: Radioisotopic
Format: Tube, Ag coated bead
Sample type: Serum, plasma
Sample pre-treatment:
  None
Sample volume: 200 µl
Number of tests: 100
Controls - standards run in assay:
  Controls: Neg (5), Pos (3)
Incubation:
  18-22 hr (RT) + 4 hr (RT)
Washes: 2

CONTENTS

Antibodies, antigens, labelled components:
  HBsAg (h) subtypes ad and ay bound to bead
  HBsAg subtypes ad and ay ^{125}I labelled
Substrate:
Controls - standards supplied:
  Controls: Neg (human serum) and Pos (human plasma)
Additional reagents:
  None
Special equipment required:
  None

INTERPRETATION

Comments on interpretation:
  Equivocal: Within cut-off ±10%; retest to confirm
  Positive: ≥ cut-off repeatably
  The use of a standard set (ABAU-STD-SET) allows
    construction of a standard curve and the assessment
    of results quantitatively
No. of references: 9

NOTES

110213.0

© *KLUWER ACADEMIC PUBLISHERS 1994, ISSN 1381-5067*

Hepatitis C virus (HCV) (Non-A, Non-B hepatitis)

Natural history

The hepatitis C virus genome was cloned in 1989, but the association of this virus with post transfusion hepatitis in which hepatitis A and B had been excluded lead to earlier use of the term non-A non-B hepatitis. HCV is classified as a distinct genus; animal pestiviruses are the closest known viruses. Infection with HCV is predominantly acquired from blood, blood products and organs, and is prevalent in all with multiple exposures to such sources before screening began in 1990–91, particularly haemophiliacs, and IV drug users. Much community-acquired hepatitis is also due to HCV, linked to household, occupational or other contact with infected blood. There is no reliable evidence that HCV is sexually transmitted, although a small proportion of infections may be acquired by this means; saliva is a possible vehicle of spread. Perinatal transmission has been shown in a few cases, especially from HIV-infected mothers. Acute infection with hepatitis C is often subclinical, following an incubation of 4–26 weeks, mean 7–8 weeks post-transfusion. The importance of HCV as a human pathogen lies in the frequently persistent infection with viraemia; 60% of cases develop a chronic hepatitis and 25% of those progress slowly to cirrhosis. There is a significant risk of hepatocellular carcinoma later. Evidence of protective immunity is lacking, with reinfection and recurrent infection common. Antiviral therapy with interferon or ribavirin has been successful in halting disease in some cases of chronic hepatitis C.

Diagnosis and markers

Cloned DNA for structural (capsid/core and envelope) and non-structural (NS) proteins of hepatitis C virus has been obtained from clinical material and recombinant proteins have been produced for use in immunoassays. First generation tests were based on the NS 4 (C 100-3) single antigen and lacked sensitivity and specificity. Second generation multiple-antigen based assays using additional NS 3 (C 33c) and core (C 22) antigens detect antibody in a greater range of infections. Third generation includes NS 5 antigen with increased concentration of other antigens, and around 95% of all infected cases can be detected. Reactive screening tests are confirmed by recombinant immunoblot assay (RIBA) or blocking (neutralisation) tests, or alternative EIAs. In the first weeks after infection, antibody will not be found; antibody to core appears earliest at about four weeks, while antibody to NS proteins appears between 6 weeks and 6 months. Tests for antibody, including IgM, do not yet distinguish current from past HCV infection; only virus detection by PCR provides that information at present. Various serotypes of hepatitis C are now known, and type-specific peptide-based assays for antibody may contribute to epidemiological studies, and to pretreatment assessment of patients. HCV cannot be isolated in cell culture; low titres of virus in circulation mean antigen detection is not generally applicable, but PCR amplification of cDNA (from reverse transcription of virion RNA) is used for virus detection and quantification.

Comment

Significant advances in knowledge of hepatitis C and the development of new immunoassays can be expected in the near future. Virus detection by PCR is advised for diagnosis in the immunocompromised host. A majority of individuals with antibody to HCV have persisting viraemia and should be considered to be a source of infection.

Reference

van der Poel CL. Hepatitis C virus: epidemiology, transmission and prevention. Reesink HW (ed). Current Studies in Hematology and Blood Transfusion. Basel: Karger. 1994;61:137–163.

Hepatitis C virus
ANTIBODY DETECTION (IgG)

Manufacturer: Boehringer Mannheim
Cat. No./Trade name: 1489 135/Enzymun-Test® Anti-HCV

SUMMARY

[Tube-strept]–[Ag-biotin]–**Ab**–[AHIgG-POD]–[ABTS]–A_{422}

Assay type: EIA (non-competitive)
Detection: Colorimetric A_{422}
Format: Tube, streptavidin coated (bought separately)
Sample type: Serum, plasma (do not heat inactivate)
Sample pre-treatment:
  None
Sample volume: 20 μl
Number of tests: Not specified
Controls - standards run in assay:
  Controls: Neg (1), Pos (1)
Incubation:
  a) 1 hr (RT) + 1 hr (RT) + 1 hr (RT)
  b) 1 hr (37°C) + 1 h r (37°C) + 30 min (37°C)
Washes: 2

CONTENTS

Antibodies, antigens, labelled components:
  Streptavidin bound to tube
  HCV Ag biotinylated
  Anti-human Fcγ Ab (sh) POD conjugated
Substrate: ABTS, H_2O_2 (bought separately)
Controls - standards supplied:
  Controls: Neg (human serum), Pos (bovine serum with human anti-HCV Ab)
Additional reagents:
  Enzymun-Test® Substrate
  Enzymun-Test® Streptavidin tubes
  Enzymun-Test® washing solution
  ES 300 cleaning solution
Special equipment required:
  None

INTERPRETATION

Comments on interpretation:
  Borderline: within 80-100% of cut-off; retest to confirm
  Repeatably borderline: retest with a confirmatory test
  Positive: ≥ cut-off repeatably and confirmed by supplemental tests
No. of references: 0

NOTES

110659.0

Hepatitis C virus
ANTIBODY DETECTION (IgG)

Manufacturer: Innogenetics SA
Cat. No./Trade name: /INNOTEST HCV Ab III

SUMMARY

[Well-Ag]–**Ab**–[AHIgG-HRP]–[TMB]–A_{450}

Assay type: EIA (non-competitive)
Detection: Colorimetric A_{450}
Format: Microtitre well, Ag coated
Sample type: Serum, plasma
Sample pre-treatment:
  None
Sample volume: 10 μl (+ 100 μl diluent)
Number of tests: 96
Controls - standards run in assay:
  Controls: Neg (1), Pos (1) per microplate strip*
Incubation:
  1 hr (37°C) + 1 hr (37°C) + 30 min (RT)
Washes:

CONTENTS

Antibodies, antigens, labelled components:
  HCV Ag (core, NS3, NS4, NS5) bound to well
  Anti-human IgG Ab (r) HRP conjugated
Substrate: TMB, H_2O_2
Controls - standards supplied:
  Controls: Neg and Pos (human serum)
Additional reagents:
  H_2SO_4
Special equipment required:
  None

INTERPRETATION

Comments on interpretation:
  Positive: ≥ cut-off repeatably and confirmed by supplemental tests
No. of references: 9

NOTES

110320.0

*If more than one strip is used, include at least 2 Neg and 2 Pos controls per strip holder

© KLUWER ACADEMIC PUBLISHERS 1994, ISSN 1381-5067

Hepatitis C virus
ANTIBODY DETECTION (IgG)

Manufacturer: Melotec S.A.
Cat. No./Trade name: /MELOTEST HCV

SUMMARY

[Well-Ag]–**Ab**–[AHIgG-HRP]–[TMB]–A_{450}

Assay type: EIA (non-competitive)
Detection: Colorimetric A_{450}
Format: Microtitre well, Ag coated
Sample type: Serum, plasma
Sample pre-treatment:
　None
Sample volume: 200 µl (of a 1:41 dilution)*
Number of tests: 96
Controls - standards run in assay:
　Controls: Neg (2), Pos (2)
Incubation:
　30 min (37°C) + 30 min (37°C) + 10 min (RT)
Washes: 2

CONTENTS

Antibodies, antigens, labelled components:
　rec HCV Ag bound to well
　Anti-human IgG Ab HRP conjugated
Substrate: TMB, H_2O_2
Controls - standards supplied:
　Controls: Neg and Pos
Additional reagents:
　None
Special equipment required:
　None

INTERPRETATION

Comments on interpretation:
　Equivocal: within cut-off and cut-off–10%; retest to
　　confirm
　Repeatably equivocal: retest a fresh sample in 1–2
　　weeks
　Positive: ≥ cut-off repeatably and confirmed by
　　supplemental tests
No. of references: 6

NOTES

110637.0

*Samples may be diluted directly into wells or prediluted in
　tubes then transferred to wells

Hepatitis C virus
ANTIBODY DETECTION (IgG)

Manufacturer: Murex Diagnostics Limited
Cat. No./Trade name: VK47/48 Murex anti-HCV

SUMMARY

[Well-Ag]–**Ab**–[AHIgG-HRP]–[TMB]–A_{450}

Assay type: EIA (non-competitive)
Detection: Colorimetric A_{450}
Format: Microtitre well, Ag coated
Sample type: Serum, plasma
Sample pre-treatment:
　None
Sample volume: 20 µl (+180 µl diluent)
Number of tests: 96, 480
Controls - standards run in assay:
　Controls: Neg (3), Pos (2)
Incubation:
　1 hr (37°C) + 30 min (37°C) + 30 min (37°C)
Washes: 2

CONTENTS

Antibodies, antigens, labelled components:
　HCV Ag (C, NS3, NS4, NS5) bound to well
　Anti-human IgG MAb (m) HRP conjugated
Substrate: TMB, H_2O_2
Controls - standards supplied:
　Controls: Neg and Pos (human serum)
Additional reagents:
　H_2SO_4
Special equipment required:
　Wellcozyme microwell plate washing system (optional)
　Wellcozyme microwell plate reader (optional)

INTERPRETATION

Comments on interpretation:
　Positive: ≥ cut-off repeatably and investigated further
No. of references: 14

NOTES

110663.0

© *KLUWER ACADEMIC PUBLISHERS 1994, ISSN 1381-5067*

Hepatitis C virus
ANTIBODY DETECTION (IgG)

Manufacturer: Sanofi Diagnostics Pasteur
Cat. No./Trade name: 72306/MONOLISA® anti-HCV
(new antigens)

SUMMARY

[Well-Ag]–**Ab**–[AHIgG-POD]–[OPD]–$A_{492/620}$

Assay type: EIA (non-competitive)
Detection: Colorimetric $A_{492/620}$
Format: Microtitre well, Ag coated
Sample type: Serum
Sample pre-treatment:
   None
Sample volume: 20 µl (+80 µl diluent)*
Number of tests: 96, 480
Controls - standards run in assay:
   Controls: Neg (2), Pos (3)
Incubation:
   1 hr (40°C) + 30 min (40°C) + 30 min (RT)
Washes: 2

CONTENTS

Antibodies, antigens, labelled components:
   rec and syn HCV Ag bound to well
   Anti-human IgG Ab (g) POD conjugated
Substrate: OPD
Controls - standards supplied:
   Controls: Neg and Pos (human serum)
Additional reagents:
   None
Special equipment required:
   None

INTERPRETATION

Comments on interpretation:
   Equivocal: within cut-off and cut-off–10%; retest to
   confirm
   Positive: ≥cut-off repeatably
No. of references: None

NOTES

110670.0

*It is also possible to dispense 100 µl of 1.5 dilution of
   sample

Hepatitis C virus
ANTIBODY DETECTION (IgG)

Manufacturer: Sorin Biomedica
Cat. No./Trade name: 3018/ETI-AB-HCVK

SUMMARY

[Well-Ag]–**Ab**–[AHIgG-HRP]–[TMB]–A_{450}

Assay type: EIA (non-competitive)
Detection: Colorimetric A_{450}
Format: Microtitre well, Ag coated
Sample type: Serum, plasma
Sample pre-treatment:
   None
Sample volume: 15 µl (+300 µl diluent)
Number of tests: 96
Controls - standards run in assay:
   Controls: Neg (3), Pos (2)
Incubation:
   30 min (37°C)* + 30 min (37°C)* + 30 min (RT)
Washes: 2

CONTENTS

Antibodies, antigens, labelled components:
   HCV Ag bound to well
   Anti-human IgG Ab (g) HRP conjugated
Substrate: TMB, H_2O_2
Controls - standards supplied:
   Controls: Neg (human serum), Pos (human plasma)
Additional reagents:
   None
Special equipment required:
   ETI-system reader and software (optional)
   ETI-system shaker/incubator (optional)
   ETI-system washer

INTERPRETATION

Comments on interpretation:
   Positive: ≥cut-off repeatably and confirmed by
      supplemental tests
No. of references: 12

NOTES

110239.0

*The first 2 incubations are on a plate shaker
This kit is not available in the UK

© KLUWER ACADEMIC PUBLISHERS 1994, ISSN 1381-5067

Hepatitis C virus
ANTIBODY DETECTION

Manufacturer: Innogenetics SA
Cat. No./Trade name: /INNO-LIA HCV Ab III

SUMMARY

[Strip-Ag]–**Ab**–[AHIgG-AP]–[BCIP]–colour

Assay type: Immunoblot assay
Detection: Visual
Format: Nylon strip, Ag coated
Sample type: Serum, plasma
Sample pre-treatment:
 None
Sample volume: 10 μl (+ 1 ml diluent)
Number of tests:
Controls - standards run in assay:
 Controls: Neg (1), Pos (1)
 Integral controls: (4) on nylon strip
Incubation:
 16 hr (RT) + 30 min (RT) + 10-30 min (RT). Use orbital
 mixer during incubation
Washes: 2

CONTENTS

Antibodies, antigens, labelled components:
 HCV Ag (core, E2/NS1, NS3, NS4, NS5) bound to nylon
 strip in 6 discrete lines
 Anti-human IgG Ab (g) AP conjugated
Substrate: BCIP
Controls - standards supplied:
 Integral controls: strong Pos, moderate Pos, weak Pos
 (human) anti-streptavidin control
 Batch controls: Neg and Pos (human serum)
Additional reagents:
 None
Special equipment required:
 Orbital mixer e.g. DENLEY OM501 or KOTTERMAN
 4010

INTERPRETATION

Comments on interpretation:
 Negative: if all HCV antigen lines have negative reactivity
 rating
 Positive: if one HCV Ag line has a reactivity rating $\geqslant$ (2+)
 or if at least two HCV Ag lines have a reactivity rating
 $\geqslant$ (1+)
 Indeterminate: if reactivity rating is (1+) or ($\pm$) advise
 patient follow-up
No. of references: 7

NOTES

110321.0

Hepatitis D virus (HDV) (Hepatitis delta)

Natural history

Infection with hepatitis delta virus is dependent on the simultaneous presence of hepatitis B virus and reaches a maximum in persons with the highest levels of HBV replication. Classification of HDV remains uncertain; distinct from any known human virus, the RNA genome of HDV is similar to that of plant viroids. The HBV DNA is necessary for synthesis of the envelope which constitutes the surface of HDV as well as of HBV particles. Hepatitis delta occurs as a co-infection with hepatitis B, or as a superinfection in around 5% of carriers of HBV, and is mainly transmitted by parenteral routes, with an incubation period of 3–7 weeks. Sexual transmission is also thought to occur. HDV is found throughout the world; it is endemic in Southern Europe and the Middle East, and causes epidemics/outbreaks in communities or groups with a high rate of HBV carriage. Acute co-infection usually leads to clearance of both HDV and HBV within a few months. There is a considerable risk of fulminant hepatitis, particularly in superinfections (20%) and a large proportion (60%) of the survivors go on to have persistent HDV in addition to their HBV. Immunity to hepatitis B is protective against HDV, however the HBV carrier is always at risk for hepatitis delta. Antiviral therapy for chronic hepatitis delta has been less successful than for the other chronic active hepatitides.

Diagnosis and markers

The great majority of HDV infections are diagnosed in patients positive for HBs antigen, but occasional cases can be HBsAg negative, IgM anti-HBcore positive. Diagnosis of current infection is based on detection of antibodies to the hepatitis delta antigen (HDAg). HDAg is produced in two forms (p22, p24), coded for by the HDV RNA, and acts as an RNA binding protein. HDAg is present in virions and can be demonstrated in serum treated to disrupt the envelope of particles. Antigenaemia and IgM anti-HDAg are found in the early phase of acute HDV infection, followed by appearance of IgG anti-HDAg. Both IgM and IgG antibodies disappear in the months after recovery, while both persist in chronic HDV infection. HD antigen can be demonstrated in hepatocytes also. HDV RNA is detectable by PCR, and mutants are known to occur.

Comment

There is no marker for past HDV infection at present since IgG antibody to HDAg disappears after recovery. Some protection is maintained however, as disease is modified in re-infections.

References

Lai MMC. Hepatitis delta virus. Webster RG and Granoff A (eds). Encyclopedia of Virology. London Academic Press. 1994;2:574–80.

© *KLUWER ACADEMIC PUBLISHERS 1994, ISSN 1381-5067*

Hepatitis D virus
ANTIGEN DETECTION

Manufacturer: Cambridge Biotech Corporation
Cat. No./Trade name: CB6496 DELTASSAY Ag EIA Kit

SUMMARY

[Well-Ab]–**Ag**–[Ab-HRP]–[TMB]–A_{450}

Assay type: EIA (non-competitive)
Detection: Colorimetric A_{450}
Format: Microtitre well, Ab coated
Sample type: Serum, plasma
Sample pre-treatment:
  None
Sample volume: 50 µl
Number of tests: 96
Controls - standards run in assay:
  Controls: Neg (3), Pos (2)
Incubation:
  Overnight (RT) + 1 hr (37°C) + 30 min (RT)
Washes: 2 (+ preliminary plate wash)

CONTENTS

Antibodies, antigens, labelled components:
  Anti-HDv IgG Ab (h) bound to well
  Anti-HDv Ab HRP conjugated
Substrate: TMB
Controls - standards supplied:
  Controls: Neg and Pos (human)
Additional reagents:
  None
Special equipment required:
  None

INTERPRETATION

Comments on interpretation:
  Positive: > cut-off repeatably
No. of references: 6

NOTES

110655.0

For research use only

Hepatitis D virus
ANTIGEN DETECTION

Manufacturer: Murex Diagnostics Limited
Cat. No./Trade name: VK32/Wellcozyme HDAg

SUMMARY

[Well-Ab]–**Ag**–[Ab-HRP]–[TMB]–A_{450}

Assay type: EIA (non-competitive)
Detection: Colorimetric A_{450}
Format: Microtitre well, Ab coated
Sample type: Serum, plasma
Sample pre-treatment:
  None
Sample volume: 50 µl
Number of tests: 96
Controls - standards run in assay:
  Controls: Neg (3), Pos (2)
Incubation:
  18-24 hr (RT) + 1 hr (37°C) + 30 min (RT)
Washes: 2 (+ preliminary plate wash)

CONTENTS

Antibodies, antigens, labelled components:
  Anti-HD Ab (h) bound to wells
  Anti-HD Ab (h) HRP conjugated
Substrate: TMB, H_2O_2
Controls - standards supplied:
  Controls: Neg and Pos (human serum)
Additional reagents:
  None
Special equipment required:
  Wellcozyme microwell plate washing system (optional)
  Wellcozyme microwell plate reader system (optional)

INTERPRETATION

Comments on interpretation:
  Classification of sample is according to cut-off; no further testing
No. of references: 8

NOTES

110162.0

Hepatitis D virus
ANTIGEN DETECTION*

Manufacturer: Organon Teknika NV
Cat. No./Trade name: 71528/Hepanostika® HDV

SUMMARY

[Well-Ab]–**Ag**–[Ab-HRP]–[TMB]–A$_{450}$

Assay type: EIA (non-competitive)
Detection: Colorimetric A$_{450}$
Format: Microtitre well, Ab coated
Sample type: Serum, plasma**
Sample pre-treatment:
  None
Sample volume: 50 µl
Number of tests: 96
Controls - standards run in assay:
  Controls: Neg (3), Pos (1)
Incubation:
  a) 1 hr (37°C) + 1 hr (37°C) + 30 min (RT)
  b) 16-24 hr (RT) + 1 hr (37°C) + 30 min (RT)
Washes: 2

CONTENTS

Antibodies, antigens, labelled components:
  Anti-HD Ab (h) bound to well
  HD Ag (chimp or human liver extract) (for Ab detection)
  Anti-HD Ab (h) HRP conjugated
Substrate: TMB, H$_2$O$_2$
Controls - standards supplied:
  Controls: Neg and Pos (human serum)
Additional reagents:
  H$_2$SO$_4$, 6% nonionic detergent
Special equipment required:
  None

INTERPRETATION

Comments on interpretation:
  Positive: ≥ cut-off repeatably and confirmed by additional
    testing for Hepatitis B virus markers on present
    sample. Retest of fresh sample taken a few weeks
    later for anti-Delta virus
No. of references: 4

NOTES

110555.0

*This kit is used for the detection of both hepatitis delta Ag
  and Ab. Details of the Ab detection are in the appropriate
  section
**Heat inactivation may give erroneous results

Hepatitis D virus
ANTIGEN DETECTION

Manufacturer: Sanofi Diagnostics Pasteur
Cat. No./Trade name: 72214/DELTASSAY® Ag

SUMMARY

[Well-Ab]–**Ag**–[Ab-POD]–[OPD]–A$_{492/620}$

Assay type: EIA (non-competitive)
Detection: Colorimetric A$_{492/620}$
Format: Microtitre well, Ab coated
Sample type: Serum, plasma
Sample pre-treatment:
  None
Sample volume: 50 µl (+50 µl extraction buffer)
Number of tests: 96
Controls - standards run in assay:
  Controls: Neg (3), Pos (2)
Incubation:
  Overnight (RT) + 1 hr (40°C) + 30 min (RT)
Washes: 2 (+ preliminary plate prewash)

CONTENTS

Antibodies, antigens, labelled components:
  Anti-HD Ab bound to well
  Anti-HD Ab POD conjugated
Substrate: OPD, H$_2$O$_2$
Controls - standards supplied:
  Controls: Neg and Pos
Additional reagents:
  None
Special equipment required:
  None

INTERPRETATION

Comments on interpretation:
  Positive: > cut-off value repeatably
No. of references: 6

NOTES

110271.0

© KLUWER ACADEMIC PUBLISHERS 1994, ISSN 1381-5067

Hepatitis D virus
ANTIGEN DETECTION

Manufacturer: Sorin Biomedica
Cat. No./Trade name: 8146/ETI-DELTAK

SUMMARY

[Well-Ab]–**Ag**–[Ab-HRP]–[TMB]–A_{450}

Assay type: EIA (non-competitive)
Detection: Colorimetric A_{450}
Format: Microtitre well, Ab coated
Sample type: Serum, plasma
Sample pre-treatment:
    None
Sample volume: 75 µl (+25 µl Tween)
Number of tests: 96
Controls - standards run in assay:
    Controls: Neg (3); Pos (2)
Incubation:
    Overnight (RT) + 2 hr (37°C) + 30 min (RT)
Washes: 2

CONTENTS

Antibodies, antigens, labelled components:
    Anti-HD IgG Ab (h) bound to well
    Anti-HD IgG Ab (h) HRP conjugated
Substrate: TMB, H_2O_2
Controls - standards supplied:
    Controls: Neg (human serum) and Pos
Additional reagents:
    None
Special equipment required:
    None

INTERPRETATION

Comments on interpretation:
    Equivocal: Within cut-off ± 10%; retest to confirm
No. of references: 8

NOTES

110227.0

Hepatitis D virus
ANTIGEN DETECTION

Manufacturer: Sorin Biomedica
Cat. No./Trade name: 5211/DELTAK

SUMMARY

[Bead-Ab]–**Ag**–[Ab-^{125}I]–radioactivity

Assay type: RIA (non-competitive)
Detection: Radioisotopic
Format: Tube, Ab coated bead
Sample type: Serum, plasma
Sample pre-treatment:
    None
Sample volume: 150 µl (+50 µl Tween)
Number of tests: 50
Controls - standards run in assay:
    Controls: Neg (3), Pos (2)
Incubation:
    18-22 hr (RT) + 2 hr (45°C)
Washes: 2

CONTENTS

Antibodies, antigens, labelled components:
    Anti-HD Ab (h) bound to beads
    Anti-HD IgG Ab (h) ^{125}I labelled
Substrate:
Controls - standards supplied:
    Controls: Neg (human serum) and Pos
Additional reagents:
    None
Special equipment required:
    Automatic rinser, PLA-2 (optional)
    Bead dispenser, MEDI-578 (optional)

INTERPRETATION

Comments on interpretation:
    Equivocal: Within cut-off ± 10%; retest to confirm
No. of references: 8

NOTES

110218.0

© KLUWER ACADEMIC PUBLISHERS 1994, ISSN 1381-5067

Hepatitis D virus
ANTIBODY DETECTION

Manufacturer: Abbott Laboratories
Cat. No./Trade name: 3018/ABBOTT ANTI-DELTA EIA

SUMMARY

$$[\text{Bead-Ag}]\bigg\langle \begin{array}{l} \textbf{Ab} \\ [\text{Ab-HRP}] \end{array} -[\text{OPD}]-A_{492}$$

Assay type: EIA (competitive)
Detection: Colorimetric A_{492}
Format: Reaction well, Ag coated bead
Sample type: Serum, plasma
Sample pre-treatment:
　None
Sample volume: 100 µl
Number of tests: 50
Controls - standards run in assay:
　Controls: Neg (3), Pos (2)
Incubation:
　20 hr (RT) + 30 min (RT)
Washes: 1

CONTENTS

Antibodies, antigens, labelled components:
　HD Ag bound to bead
　Anti-HD Ab (h) HRP conjugated
Substrate: OPD, H_2O_2
Controls - standards supplied:
　Controls: Neg and Pos (human plasma)
Additional reagents:
　H_2SO_4
Special equipment required:
　None

INTERPRETATION

Comments on interpretation:
　Equivocal: within cut-off ±5%; retest to confirm
No. of references: 15

NOTES

110032.0

Hepatitis D virus
ANTIBODY DETECTION

Manufacturer: Cambridge Biotech Corporation
Cat. No./Trade name: CB6296 DELTASSAY Ab EIA Kit

SUMMARY

$$[\text{Well-Ag}]\bigg\langle \begin{array}{l} \textbf{Ab} \\ [\text{Ab-HRP}] \end{array} -[\text{TMB}]-A_{450}$$

Assay type: EIA (competitive)
Detection: Colorimetric A_{450}
Format: Microtitre well, Ag coated
Sample type: Serum, plasma
Sample pre-treatment:
　None
Sample volume: 100 µl
Number of tests: 96
Controls - standards run in assay:
　Controls: Neg (3), Pos (2)
Incubation:
　(a)Overnight (RT)* + 1 hr (37°C) + 30 min (RT)
　(b)2 hr (37°C) + 1 hr (37°C) + 30 min (RT)
Washes: 2

CONTENTS

Antibodies, antigens, labelled components:
　HD Ag bound to well
　Anti-HD Ab HRP conjugated
Substrate: TMB
Controls - standards supplied:
　Controls: Neg and Pos (human serum)
Additional reagents:
　None
Special equipment required:
　None

INTERPRETATION

Comments on interpretation:
　Positive: < cut-off repeatably
No. of references: 5

NOTES

110657.0

For research use only
*Overnight incubation gives maximum sensitivity

Hepatitis D virus
ANTIBODY DETECTION

Manufacturer: Murex Diagnostics Limited
Cat. No./Trade name: VK31/Wellcozyme anti-HD

SUMMARY

$$[\text{Well-Ag}] \Big\langle {}^{\textbf{Ab}}_{[\text{Ab-HRP}]} - [\text{TMB}] - A_{450}$$

Assay type: EIA (competitive)
Detection: Colorimetric A_{450}
Format: Microtitre well, Ag coated
Sample type: Serum, plasma
Sample pre-treatment:
　None
Sample volume: 100 µl
Number of tests: 96
Controls - standards run in assay:
　Controls: Neg (3), Pos (2)
Incubation:
　2 hr (37°C) + 1 hr (37°C) + 30 min (RT)
Washes: 2

CONTENTS

Antibodies, antigens, labelled components:
　HD Ag bound to wells
　Anti-HD Ab (h) HRP conjugated
Substrate: TMB, H_2O_2
Controls - standards supplied:
　Controls: Neg and Pos (human serum)
Additional reagents:
　None
Special equipment required:
　Wellcozyme microwell plate washing system (optional)
　Wellcozyme microwell plate reader system (optional)

INTERPRETATION

Comments on interpretation:
　Classification of sample is according to cut-off; no further
　　testing
No. of references: 7

NOTES

110163.0

Hepatitis D virus
*ANTIBODY DETECTION**

Manufacturer: Organon Teknika NV
Cat. No./Trade name: 71528/Hepanostika® HDV

SUMMARY

$$\Big\langle {}^{\textbf{Ab}}_{[\text{Well-Ab}]} [\text{Ag}] - [\text{Ab-HRP}] - [\text{TMB}] - A_{450}$$

Assay type: EIA (competitive)
Detection: Colorimetric A_{450}
Format: Microtitre well, Ab coated
Sample type: Serum, plasma**
Sample pre-treatment:
　None
Sample volume: 50 µl
Number of tests: 96
Controls - standards run in assay:
　Controls:
　Neg (1), Pos (1) (one strip)
　Neg (2), Pos (2) (two or more strips)
Incubation:
　1 hr (37°C) + 1 hr (37°C) + 30 min (RT)
Washes: 2

CONTENTS

Antibodies, antigens, labelled components:
　Anti-HD Ab (h) bound to well
　HD Ag (chimp or human liver extract) (for Ab detection)
　Anti-HD Ab (h) HRP conjugated
Substrate: TMB, H_2O_2
Controls - standards supplied:
　Controls: Neg and Pos (human serum)
Additional reagents:
　H_2SO_4
Special equipment required:
　None

INTERPRETATION

Comments on interpretation:
　Positive: ⩽ cut-off repeatably and confirmed by
　　supplemental tests (e.g. Hepanostika® HDV direct
　　test)
　Semi-quantitative procedure available
No. of references: 4

NOTES

110554.0

*This kit is used for the detection of both hepatitis delta Ag
　and Ab. Details of the Ag detection are in the appropriate
　section
**Heat inactivation may give erroneous results

Hepatitis D virus
ANTIBODY DETECTION

Manufacturer: Sanofi Diagnostics Pasteur
Cat. No./Trade name: 72215/DELTASSAY® Ac Ab AK

SUMMARY

$$[\text{Well-Ag}]\Big\langle\begin{matrix}\textbf{Ab}\\ [\text{Ab-HRP}]\end{matrix}-[\text{OPD}]-A_{492/620}$$

Assay type: EIA (competitive)
Detection: Colorimetric $A_{492/620}$
Format: Microtitre well, Ag coated
Sample type: Serum, plasma
Sample pre-treatment:
  None
Sample volume: 100 µl
Number of tests: 96
Controls - standards run in assay:
  Controls: Neg (3), Pos (2)
Incubation:
  a) overnight (RT) + 1 hr (40°C) + 30 min (RT)
  b) 2 hr (40°C) + 1 hr (40°C) + 30 min (RT)
Washes: 2

CONTENTS

Antibodies, antigens, labelled components:
  HD Ag bound to well
  Anti-HD Ab POD conjugated
Substrate: OPD, H_2O_2
Controls - standards supplied:
  Controls: Neg and Pos (human serum)
Additional reagents:
  None
Special equipment required:
  None

INTERPRETATION

Comments on interpretation:
  Positive: < cut-off value repeatably
No. of references: 4

NOTES

110272.0

Hepatitis D virus
ANTIBODY DETECTION

Manufacturer: Sorin Biomedica
Cat. No./Trade name: P2808/ETI-AB-DELTAK-2

SUMMARY

$$[\text{Well-Ag}]\Big\langle\begin{matrix}\textbf{Ab}\\ [\text{Ab-HRP}]\end{matrix}-[\text{TMB}]-A_{450}$$

Assay type: EIA (competitive)
Detection: Colorimetric A_{450}
Format: Microtitre well, Ag coated
Sample type: Serum, plasma
Sample pre-treatment:
  None
Sample volume: 50 µl
Number of tests: 96
Controls - standards run in assay:
  Controls: Neg (3), Pos (2)
Incubation:
  3 hr (37°C) + 30 min (RT)
Washes: 1

CONTENTS

Antibodies, antigens, labelled components:
  rec HD Ag
  Anti-HD IgG Ab HRP conjugated
Substrate: TMB, H_2O_2
Controls - standards supplied:
  Controls: Neg (human serum) and Pos
Additional reagents:
  None
Special equipment required:
  ETI-system reader and software (optional)

INTERPRETATION

Comments on interpretation:
  Equivocal: Within cut-off ± 10%; retest to confirm
No. of references: 9

NOTES

110231.0

Hepatitis D virus
ANTIBODY DETECTION

Manufacturer: Sorin Biomedica
Cat. No./Trade name: 2415/AB-DELTAK eia

SUMMARY

$$[Bead-Ag] \begin{cases} Ab \\ [Ab-HRP] \end{cases} -[OPD]-A_{492}$$

Assay type: EIA (competitive)
Detection: Colorimetric A_{492}
Format: Tray/Tube, Ag coated bead
Sample type: Serum, plasma
Sample pre-treatment:
    None
Sample volume: 100 µl
Number of tests: 50
Controls - standards run in assay:
    Controls: Neg (3), Pos (2)
Incubation:
    18-22 hr (RT) + 30 min (RT)
Washes: 1

CONTENTS

Antibodies, antigens, labelled components:
    HD Ag bound to bead
    Anti-HD Ag IgG Ab (h) HRP conjugated
Substrate: OPD; H_2O_2
Controls - standards supplied:
    Controls: Neg and Pos (human serum)
Additional reagents:
    None
Special equipment required:
    Automatic rinsing device, PLA-2 (optional)
    Bead dispenser, MEDI-578 (optional)

INTERPRETATION

Comments on interpretation:
    Equivocal: Within cut-off ± 10%; retest to confirm
No. of references: 9

NOTES

110241.0

This kit will be discontinued in December 1994

Hepatitis D virus
ANTIBODY DETECTION (IgM)

Manufacturer: Cambridge Biotech Corporation
Cat. No./Trade name: CB6596 DELTASSAY IgM EIA Kit

SUMMARY

$$[Well-AHIgM]-Ab-[Ag]-[Ab-HRP]-[TMB]-A_{450}$$

Assay type: EIA (non-competitive)
Detection: Colorimetric A_{450}
Format: Microtitre well, Ab coated
Sample type: Serum, plasma
Sample pre-treatment:
    None
Sample volume: 10 µl (+1 ml diluent)*
Number of tests: 96
Controls - standards run in assay:
    Controls: Neg (2), Pos (2)
Incubation:
    1 hr (37°C) + overnight (RT) + 1 hr (37°C) + 30 min (RT)
Washes: 3 (+ preliminary plate wash)

CONTENTS

Antibodies, antigens, labelled components:
    Anti-human IgM Ab (r) bound to well
    HD Ag
    Anti-HD Ab HRP conjugated
Substrate: TMB
Controls - standards supplied:
    Controls: Neg and Pos (human serum); Antigen control (human serum)
Additional reagents:
    None
Special equipment required:
    None

INTERPRETATION

Comments on interpretation:
    Positive: > cut-off repeatably
No. of references: 4

NOTES

110654.0

For research use only
*Samples are tested in duplicate

© KLUWER ACADEMIC PUBLISHERS 1994, ISSN 1381-5067

Hepatitis D virus
ANTIBODY DETECTION (IgM)

Manufacturer: Murex Diagnostics Limited
Cat. No./Trade name: VK33/Wellcozyme anti-HD IgM

SUMMARY

[Well-AHIgM]–**Ab**–[Ag]–[Ab-HRP]–[TMB]–A_{450}

Assay type: EIA (non-competitive)
Detection: Colorimetric A_{450}
Format: Microtitre well, Ab coated
Sample type: Serum, plasma
Sample pre-treatment:
  None
Sample volume: 10 μl (+ 1 ml diluent)*
Number of tests: 96
Controls - standards run in assay:
  Controls: Neg (2), Pos (2)
Incubation:
  1 hr (37°C) + 18 hr (RT) + 1 hr (37°C) + 30 min (RT)
Washes: 3 (+ preliminary plate wash)

CONTENTS

Antibodies, antigens, labelled components:
  Anti-human IgM Ab (r) bound to well
  HD Ag
  Anti-HD Ab (h) HRP conjugated
Substrate: TMB, H_2O_2
Controls - standards supplied:
  Controls: Neg and Pos (human serum)
Additional reagents:
  None
Special equipment required:
  Wellcozyme microwell plate washing system (optional)
  Wellcozyme microwell plate reader system (optional)

INTERPRETATION

Comments on interpretation:
  Positive: ⩾cut-off repeatably
No. of references: 6

NOTES

110164.0

*Sample assayed in duplicate wells (test and control wells);
  Delta antigen is added to test well and antigen control is
  added to control well

Hepatitis D virus
ANTIBODY DETECTION (IgM)

Manufacturer: Sanofi Diagnostics Pasteur
Cat. No./Trade name: 72216/DELTASSAY® IgM

SUMMARY

[Well-AHIgM]–**Ab**–[Ag]–[Ab-POD]–[TMB]–$A_{450/620}$

Assay type: EIA (non-competitive)
Detection: Colorimetric $A_{492/620}$
Format: Microtitre well, Ab coated
Sample type: Serum, plasma
Sample pre-treatment:
  None
Sample volume: 100 μl of 1:100 dilution x 2*
Number of tests: 96
Controls - standards run in assay:
  Controls: Neg (2), Pos (2)
Incubation:
  1 hr (40°C) + overnight (RT) + 1 hr (40°C) + 30 min
  (RT)
Washes: 3 (+ preliminary plate prewash)

CONTENTS

Antibodies, antigens, labelled components:
  Anti-human IgM Ab bound to well
  HD Ag and control Ag
  Anti-HD Ab POD conjugated
Substrate: TMB, H_2O_2
Controls - standards supplied:
  Controls: Ab Neg and Pos (human serum); Ag control
  (human serum)
Additional reagents:
  None
Special equipment required:
  None

INTERPRETATION

Comments on interpretation:
  Positive: sample OD corrected value ⩾0.08 repeatably
No. of references: 4

NOTES

110270.0

*Duplicate wells are incubated in parallel with Delta Ag or
  control Ag

Hepatitis D virus
ANTIBODY DETECTION (IgM)

Manufacturer: Sorin Biomedica
Cat. No./Trade name: 8148/ETI-DELTA-IGMK

SUMMARY

$$[\text{Well-AHIgM}]-\textbf{Ab}-[\text{Ag}]-[\text{Ab-HRP}]-[\text{TMB}]-A_{450}$$

Assay type: EIA (non-competitive)
Detection: Colorimetric A_{450}
Format: Microtitre well, Ab coated
Sample type: Serum, plasma
Sample pre-treatment:
    None
Sample volume: 10 µl (+ 1 ml diluent)
Number of tests: 96
Controls - standards run in assay:
    Controls: Neg (3), Pos (2)
Incubation:
    1 hr (37°C) + overnight (RT) + 1 hr (37°C) + 30 min
       (RT)
Washes: 3

CONTENTS

Antibodies, antigens, labelled components:
    Anti-human IgM IgG MAb (m) bound to well
    HD Ag
    Anti-HD IgG Ab (h) HRP conjugated
Substrate: TMB, H_2O_2
Controls - standards supplied:
    Controls: Neg and Pos (human serum)
Additional reagents:
    None
Special equipment required:
    None

INTERPRETATION

Comments on Interpretation:
    Equivocal: Within cut-off ± 10%; retest to confirm
No. of references: 6

NOTES

110230.0

Hepatitis D virus
ANTIBODY DETECTION

Manufacturer: Sorin Biomedica
Cat. No./Trade name: 2908/Ab-DELTAK

SUMMARY

$$[\text{Bead-Ag}]\left\langle\begin{array}{l}\textbf{Ab}\\ [\text{Ab}^{125}\text{I}]\end{array}\right. \rightarrow\text{radioactivity}$$

Assay type: RIA (competitive)
Detection: Radioisotopic
Format: Tray/Tube, Ag coated bead
Sample type: Serum, plasma
Sample pre-treatment:
    None
Sample volume: 100 µl
Number of tests: 50
Controls - standards run in assay:
    Controls: Neg (3), Pos (2)
Incubation:
    Overnight (RT)
Washes: 1

CONTENTS

Antibodies, antigens, labelled components:
    Anti-HD Ab bound to beads
    Anti-HD IgG Ab (h) ^{125}I labelled
Substrate:
Controls - standards supplied:
    Controls: Neg and Pos (human serum)
Additional reagents:
    None
Special equipment required:
    Automatic rinser, PLA-2 (optional)
    Bead dispenser, MEDI-578

INTERPRETATION

Comments on Interpretation:
    Equivocal: Within cut-off ± 10%; retest to confirm
No. of references: 9

NOTES

110220.0

Hepatitis D virus
ANTIBODY DETECTION (IgM)

Manufacturer: Sorin Biomedica
Cat. No./Trade name: 5209/DELTA-IGMK

SUMMARY

[Bead-AHIgM]–**Ab**–[Ag]–[Ab-^{125}I]–radioactivity

Assay type: RIA (non-competitive)
Detection: Radioisotopic
Format: Tray/Tube, Ab coated bead
Sample type: Serum, plasma
Sample pre-treatment:
   None
Sample volume: 10 µl (+1 ml diluent)
Number of tests: 50
Controls - standards run in assay:
   Controls: Neg (3), Pos (2)
Incubation:
   1 hr (45°C) + 18-22 hr (RT) + 2 hr (45°C)
Washes: 3

CONTENTS

Antibodies, antigens, labelled components:
   Anti-human IgM Ab bound to beads
   Hepatitis HD Ag
   Anti-HD Ab (h) ^{125}I labelled
Substrate:
Controls - standards supplied:
   Controls: Neg and Pos (human serum)
Additional reagents:
   None
Special equipment required:
   Automatic rinser, PLA-2 (optional)
   Bead dispenser, MEDI-578 (optional)

INTERPRETATION

Comments on interpretation:
   Equivocal: Within cut-off ± 10%; retest to confirm
   Positive: ≥cut-off repeatably
No. of references: None

NOTES

110219.0

Herpes simplex virus (HSV-1; HSV-2) (Genital herpes)

Natural history

Either serotype of herpes simplex virus may infect any mucosal or cutaneous site, producing painful red papules progressing to intra-epithelial vesicles which rapidly ulcerate prior to gradual re-epithelialisation. However many infections are sub-clinical or not recognised as herpetic. HSV type 1 oral infection (gingivo-stomatitis) is often acquired in childhood, and latent virus is established in the trigeminal ganglion, from where it may reactivate and lead to recurrent muco-cutaneous lesions. Genital tract infection with HSV is mainly acquired after puberty by sexual contact, including oro-genital contact. Genital herpes as a primary (first-ever) HSV infection is more severe than a non-primary (initial genital) infection with HSV-2 in someone with previous HSV-1 as there is some cross-protection. Systemic symptoms occur and recovery takes 3–4 weeks; complications include sacral radiculopathy and rarely disseminated or CNS disease. HSV from genital lesions becomes latent in the sacral nerve ganglia, with the recognised potential for reactivation, asymptomatic shedding and recurrent disease in the area innervated. HSV-2 recurs more frequently than HSV-1 at this site; recurrent episodes are shorter, lasting 7–10 days. Transmission may occur during any period of active virus shedding, which may not be recognised. Persistent ulcerative disease is seen in severe immune deficiency. Infants exposed to primary maternal HSV during birth are at high risk of life-threatening neonatal herpes simplex.

Diagnosis and markers

Acute genital herpes is readily diagnosed by virus isolation from swabs of vesicles or early ulcers. Fluorescent-labelled monoclonal antibodies to common or type-specific epitopes on glycoprotein or other antigens can be applied directly to cell smears from ulcer bases for virus identification, or to cells showing a characteristic cytopathic effect (cpe) in culture for confirmation and serotyping. Centrifugation-enhanced cultures can be stained for antigen prior to development of cpe. Enzyme immunoassays used in the direct detection of virus antigen offer earlier results but do not achieve the sensitivity of culture in asymptomatic cases. HSV DNA detection by PCR amplifica-tion has a place when isolation is a problem, as in investigation of neonatal herpes, herpes encephalitis and asymptomatic shedding. Serological diagnosis of a primary HSV infection is generally straightforward, although seroconversion may be delayed after antiviral therapy. EIAs for antibody are used as well as the traditional complement fixation test (CFT) which is not type-specific. Truly type-specific antibody assays have not been available commercially. Surveys by investigators using EIA for antibody to type-specific glycoproteins (gG1, gG2) or immunoblotting have shown that many women without any history of clinical genital herpes have antibody to HSV-2.

Comment

Genital herpes is a significant diagnosis, with implications for recurrence and transmissibility. Effective safe antiviral treatment for acute episodes and suppression of recurrences has been available for more than ten years, but does not affect latent virus. Laboratory confirmation of a first clinical diagnosis of genital herpes should be undertaken. Serology is useful in confirming primary infection, and type-specific antibody immunoassays will be increasingly important to establish if either virus is latent.

Reference

Corey L. Herpes simplex virus infections during the decade since the licensure of acyclovir. Journal of Medical Virology. 1993;Supplement 1:7–12.

Herpes simplex virus
ANTIGEN DETECTION

Manufacturer: Dako A/S
Cat. No./Trade name: K6000/IDEIA® HERPES SIMPLEX VIRUS Test

SUMMARY

[Well-MAb]–**Ag**–[MAb-AP]–[NADP + ampl]–A_{492}

Assay type: EIA (non-competitive, amplified)
Detection: Colorimetric A_{492}
Format: Microtitre well, Ab coated
Sample type: Swabs: lesions, cervix, in transport medium
Sample pre-treatment:
   Vortex (15 sec)
Sample volume: 200 µl
Number of tests: 96
Controls - standards run in assay:
   Controls: Neg (3), Pos (1)
Incubation:
   3 hr (RT) + 40 min (RT) + 10 min (RT)
Washes: 1

CONTENTS

Antibodies, antigens, labelled components:
   Anti-HSV MAb (m) bound to wells
   Anti-HSV (Fab) MAb (m) AP conjugated
Substrate: NADP + amplifier
Controls - standards supplied:
   Controls: Neg (transport medium), Pos
Additional reagents:
   None
Special equipment required:
   IDEIA® HSV Specimen Collection Kit (optional)

INTERPRETATION

Comments on interpretation:
   Classification of samples is according to cut-off; no further testing
No. of references: 13

NOTES

110037.0

Herpes simplex virus
ANTIGEN DETECTION

Manufacturer: Kodak Clinical Diagnostics
Cat. No./Trade name: 805 7085/KODAK SURECELL® Herpes (HSV) Test

SUMMARY

[Treated membrane]–**Ag**–[MAb-enzyme]–[dye]–
red dot

Assay type: EIA (non-competitive)
Detection: Visual
Format: Test cell membrane treated to bind HSV Ag
Sample type: Swabs* (genital, rectal, oral dermal), transport medium from swabs, tissue culture cells
Sample pre-treatment:
   Sample extraction in buffer provided
Sample volume: Not specified
Number of tests: 10, 25
Controls - standards run in assay:
   Controls: Neg (1), Integral Pos (1)
Incubation:
   Read results 5 min after adding the final reagent (dye) to wells
Washes: 3

CONTENTS

Antibodies, antigens, labelled components:
   Anti-HSV MAb enzyme conjugated
Substrate: Not specified
Controls - standards supplied:
   Controls: Neg control conjugate, Integral Pos (HSV-1, HSV-2 bound to membrane in Pos control well)
Additional reagents:
   None
Special equipment required:
   None

INTERPRETATION

Comments on interpretation:
   Negative: colour in sample well equal to colour in Neg control well
   Positive: uniform pink/red colour in sample well greater than colour in Neg control well
   Invalid: red/pink colour in Neg control well or no colour in Pos control well; repeat test
No. of references: 0

NOTES

110660.0

*It is preferable to use special swabs provided. Do not use calcium alginate swabs

© KLUWER ACADEMIC PUBLISHERS 1994, ISSN 1381-5067

Herpes simplex virus
ANTIGEN DETECTION

Manufacturer: Murex Diagnostics Limited
Cat. No./Trade name: WZ02/Wellcozyme HSV

SUMMARY

[Well-MAb]–**Ag**–[MAb-AP]–[NADP-ampl]–A_{492}

Assay type: EIA (non-competitive, amplified)
Detection: Colorimetric A_{492}
Format: Microtitre well, Ab coated
Sample type: Dry swabs, swabs in transport medium/ extraction buffer*, cell culture lysate
Sample pre-treatment:
Dry swab: add 1 ml extraction buffer; vortex 10 sec
Swabs in fluid: vortex 10 sec
Cell culture: dilute fluid with extraction buffer
Sample volume: 150 µl
Number of tests: 96
Controls - standards run in assay:
Controls: Neg (3), Pos (2)
Incubation:
2 hr (37°C) + 30 min (37°C) + 10 min (RT)
Washes: 1

CONTENTS

Antibodies, antigens, labelled components:
Anti-HSV MAb (m) bound to wells
Anti-HSV MAb (m) AP conjugated
Substrate: NADP + amplifier
Controls - standards supplied:
Controls: Neg (diluted extraction buffer or transport medium); Pos (HSV-1 and HSV-2)
Additional reagents:
H_2SO_4
Special equipment required:
Wellcozyme microwell plate washing system (optional)
Wellcozyme microwell plate reader (optional)

INTERPRETATION

Comments on interpretation:
Positive: ⩾cut-off repeatably and confirmed by Wellcozyme HSV confirmatory test
Visual interpretation is possible
No. of references: 15

NOTES

110169.0

*Swabs collected in extraction buffer give higher HSV detection rate. Swabs in transport medium should be innoculated concurrently into cell culture to ensure no positive sample are missed

Herpes simplex virus
ANTIGEN DETECTION

Manufacturer: Savyon Diagnostics Ltd
Cat. No./Trade name: 250-01/HerpELISA Kit

SUMMARY

[Well-Ab]–**Ag**–[Ab-HRP]–[TMB]–A_{450}

Assay type: EIA (non-competitive)
Detection: Colorimetric A_{450}
Format: Microtitre well, Ab coated
Sample type: Swabs from vesicles, ulcers, endocervix
Sample pre-treatment:
Extraction of swab sample into specimen diluent
Sample volume: 200 µl of extract
Number of tests: 96
Controls - standards run in assay:
Controls: Neg (3), Pos (1)
Incubation:
3 hr (37°C) + 45 min (37°C) + 20 min (RT)
Washes: 1

CONTENTS

Antibodies, antigens, labelled components:
Anti-HSV-1 and HSV-2 PAb bound to well
Anti-HSV-1 and HSV-2 Ab HRP conjugated
Substrate: TMB
Controls - standards supplied:
Controls: Neg and Pos
Additional reagents:
Washing solution, sample diluent
Special equipment required:
HerpELISA collection and transport system*

INTERPRETATION

Comments on interpretation:
Classification of samples is according to cut-off; no further testing
No. of references: 7

NOTES

110596.0

*If not using recommended collection and transport system, use only cotton and dacron tipped swabs

© **KLUWER ACADEMIC PUBLISHERS 1994, ISSN 1381-5067**

Herpes simplex virus
ANTIGEN DETECTION

Manufacturer: Baxter Diagnostics Inc (Bartels Division)
Cat. No./Trade name: B1029-47/HSV Monoclonal FA Kit

SUMMARY

[Slide]–**Ag**–[MAb-FITC]–fluorescence

Assay type: Immunofluorescence assay (direct)
Detection: Fluorescence microscopy
Format: Slide well, or vial with fixed cell monolayer
Sample type: Cell culture cells showing HSV cytopathogenic effect*
Sample pre-treatment:
  Vials: remove culture medium, rinse with PBS, add acetone
  Tubes: remove culture medium, rinse with PBS, spot cells onto slide, dry, fix with acetone
Sample volume: One vial monolayer or 1 drop from tube culture
Number of tests: 100, 200
Controls - standards run in assay:
  Controls: Neg (1), Pos (1)
Incubation:
  30 min (37°C)
Washes: 2

CONTENTS

Antibodies, antigens, labelled components:
  Anti-HSV MAb FITC conjugated
Substrate:
Controls - standards supplied:
  Controls: Neg and Pos (Ag control slides with Neg and Pos wells)
Additional reagents:
  None
Special equipment required:
  None

INTERPRETATION

Comments on interpretation:
  Negative: uninfected cells stained dull red and no fluorescence
  Positive: bright green fluorescence in cytoplasm of infected cells
No. of references: 5

NOTES

110357.0

*Clinical specimens are vesicular fluid, basal cells from ulcerated or crusted lesions, cervical, vulval, or conjunctival scrapings, CSF (all vortexed and centrifuged prior to innoculation into tissue culture vials/tubes)

Herpes simplex virus
ANTIGEN DETECTION

Manufacturer: Syva Company
Cat. No./Trade name: 8H529/MicroTrak® HSV culture identification test

SUMMARY

[Slide]–**Ag**–[MAb-FITC]–fluorescence

Assay type: Immunofluorescence assay (direct)
Detection: Fluorescence microscopy
Format: Slide/well specimen coated
Sample type: Infected tissue culture cell*
Sample pre-treatment:
  Acetone fix air-dried smear or washed coverslip (10 min)
Sample volume:
Number of tests: 60-300**
Controls - standards run in assay:
  Controls: Neg (1), Pos (2)
Incubation:
  30 min (37°C)
Washes: 1

CONTENTS

Antibodies, antigens, labelled components:
  Anti-HSV MAb (3) (m) FITC conjugated
Substrate:
Controls - standards supplied:
  None
Additional reagents:
  Pos and Neg controls. Microscope slides/wells or shell vials with 12 mm coverslips seeded with MRC-5 cells
Special equipment required:
  None

INTERPRETATION

Comments on interpretation:
  Negative: no fluorescent staining of at least 50 cells; confirm by repeating isolation procedure if necessary
  Positive: fluorescent staining of cytoplasm in at least one intact cell
No. of references: 12

NOTES

110521.0

*Test can be done on conventional cell culture and shell-vial cultures (MRC-5 cells)
**depending on sample format (smear or coverslip)

Herpes simplex virus
ANTIBODY DETECTION (IgG)

Manufacturer: Amico Laboratories Inc
Cat. No./Trade name: 5100G/AMIZYME® HSV IgG

SUMMARY

[Well-Ag]–**Ab**–[AHIgG-HRP]–[ABTS]–A_{405}

Assay type: EIA (non-competitive)
Detection: Colorimetric A_{405}
Format: Microtitre well, Ag coated
Sample type: Serum
Sample pre-treatment:
   None
Sample volume: 10 µl (+490 µl diluent)
Number of tests: 96
Controls - standards run in assay:
   Controls: Neg (1), Pos (1)
Incubation:
   25 min (RT) + 25 min (RT) + 25 min (RT)
Washes: 2

CONTENTS

Antibodies, antigens, labelled components:
   HSV Ag bound to well
   Anti-human IgG Ab (g) HRP conjugated
Substrate: ABTS
Controls - standards supplied:
   Controls: Pos and Neg
Additional reagents:
   None
Special equipment required:
   None

INTERPRETATION

Comments on interpretation:
   Classification of sample is according to cut-off; no further
   testing
No. of references: 18

NOTES

110288.0

Herpes simplex virus
ANTIBODY DETECTION (IgG)

Manufacturer: Behringwerke AG
Cat. No./Trade name: OWMX/Enzygnost® Anti-HSV/
IgG

SUMMARY

[Well-Ag]–**Ab**–[AHIgG-POD]–[TMB]–A_{450}

Assay type: EIA (non-competitive)
Detection: Colorimetric A_{450} or visual
Format: Microtitre well, Ag coated
Sample type: Serum, plasma, Ig preparations
Sample pre-treatment:
   None
Sample volume: 20 µl of 1:21 dilution (+200 µl diluent) x 2*
Number of tests: 48
Controls - standards run in assay:
   Controls: Pos (2) per plate
Incubation:
   1 hr (37°C) + 1 hr (37°C) + 30 min (RT)
Washes: 2

CONTENTS

Antibodies, antigens, labelled components:
   HSV Ag or control tissue culture Ag bound to well
   Anti-human IgG (r), Fab', POD conjugated
Substrate: TMB, H_2O_2
Controls - standards supplied:
   Controls: Pos (human IgG)
Additional reagents:
   Substrate and H_2SO_4
Special equipment required:
   Behring ELISA processor (optional)

INTERPRETATION

Comments on interpretation:
   Equivocal: within range of cut-off value and retest limit;
   retest to confirm. Interpretation of a repeatably
   equivocal result depends on patient group
   A method is available for the comparison of paired sera
   based on a quantitative procedure
No. of references: 23

NOTES

110106.0

*Samples are tested in parallel in Ag and control-Ag coated
   wells

© *KLUWER ACADEMIC PUBLISHERS 1994, ISSN 1381-5067*

Herpes simplex virus
ANTIBODY DETECTION (IgG)

Manufacturer: Biowhittaker
Cat. No./Trade name: 30-637 U/HSV ELISA II

SUMMARY

[Well-Ag]-**Ab**-[AHIgG-AP]-[PMP]-A_{550}

Assay type: EIA (non-competitive)
Detection: Colorimetric A_{550}
Format: Microtitre well, Ag coated
Sample type: Serum (do not heat inactivate)
Sample pre-treatment:
  None
Sample volume: 10 µl (+200 µl diluent)
Number of tests: 192
Controls - standards run in assay:
  Controls: Neg (1), Pos (1)
  Calibrators: (3)
Incubation:
  45 min (RT) + 45 min (RT) + 45 min (RT)
Washes: 2 (+ preliminary plate wash)

CONTENTS

Antibodies, antigens, labelled components:
  HSV Ag (partially purified) bound to well
  Anti-human IgG Ab AP conjugated
Substrate: PMP
Controls - standards supplied:
  Controls: Neg and Pos (human)
  Calibrators: (3) (human) with assigned HSV Elisa values
Additional reagents:
  None
Special equipment required:
  Wellwash 4 automated washer (optional)
  Biowhittaker automated system and software (optional)

INTERPRETATION

Comments on interpretation:
  Equivocal: HSV Elisa Value 0.18-0.19. Retest to
  confirm
No. of references: 3

NOTES

110186.0

Herpes simplex virus
ANTIBODY DETECTION (IgG)

Manufacturer: Biowhittaker
Cat. No./Trade name: 30-337/Herpes STAT

SUMMARY

[Well-Ag]-**Ab**-[AHIgG-AP]-A_{550}

Assay type: EIA (non-competitive)
Detection: Colorimetric A_{550}
Format: Microtitre well, Ag coated
Sample type: Serum
Sample pre-treatment:
  None
Sample volume: 10 µl (+200 µl diluent)
Number of tests: 192
Controls - standards run in assay:
  Controls: Neg (1), Pos (1)
  Standards: low Pos (3), high Pos (1), Neg (1)
Incubation:
  15 min (RT) + 15 min (RT) + 15 min (RT) on plate
  shaker
Washes: 2 (+ preliminary plate wash)

CONTENTS

Antibodies, antigens, labelled components:
  HSV group antigen bound to well
  Anti-human IgG Ab AP conjugated
Substrate: PMP
Controls - standards supplied:
  Controls: Neg and Pos (human)
  Standards: Low Pos, high Pos and Neg (human) with
  assigned index values
Additional reagents:
  None
Special equipment required:
  Biowhittaker automated systems and software (optional)

INTERPRETATION

Comments on interpretation:
  Predicted Index Value (PIV) 0.8-0.99. Retest to confirm
  Repeatably equivocal: retest with an alternative method
  or repeat with a fresh sample
  A method is available for the comparison of acute and
  convalescent sera
No. of references: 3

NOTES

110189.0

© KLUWER ACADEMIC PUBLISHERS 1994, ISSN 1381-5067

Herpes simplex virus
ANTIBODY DETECTION (IgG)

Manufacturer: Laboratoire Eurobio
Cat. No./Trade name: 900279/HERPES IgG ELIT®

SUMMARY

[Well-Ag]–**Ab**–[AHIgG-POD]–[OPD]–$A_{492/630}$

Assay type: EIA (non-competitive)
Detection: Colorimetric $A_{492/630}$
Format: Microtitre well, Ag coated
Sample type: Serum, plasma
Sample pre-treatment:
  None
Sample volume: 10 µl of 1:101 dilution
Number of tests: 96
Controls - standards run in assay:
  Standards: I (1), II (2), III (1), IV (1)
Incubation:
  1 hr (RT) + 1 hr (RT) + 30 min (RT)
Washes: 2

CONTENTS

Antibodies, antigens, labelled components:
  HSV Ag bound to well
  Anti-human IgG PAb (g) POD conjugated
Substrate: OPD, H_2O_2
Controls - standards supplied:
  Standards: 4 (human serum with defined EIA values)
Additional reagents:
  None
Special equipment required:
  None

INTERPRETATION

Comments on interpretation:
  Negative: ratio of sample: standard II absorbance < 0.5;
    retest a fresh sample 1-2 weeks later
  Indeterminate: ratio of sample: standard absorbance
    > 0.5 and < 1.0
  Positive: ratio of sample: standard absorbance > 1.0
  A quantitative assay can also be performed
No. of references: None

NOTES

110528.0

Herpes simplex virus
ANTIBODY DETECTION (IgG)

Manufacturer: Menarini Diagnostics
Cat. No./Trade name: M6238/HF Herpes 1/2 IgG

SUMMARY

[Well-Ag]–**Ab**–[AHIgG-POD]–[TMB]–A_{450}

Assay type: EIA (non-competitive)
Detection: Colorimetric A_{450}
Format: Microtitre well, Ag coated
Sample type: Serum
Sample pre-treatment:
  None
Sample volume: 100 µl (of a 1:101 dilution)
Number of tests: 96
Controls - standards run in assay:
  Controls: Neg (1), Pos (1), cut-off (1)
Incubation:
  45 min (37°C) + 45 min (37°C) + 15 min (RT)
Washes: 2

CONTENTS

Antibodies, antigens, labelled components:
  HSV-1 and HSV-2 Ag bound to well
  Anti-human IgG MAb POD conjugated
Substrate: TMB, H_2O_2
Controls - standards supplied:
  Controls: Neg, Pos and cut-off (serum)
Additional reagents:
  None
Special equipment required:
  Not specified

INTERPRETATION

Comments on interpretation:
  Not specified
No. of references: None

NOTES

110355.0

© KLUWER ACADEMIC PUBLISHERS 1994, ISSN 1381-5067

Herpes simplex virus
ANTIBODY DETECTION (IgM)

Manufacturer: Amico Laboratories Inc
Cat. No./Trade name: 5100M/AMIZYME® HSV IgM

SUMMARY

[Well-Ag]–**Ab**–[AHIgM-HRP]–[ABTS]–A$_{405}$

Assay type: EIA (non-competitive)
Detection: Colorimetric A$_{405}$
Format: Microtitre well, Ag coated
Sample type: Serum
Sample pre-treatment:
  None
Sample volume: 5 µl (+450 µl diluent)
Number of tests: 96
Controls - standards run in assay:
  Controls: Neg (1), weak Pos (1)
  Calibrator: (1)
Incubation:
  25 min (RT) + 25 min (RT) + 25 min (RT)
Washes: 2

CONTENTS

Antibodies, antigens, labelled components:
  HSV Ag bound to well
  Anti-human IgM Ab HRP conjugated
Substrate: ABTS
Controls - standards supplied:
  Controls: Neg and weak Pos
  Calibrator: (1) with assigned concentration
Additional reagents:
  None
Special equipment required:
  None

INTERPRETATION

Comments on interpretation:
  Equivocal: 31-69 U/ml at 1:50 dilution; retest
  Repeatably equivocal: repeat with a fresh sample
No. of references: 18

NOTES

110289.0

Herpes simplex virus
ANTIBODY DETECTION (IgM)

Manufacturer: Behringwerke AG
Cat. No./Trade name: OWNX/Enzygnost® Anti-HSV IgM

SUMMARY

[Well-Ag]–**Ab**–[AHIgM-POD]–[TMB}–A$_{450}$

Assay type: EIA (non-competitive)
Detection: Colorimetric A$_{450}$ or visual
Format: Microtitre well, Ag coated
Sample type: Serum, plasma
Sample pre-treatment:
  Incubate 1:21 pre-diluted sample with RF absorbent 15
    min (RT) or overnight (4°C)
Sample volume: 150 µl of 1:42 dilution
Number of tests: 48
Controls - standards run in assay:
  Controls: Neg (1) and Pos (2) per plate
Incubation:
  1 hr (37°C) + 1 hr (37°C) + 30 min (RT)
Washes: 2

CONTENTS

Antibodies, antigens, labelled components:
  HSV Ag or control tissue culture Ag bound to well
  Anti-human IgM (g) POD conjugated
Substrate: TMB, H$_2$O$_2$
Controls - standards supplied:
  Controls: Neg and Pos (human Ig)
Additional reagents:
  Substrate and H$_2$SO$_4$
Special equipment required:
  Behring ELISA processor (optional)

INTERPRETATION

Comments on interpretation:
  Equivocal: within range of cut-off value and retest limit;
    retest to confirm
  Quantitative procedure available
No. of references: 15

NOTES

110109.0

*Samples are tested in parallel in Ag and control-Ag coated
  wells

Herpes simplex virus
ANTIBODY DETECTION (IgM)

Manufacturer: Bio-Stat Diagnostics
Cat. No./Trade name: 851126/ELISA IgM Antibody Test

SUMMARY

[Well-Ag]–**Ab**–[AHIgM-HRP]–[TMB]–A_{450}

Assay type: EIA (non-competitive)
Detection: Colorimetric A_{450}
Format: Microtitre well, Ag coated
Sample type: Serum
Sample pre-treatment:
    None
Sample volume: 10 µl (+ 1 ml diluent)
Number of tests: 96
Controls - standards run in assay:
    Controls: Neg (2), Pos (2)
Incubation:
    30 min (RT) + 30 min (RT) + 15 min (RT)
Washes: 2

CONTENTS

Antibodies, antigens, labelled components:
    HSV Ag bound to wells
    Anti-human IgM Ab (r) HRP conjugated
Substrate: TMB, H_2O_2
Controls - standards supplied:
    Controls: Neg and Pos
Additional reagents:
    None
Special equipment required:
    None

INTERPRETATION

Comments on interpretation:
    Classification of samples is according to cut-off; no
        further testing
    Visual interpretation is possible
No. of references: 5

NOTES

110087.0

Herpes simplex virus
ANTIBODY DETECTION (IgM)

Manufacturer: E. Merck
Cat. No./Trade name: 14485/Herpes Simplex Virus IgM

SUMMARY

[Well-Ag]–**Ab**–[AHIgM-HRP]–[TMB]–A_{450}

Assay type: EIA (non-competitive)
Detection: Colorimetric A_{450}
Format: Microtitre well, Ag coated
Sample type: Serum
Sample pre-treatment:
    None
Sample volume: 10 µl (+ 1 ml diluent)*
Number of tests: 96
Controls - standards run in assay:
    Controls: Neg (2), Pos (2)
Incubation:
    30 min (RT) + 30 min (RT) + 15 min (RT)
Washes: 2

CONTENTS

Antibodies, antigens, labelled components:
    HSV Ag bound to well
    Anti-human IgM PAb (r) HRP conjugated
Substrate: TMB
Controls - standards supplied:
    Controls: Neg and Pos
Additional reagents:
    None
Special equipment required:
    None

INTERPRETATION

Comments on interpretation:
    Classification of samples is according to cut-off; no
        further testing
No. of references: 5

NOTES

110314.0

*Dilution buffer contains anti-human IgG to prevent
    interference of rheumatoid factors or specific IgG

© KLUWER ACADEMIC PUBLISHERS 1994, ISSN 1381-5067

Herpes simplex virus
ANTIBODY DETECTION (IgM)

Manufacturer: Eurogenetics
Cat. No./Trade name: /Eurogenetics® Herpes IgM ELISA

SUMMARY

[Well-Ag]–**Ab**–[AHIgM-POD]–[OPD]–A$_{492}$

Assay type: EIA (non-competitive)
Detection: Colorimetric A$_{492}$
Format: Microtitre well, Ag coated
Sample type: Serum
Sample pre-treatment:
   None
Sample volume: 100 µl of 1:300 dilution x 2
Number of tests: 96
Controls - standards run in assay:
   Controls: Neg (2), Pos (2)
Incubation:
   1 hr (37°C) + 30 min (37°C) + 20 min (RT)
Washes: 2 (+ preliminary plate wash)

CONTENTS

Antibodies, antigens, labelled components:
   Herpes Ag bound to wells
   Anti-human IgM Ab POD conjugated
Substrate: OPD, H$_2$O$_2$
Controls - standards supplied:
   Controls: Neg and Pos (human serum)
Additional reagents:
   None
Special equipment required:
   Eurogenetics Microtitre plate reader (or similar)

INTERPRETATION

Comments on interpretation:
   Equivocal: within cut-off and cut-off + 0.1; retest a
   fresh sample
No. of references: 3

NOTES

110036.0

Herpes simplex virus
ANTIBODY DETECTION (IgM)

Manufacturer: Gamma SA
Cat. No./Trade name: /HERPES SIMPLEX VIRUS IgM ELISA

SUMMARY

[Well-Ag]–**Ab**–[AHIgM-HRP]–[TMB]–A$_{450}$

Assay type: EIA (non-competitive)
Detection: Colorimetric A$_{450}$
Format: Microtitre well, Ag coated
Sample type: Serum
Sample pre-treatment:
   Pre-dilution of sera (1:100) with dilution buffer to prevent
   interference due to IgG and RF
Sample volume: 100 µl (of pre-diluted sample)
Number of tests: 96
Controls - standards run in assay:
   Controls: Neg (2), Pos (2)
Incubation:
   30 min (RT) + 30 min (RT) + 15 min (RT)
Washes: 2

CONTENTS

Antibodies, antigens, labelled components:
   HSV Ag bound to well
   Anti-human IgM conjugated
Substrate: TMB
Controls - standards supplied:
   Controls: Neg and Pos
Additional reagents:
   None
Special equipment required:
   None

INTERPRETATION

Comments on interpretation:
   Classification of results is according to cut-off; no further
   testing
   Visual interpretation is possible
No. of references: 0

NOTES

110586.0

© *KLUWER ACADEMIC PUBLISHERS 1994, ISSN 1381-5067*

Herpes simplex virus
ANTIBODY DETECTION (IgM)

Manufacturer: Human GmbH
Cat. No./Trade name: 51 126/HERPES SIMPLEX VIRUS IgM ELISA

SUMMARY

[Well-Ag]–**Ab**–[AHIgM-HRP]–[TMB]–A_{450}

Assay type: EIA (non-competitive)
Detection: Colorimetric A_{450}
Format: Microtitre well, Ag coated
Sample type: Serum
Sample pre-treatment:
   Removal of IgG - 5 min incubation with sample diluent
Sample volume: 100 µl of 1:101 dilution
Number of tests: 96
Controls - standards run in assay:
   Controls: Neg (2), Pos (2)
Incubation:
   30 min (RT) + 30 min (RT) + 15 min (RT)
Washes: 2

CONTENTS

Antibodies, antigens, labelled components:
   HSV Ag bound to well
   Anti-human IgM Ab (r) HRP conjugated
Substrate: TMB, H_2O_2
Controls - standards supplied:
   Controls: Neg, Pos (human serum)
Additional reagents:
   None
Special equipment required:
   None

INTERPRETATION

Comments on interpretation:
   Equivocal: within cut-off ± 15%; retest in parallel with sample taken 7-14 days later
   The result may be read visually in comparison with the negative controls
No. of references: 5

NOTES

110515.0

Herpes simplex virus
ANTIBODY DETECTION (IgM)

Manufacturer: Laboratoire Eurobio
Cat. No./Trade name: 900280/HERPES IgM ELIT®

SUMMARY

[Well-AHIgM]–**Ab**–[Ag]–[Ab-POD]–[OPD]–$A_{492/630}$

Assay type: EIA (non-competitive)
Detection: Colorimetric $A_{492/630}$
Format: Microtitre well, Ab coated
Sample type: Serum, plasma
Sample pre-treatment:
   None
Sample volume: 50 µl of 1:101 dilution
Number of tests: 96
Controls - standards run in assay:
   Standards: I (1), II (2), III (1)
Incubation:
   1 hr (RT) + 1 hr (RT) + 1 hr (RT) + 30 min (RT)
Washes: 3

CONTENTS

Antibodies, antigens, labelled components:
   Anti-human IgM MAb bound to well
   HSV Ag
   Anti-HSV Ab POD conjugated
Substrate: OPD, H_2O_2
Controls - standards supplied:
   Standards: 3 (human serum with defined EIA values)
Additional reagents:
   None
Special equipment required:
   None

INTERPRETATION

Comments on interpretation:
   Indeterminate: ratio of sample: standard II absorbaance >0.8 and <1.2; retest a fresh sample 1-2 weeks later
   Positive: ratio of sample: standard absorbance >1.2
No. of references: None

NOTES

110529.0

© KLUWER ACADEMIC PUBLISHERS 1994, ISSN 1381-5067

Herpes simplex virus
ANTIBODY DETECTION (IgM)

Manufacturer: Menarini Diagnostics
Cat. No./Trade name: M6238/HF HERPES 1/2 IgM

SUMMARY

[Well-AHIgM]–**Ab**–[Ag-POD]–[TMB]–A_{450}

Assay type: EIA (non-competitive)
Detection: Colorimetric A_{450}
Format: Microtitre well, Ab coated
Sample type: Serum
Sample pre-treatment:
  None
Sample volume: 100 µl (of a 1:101 dilution)
Number of tests: 96
Controls - standards run in assay:
  Controls: Neg (1), Pos (1), cut-off (1)
Incubation:
  45 min (37°C) + 45 min (37°C) + 15 min (RT)
Washes: 2

CONTENTS

Antibodies, antigens, labelled components:
  Anti-human IgM MAb bound to well
  HSV Ag
  Anti-HSV MAb POD conjugated
Substrate: TMB, H_2O_2
Controls - standards supplied:
  Controls: Neg, Pos and cut-off (serum)
Additional reagents:
  None
Special equipment required:
  Not specified

INTERPRETATION

Comments on interpretation:
  Not specified
No. of references: 0

NOTES

110354.0

Herpes simplex virus
ANTIBODY DETECTION (IgM)

Manufacturer: Radim
Cat. No./Trade name: KHM/HSV IgM EIA WELL

SUMMARY

[Well-Ag]–**Ab**–[AHIgM-HRP]–[TMB]–A_{450}

Assay type: EIA (non-competitive)
Detection: Colorimetric A_{450}
Format: Microtitre well, Ag coated
Sample type: Serum or plasma
Sample pre-treatment:
  None
Sample volume: 100 µl of 1:300 dilution x 2
Number of tests: 96
Controls - standards run in assay:
  Controls: Neg (2), Pos (2), cut-off (2)
Incubation:
  1 hr (37°C) + 30 min (37°C) + 10 min (37°C) or 15 min
  (RT)
Washes: 2

CONTENTS

Antibodies, antigens, labelled components:
  HSV bound to well
  Anti-human IgM (g) HRP conjugated
Substrate: TMB, H_2O_2
Controls - standards supplied:
  Controls: Neg, Pos, cut-off (serum)
Additional reagents:
  None
Special equipment required:
  None

INTERPRETATION

Comments on interpretation:
  Grey area: within cut-off value $\pm 10\%$; retest to confirm
No. of references: 5

NOTES

110449.0

© KLUWER ACADEMIC PUBLISHERS 1994, ISSN 1381-5067

Herpes simplex virus
ANTIBODY DETECTION (IgM)

Manufacturer: Schiapparelli Biosystems Inc
Cat. No./Trade name: 5772918/HERPES IgM ELISA SYSTEM

SUMMARY

[Well-Ag]–**Ab**–[AHIgM-HRP]–[OPD]–A$_{492}$

Assay type: EIA (non-competitive)
Detection: Colorimetric A$_{492}$
Format: Microtitre well, Ag coated
Sample type: Serum (do not heat inactivate)
Sample pre-treatment:
　None
Sample volume: 100 μl of 1:300 dilution x 2
Number of tests: 96
Controls - standards run in assay:
　Controls: Neg (2), Pos (2)
Incubation:
　1 hr (37°C) + 30 min (37°C) + 10 min (37°C)
Washes: 3

CONTENTS

Antibodies, antigens, labelled components:
　HSV specific Ag bound to well
　Anti-human IgM Ab (g) HRP conjugated
Substrate: OPD, H$_2$O$_2$
Controls - standards supplied:
　Controls: Neg and Pos (human serum)
Additional reagents:
　None
Special equipment required:
　None

INTERPRETATION

Comments on interpretation:
　Doubtful range:　within cut-off value and cut-off +
　　0.100; retest to confirm
No. of references: 5

NOTES

110418.0

Herpes simplex virus
ANTIBODY DETECTION (IgG)

Manufacturer: Gen Bio
Cat. No./Trade name: 4110/ImmunoDOT® TORCH TEST*

SUMMARY

[Membrane-Ag]–**Ab**–[AHIgG-AP]–[BCIP]–violet dot

Assay type: Immunoblot assay
Detection: Visual
Format: Reaction vessel, membrane strip, Ag coated
Sample type: Serum, whole blood
Sample pre-treatment:
　None
Sample volume: 10 μl (serum), 20 μl (whole blood)
Number of tests: 10, 50, 100
Controls - standards run in assay:
　Controls: Neg integral (1), Pos integral (1), Pos (1)
Incubation:
　5 x 4 min standing time in controlled temperature
　　workstation
Washes: 4

CONTENTS

Antibodies, antigens, labelled components:
　HSV-1, HSV-2 Ag bound as a discrete dot on membrane
　　strip (one of 4 separate antigen dots)*
　Anti-human IgG Ab (g) AP conjugated
Substrate: BCIP
Controls - standards supplied:
　Controls: Integral Neg, Integral Pos
Additional reagents:
　Pos control serum (for all antigens) (no. 2215)
Special equipment required:
　Gen Bio workstation (Cat. no. 4001 or 4990)

INTERPRETATION

Comments on interpretation:
　Negative: no dot or indistinct dot in HSV Ag window
　Positive: blue-violet dot in HSV Ag window
No. of references: 17

NOTES

110379.0

*Simultaneous testing for T. gondii, Rubella virus, CMV and
　HSV with the ImmunoDOT® TORCH test system.
　Designed for preconception/postnatal screening

© KLUWER ACADEMIC PUBLISHERS 1994, ISSN 1381-5067

Herpes simplex virus
ANTIBODY DETECTION (IgG)

Manufacturer: Gen Bio
Cat. No./Trade name: 2210/ImmunoDOT® T.E.C.H. TEST*

SUMMARY

[Membrane-Ag]–**Ab**–[AHIgG-AP]–{BCIP}–violet dot

Assay type: Immunoblot assay
Detection: Visual
Format: Reaction vessel, membrane strip, Ag coated
Sample type: Serum, whole blood
Sample pre-treatment:
  None
Sample volume: 10 μl (serum), 20 μl (whole blood)
Number of tests: 10, 50, 100
Controls - standards run in assay:
  Controls: Neg integral (1), Pos integral (1), Pos (1)
Incubation:
  5 x 4 min standing time in controlled temperature workstation
Washes: 4

CONTENTS

Antibodies, antigens, labelled components:
  HSV-1, HSV-2 Ag bound as a discrete dot on membrane strip (one of 4 separate antigen dots)*
  Anti-human IgG Ab (g) AP conjugated
Substrate: BCIP
Controls - standards supplied:
  Controls: Integral Neg, Integral Pos
Additional reagents:
  Pos control serum (for all antigens) (no. 2215)
Special equipment required:
  Gen Bio workstation (Cat. no. 4001 or 4990)

INTERPRETATION

Comments on interpretation:
  Negative: no dot or indistinct dot in HSV Ag window
  Positive: distinct blue-violet dot in HSV Ag window
No. of references: 17

NOTES

110361.0

*Simultaneous testing for T. gondii, EBV, CMV and HSV with the ImmunoDOT® TECH Test system

Herpes simplex virus
ANTIBODY DETECTION

Manufacturer: Gull Laboratories
Cat. No./Trade name: HS 100/HSV Test

SUMMARY

[Slide well-Ag]–**Ab**–[AHIg-FITC]–fluorescence

Assay type: Immunofluorescence assay (indirect)
Detection: Fluorescence microscopy
Format: Slide well, Ag coated
Sample type: Serum
Sample pre-treatment:
  None
Sample volume: 15 μl of a 1:10 dilution*
Number of tests: 100
Controls - standards run in assay:
  Controls: Neg (1), Pos (1)
Incubation:
  30 min (RT) + 30 min (RT)
Washes: 2

CONTENTS

Antibodies, antigens, labelled components:
  HSV Ag infected and uninfected cells bound to slide well
  Anti-human Ig Ab (g) FITC conjugated
Substrate:
Controls - standards supplied:
  Controls: Neg and Pos (human serum - titre stated on label)
Additional reagents:
  None
Special equipment required:
  None

INTERPRETATION

Comments on interpretation:
  Negative: cells show red counterstain and no fluorescence
  Positive: fluorescence in ⩾10% of infected cells per field at 1:10 or greater dilution
  A method is available for the comparison of acute and convalescent sera
No. of references: 17

NOTES

110110.0

*Sera found Pos at 1:10 can be titrated using serial two fold dilutions

© KLUWER ACADEMIC PUBLISHERS 1994, ISSN 1381-5067

Herpes simplex virus
ANTIBODY DETECTION (IgG)

Manufacturer: Amico Laboratories Inc
Cat. No./Trade name: 5100FG/IFA HSV IgG Antibody Test

SUMMARY

[Slide-Ag]–**Ab**–[AHIgG-FITC]–fluorescence

Assay type: Immunofluorescence assay (indirect)
Detection: Fluorescence microscopy
Format: Slide well, Ag coated
Sample type: Serum
Sample pre-treatment:
  Dilute patient serum: 100 µl (+900 µl diluent)
Sample volume: 1 drop of diluted sample
Number of tests: 100
Controls - standards run in assay:
  Controls: Neg (1), Pos (1)
Incubation:
  25 min (RT) + 25 min (RT)
Washes: 1

CONTENTS

Antibodies, antigens, labelled components:
  HSV Ag bound to slide well
  Anti-human IgG Ab FITC conjugated
Substrate:
Controls - standards supplied:
  Controls: Neg and Pos (slides)
Additional reagents:
  None
Special equipment required:
  None

INTERPRETATION

Comments on interpretation:
  At test dilution of 1:10:
  Negative: red counterstained cells and no fluorescence
  Equivocal: colour intensity of apple green fluorescence
    (+/-)
  Positive: colour intensity of apple green fluorescence
    (+1) to (+4)
  Semiquantitative procedure is available using serial
    dilutions of samples
No. of references: 15

NOTES

110578.0

Herpes simplex virus
ANTIBODY DETECTION (IgM)

Manufacturer: Amico Laboratories Inc
Cat. No./Trade name: 5100FM/IFA HSV IgM Antibody Test

SUMMARY

[Slide-Ag]–**Ab**–[AHIgM-FITC]–fluorescence

Assay type: Immunofluorescence assay (indirect)
Detection: Fluorescence microscopy
Format: Slide well, Ag coated
Sample type: Serum
Sample pre-treatment:
  Dilute patient serum: 100 µl (+900 µl diluent)
Sample volume: 1 drop of diluted sample
Number of tests: 100
Controls - standards run in assay:
  Controls: Neg (1), Pos (1)
Incubation:
  25 min (RT) + 25 min (RT)
Washes: 1

CONTENTS

Antibodies, antigens, labelled components:
  HSV Ag bound to slide well
  Anti-human IgM Ab FITC conjugated
Substrate:
Controls - standards supplied:
  Controls: Neg and Pos (slides)
Additional reagents:
  None
Special equipment required:
  None

INTERPRETATION

Comments on interpretation:
  At test dilution of 1:10:
  Negative: red counterstained cells and no fluorescence
  Equivocal: colour intensity of apple green fluorescence
    (+/-)
  Positive: colour intensity of apple green fluorescence
    (+1) to (+4)
  Semiquantitative procedure is available using serial
    dilutions of samples
No. of references: 15

NOTES

110577.0

© *KLUWER ACADEMIC PUBLISHERS 1994, ISSN 1381-5067*

Herpes simplex virus
ANTIBODY DETECTION (IgM)

Manufacturer: Gull Laboratories
Cat. No./Trade name: HS 140/HSV IgM Test

SUMMARY

[Slide-Ag]–**Ab**–[AHIgM-FITC]–fluorescence

Assay type: Immunofluorescence assay (indirect)
Detection: Fluorescence microscopy
Format: Slide well, Ag coated
Sample type: Serum
Sample pre-treatment:
   May treat with GULLSORB Reagent to remove IgG and RF
Sample volume: 15 µl of 1:10 and 1:40 dilution*
Number of tests: 50, 100
Controls - standards run in assay:
   Controls: Neg (1), Pos (1)
Incubation:
   1 hr (37°C) + 30 min (37°C)
Washes: 2

CONTENTS

Antibodies, antigens, labelled components:
   HSV Ag and uninfected control cells bound to slide well
   Anti-human IgM Ab FITC conjugated
Substrate:
Controls - standards supplied:
   Controls: Neg and Pos (human serum)
Additional reagents:
   None
Special equipment required:
   None

INTERPRETATION

Comments on interpretation:
   Negative: cells show red counterstain but no fluorescence
   Positive: fluorescence in 10-20% of infected cells per field at 1:10 or greater dilution
No. of references: 4

NOTES

110114.0

*If treated with GULLSORB reagent only 1:10 dilution required in assay

Herpes simplex virus (HSV-1)
ANTIGEN DETECTION

Manufacturer: Bio-Stat Diagnostics
Cat. No./Trade name: 851101/ELISA Antigen Test

SUMMARY

[Well-Ab]–**Ag**–[Ab-HRP]–[TMB]–A_{450}

Assay type: EIA (non-competitive)
Detection: Colorimetric A_{450}
Format: Microtitre well, Ab
Sample type: Swab of vesicle, vesicle fluid, cell culture
Sample pre-treatment:
   Swab, vesicle fluid: extraction (+1 ml diluent). Cell culture: freeze and thaw x 2 (+1:10 dilution)*
Sample volume: 100 µl x 2
Number of tests: 96
Controls - standards run in assay:
   Controls: Neg (one per sample); Pos (1) x 2*
Incubation:
   a) 1 hr (37°C) + 15 min (37°C) + 15 min (RT)
   b) 2 hr (RT) + 30 min (RT) + 15 min (RT)
Washes: 2

CONTENTS

Antibodies, antigens, labelled components:
   Anti-HSV-1 Ab bound to wells
   Neg control coated wells
   Anti-HSV-1 Ab HRP congugated
Substrate: TMB, H_2O_2
Controls - standards supplied:
   Controls: Neg (coated on microtitre wells), Pos
Additional reagents:
   None
Special equipment required:
   None

INTERPRETATION

Comments on interpretation:
   Classification of samples is according to cut-off; no further testing
   Visual interpretation is possible
No. of references: 5

NOTES

110079.0

*Sample and Pos control assayed in parallel in antibody coated and Neg control coated microtitre wells
Assay may be run in parallel with HSV-2 ELISA Antigen Test for HSV classification

© *KLUWER ACADEMIC PUBLISHERS 1994, ISSN 1381-5067*

Herpes simplex virus (HSV-1)
ANTIBODY DETECTION (IgG)

Manufacturer: Biologische Analysensystem GmbH
Cat. No./Trade name: 5210/BAG-HSV-1-EIA-G

SUMMARY

[Well-Ag]–**Ab**–[AHIgG-HRP]–[TMB]–A$_{450}$

Assay type: EIA (non-competitive)
Detection: Colorimetric A$_{450}$
Format: Microtitre well, Ag coated
Sample type: Serum
Sample pre-treatment:
    None
Sample volume: 10 µl (+1 ml diluent)
Number of tests: 96
Controls - standards run in assay:
    Controls: Neg (1), Cut-off (2), Pos (1)
Incubation:
    30 min (RT) + 30 min (RT) + 10 min (RT)
Washes: 2

CONTENTS

Antibodies, antigens, labelled components:
    HSV-1 Ag bound to well
    Anti-human IgG Ab (sh) HRP conjugated
Substrate: TMB
Controls - standards supplied:
    Controls: Neg, Pos and cut-off
Additional reagents:
    None
Special equipment required:
    None

INTERPRETATION

Comments on interpretation:
    Equivocal: within cut-off ± 20%; retest to confirm
No. of references: 0

NOTES

110263.0

Herpes simplex virus (HSV-1)
ANTIBODY DETECTION (IgG)

Manufacturer: Cambridge Biotech Corporation
Cat. No./Trade name: /HSV-1 IgG EIA Test

SUMMARY

[Well-Ag]–**Ab**–[AHIgG-AP]–[PNP]–A$_{405}$

Assay type: EIA (non-competitive)
Detection: Colorimetric A$_{405}$
Format: Microtitre well, Ag coated
Sample type: Serum
Sample pre-treatment:
    None
Sample volume: 100 µl of 1:21 dilution
Number of tests: 96
Controls - standards run in assay:
    Controls: Neg (1), Pos (1), Reference serum (3)
Incubation:
    30 min (37°C) + 30 min (37°C) + 30 min (37°C)
Washes: 2

CONTENTS

Antibodies, antigens, labelled components:
    HSV-1 Ag bound to well
    Anti-human IgG Ab (g) AP conjugated
Substrate: PNP
Controls - standards supplied:
    Controls: Neg and Pos (human serum); Reference serum (human)
Additional reagents:
    None
Special equipment required:
    None

INTERPRETATION

Comments on interpretation:
    Equivocal: samples within specified range; retest to confirm
    Repeatably equivocal: retest using an alternative method
No. of references: 12

NOTES

110647.0

© KLUWER ACADEMIC PUBLISHERS 1994, ISSN 1381-5067

Herpes simplex virus (HSV-1)
ANTIBODY DETECTION (IgG)

Manufacturer: Chimica Diagnostica
Cat. No./Trade name: COD.41600/Herpes Simplex Virus I IgG

SUMMARY

$[Well-Ag]-\textbf{Ab}-[AHIgG-POD]-[TMB]-A_{450}$

Assay type: EIA (non-competitive)
Detection: Colorimetric A_{450}
Format: Microtitre well, Ag coated
Sample type: Serum
Sample pre-treatment:
   None
Sample volume: 10 µl (+1 ml diluent)
Number of tests: 96
Controls - standards run in assay:
   Controls: Neg (1), cut-off (1), Pos (1)
Incubation:
   30 min (RT) + 30 min (RT) + 15 min (RT)
Washes: 2

CONTENTS

Antibodies, antigens, labelled components:
   HSV-1 Ag bound to well
   Anti-human IgG PAb (g) POD conjugated
Substrate: TMB
Controls - standards supplied:
   Controls: Neg, cut-off and Pos
Additional reagents:
   None
Special equipment required:
   None

INTERPRETATION

Comments on interpretation:
   Equivocal: Sample index (ratio of O.D. sample: cut-off)
      > 0.9 < 1.1; retest to confirm
No. of references: 2

NOTES

110310.0

Herpes simplex virus (HSV-1)
ANTIBODY DETECTION (IgG)

Manufacturer: Diamedix Corporation
Cat. No./Trade name: 783-340/HERPES 1 Microassay

SUMMARY

$[Well-Ag]-\textbf{Ab}-[AHIgG-AP]-[PNP]-A_{405}$

Assay type: EIA (non-competitive)
Detection: Colorimetric A_{405}
Format: Microtitre well, Ag coated
Sample type: Serum (do not heat inactivate)
Sample pre-treatment:
   None
Sample volume: 100 µl of 1:41 dilution
Number of tests: 96
Controls - standards run in assay:
   Controls: Neg (1), Pos (1)
   Calibrator: (1)
Incubation:
   30 min (RT) + 30 min (RT) + 30 min (RT)
Washes: 2

CONTENTS

Antibodies, antigens, labelled components:
   HSV-1 Ag bound to well
   Anti-human IgG Ab (g) AP conjugated
Substrate: PNP
Controls - standards supplied:
   Controls: Neg and Pos (human serum)
   Calibrators: (1) human serum
Additional reagents:
   None
Special equipment required:
   None

INTERPRETATION

Comments on interpretation:
   Positive: ⩾ 20 ELISA unit (EU)/ml
No. of references: 2

NOTES

110493.0

This test is designed to be run in parallel with the Herpes 2
   Microassay

Herpes simplex virus (HSV-1)
ANTIBODY DETECTION (IgG)

Manufacturer: E. Merck
Cat. No./Trade name: 14455/Herpes Simplex Virus 1 IgG

SUMMARY

[Well-Ag]–**Ab**–[AHIgG-HRP]–[TMB]–A$_{450}$

Assay type: EIA (non-competitive)
Detection: Colorimetric A$_{450}$
Format: Microtitre well, Ag coated
Sample type: Serum
Sample pre-treatment:
  None
Sample volume: 10 µl (+1 ml diluent)
Number of tests: 96
Controls - standards run in assay:
  Controls: Neg (2), Pos (2)
Incubation:
  30 min (RT) + 30 min (RT) + 15 min (RT)
Washes: 2

CONTENTS

Antibodies, antigens, labelled components:
  HSV-1 Ag bound to well
  Anti-human IgG PAb (r) HRP conjugated
Substrate: TMB
Controls - standards supplied:
  Controls: Neg and Pos
Additional reagents:
  None
Special equipment required:
  None

INTERPRETATION

Comments on interpretation:
  Classification of samples is according to cut-off; no
  further testing
No. of references: 5

NOTES

110315.0

Herpes simplex virus (HSV-1)
ANTIBODY DETECTION (IgG)

Manufacturer: Eurogenetics
Cat. No./Trade name: /Eurogenetics® Herpes I IgG ELISA

SUMMARY

[Well-Ag]–**Ab**–[AHIgG-POD]–[OPD]–A$_{492}$

Assay type: EIA (non-competitive)
Detection: Colorimetric A$_{492}$
Format: Microtitre well, Ag coated
Sample type: Serum
Sample pre-treatment:
  None
Sample volume: 100 µl of 1:300 dilution x 2
Number of tests: 96
Controls - standards run in assay:
  Controls: Neg (2), Pos (2)
Incubation:
  1 hr (37°C) + 30 min (37°C) + 20 min (RT)
Washes: 2 (+ preliminary plate wash)

CONTENTS

Antibodies, antigens, labelled components:
  HSV-1 Ag bound to wells
  Anti-human IgG Ab POD conjugated
Substrate: OPD, H$_2$O$_2$
Controls - standards supplied:
  Controls: Neg and Pos (human serum)
Additional reagents:
  None
Special equipment required:
  Eurogenetics Microtitre plate reader (or similar)

INTERPRETATION

Comments on interpretation:
  Equivocal: within cut-off + 0.1; retest a fresh sample
No. of references: 12

NOTES

110035.0

Herpes simplex virus (HSV-1)
ANTIBODY DETECTION (IgG)

Manufacturer: Gamma SA
Cat. No./Trade name: /HERPES SIMPLEX VIRUS 1 IgG
ELISA

SUMMARY

[Well-Ag]–**Ab**–[AHIgG-HRP]–[TMB]–A_{450}

Assay type: EIA (non-competitive)
Detection: Colorimetric A_{450}
Format: Microtitre well, Ag coated
Sample type: Serum
Sample pre-treatment:
    None
Sample volume: 100 µl of 1:100 diluted sample
Number of tests: 96
Controls - standards run in assay:
    Controls: Neg (2), Pos (2)
Incubation:
    30 min (RT) + 30 min (RT) + 15 min (RT)
Washes: 2

CONTENTS

Antibodies, antigens, labelled components:
    HSV-1 Ag bound to well
    Anti-human IgG Ab (r) HRP conjugated
Substrate: TMB
Controls - standards supplied:
    Controls: Neg and Pos
Additional reagents:
    None
Special equipment required:
    None

INTERPRETATION

Comments on interpretation:
    Classification of sample is according to cut-off; no further
        testing. (Results may be expressed in units based on
        the positive control)
    Visual interpretation is possible
No. of references: 0

NOTES

110587.0

Herpes simplex virus (HSV-1)
ANTIBODY DETECTION (IgG)

Manufacturer: Human GmbH
Cat. No./Trade name: 51 216/HERPES SIMPLEX
VIRUS 1 IgG ELISA

SUMMARY

[Well-Ag]–**Ab**–[AHIgG-HRP]–[TMB]–A_{450}

Assay type: EIA (non-competitive)
Detection: Colorimetric A_{450}
Format: Microtitre well, Ag coated
Sample type: Serum
Sample pre-treatment:
    None
Sample volume: 100 µl of 1:101 dilution
Number of tests: 96
Controls - standards run in assay:
    Controls: Neg (2), Pos (2)
Incubation:
    30 min (RT) + 30 min (RT) + 15 min (RT)
Washes: 2

CONTENTS

Antibodies, antigens, labelled components:
    HSV-1 Ag bound to well
    Anti-human IgG Ab (r) HRP conjugated
Substrate: TMB, H_2O_2
Controls - standards supplied:
    Controls: Neg, Pos (human serum)
Additional reagents:
    None
Special equipment required:
    None

INTERPRETATION

Comments on interpretation:
    Equivocal: within cut-off $\pm 15\%$; retest in parallel with
        sample taken 7-14 days later
    The result may be read visually in comparison with the
        negative controls
No. of references: 5

NOTES

110513.0

© *KLUWER ACADEMIC PUBLISHERS 1994, ISSN 1381-5067*

Herpes simplex virus (HSV-1)
ANTIBODY DETECTION (IgG)

Manufacturer: Immunobiological Laboratories
Cat. No./Trade name: VE57111/Herpes 1 Virus IgG

SUMMARY

[Well-Ag]–**Ab**–[AHIgG-HRP]–[TMB]–A_{450}

Assay type: EIA (non-competitive)
Detection: Colorimetric A_{450}
Format: Microtitre well, Ag coated
Sample type: Serum
Sample pre-treatment:
 None
Sample volume: 100 µl of a 1:100 dilution x 2
Number of tests: 96
Controls - standards run in assay:
 Controls: Neg (2), low Pos (2), high Pos (2)
Incubation:
 1 hr(RT) + 30 min (RT) + 15 min (RT)
Washes: 2

CONTENTS

Antibodies, antigens, labelled components:
 HSV-1 Ag bound to well
 Anti-human IgG Ab HRP conjugated
Substrate: TMB, H_2O_2
Controls - standards supplied:
 Controls: Neg, low Pos, high Pos
Additional reagents:
 None
Special equipment required:
 None

INTERPRETATION

Comments on interpretation:
 Classification of samples is according to cut-off; no further testing
No. of references: 8

NOTES

110327.0

Herpes simplex virus (HSV-1)
ANTIBODY DETECTION (IgG)

Manufacturer: Incstar
Cat. No./Trade name: 4510/Clin-ELISA HSV-1 IgG

SUMMARY

[Well-Ag]–**Ab**–[AHIgG-AP]–[PNP]–A_{405}

Assay type: EIA (non-competitive)
Detection: Colorimetric A_{405}
Format: Microtitre well, Ag coated
Sample type: Serum
Sample pre-treatment:
 None
Sample volume: 10 µl (+500 µl diluent)
Number of tests: 96
Controls - standards run in assay:
 Controls: low Pos (1), high Pos (1)
 Calibrators: Neg (2), low Pos (2), high Pos (2)
Incubation:
 30 min (RT) + 30 min (RT) + 45 min (RT)
Washes: 2

CONTENTS

Antibodies, antigens, labelled components:
 HSV-1 Ag bound to well
 Anti-human IgG Ab AP conjugated
Substrate: PNP
Controls - standards supplied:
 Controls: Low Pos, high Pos (human serum)
 Calibrators (3) with assigned ELISA values
Additional reagents:
 None
Special equipment required:
 Clin-ELISA reader (optional)

INTERPRETATION

Comments on interpretation:
 Equivocal: ELISA value 21-29; retest to confirm and/or test a fresh sample in 2-3 weeks
No. of references: 23

NOTES

110252.0

© KLUWER ACADEMIC PUBLISHERS 1994, ISSN 1381-5067

Herpes simplex virus (HSV-1)
ANTIBODY DETECTION (IgG)

Manufacturer: International Immunodiagnostics
Cat. No./Trade name: 108 140/HSV-Typ 1 IgG

SUMMARY

[Well-Ag]–**Ab**–[AHIgG-HRP]–[TMB]–A_{450}

Assay type: EIA (non-competitive)
Detection: Colorimetric A_{450}
Format: Microtitre well, Ag coated
Sample type: Serum
Sample pre-treatment:
 None
Sample volume: 10 µl (+ 1 ml diluent)*
Number of tests: 96
Controls - standards run in assay:
 Controls: Neg (2), Pos (2)
Incubation:
 30 min (RT) + 30 min (RT) + 15 min (RT) (first two
  incubations on plate shaker)
Washes: 2

CONTENTS

Antibodies, antigens, labelled components:
 HSV-1 Ag bound to well
 Anti-human IgG Ab HRP conjugated
Substrate: TMB, H_2O_2
Controls - standards supplied:
 Controls: Neg and Pos (human serum)
Additional reagents:
 None
Special equipment required:
 None

INTERPRETATION

Comments on Interpretation:
 Classification of results is according to cut-off; no further
  testing
 Quantitative interpretation also available
No. of references: 0

NOTES

110334.0

*Samples assayed in duplicate

Herpes simplex virus (HSV-1)
ANTIBODY DETECTION (IgG)

Manufacturer: Melja Diagnostik GmbH
Cat. No./Trade name: HSV-E01/Herpes Simplex Virus
Type 1 IgG EIA Kit

SUMMARY

[Well-Ag]–**Ab**–[AHIgG-HRP]–[TMB]–A_{450}

Assay type: EIA (non-competitive)
Detection: Colorimetric A_{450}
Format: Microtitre well, Ag coated
Sample type: Serum, plasma
Sample pre-treatment:
 None
Sample volume: 100 µl of 1:100 dilution x 2
Number of tests: 96
Controls - standards run in assay:
 Controls: low Pos (2), high Pos (2), Neg (2)
Incubation:
 1 hr (RT) + 30 min (RT) + 15 min (RT)
Washes: 2

CONTENTS

Antibodies, antigens, labelled components:
 HSV-1 Ag bound to well
 Anti-human IgG PAb HRP conjugated
Substrate: TMB
Controls - standards supplied:
 Controls: low Pos, high Pos and Neg
Additional reagents:
 None
Special equipment required:
 None

INTERPRETATION

Comments on interpretation:
 Positive: > cut-off + 20%
 Negative: < cut-off - 20%
 A MELJA titre may be calculated from a single sample
  dilution
No. of references: 8

NOTES

110361.0

© *KLUWER ACADEMIC PUBLISHERS 1994, ISSN 1381-5067*

Herpes simplex virus (HSV-1)
ANTIBODY DETECTION (IgG)

Manufacturer: Melotec S.A.
Cat. No./Trade name: MHIG/MELOTEST HSV-1 IgG

SUMMARY

[Well-Ag]–**Ab**–[AHIgG-HRP]–[TMB]–A_{450}

Assay type: EIA (non-competitive)
Detection: Colorimetric A_{450}
Format: Microtitre well, Ag coated
Sample type: Serum, plasma
Sample pre-treatment:
   None
Sample volume: 10 µl (+ 190 µl diluent)
Number of tests: 96
Controls - standards run in assay:
   Controls: Neg (1), low Pos (2), high Pos (1)
Incubation:
   20 min (RT) + 20 min (RT) + 10 min (RT)
Washes: 2

CONTENTS

Antibodies, antigens, labelled components:
   HSV-1 Ag bound to well
   Anti-human IgG Ab HRP conjugated
Substrate: TMB, H_2O_2
Controls - standards supplied:
   Controls: Neg, low Pos, high Pos (human serum)
Additional reagents:
   None
Special equipment required:
   None

INTERPRETATION

Comments on interpretation:
   Equivocal: ratio of OD of sample to low Pos control is
      within the range 0.9 to 1.1; retest fresh sample
   Repeatably equivocal: retest fresh sample in 4-6 weeks
No. of references: 9

NOTES

110068.0

Herpes simplex virus (HSV-1)
ANTIBODY DETECTION (IgG)

Manufacturer: Radim
Cat. No./Trade name: KH1G/HSV1 IgG EIA WELL

SUMMARY

[Well-Ag]–**Ab**–[AHIgG-HRP]–[TMB]–A_{450}

Assay type: EIA (non-competitive)
Detection: Colorimetric A_{450}
Format: Microtitre well, Ag coated
Sample type: Serum or plasma
Sample pre-treatment:
   None
Sample volume: 100 µl of 1:300 dilution x 2
Number of tests: 96, 192
Controls - standards run in assay:
   Controls: Neg (2), Pos (2), Cut-off (2)
Incubation:
   1 hr (37°C) + 30 min (37°C) + 10 min (37°C) or 15 min
      (RT)
Washes: 2

CONTENTS

Antibodies, antigens, labelled components:
   HSV-1 Ag bound to well
   Anti-human IgG (g) HRP conjugated
Substrate: TMB, H_2O_2
Controls - standards supplied:
   Controls: Neg, Pos, Cut-off (serum)
Additional reagents:
   None
Special equipment required:
   None

INTERPRETATION

Comments on interpretation:
   Grey area: within cut-off value ± 10%; retest to confirm
No. of references: 5

NOTES

110447.0

© *KLUWER ACADEMIC PUBLISHERS 1994, ISSN 1381-5067*

Herpes simplex virus (HSV-1)
ANTIBODY DETECTION (IgG)

Manufacturer: Schiapparelli Biosystems Inc
Cat. No./Trade name: 5772916/HERPES 1 IgG ELISA SYSTEM

SUMMARY

[Well-Ag]–**Ab**–[AHIgG-HRP]–[OPD]–A$_{492}$

Assay type: EIA (non-competitive)
Detection: Colorimetric A$_{492}$
Format: Microtitre well, Ag coated
Sample type: Serum (do not heat inactivate)
Sample pre-treatment:
    None
Sample volume: 100 µl of 1:300 dilution x 2
Number of tests: 96
Controls - standards run in assay:
    Controls: Neg (2), Pos (2)
Incubation:
    1 hr (37°C) + 30 min (37°C) + 10 min (37°C)
Washes: 3

CONTENTS

Antibodies, antigens, labelled components:
    HSV-1 specific Ag bound to well
    Anti-human IgG Ab (g) HRP conjugated
Substrate: OPD, H$_2$O$_2$
Controls - standards supplied:
    Controls: Neg and Pos (human serum)
Additional reagents:
    None
Special equipment required:
    None

INTERPRETATION

Comments on interpretation:
    Doubtful range: within cut-off value and cut-off +0.100; retest to confirm
No. of references: 5

NOTES

110419.0

Herpes simplex virus (HSV-1)
ANTIBODY DETECTION (IgG)

Manufacturer: Sigma Diagnostics
Cat. No./Trade name: SIA 411-A (Herpes-1)*/SIA Herpes 1 kit

SUMMARY

[Well-Ag]–**Ab**–[AHIgG-AP]–[PMP]–A$_{550}$

Assay type: EIA (non-competitive)
Detection: Colorimetric A$_{550}$
Format: Microtitre well, Ag coated
Sample type: Serum (do not heat inactivate)
Sample pre-treatment:
    None
Sample volume: 10 µl (+200 µl diluent)
Number of tests: 96
Controls - standards run in assay:
    Controls: Pos (1), Neg (1)
    Calibrator: (3)
Incubation:
    45 min (RT) + 45 min (RT) + 45 min (RT)
Washes: 2

CONTENTS

Antibodies, antigens, labelled components:
    HSV Type 1 bound to well
    Anti-human IgG PAb (g) AP conjugated
Substrate: PMP
Controls - standards supplied:
    Controls: Neg and Pos, human serum
    Calibrator (3), human serum with assigned value
Additional reagents:
    None
Special equipment required:
    Sigma EIA microwell plate or strip reader (optional)

INTERPRETATION

Comments on interpretation:
    Results expressed as S.I.A HERPES IgG Value
    Equivocal: 0.92-0.99; retest to confirm
No. of references: 3

NOTES

110116.0

*The assay is designed to be run in parallel with SIA Herpes Type 2 kit

© *KLUWER ACADEMIC PUBLISHERS 1994, ISSN 1381-5067*

Herpes simplex virus (HSV-1)
ANTIBODY DETECTION (IgG)

Manufacturer: United Biotech Inc
Cat. No./Trade name: IA-401/MAGIWEL® HSV-1 IgG

SUMMARY

[Well-Ag]–**Ab**–[AHIgG-HRP]–[TMB]–A_{450}

Assay type: EIA (non-competitive)
Detection: Colorimetric A_{450}
Format: Microtitre well, Ag coated
Sample type: Serum
Sample pre-treatment:
  None
Sample volume: 100 µl of 1:101 dilution
Number of tests: 96
Controls - standards run in assay:
  Reference standard set: Neg (1), Pos (1), Calibrator (1)
Incubation:
  30 min (RT) + 30 min (RT) + 15 min (RT)
Washes: 2

CONTENTS

Antibodies, antigens, labelled components:
  HSV Type 1 Ag bound to well
  Anti-human IgG Ab (g) HRP conjugated
Substrate: TMB, H_2O_2
Controls - standards supplied:
  Reference standard set: Neg, Pos, Calibrator (100 EU/
  ml)
Additional reagents:
  H_2SO_4
Special equipment required:
  None

INTERPRETATION

Comments on interpretation:
  Positive: ⩾20 EU/ml
No. of references: 5

NOTES

110500.0

Herpes simplex virus (HSV-1)
ANTIBODY DETECTION (IgM)

Manufacturer: Baxter Diagnostics Inc (Bartels Division)
Cat. No./Trade name: B1029-345/Herpes Simplex Virus 1 IgM EIA

SUMMARY

[Well-Ag]–**Ab**–[AHIgM-Enzyme]–[PNP]–A_{405}

Assay type: EIA (non-competitive)
Detection: Colorimetric A_{405}
Format: Microtitre well, Ag coated
Sample type: Serum
Sample pre-treatment:
  None
Sample volume: 100 µl 1:11 dilution*
Number of tests: 96
Controls - standards run in assay:
  Controls: not specified)
Incubation:
  30 min (37°C) + 30 min (37°C) + 30 min (37°C)
Washes: 2

CONTENTS

Antibodies, antigens, labelled components:
  HSV-1 Ag bound to well
  Anti-human IgM Ab enzyme conjugated**
Substrate: PNP
Controls - standards supplied:
  Controls: Neg, Pos and reference serum
Additional reagents:
  None
Special equipment required:
  None

INTERPRETATION

Comments on interpretation:
  Classification of samples according to cut-off; further
  details not specified
No. of references: 6

NOTES

110827.0

*Diluent contains an absorbant to remove IgG and prevent
  IgG/rheumatoid factor complexes interfering with assay
**Enzyme label not specified

© KLUWER ACADEMIC PUBLISHERS 1994, ISSN 1381-5067

Herpes simplex virus (HSV-1)
ANTIBODY DETECTION (IgM)

Manufacturer: Biologische Analysensystem GmbH
Cat. No./Trade name: 5211/BAG-HSV-1-EIA-M

SUMMARY

[Well-Ag]–**Ab**–[AHIgM-HRP]–[TMB]–A_{450}

Assay type: EIA (non-competitive)
Detection: Colorimetric A_{450}
Format: Microtitre well, Ag coated
Sample type: Serum
Sample pre-treatment:
  None
Sample volume: 10 μl (+ 1 ml diluent)
Number of tests: 96
Controls - standards run in assay:
  Controls: Neg (1), Cut-off (2), Pos (1)
Incubation:
  30 min (RT) + 30 min (RT) + 10 min (RT)
Washes: 2

CONTENTS

Antibodies, antigens, labelled components:
  HSV-1 Ag bound to well
  Anti-human IgM Ab (sh) HRP conjugated
Substrate: TMB
Controls - standards supplied:
  Controls: Neg, Pos and cut-off
Additional reagents:
  None
Special equipment required:
  None

INTERPRETATION

Comments on interpretation:
  Equivocal: within cut-off ± 10%; retest to confirm
No. of references: 0

NOTES

110284.0

Herpes simplex virus (HSV-1)
ANTIBODY DETECTION (IgM)

Manufacturer: Cambridge Biotech Corporation
Cat. No./Trade name: /HSV-1 IgM EIA Test

SUMMARY

[Well-Ag]–**Ab**–[AHIgM-AP]–[PNP]–A_{405}

Assay type: EIA (non-competitive)
Detection: Colorimetric A_{405}
Format: Microtitre well, Ag coated
Sample type: Serum
Sample pre-treatment:
  None
Sample volume: 100 μl of 1:11 dilution*
Number of tests: 96
Controls - standards run in assay:
  Controls: Neg (1), Pos (1), Reference serum (3)
Incubation:
  30 min (37°C) + 30 min (37°C) + 30 min (37°C)
Washes: 2

CONTENTS

Antibodies, antigens, labelled components:
  HSV-1 Ag bound to well
  Anti-human IgM Ab (g) AP conjugated
Substrate: PNP
Controls - standards supplied:
  Controls: Neg and Pos (human serum); Reference serum (human)
Additional reagents:
  None
Special equipment required:
  None

INTERPRETATION

Comments on interpretation:
  Equivocal: samples within specified range; retest to confirm
  Repeatably equivocal: retest using an alternative method
No. of references: 13

NOTES

110648.0

*Diluent contains an absorbant to remove IgG/RF complexes from patient serum

Herpes simplex virus (HSV-1)
ANTIBODY DETECTION (IgM)

Manufacturer: Chimica Diagnostica
Cat. No./Trade name: 41750/Herpes Simplex Virus 1 IgM

SUMMARY

[Well-Ag]–**Ab**–[AHIgM-POD]–[TMB]–A_{450}

Assay type: EIA (non-competitive)
Detection: Colorimetric A_{450}
Format: Microtitre well, Ag coated
Sample type: Serum
Sample pre-treatment:
  None
Sample volume: 10 µl (+1 ml diluent)
Number of tests: 96
Controls - standards run in assay:
  Controls: Neg (1), cut-off (1), Pos (1)
Incubation:
  30 min (RT) + 30 min (RT) + 15 min (RT)
Washes: 2

CONTENTS

Antibodies, antigens, labelled components:
  HSV-1 Ag bound to well
  Anti-human IgM PAb (g) POD conjugated
Substrate: TMB
Controls - standards supplied:
  Controls: Neg, cut-off and Pos
Additional reagents:
  None
Special equipment required:
  None

INTERPRETATION

Comments on interpretation:
  Equivocal: Sample index (ratio of O.D. sample: cut-off) >0.9<1.1; retest to confirm
No. of references: 2

NOTES

110312.0

Herpes simplex virus (HSV-1)
ANTIBODY DETECTION (IgM)

Manufacturer: Gull Laboratories
Cat. No./Trade name: HIE 150/HSV-1 IgM ELISA Test

SUMMARY

[Well-Ag]–**Ab**–[AHIgM-AP]–[PNP]–A_{405}

Assay type: EIA (non-competitive)
Detection: Colorimetric A_{405}
Format: Microtitre well, Ag coated
Sample type: Serum
Sample pre-treatment:
  None
Sample volume: 15 µl (+150 µl diluent)*
Number of tests: 96
Controls - standards run in assay:
  Controls: Neg (1), Pos (1)
  Reference serum (3)
Incubation:
  30 min (37°C) + 30 min (37°C) + 30 min (37°C)
Washes: 2

CONTENTS

Antibodies, antigens, labelled components:
  HSV-1 Ag bound to well
  Anti-human IgM Ab (g) AP conjugated
Substrate: PNP
Controls - standards supplied:
  Controls: Neg and Pos (human serum)
  Reference serum (human)
Additional reagents:
  None
Special equipment required:
  None

INTERPRETATION

Comments on interpretation:
  Equivocal: within cut-off and cut-off x 0.9; retest
  Repeatably equivocal: retest with alternative method
No. of references: 13

NOTES

110113.0

*Sample diluent contains an absorbant to remove IgG and RF

Herpes simplex virus (HSV-1)
ANTIBODY DETECTION (IgM)

Manufacturer: Immunobiological Laboratories
Cat. No./Trade name: VE57131/Herpes 1 Virus IgM

SUMMARY

[Well-Ag]–**Ab**–[AHIgM-HRP]–[TMB]–A$_{450}$

Assay type: EIA (non-competitive)
Detection: Colorimetric A$_{450}$
Format: Microtitre well, Ag coated
Sample type: Serum
Sample pre-treatment:
  None
Sample volume: 100 µl of a 1:100 dilution x 2
Number of tests: 96
Controls - standards run in assay:
  Controls: Neg (2), low Pos (2), high Pos (2)
Incubation:
  1 hr (RT) + 30 min (RT) + 15 min (RT)
Washes: 2

CONTENTS

Antibodies, antigens, labelled components:
  HSV-1 Ag bound to well
  Anti-human IgM Ab HRP conjugated
Substrate: TMB, H$_2$O$_2$
Controls - standards supplied:
  Controls: Neg, low Pos, high Pos
Additional reagents:
  None
Special equipment required:
  None

INTERPRETATION

Comments on interpretation:
  Classification of samples is according to cut-off; no further testing
No. of references: 8

NOTES

110329.0

Herpes simplex virus (HSV-1)
ANTIBODY DETECTION (IgM)

Manufacturer: International Immunodiagnostics
Cat. No./Trade name: 108 141/HSV-Typ 1 IgM

SUMMARY

[Well-Ag]–**Ab**–[AHIgM-HRP]–[TMB]–A$_{450}$

Assay type: EIA (non-competitive)
Detection: Colorimetric A$_{450}$
Format: Microtitre well, Ag coated
Sample type: Serum
Sample pre-treatment:
  None
Sample volume: 10 µl (+ 1 ml diluent)*
Number of tests: 96
Controls - standards run in assay:
  Controls: Neg (2), Pos (2)
Incubation:
  30 min (RT) + 30 min (RT) + 15 min (RT) (first two incubations on plate shaker)
Washes: 2

CONTENTS

Antibodies, antigens, labelled components:
  HSV-1 Ag bound to well
  Anti-human IgM Ab HRP conjugated
Substrate: TMB, H$_2$O$_2$
Controls - standards supplied:
  Controls: Neg and Pos (human serum)
Additional reagents:
  None
Special equipment required:
  None

INTERPRETATION

Comments on interpretation:
  Classification of results is according to cut-off; no further testing
  Quantitative interpretation also available
No. of references: 0

NOTES

110335.0

*Samples assayed in duplicate

© *KLUWER ACADEMIC PUBLISHERS 1994, ISSN 1381-5067*

Herpes simplex virus (HSV-1)
ANTIBODY DETECTION (IgM)

Manufacturer: Melja Diagnostik GmbH
Cat. No./Trade name: HSV-E03/Herpes Simplex Virus ype 1 IgM EIA Kit

SUMMARY

[Well-Ag]–**Ab**–[AHIgM-HRP]–[TMB]–A_{450}

Assay type: EIA (non-competitive)
Detection: Colorimetric A_{450}
Format: Microtitre well, Ag coated
Sample type: Serum, plasma
Sample pre-treatment:
None
Sample volume: 100 μl of 1:100 dilution x 2
Number of tests: 96
Controls - standards run in assay:
Controls: low Pos (2), high Pos (2), Neg (2)
Incubation:
1 hr (RT) + 30 min (RT) + 15 min (RT)
Washes: 2

CONTENTS

Antibodies, antigens, labelled components:
HSV-1 Ag bound to well
Anti-human IgM Ab HRP conjugated
Substrate: TMB
Controls - standards supplied:
Controls: low Pos, high Pos and Neg
Additional reagents:
None
Special equipment required:
None

INTERPRETATION

Comments on interpretation:
Positive: >cut-off + 20%
Negative: <cut-off - 20%
A MELJA titre may be calculated from a single sample dilution
No. of references: 8

NOTES

110363.0

Herpes simplex virus (HSV-1)
ANTIBODY DETECTION (IgM)

Manufacturer: Melotec S.A.
Cat. No./Trade name: MH1M/MELOTEST HSV-1 IgM

SUMMARY

[Well-Ag]–**Ab**–[AHIgM-HRP]–[TMB]–A_{450}

Assay type: EIA (non-competitive)
Detection: Colorimetric A_{450}
Format: Microtitre well, Ag coated*
Sample type: Serum, plasma
Sample pre-treatment:
Incubation with absorbant 20 min (RT) to remove IgG
Sample volume: 5 μl (+ 195 μl diluent)**
Number of tests: 96
Controls - standards run in assay:
Controls: Neg (1), low Pos (2), high Pos (1)**
Incubation:
20 min (RT) + 20 min (RT) + 10 min (RT)
Washes: 2

CONTENTS

Antibodies, antigens, labelled components:
HSV-1 Ag bound to well
Control Ag coated well
Anti-human IgM Ab HRP conjugated
Substrate: TMB, H_2O_2
Controls - standards supplied:
Controls: Neg, low Pos, high Pos (human serum)
Additional reagents:
None
Special equipment required:
None

INTERPRETATION

Comments on interpretation:
Equivocal: ratio of OD sample to low Pos control is within the range 0.9 to 1.1; retest fresh sample
Repeatably equivocal: retest fresh sample in 1 week
No. of references: 14

NOTES

110131.0

*Samples and controls assayed simultaneously in antigen and control coated wells (control wells eliminate any anti-nuclear antibody interference not neutralised by the absorbant)
**It is recommended to run duplicates of samples and controls for greater precision

© KLUWER ACADEMIC PUBLISHERS 1994, ISSN 1381-5067

Herpes simplex virus (HSV-1)
ANTIBODY DETECTION (IgM)

Manufacturer: United Biotech Inc
Cat. No./Trade name: IA-402/MAGIWEL® HSV-1 IgM

SUMMARY

[Well-Ag]–**Ab**–[AHIgM-HRP]–[TMB]–A_{450}

Assay type: EIA (non-competitive)
Detection: Colorimetric A_{450}
Format: Microtitre well, Ag coated
Sample type: Serum
Sample pre-treatment:
　None
Sample volume: 100 µl of 1:101 dilution
Number of tests: 96
Controls - standards run in assay:
　Controls: Neg (1)
　Calibrator: (1)
Incubation:
　30 min (RT) + 30 min (RT) + 15 min (RT)
Washes: 2

CONTENTS

Antibodies, antigens, labelled components:
　HSV-1 Ag bound to well
　Anti-human IgM Ab (g) HRP conjugated
Substrate: TMB, H_2O_2
Controls - standards supplied:
　Controls: Neg
　Calibrator: IgM Pos (100 EU/ml)
Additional reagents:
　H_2SO_4
Special equipment required:
　None

INTERPRETATION

Comments on interpretation:
　Positive: $\geqslant$100 EU/ml
No. of references: 5

NOTES

110499.0

Herpes simplex virus (HSV-1)
ANTIBODY DETECTION

Manufacturer: Incstar
Cat. No./Trade name: 1810/HSV-1 Fluoro Kit®

SUMMARY

[Slide-Ag]–**Ab**–[AHIg-FITC]–fluorescence

Assay type: Immunofluorescence assay (indirect)
Detection: Fluorescence microscopy
Format: Slide well, Ag coated
Sample type: Serum, plasma
Sample pre-treatment:
　None
Sample volume: 20 µl of 1:10 and 1:20 dilution*
Number of tests: 60,120
Controls - standards run in assay:
　Controls: Neg (1), Pos (1)
Incubation:
　30 min (RT) + 30 min (RT)
Washes: 2

CONTENTS

Antibodies, antigens, labelled components:
　HSV-1 infected and uninfected tissue culture cells bound
　　to slide well
　Anti-human Ig (g or sh) FITC conjugated
Substrate:
Controls - standards supplied:
　Positive and negative (human serum)
Additional reagents:
　None
Special equipment required:
　None

INTERPRETATION

Comments on interpretation:
　Positive: $\geqslant$(1+) specific apple-green fluorescence of
　　the nucleus and/or cytoplasm of at least 10% to 75%
　　of the cells
No. of references: 14

NOTES

110253.0

*Previously screened positive sera should be titred to end-
　point
The assay can be run in parallel with the HSV-2 Fluoro Kit®

© KLUWER ACADEMIC PUBLISHERS 1994, ISSN 1381-5067

Herpes simplex virus (HSV-1)
ANTIBODY DETECTION (IgG)

Manufacturer: Bion Enterprises Ltd
Cat. No./Trade name: HS1G-60/Herpes Simplex Virus Type 1 IgG

SUMMARY

[Well-Ag]–Ab–[AHIgG-FITC]–fluorescence

Assay type: Immunofluorescence assay (indirect)
Detection: Fluorescence microscopy
Format: Slide/well Ag coated
Sample type: Serum
Sample pre-treatment:
   None
Sample volume: 50 µl (+450 µl diluent)
Number of tests: 60, 120
Controls - standards run in assay:
   Controls: Neg (1), Pos (1)
Incubation:
   30 min (RT) + 30 min (RT)
Washes: 2

CONTENTS

Antibodies, antigens, labelled components:
   HSV-1 (Strain F) infected and uninfected diploid
      fibroblasts fixed to slide well
   Anti-human IgG Ab (g) FITC conjugated
Substrate:
Controls - standards supplied:
   Controls: Pos and Neg (human serum)
Additional reagents:
   None
Special equipment required:
   None

INTERPRETATION

Comments on interpretation:
   Positive: > (+1) grade fluorescence with well-defined
      nuclear inclusions and/or homogeneous nuclear and
      cytoplasmic fluorescence in 10-50% cells at dilution
      ≥1:10
   Serial dilutions (1:10-1:2560) tested for a quantitative
      assay
No. of references: 27

NOTES

110208.0

Herpes simplex virus (HSV-1)
ANTIBODY DETECTION (IgG)

Manufacturer: Biowhittaker
Cat. No./Trade name: 1242/FIAX®

SUMMARY

[Solid phase Ag]–Ab–[AHIgG-FITC]–fluorescence

Assay type: Immunofluorescence assay (indirect)
Detection: Fluorometric
Format: FIAX sampler, Ag coated
Sample type: Serum
Sample pre-treatment:
   None
Sample volume: 5 µl (+500 µl diluent)
Number of tests: 60
Controls - standards run in assay:
   Controls: Neg (1), low Pos (1), high Pos (1)
   Standards: (4)
Incubation:
   1 hr (RT) + 30 min (RT)
Washes: 2 (each wash involves a 5 min incubation)

CONTENTS

Antibodies, antigens, labelled components:
   HSV-1 Ag bound to side 1 of the FIAX sampler (Side 2
      contains no antigen and serves as a blank)
   Anti-human IgG Ab (g) FITC conjugated
Substrate:
Controls - standards supplied:
   Controls: Neg and Pos (human sera)
   Standards: 4 (human sera) with assigned titre values
Additional reagents:
   None
Special equipment required:
   FIAX fluorometer, shaker, diluter

INTERPRETATION

Comments on interpretation:
   Equivocal: FIAX titre 8-12. Retest to confirm
No. of references: 24

NOTES

110185.0

© KLUWER ACADEMIC PUBLISHERS 1994, ISSN 1381-5067

Herpes simplex virus (HSV-1)
ANTIBODY DETECTION (IgG)

Manufacturer: Gen Bio
Cat. No./Trade name: 1401 EB/Herpes 1 IgG Test Kit

SUMMARY

[Slide-Ag]–**Ab**–[AHIgG-FITC]–fluorescence

Assay type: Immunofluorescence assay (indirect)
Detection: Fluorescence microscopy
Format: Slide well, Ag coated
Sample type: Serum
Sample pre-treatment:
　　None
Sample volume: 30 µl of 1:10 and 1:100 dilutions*
Number of tests: 100
Controls - standards run in assay:
　　Controls: Neg (1), Pos (4) (serial dilutions 1:10 to 1:200)*
Incubation:
　　30 min (37°C) + 30 min (37°C)
Washes: 2

CONTENTS

Antibodies, antigens, labelled components:
　　HSV-1 infected and uninfected cells bound to slide well
　　Anti-human IgG Ab (g) FITC conjugated
Substrate:
Controls - standards supplied:
　　Controls: Neg and Pos (human serum)
Additional reagents:
　　None
Special equipment required:
　　None

INTERPRETATION

Comments on interpretation:
　　Negative: no specific fluorescence at 1:10 dilution
　　Positive: specific apple green cytoplasmic/nuclear
　　　fluorescence at intensity (1+) to (4+). The endpoint
　　　is considered to be the highest dilution showing a
　　　(2+) fluorescence in infected cells
　　Antibody titre of samples may be obtained by testing
　　　further serial sample dilutions
　　Non-specific reaction: fluorescence in infected and
　　　uninfected cells usually due to antinuclear antibody in
　　　test serum
No. of references: 11

NOTES

110374.0

*The choice of sample dilution and the number of control
　dilutions run is at the discretion of the user. The example
　given is suggested by the manufacturer

Herpes simplex virus (HSV-1)
ANTIBODY DETECTION (IgG)

Manufacturer: Schiapparelli Biosystems Inc
Cat. No./Trade name: 2500/VIRGO HSV-1 IgG IFA

SUMMARY

[Slide-Ag]–**Ab**–[AHIgG-FITC]–fluorescence

Assay type: Immunofluorescence assay (indirect)
Detection: Fluorescence microscopy
Format: Slide well, Ag coated
Sample type: Serum
Sample pre-treatment:
　　None
Sample volume: 20 µl of 1:10 and 1:100 dilution
Number of tests: 96, 200
Controls - standards run in assay:
　　Controls: Neg (1), Pos (1)
Incubation:
　　30 min (RT) + 30 min (RT)
Washes: 2

CONTENTS

Antibodies, antigens, labelled components:
　　HSV-1 infected and uninfected tissue culture cells bound
　　　to slide well
　　Anti-human IgG Ab (g) FITC conjugated
Substrate:
Controls - standards supplied:
　　Controls: Neg and Pos (human serum)
Additional reagents:
　　None
Special equipment required:
　　None

INTERPRETATION

Comments on interpretation:
　　Positive: ≥(1+) specific apple green fluorescence at
　　　1:10 dilution or greater OR little or no fluorescence at
　　　1:10 but ≥(1+) at 1:100 dilution or greater
　　Acute and convalescent sera should be tested together
　　　to diagnose recent or current infection
　　Serial dilutions for quantitative assay
No. of references: 32

NOTES

110412.0

Herpes simplex virus (HSV-1)
ANTIBODY DETECTION (IgG)

Manufacturer: Zeus Scientific Inc
Cat. No./Trade name: 9051-10

SUMMARY

[Slide-Ag]–**Ab**–[AHIgG-FITC]–fluorescence

Assay type: Immunofluorescence assay (indirect)
Detection: Fluorescence microscopy
Format: Slide well, Ag coated
Sample type: Serum
Sample pre-treatment:
  None
Sample volume: 20 µl of 1:10 and 1:100 dilutions (for screening)*
Number of tests: 100
Controls - standards run in assay:
  Controls: Pos (1), Neg (1)
Incubation:
  30 min (RT) + 30 min (RT)
Washes: 2

CONTENTS

Antibodies, antigens, labelled components:
  HSV-1 infected substrate cells fixed to slide well
  Anti-human IgG Ab (r or g) FITC conjugated**
Substrate:
Controls - standards supplied:
  Controls: Pos and Neg (human serum)
Additional reagents:
  None
Special equipment required:
  None

INTERPRETATION

Comments on interpretation:
  Positive: (1+) to (4+) apple green fluorescence in the nucleus and/or cytoplasm of infected cells. Serum titre ⩾ 1:10
No. of references: 13

NOTES

110294.0

*Positive sera are titred to end-point
**Anti-human IgM Ab-FITC conjugated is also available

Herpes simplex virus (HSV-1)
ANTIBODY DETECTION (IgM)

Manufacturer: Gen Bio
Cat. No./Trade name: 1501 EB/Herpes 1 IgM Test Kit

SUMMARY

[Slide-Ag]–**Ab**–[AHIgM-FITC]–fluorescence

Assay type: Immunofluorescence assay (indirect)
Detection: Fluorescence microscopy
Format: Slide well, Ag coated
Sample type: Serum
Sample pre-treatment:
  None
Sample volume: 30 µl serial dilutions 1:5 to 1:160*
Number of tests: 100
Controls - standards run in assay:
  Controls: Neg (1), Pos (5) (serial dilutions 1:10 to 1:160)*
Incubation:
  1 hr (37°C) + 30 min (37°C)
Washes: 2

CONTENTS

Antibodies, antigens, labelled components:
  HSV-1 infected and uninfected cells bound to slide well
  Anti-human IgM Ab (g) FITC conjugated
Substrate:
Controls - standards supplied:
  Controls: Neg and Pos (human serum)
Additional reagents:
  None
Special equipment required:
  None

INTERPRETATION

Comments on interpretation:
  Negative: no specific fluorescence at 1:5 dilution
  Positive: specific apple green cytoplasmic/nuclear fluorescence at intensity (1+) to (4+)
  Antibody titre of samples may be obtained by testing further serial sample dilutions
  Non-specific reaction: fluorescence in infected and uninfected cells usually due to antinuclear antibody in test serum
No. of references: 12

NOTES

110376.0

*The choice of sample dilution and the number of control dilutions run is at the discretion of the user. The example given is suggested by the manufacturer
It is recommended that HSV-IgG antibody testing be performed simultaneously with HSV-IgM antibody tests

© *KLUWER ACADEMIC PUBLISHERS 1994, ISSN 1381-5067*

Herpes simplex virus (HSV-1 and HSV-2)
ANTIGEN DETECTION

Manufacturer: Baxter Diagnostics Inc (Bartels Division)
Cat. No./Trade name: B-029-44/HSV Type 1 + 2 Direct FA Kit

SUMMARY

[Slide/vial]–**Ag**–[Ab-FITC]–fluorescence

Assay type: Immunofluorescence assay (direct)
Detection: Fluorescence microscopy
Format: Slide well or cell culture vial
Sample type: Cell culture cells showing cytopathogenic effect*
Sample pre-treatment:
　Vials: remove culture medium, fix with acetone, air dry, rinse with PBS
　Tubes: spot cells on slides, fix with acetone, air dry, rinse with PBS
Sample volume: 2 vials or cells spotted onto 2 slide wells
Number of tests: 10
Controls - standards run in assay:
　Controls: Neg (1), Pos (2) (every time staining procedure is performed)
Incubation:
　30 min (37°C)
Washes: 1

CONTENTS

Antibodies, antigens, labelled components:
　Anti-HSV-1 MAb FITC conjugated
　Anti-HSV-2 MAb FITC conjugated
Substrate:
Controls - standards supplied:
　Controls: Neg and Pos (control slides)
Additional reagents:
　None
Special equipment required:
　None

INTERPRETATION

Comments on interpretation:
　HSV-1 Positive: bright green fluorescence with HSV-1 conjugate and no fluorescence with HSV-2 conjugate
　HSV-2 Positive: bright green fluorescence with HSV-2 conjugate and no fluorescence with HSV-1 conjugate
No. of references: 6

NOTES

110630.0

*Specimens from vesicular fluid, basal cells from ulcerated/crusted lesions, cervical/vulvar scrapings, conjunctival scrapings, CSF (all centrifuged prior to innoculation into vials or tubes)

Herpes simplex virus (HSV-1 and HSV-2)
ANTIGEN DETECTION

Manufacturer: Dako A/S
Cat. No./Trade name: K6106/IMAGEN® Herpes Simplex Virus Type 1 and 2

SUMMARY

[Slide well]–**Ag**–[MAb-FITC]–fluorescence

Assay type: Immunofluorescence assay (direct)
Detection: Fluorescence microscopy
Format: Slide well
Sample type: Cell culture
Sample pre-treatment:
　Harvest cell culture; centrifuge (10 min); remove supernatant; resuspend in PBS
Sample volume: 25 µl x 2
Number of tests: 50
Controls - standards run in assay:
　Controls: Pos (2)
Incubation:
　30 min (37°C)
Washes: 1

CONTENTS

Antibodies, antigens, labelled components:
　Anti-HSV-1 MAb (m) FITC conjugated
　Anti-HSV-2 MAb (m) FITC conjugated
Substrate:
Controls - standards supplied:
　Controls: Pos (slides coated with fibroblasts Pos for HSV type 1 or HSV type 2)
Additional reagents:
　None
Special equipment required:
　None

INTERPRETATION

Comments on interpretation:
　Negative: at least 50 visible cells and no fluorescence
　Positive: ≥ one cell showing green intracellular fluorescence
No. of references: 14

NOTES

110033.0

© KLUWER ACADEMIC PUBLISHERS 1994, ISSN 1381-5067

Herpes simplex virus (HSV-1 and HSV-2)
ANTIGEN DETECTION

Manufacturer: Syva Company
Cat. No./Trade name: 8H349/MicroTrak® HSV 1/HSV 2 Direct Specimen Identification/Typing Test

SUMMARY

[Slide]–**Ag**–[MAb-FITC]–fluorescence

Assay type: Immunofluorescence assay (direct)
Detection: Fluorescence microscopy
Format: Slide well, specimen coated
Sample type: Direct specimen swab
Sample pre-treatment:
    Prepare smear, air-dry and acetone fix
Sample volume:
Number of tests: 60
Controls - standards run in assay:
    Controls: Neg (1), Pos (1)
Incubation:
    15 min (37°C) or 30 min (RT)
Washes: 1

CONTENTS

Antibodies, antigens, labelled components:
    Anti-HSV-1 MAb (m) FITC conjugated
    Anti-HSV-2 MAbs (3) (m) FITC conjugated
Substrate:
Controls - standards supplied:
    None
Additional reagents:
    HSV-1 and HSV-2 Ag control slides (Cat no. 8H399)
Special equipment required:
    Syva MicroTrak® HSV-1/HSV-2 specimen collection kit
    (Cat. no. 8H319)

INTERPRETATION

Comments on interpretation:
    Negative: no fluorescent staining of at least 20 intact
        nonsuperficial epithelial cells; confirm by culturing
        separate viral isolation sample*
    Positive: fluorescent staining of at least one intact cell
No. of references: 12

NOTES
110519.0

*Syva MicroTrak® HSV-1/HSV-2 culture identification/typing
    test available (Cat. no. 8H219)

Herpes simplex virus (HSV-1 and HSV-2)
ANTIGEN DETECTION

Manufacturer: Syva Company
Cat. No./Trade name: 8H219/MicroTrak® HSV 1/HSV 2 Culture Identification/Typing Test

SUMMARY

[Slide]–**Ag**–[MAb-FITC]–fluorescence

Assay type: Immunofluorescence assay (direct)
Detection: Fluorescence microscopy
Format: Slide well, specimen coated
Sample type: Infected tissue culture cell*
Sample pre-treatment:
    Acetone fix air-dried smear or washed coverslip (10 min)
Sample volume:
Number of tests: 18-25**
Controls - standards run in assay:
    Controls: Neg (1), Pos (1)
Incubation:
    30 min (37°C)
Washes: 1

CONTENTS

Antibodies, antigens, labelled components:
    Anti-HSV-1 MAb (m) FITC conjugated
    Anti-HSV-2 MAbs (2) (m) FITC conjugated
Substrate:
Controls - standards supplied:
    None
Additional reagents:
    Pos and Neg controls. Microscope slides/wells or shell
        vials with 12 mm coverslips seeded with MRC-5 cells
Special equipment required:
    None

INTERPRETATION

Comments on interpretation:
    Negative: no fluorescent staining of at least 50 cells;
        confirm by repeating isolation procedure if necessary
    Positive: fluorescent staining of cytoplasm in at least one
        intact cell
No. of references: 15

NOTES
110520.0

*Test can be done on conventional cell culture and shell-vial
    cultures (MRC-5 cells)
**depending on sample format (smear or coverslip)

Herpes simplex virus (HSV-1 and HSV-2)
ANTIBODY DETECTION (IgG)

Manufacturer: Biowhittaker
Cat. No./Trade name: 30-629 U/HERPELISA II

SUMMARY

[Well-Ag]–**Ab**–[AHIgG-AP]–[PMP]–A_{550}

Assay type: EIA (non-competitive)
Detection: Colorimetric A_{550}
Format: Microtitre well, Ag coated
Sample type: Serum (do not heat inactivate)
Sample pre-treatment:
   None
Sample volume: 10 µl (+200 µl diluent)
Number of tests: 192*
Controls - standards run in assay:
   Controls: Neg (1), Pos (1)
   Calibrators: (3)
Incubation:
   45 min (RT) + 45 min (RT) + 45 min (RT)
Washes: 2 (+ preliminary plate wash)

CONTENTS

Antibodies, antigens, labelled components:
   HSV-1 Ag (partially purified) bound to well
   HSV-2 Ag (partially purified) bound to well
   Anti-human IgG Ab AP conjugated
Substrate: PMP
Controls - standards supplied:
   Controls: Neg and Pos (human serum)
   Calibrators: 3 (human) with assigned HERPELISA value
Additional reagents:
   None
Special equipment required:
   Biowhittaker automated system and software (optional)

INTERPRETATION

Comments on interpretation:
   Equivocal: Herpelisa I value 0.23-0.24
      Herpelisa II value 0.20-0.21; retest to confirm
   Repeatably equivocal: retest with an alternative method
      or repeat with a fresh sample
   A method is available for the comparison of acute and
      convalescent sera
No. of references: 3

NOTES

110187.0

*96 for each of type 1 and type 2

Herpes simplex virus (HSV-1 and HSV-2)
ANTIBODY DETECTION (IgG)

Manufacturer: Biowhittaker
Cat. No./Trade name: 30-367 U/HERPES 1 & 2 STAT

SUMMARY

[Well-Ag]–**Ab**–[AHIgG-AP]–[PMP]–A_{550}

Assay type: EIA (non-competitive)
Detection: Colorimetric A_{550}
Format: Microtitre well, Ag coated
Sample type: Serum (do not heat inactivate)
Sample pre-treatment:
   None
Sample volume: 10 µl
Number of tests: 192*
Controls - standards run in assay:
   Controls: Neg (1), Pos (1)
   Standards: low Pos (3), high Pos (1), Neg (1)
Incubation:
   15 min (RT) + 15 min (RT) + 15 min (RT) on plate
      shaker
Washes: 2 (+ preliminary plate wash)

CONTENTS

Antibodies, antigens, labelled components:
   HSV-1 Ag bound to plate
   HSV-2 Ag bound to plate
   Anti-human IgG Ab AP conjugated
Substrate: PMP
Controls - standards supplied:
   Controls: Neg and Pos (human)
   Calibrators: low Pos, high Pos and Neg (human) with
      assigned index values
Additional reagents:
   None
Special equipment required:
   Biowhittaker automated system and software (optional)

INTERPRETATION

Comments on interpretation:
   Equivocal: Predicted Index Value (PIV) 0.8-0.99.
      Retest to confirm
   Repeatably equivocal: Retest with a fresh sample or
      using an alternative method
   A method is available for the comparison of acute and
      convalescent sera
No. of references: 3

NOTES

110188.0

*96 of each for type 1 and type 2

Herpes simplex virus (HSV-1 and HSV-2)
ANTIBODY DETECTION (IgG)

Manufacturer: Zeus Scientific Inc
Cat. No./Trade name: Series 9700G*

SUMMARY

[Well-Ag]–**Ab**–[AHIgG-HRP]–[OPD]–A_{490}

Assay type: EIA (non-competitive)
Detection: Colorimetric A_{490}
Format: Microtitre well, Ag coated
Sample type: Serum
Sample pre-treatment:
   None
Sample volume: 10 μl (+200 μl diluent)
Number of tests: 96
Controls - standards run in assay:
   Controls: Neg (1), low Pos (3), high Pos (1)
Incubation:
   20 min (RT) + 20 min (RT) + 10 min (RT)
Washes: 2

CONTENTS

Antibodies, antigens, labelled components:
   HSV-1 Ag (strain E) bound to well
   HSV-2 Ag (strain G) bound to well
   Anti-human IgG Ab HRP conjugated
Substrate: OPD
Controls - standards supplied:
   Controls: Neg, low Pos and high Pos (human serum)
Additional reagents:
   None
Special equipment required:
   None

INTERPRETATION

Comments on Interpretation:
   Equivocal: OD ratio of sample: cut-off between 0.91
      and 1.09; retest to confirm
   Repeatably equivocal: re-test using a fresh sample or an
      alternative method
No. of references: 18

NOTES

110297.0

*Component parts bought separately

Herpes simplex virus (HSV-1 and HSV-2)
ANTIBODY DETECTION (IgM)

Manufacturer: Zeus Scientific Inc
Cat. No./Trade name: 9700M Series

SUMMARY

[Well-Ag]–**Ab**–[AHIgM-HRP]–[TMB]–A_{450}

Assay type: EIA (non-competitive)
Detection: Colorimetric A450
Format: Microtitre well, Ag coated
Sample type: Serum
Sample pre-treatment:
   Incubation with absorbent to remove IgG (20 min RT)
Sample volume: 10 μl (+200 μl diluent)
Number of tests: 96
Controls - standards run in assay:
   Controls: Neg (1), low Pos (3), high Pos (1)
Incubation:
   20 min (RT) + 20 min (RT) + 10 min (RT)
Washes: 2

CONTENTS

Antibodies, antigens, labelled components:
   HSV-1 Ag (strain E) bound to well
   HSV-2 Ag (strain G) bound to well
   Anti-human IgM Ab HRP conjugated
Substrate: TMB, H_2O_2
Controls - standards supplied:
   Controls: Neg, low Pos and high Pos (human serum)
Additional reagents:
   None
Special equipment required:
   None

INTERPRETATION

Comments on Interpretation:
   Equivocal: OD ratio of sample: cut-off between 0.91-
      1.09; repeat to confirm
   Repeatably equivocal: re-test using a fresh sample or an
      alternative method
No. of references: 23

NOTES

110298.0

Herpes simplex virus (HSV-2)
ANTIGEN DETECTION

Manufacturer: Bio-Stat Diagnostics
Cat. No./Trade name: 851102/ELISA Antigen Test

SUMMARY

[Well-Ab]–**Ag**–[Ab-HRP]–[TMB]–A_{450}

Assay type: EIA (non-competitive)
Detection: Colorimetric A_{450}, visual
Format: Microtitre well, Ab coated
Sample type: Swab of vesicle, vesicle fluid, cell culture
Sample pre-treatment:
Swab, vesicle fluid: extraction (+1 ml diluent). Cell culture: freeze and thaw x 2 (+1:10 dilution)*
Sample volume: 100 μl x 2
Number of tests: 96
Controls - standards run in assay:
Controls: Neg (one per sample); Pos (1) x 2*
Incubation:
a) 1 hr (37°C) + 15 min (37°C) + 15 min (RT)
b) 2 hr (RT) + 30 min (RT) + 15 min (RT)
Washes: 2

CONTENTS

Antibodies, antigens, labelled components:
Anti-HSV-2 Ab bound to wells
Anti-HSV-2 Ab HRP conjugated
Substrate: TMB, H_2O_2
Controls - standards supplied:
Controls: Neg (coated on microtitre wells), Pos
Additional reagents:
None
Special equipment required:
None

INTERPRETATION

Comments on interpretation:
Classification of samples is according to cut-off; no further testing
Visual interpretation is possible
No. of references: None

NOTES

110077.0

*Sample and Pos control assayed in parallel in antibody coated and Neg control coated microtitre wells
Assay may be run in parallel with HSV-I ELISA Antigen Test for HSV classification

Herpes simplex virus (HSV-2)
ANTIBODY DETECTION (IgG)

Manufacturer: Baxter Diagnostics Inc (Bartels Division)
Cat. No./Trade name: B1029-350/Herpes Simplex Virus-2 IgG EIA

SUMMARY

[Well-Ag]–**Ab**–[AHIgG-Enzyme]–[PNP]–A_{405}

Assay type: EIA (non-competitive)
Detection: Colorimetric A_{405}
Format: Microtitre well, Ag coated
Sample type: Serum
Sample pre-treatment:
None
Sample volume: 100 μl of 1:21 dilution
Number of tests: 96
Controls - standards run in assay:
Controls: not specified
Incubation:
30 min (37°C) + 30 min (37°C) + 30 min (37°C)
Washes: 2

CONTENTS

Antibodies, antigens, labelled components:
HSV-2 Ag bound to well
Anti-human IgG Ab enzyme conjugated*
Substrate: PNP
Controls - standards supplied:
Controls: Neg, Pos, reference serum
Additional reagents:
None
Special equipment required:
None

INTERPRETATION

Comments on interpretation:
Classification of samples is according to cut-off; further details not specified
No. of references: 6

NOTES

110826.0

*Enzyme label not specified

© *KLUWER ACADEMIC PUBLISHERS 1994, ISSN 1381-5067*

Herpes simplex virus (HSV-2)
ANTIBODY DETECTION (IgG)

Manufacturer: Bio-Stat Diagnostics
Cat. No./Trade name: 851226/ELISA IgG Antibody Test

SUMMARY

[Well-Ag]–**Ab**–[AHIgG-HRP]–[TMB]–A$_{450}$

Assay type: EIA (non-competitive)
Detection: Colorimetric A$_{450}$
Format: Microtitre well, Ag coated
Sample type: Serum
Sample pre-treatment:
  None
Sample volume: 10 µl (+ 1 ml diluent)
Number of tests: 96
Controls - standards run in assay:
  Controls: Neg (2), Pos (2)
Incubation:
  30 min (RT) + 30 min (RT) + 15 min (RT)
Washes: 2

CONTENTS

Antibodies, antigens, labelled components:
  HSV-2 Ag bound to wells
  Anti-human IgG Ab HRP conjugated
Substrate: TMB, H$_2$O$_2$
Controls - standards supplied:
  Controls: Neg and Pos
Additional reagents:
  None
Special equipment required:
  None

INTERPRETATION

Comments on interpretation:
  Classification of samples is according to cut-off; no
    further testing
  Visual interpretation is possible
No. of references: 5

NOTES

110086.0

Herpes simplex virus (HSV-2)
ANTIBODY DETECTION (IgG)

Manufacturer: Biologische Analysensystem GmbH
Cat. No./Trade name: 5212/BAG-HSV-2-EIA-G

SUMMARY

[Well-Ag]–**Ab**–[AHIgG-HRP]–[TMB]–A$_{450}$

Assay type: EIA (non-competitive)
Detection: Colorimetric A$_{450}$
Format: Microtitre well, Ag coated
Sample type: Serum
Sample pre-treatment:
  None
Sample volume: 10 µl (+ 1 ml diluent)
Number of tests: 96
Controls - standards run in assay:
  Controls: Neg (1), Cut-off (2), Pos (1)
Incubation:
  30 min (RT) + 30 min (RT) + 10 min (RT)
Washes: 2

CONTENTS

Antibodies, antigens, labelled components:
  HSV-2 Ag bound to well
  Anti-human IgG Ab (sh) HRP conjugated
Substrate: TMB
Controls - standards supplied:
  Controls: Neg, Pos and cut-off
Additional reagents:
  None
Special equipment required:
  None

INTERPRETATION

Comments on interpretation:
  Equivocal: within cut-off ± 20%; retest to confirm
No. of references: 0

NOTES

110285.0

© KLUWER ACADEMIC PUBLISHERS 1994, ISSN 1381-5067

Herpes simplex virus (HSV-2)
ANTIBODY DETECTION (IgG)

Manufacturer: Cambridge Biotech Corporation
Cat. No./Trade name: /HSV-2 IgG EIA Test

SUMMARY

[Well-Ag]–**Ab**–[AHIgG-AP]–[PNP]–A_{405}

Assay type: EIA (non-competitive)
Detection: Colorimetric A_{405}
Format: Microtitre well, Ag coated
Sample type: Serum
Sample pre-treatment:
    None
Sample volume: 100 µl of 1:21 dilution
Number of tests: 96
Controls - standards run in assay:
    Controls: Neg (1), Pos (1), Reference serum (3)
Incubation:
    30 min (37°C) + 30 min (37°C) + 30 min (37°C)
Washes: 2

CONTENTS

Antibodies, antigens, labelled components:
    HSV-2 Ag bound to well
    Anti-human IgG Ab (g) AP conjugated
Substrate: PNP
Controls - standards supplied:
    Controls: Neg and Pos (human serum); Reference serum (human)
Additional reagents:
    None
Special equipment required:
    None

INTERPRETATION

Comments on interpretation:
    Equivocal: samples within specified range; retest to confirm
    Repeatably equivocal: retest using an alternative method
No. of references: 12

NOTES

110649.0

Herpes simplex virus (HSV-2)
ANTIBODY DETECTION (IgG)

Manufacturer: Chimica Diagnostica
Cat. No./Trade name: 41700/Herpes Simplex Virus 2 IgG

SUMMARY

[Well-Ag]–**Ab**–[AHIgG-POD]–[TMB]–A_{450}

Assay type: EIA (non-competitive)
Detection: Colorimetric A_{450}
Format: Microtitre well, Ag coated
Sample type: Serum
Sample pre-treatment:
    None
Sample volume: 10 µl (+ 1 ml diluent)
Number of tests: 96
Controls - standards run in assay:
    Controls: Neg (1), cut-off (1), Pos (1)
Incubation:
    30 min (RT) + 30 min (RT) + 15 min (RT)
Washes: 2

CONTENTS

Antibodies, antigens, labelled components:
    HSV-2 Ag bound to well
    Anti-human IgG PAb (g) POD conjugated
Substrate: TMB
Controls - standards supplied:
    Controls: Neg, cut-off and Pos (100 IU/ml)
Additional reagents:
    None
Special equipment required:
    None

INTERPRETATION

Comments on interpretation:
    Equivocal: Sample index (ratio of O.D. sample: cut-off) > 0.9 < 1.1; retest to confirm
No. of references: 2

NOTES

110311.0

© *KLUWER ACADEMIC PUBLISHERS 1994, ISSN 1381-5067*

Herpes simplex virus (HSV-2)
ANTIBODY DETECTION (IgG)

Manufacturer: Diamedix Corporation
Cat. No./Trade name: 783-350/HERPES 2 Microassay

SUMMARY

[Well-Ag]–**Ab**–[AHIgG-AP]–[PNP]–A_{405}

Assay type: EIA (non-competitive)
Detection: Colorimetric A_{405}
Format: Microtitre well, Ag coated
Sample type: Serum (do not heat inactivate)
Sample pre-treatment:
 None
Sample volume: 100 µl of 1:41 dilution
Number of tests: 96
Controls - standards run in assay:
 Controls: Neg (1), Pos (1)
 Calibrator: (1)
Incubation:
 30 min (RT) + 30 min (RT) + 30 min (RT)
Washes: 2

CONTENTS

Antibodies, antigens, labelled components:
 HSV-2 Ag bound to well
 Anti-human IgG Ab (g) AP conjugated
Substrate: PNP
Controls - standards supplied:
 Controls: Neg and Pos (human serum)
 Calibrators: (1) (human serum)
Additional reagents:
 None
Special equipment required:
 None

INTERPRETATION

Comments on interpretation:
 Positive: ≥ 20 ELISA unit (EU)/ml
No. of references: 2

NOTES

110494.0

This test is designed to be run in parallel with the Herpes 1
 Microassay

Herpes simplex virus (HSV-2)
ANTIBODY DETECTION (IgG)

Manufacturer: E. Merck
Cat. No./Trade name: 14457/Herpes Simplex Virus 2 IgG

SUMMARY

[Well-Ag]–**Ab**–[AHIgG-HRP]–[TMB]–A_{450}

Assay type: EIA (non-competitive)
Detection: Colorimetric A_{450}
Format: Microtitre well, Ag coated
Sample type: Serum
Sample pre-treatment:
 None
Sample volume: 10 µl (+ 1 ml diluent)
Number of tests: 96
Controls - standards run in assay:
 Controls: Neg (2), Pos (2)
Incubation:
 30 min (RT) + 30 min (RT) + 15 min (RT)
Washes: 2

CONTENTS

Antibodies, antigens, labelled components:
 HSV-2 Ag bound to well
 Anti-human IgG PAb (r) HRP conjugated
Substrate: TMB
Controls - standards supplied:
 Controls: Neg and Pos
Additional reagents:
 None
Special equipment required:
 None

INTERPRETATION

Comments on interpretation:
 Classification of samples is according to cut-off; no
 further testing
No. of references: 5

NOTES

110316.0

Herpes simplex virus (HSV-2)
ANTIBODY DETECTION (IgG)

Manufacturer: Eurogenetics
Cat. No./Trade name: /Eurogenetics® Herpes 2 IgG ELISA

SUMMARY

$$[\text{Well-Ag}]–\textbf{Ab}–[\text{AHIgG-POD}]–[\text{OPD}]–A_{492}$$

Assay type: EIA (non-competitive)
Detection: Colorimetric A_{492}
Format: Microtitre well, Ag coated
Sample type: Serum
Sample pre-treatment:
    None
Sample volume: 100 µl of 1:300 dilution x 2
Number of tests: 96
Controls - standards run in assay:
    Controls: Neg (2), Pos (2)
Incubation:
    1 hr (37°C) + 30 min (37°C) + 20 min (RT)
Washes: 2 (+ preliminary plate wash)

CONTENTS

Antibodies, antigens, labelled components:
    HSV-2 Ag bound to wells
    Anti-human IgG Ab POD conjugated
Substrate: OPD, H_2O_2
Controls - standards supplied:
    Controls: Neg and Pos (human serum)
Additional reagents:
    None
Special equipment required:
    Eurogenetics Microtitre plate reader (or similar)

INTERPRETATION

Comments on interpretation:
    Equivocal: within cut-off + 0.1; retest a fresh sample
No. of references: 12

NOTES

110034.0

Herpes simplex virus (HSV-2)
ANTIBODY DETECTION (IgG)

Manufacturer: Gamma SA
Cat. No./Trade name: /HERPES SIMPLEX VIRUS 2 IgG ELISA

SUMMARY

$$[\text{Well-Ag}]–\textbf{Ab}–[\text{AHIgG-HRP}]–[\text{TMB}]–A_{450}$$

Assay type: EIA (non-competitive)
Detection: Colorimetric A_{450}
Format: Microtitre well, Ag coated
Sample type: Serum
Sample pre-treatment:
    None
Sample volume: 100 µl of 1:100 dilution
Number of tests: 96
Controls - standards run in assay:
    Controls: Neg (2), Pos (2)
Incubation:
    30 min (RT) + 30 min (RT) + 15 min (RT)
Washes: 2

CONTENTS

Antibodies, antigens, labelled components:
    HSV-2 Ag bound to well
    Anti-human IgG Ab (r) HRP conjugated
Substrate: TMB
Controls - standards supplied:
    Controls: Neg and Pos
Additional reagents:
    None
Special equipment required:
    None

INTERPRETATION

Comments on interpretation:
    Classification of sample is according to cut-off; no further testing. (Results may be expressed in units based on the positive control)
    Visual interpretation is possible
No. of references: 0

NOTES

110588.0

© KLUWER ACADEMIC PUBLISHERS 1994, ISSN 1381-5067

Herpes simplex virus (HSV-2)
ANTIBODY DETECTION (IgG)

Manufacturer: Gull Laboratories
Cat. No./Trade name: H2E 100-E/HSV-2 IgG ELISA Test

SUMMARY

[Well-Ag]–**Ab**–[AHIgG-AP]–[PNP]–A_{405}

Assay type: EIA (non-competitive)
Detection: Colorimetric A_{405}
Format: Microtitre well, Ag coated
Sample type: Serum
Sample pre-treatment:
   None
Sample volume: 10 µl (+200 µl diluent)
Number of tests: 96
Controls - standards run in assay:
   Controls: Neg (1), Pos (1)
   Reference serum: (3)
Incubation:
   30 min (37°C) + 30 min (37°C) + 30 min (37°C)
Washes: 2

CONTENTS

Antibodies, antigens, labelled components:
   HSV-2 Ag bound to well
   Anti-human IgG Ab (g) AP conjugated
Substrate: PNP
Controls - standards supplied:
   Controls: Neg and Pos (human serum)
   Reference serum (human)
Additional reagents:
   None
Special equipment required:
   None

INTERPRETATION

Comments on interpretation:
   Equivocal: within cut-off and cut-off x 0.9; retest
   Repeatably equivocal: retest with alternative method
No. of references: 12

NOTES

110111.0

Herpes simplex virus (HSV-2)
ANTIBODY DETECTION (IgG)

Manufacturer: Human GmbH
Cat. No./Trade name: 51 226/HERPES SIMPLEX VIRUS 2 IgG ELISA

SUMMARY

[Well-Ag]–**Ab**–[AHIgG-HRP]–[TMB]–A_{450}

Assay type: EIA (non-competitive)
Detection: Colorimetric A_{450}
Format: Microtitre well, Ag coated
Sample type: Serum
Sample pre-treatment:
   None
Sample volume: 100 µl of 1:101 dilution
Number of tests: 96
Controls - standards run in assay:
   Controls: Neg (2), Pos (2)
Incubation:
   30 min (RT) + 30 min (RT) + 15 min (RT)
Washes: 2

CONTENTS

Antibodies, antigens, labelled components:
   HSV-2 Ag bound to well
   Anti-human IgG Ab (r) HRP conjugated
Substrate: TMB, H_2O_2
Controls - standards supplied:
   Controls: Neg, Pos (human serum)
Additional reagents:
   None
Special equipment required:
   None

INTERPRETATION

Comments on interpretation:
   Equivocal: within cut-off ±15%; retest in parallel with
     sample taken 7-14 days later
   The result may be read visually in comparison with the
     negative controls
No. of references: 5

NOTES

110514.0

Herpes simplex virus (HSV-2)
ANTIBODY DETECTION (IgG)

Manufacturer: Immunobiological Laboratories
Cat. No./Trade name: VE57121/Herpes 2 Virus IgG EIA test

SUMMARY

$[Well-Ag]$–**Ab**–$[AHIgG-HRP]$–$[TMB]$–A_{450}

Assay type: EIA (non-competitive)
Detection: Colorimetric A_{450}
Format: Microtitre well, Ag coated
Sample type: Serum
Sample pre-treatment:
    None
Sample volume: 100 μl of a 1:100 dilution x 2
Number of tests: 96
Controls - standards run in assay:
    Controls: Neg (2), low Pos (2), high Pos (2)
Incubation:
    1 hr (RT) + 30 min (RT) + 15 min (RT)
Washes: 2

CONTENTS

Antibodies, antigens, labelled components:
    HSV-2 virus Ag bound to well
    Anti-human IgG Ab HRP conjugated
Substrate: TMB, H_2O_2
Controls - standards supplied:
    Controls: Neg, low Pos, high Pos
Additional reagents:
    None
Special equipment required:
    None

INTERPRETATION

Comments on interpretation:
    Classification of samples is according to cut-off; no further testing
No. of references: 0

NOTES

110328.0

Herpes simplex virus (HSV-2)
ANTIBODY DETECTION (IgG)

Manufacturer: Incstar
Cat. No./Trade name: 4512/Clin-ELISA HSV-2 IgG

SUMMARY

$[Well-Ag]$–**Ab**–$[AHIgG-AP]$–$[PNP]$–A_{405}

Assay type: EIA (non-competitive)
Detection: Colorimetric A_{405}
Format: Microtitre well, Ag coated
Sample type: Serum
Sample pre-treatment:
    None
Sample volume: 10 μl (+500 μl diluent)
Number of tests: 96
Controls - standards run in assay:
    Controls: Low pos (1), high Pos (1)
    Calibrators: Neg (2), low Pos (2), high Pos (2)
Incubation:
    30 min (RT) + 30 min (RT) + 45 min (RT)
Washes: 2

CONTENTS

Antibodies, antigens, labelled components:
    HSV-2 Ag bound to well
    Anti-human IgG Ab AP conjugated
Substrate: PNP
Controls - standards supplied:
    Controls: Low Pos, high Pos (human serum)
    Calibrators: (3) with assigned ELISA values
Additional reagents:
    None
Special equipment required:
    Clin-ELISA reader (optional)

INTERPRETATION

Comments on interpretation:
    Equivocal: ELISA value 31-39; retest to confirm and/or test a fresh sample in 2-3 weeks
No. of references: 23

NOTES

110276.0

© *KLUWER ACADEMIC PUBLISHERS 1994, ISSN 1381-5067*

Herpes simplex virus (HSV-2)
ANTIBODY DETECTION (IgG)

Manufacturer: International Immunodiagnostics
Cat. No./Trade name: 108 142/HSV-Typ 2 IgG

SUMMARY

[Well-Ag]–**Ab**–[AHIgG-HRP]–[TMB]–A$_{450}$

Assay type: EIA (non-competitive)
Detection: Colorimetric A$_{450}$
Format: Microtitre well, Ag coated
Sample type: Serum
Sample pre-treatment:
   None
Sample volume: 10 μl (+ 1 ml diluent)*
Number of tests: 96
Controls - standards run in assay:
   Controls: Neg (2), Pos (2)
Incubation:
   30 min (RT) + 30 min (RT) + 15 min (RT) (first two incubations on plate shaker)
Washes: 2

CONTENTS

Antibodies, antigens, labelled components:
   HSV-2 Ag bound to well
   Anti-human IgG Ab HRP conjugated
Substrate: TMB, H$_2$O$_2$
Controls - standards supplied:
   Controls: Neg and Pos (human serum)
Additional reagents:
   None
Special equipment required:
   None

INTERPRETATION

Comments on interpretation:
   Classification of results is according to cut-off; no further testing
   Quantitative interpretation also available
No. of references: 0

NOTES

110336.0

*Samples assayed in duplicate

Herpes simplex virus (HSV-2)
ANTIBODY DETECTION (IgG)

Manufacturer: Melja Diagnostik GmbH
Cat. No./Trade name: HSV-E02/Herpes Simplex Virus Type 2 IgG EIA Kit

SUMMARY

[Well-Ag]–**Ab**–[AHIgG-HRP]–[TMB]–A$_{450}$

Assay type: EIA (non-competitive)
Detection: Colorimetric A$_{450}$
Format: Microtitre well, Ag coated
Sample type: Serum, plasma
Sample pre-treatment:
   None
Sample volume: 100 μl of 1:100 dilution x 2
Number of tests: 96
Controls - standards run in assay:
   Controls: low Pos (2), high Pos (2), Neg (2)
Incubation:
   1 hr (RT) + 30 min (RT) + 15 min (RT)
Washes: 2

CONTENTS

Antibodies, antigens, labelled components:
   HSV-2 Ag bound to well
   Anti-human IgG PAb HRP conjugated
Substrate: TMB
Controls - standards supplied:
   Controls: low Pos, high Pos and Neg
Additional reagents:
   None
Special equipment required:
   None

INTERPRETATION

Comments on interpretation:
   Positive: > cut-off + 20%
   Negative: < cut-off - 20%
   A MELJA titre may be calculated from a single sample dilution
No. of references: 8

NOTES

110362.0

Herpes simplex virus (HSV-2)
ANTIBODY DETECTION (IgG)

Manufacturer: Melotec S.A.
Cat. No./Trade name: MH2G/MELOTEST HSV-2 IgG

SUMMARY

[Well-Ag]–**Ab**–[AHIgG-HRP]–[TMB]–A_{450}

Assay type: EIA (non-competitive)
Detection: Colorimetric A_{450}
Format: Microtitre well, Ag coated
Sample type: Serum, plasma
Sample pre-treatment:
None
Sample volume: 10 µl (+ 190 µl diluent)
Number of tests: 96
Controls - standards run in assay:
Controls: Neg (1), low Pos (2), high Pos (1)
Incubation:
20 min (RT) + 20 min (RT) + 10 min (RT)
Washes: 2

CONTENTS

Antibodies, antigens, labelled components:
HSV-2 Ag bound to well
Anti-human IgG Ab HRP conjugated
Substrate: TMB, H_2O_2
Controls - standards supplied:
Controls: Neg, low Pos, high Pos (human serum)
Additional reagents:
None
Special equipment required:
None

INTERPRETATION

Comments on interpretation:
Equivocal: ratio of OD of sample to low Pos control is
within the range 0.9 to 1.1; retest fresh sample
Repeatably equivocal: retest fresh sample in 4-6 weeks
No. of references: 9

NOTES

110133.0

Herpes simplex virus (HSV-2)
ANTIBODY DETECTION (IgG)

Manufacturer: Radim
Cat. No./Trade name: KH2G/HSV2 IgG

SUMMARY

[Well-Ag]–**Ab**–[AHIgG-HRP]–[TMB]–A_{450}

Assay type: EIA (non-competitive)
Detection: Colorimetric A_{450}
Format: Microtitre well, Ag coated
Sample type: Serum or plasma
Sample pre-treatment:
None
Sample volume: 100 µl of 1:300 dilution x 2
Number of tests: 96, 192
Controls - standards run in assay:
Controls: Neg (2), Pos (2), cut-off (2)
Incubation:
1 hr (37°C) + 30 min (37°C) + 10 min (37°C) or 15 min
(RT)
Washes: 2

CONTENTS

Antibodies, antigens, labelled components:
HSV-2 specific glycoprotein bound to well
Anti-human IgG (g) HRP conjugated
Substrate: TMB, H_2O_2
Controls - standards supplied:
Controls: Neg, Pos, cut-off (serum)
Additional reagents:
None
Special equipment required:
None

INTERPRETATION

Comments on interpretation:
Grey area: within cut-off value ±10%; retest to confirm
No. of references: 5

NOTES

110448.0

© KLUWER ACADEMIC PUBLISHERS 1994, ISSN 1381-5067

Herpes simplex virus (HSV-2)
ANTIBODY DETECTION (IgG)

Manufacturer: Schiapparelli Biosystems Inc
Cat. No./Trade name: 5772917/HERPES 2 IgG ELISA SYSTEM

SUMMARY

[Well-Ag]–**Ab**–[AHIgG-HRP]–[OPD]–A_{492}

Assay type: EIA (non-competitive)
Detection: Colorimetric A_{492}
Format: Microtitre well, Ag coated
Sample type: Serum (do not heat inactivate)
Sample pre-treatment:
   None
Sample volume: 100 µl of 1:300 dilution x 2
Number of tests: 96
Controls - standards run in assay:
   Controls: Neg (2), Pos (2)
Incubation:
   1 hr (37°C) + 30 min (37°C) + 10 min (37°C)
Washes: 3

CONTENTS

Antibodies, antigens, labelled components:
   HSV-2 specific Ag bound to well
   Anti-human IgG Ab (g) HRP conjugated
Substrate: OPD, H_2O_2
Controls - standards supplied:
   Controls: Neg and Pos (human serum)
Additional reagents:
   None
Special equipment required:
   None

INTERPRETATION

Comments on interpretation:
   Doubtful range: within cut-off value and cut-off +0.100; retest to confirm
No. of references: 5

NOTES

110420.0

Herpes simplex virus (HSV-2)
ANTIBODY DETECTION (IgG)

Manufacturer: Sigma Diagnostics
Cat. No./Trade name: SIA 412-A (Herpes-2)*/SIA Herpes 2 Kit

SUMMARY

[Well-Ag]–**Ab**–[AHIgG-AP]–[PMP]–A_{550}

Assay type: EIA (non-competitive)
Detection: Colorimetric A_{550}
Format: Microtitre well, Ag coated
Sample type: Serum (do not heat inactivate)
Sample pre-treatment:
   None
Sample volume: 10 µl (+200 µl diluent)
Number of tests: 96
Controls - standards run in assay:
   Controls: Pos (1), Neg (1)
   Calibrator: (3)
Incubation:
   45 min (RT) + 45 min (RT) + 45 min (RT)
Washes: 2 (+ preliminary plate wash)

CONTENTS

Antibodies, antigens, labelled components:
   HSV-2 Ag bound to well
   Anti-human IgG PAb (g) AP conjugated
Substrate: PMP
Controls - standards supplied:
   Controls: Neg and Pos, human serum
   Calibrator (3), human serum with assigned value
Additional reagents:
   None
Special equipment required:
   Sigma EIA microwell plate or strip reader (optional)

INTERPRETATION

Comments on interpretation:
   Results expressed as S.I.A. HERPES IgG values
   Equivocal: 0.92-0.99; retest to confirm
No. of references: 3

NOTES

110115.0

*The assay is designed to be run in parallel with SIA Herpes Type 1 kit

Herpes simplex virus (HSV-2)
ANTIBODY DETECTION (IgG)

Manufacturer: United Biotech Inc
Cat. No./Trade name: IA-403/MAGIWEL® HSV-2 IgG

SUMMARY

[Well-Ag]–**Ab**–[AHIgG-HRP]–[TMB]–A_{450}

Assay type: EIA (non-competitive)
Detection: Colorimetric A_{450}
Format: Microtitre well, Ag coated
Sample type: Serum
Sample pre-treatment:
　None
Sample volume: 100 µl of 1:101 dilution
Number of tests: 96
Controls - standards run in assay:
　Reference standard set: Neg (1), Pos (1), Calibrator (1)
Incubation:
　30 min (RT) + 30 min (RT) + 15 min (RT)
Washes: 2

CONTENTS

Antibodies, antigens, labelled components:
　HSV-2 Ag bound to well
　Anti-human IgG Ab (g) HRP conjugated
Substrate: TMB, H_2O_2
Controls - standards supplied:
　Reference standard set: Neg, Pos, Calibrator (100 EU/
　ml)
Additional reagents:
　H_2SO_4
Special equipment required:
　None

INTERPRETATION

Comments on interpretation:
　Positive: $\geqslant 20$ EU/ml
No. of references: 5

NOTES

110502.0

Herpes simplex virus (HSV-2)
ANTIBODY DETECTION (IgM)

Manufacturer: Biologische Analysensystem GmbH
Cat. No./Trade name: 5213/BAG-HSV-2-EIA-M

SUMMARY

[Well-Ag]–**Ab**–[AHIgM-HRP]–[TMB]–A_{450}

Assay type: EIA (non-competitive)
Detection: Colorimetric A_{450}
Format: Microtitre well, Ag coated
Sample type: Serum
Sample pre-treatment:
　None
Sample volume: 10 µl (+1 ml diluent)
Number of tests: 96
Controls - standards run in assay:
　Controls: Neg (1), Cut-off (2), Pos (1)
Incubation:
　30 min (RT) + 30 min (RT) + 10 min (RT)
Washes: 2

CONTENTS

Antibodies, antigens, labelled components:
　HSV-2 Ag bound to well
　Anti-human IgM Ab (sh) HRP conjugated
Substrate: TMB
Controls - standards supplied:
　Controls: Neg, Pos and cut-off
Additional reagents:
　None
Special equipment required:
　None

INTERPRETATION

Comments on interpretation:
　Equivocal: within cut-off ± 10%; retest to confirm
No. of references: 0

NOTES

110286.0

Herpes simplex virus (HSV-2)
ANTIBODY DETECTION (IgM)

Manufacturer: Cambridge Biotech Corporation
Cat. No./Trade name: /HSV-2 IgM EIA Test

SUMMARY

[Well-Ag]–**Ab**–[AHIgM-AP]–[PNP]–A_{405}

Assay type: EIA (non-competitive)
Detection: Colorimetric A_{405}
Format: Microtitre well, Ag coated
Sample type: Serum
Sample pre-treatment:
  None
Sample volume: 100 µl of 1:11 dilution*
Number of tests: 96
Controls - standards run in assay:
  None
Incubation:
  30 min (37°C) + 30 min (37°C) + 30 min (37°C)
Washes: 2

CONTENTS

Antibodies, antigens, labelled components:
  HSV-2 Ag bound to well
  Anti-human IgM Ab (g) AP conjugated
Substrate: PNP
Controls - standards supplied:
  Controls: Neg and Pos (human serum); Reference serum (human)
Additional reagents:
  None
Special equipment required:
  None

INTERPRETATION

Comments on interpretation:
  Equivocal: samples within specified range; retest to confirm
  Repeatably equivocal: retest using an alternative method
No. of references: 13

NOTES

110650.0

*Diluent contains an absorbant to remove IgG/RF complexes from patient serum

Herpes simplex virus (HSV-2)
ANTIBODY DETECTION (IgM)

Manufacturer: Chimica Diagnostica
Cat. No./Trade name: 41760/Herpes Simplex Virus 2 IgM

SUMMARY

[Well-Ag]–**Ab**–[AHIgM-POD]–[TMB]–A_{450}

Assay type: EIA (non-competitive)
Detection: Colorimetric A_{450}
Format: Microtitre well, Ag coated
Sample type: Serum
Sample pre-treatment:
  None
Sample volume: 10 µl (+1 ml diluent)
Number of tests: 96
Controls - standards run in assay:
  Controls: Neg (1), cut-off (1), Pos (1)
Incubation:
  30 min (RT) + 30 min (RT) + 15 min (RT)
Washes: 2

CONTENTS

Antibodies, antigens, labelled components:
  HSV-2 Ag bound to well
  Anti-human IgM PAb (g) POD conjugated
Substrate: TMB
Controls - standards supplied:
  Controls: Neg, cut-off and Pos
Additional reagents:
  None
Special equipment required:
  None

INTERPRETATION

Comments on interpretation:
  Equivocal: Sample index (ratio of O.D. sample: cut-off) >0.9<1.1; retest to confirm
No. of references: 2

NOTES

110313.0

© *KLUWER ACADEMIC PUBLISHERS 1994, ISSN 1381-5067*

Herpes simplex virus (HSV-2)
ANTIBODY DETECTION (IgM)

Manufacturer: Gull Laboratories
Cat. No./Trade name: H2E 150/HSV-2 IgM ELISA Test

SUMMARY

[Well-Ag]–**Ab**–[AHIgM-AP]–[PNP]–A_{405}

Assay type: EIA (non-competitive)
Detection: Colorimetric A_{405}
Format: Microtitre well, Ag coated
Sample type: Serum
Sample pre-treatment:
   None
Sample volume: 15 µl (+ 150 µl diluent)*
Number of tests: 96
Controls - standards run in assay:
   Controls: Neg (1), Pos (1)
   Reference serum: (3)
Incubation:
   30 min (37°C) + 30 min (37°C) + 30 min (37°C)
Washes: 2

CONTENTS

Antibodies, antigens, labelled components:
   HSV-2 Ag bound to well
   Anti-human IgM Ab (g) AP conjugated
Substrate: PNP.
Controls - standards supplied:
   Controls: Neg and Pos (human serum)
   Reference serum (human)
Additional reagents:
   None
Special equipment required:
   None

INTERPRETATION

Comments on interpretation:
   Equivocal: within cut-off and cut-off x 0.9; retest
   Repeatably equivocal: retest with alternative method
No. of references: 13

NOTES

110112.0

*Sample diluent contains an absorbent to remove IgG and RF

Herpes simplex virus (HSV-2)
ANTIBODY DETECTION (IgM)

Manufacturer: Immunobiological Laboratories
Cat. No./Trade name: VE57231/Herpes 2 Virus IgM EIA test

SUMMARY

[Well-Ag]–**Ab**–[AHIgM-POD]–[TMB]–A_{450}

Assay type: EIA (non-competitive)
Detection: Colorimetric A_{450}
Format: Microtitre well, Ag coated
Sample type: Serum
Sample pre-treatment:
   None
Sample volume: 100 µl of a 1:100 dilution x 2
Number of tests: 96
Controls - standards run in assay:
   Controls: Neg (2), low Pos (2), high Pos (2)
Incubation:
   1 hr (RT) + 30 min (RT) + 15 min (RT)
Washes: 2

CONTENTS

Antibodies, antigens, labelled components:
   HSV-2 Ag bound to well
   Anti-human IgM Ab HRP conjugated
Substrate: TMB, H_2O_2
Controls - standards supplied:
   Controls: Neg, low Pos, high Pos
Additional reagents:
   None
Special equipment required:
   None

INTERPRETATION

Comments on interpretation:
   Classification of samples is according to cut-off; no further testing
No. of references: 0

NOTES

110330.0

© *KLUWER ACADEMIC PUBLISHERS 1994, ISSN 1381-5067*

Herpes simplex virus (HSV-2)
ANTIBODY DETECTION (IgM)

Manufacturer: International Immunodiagnostics
Cat. No./Trade name: 108 143/HSV-Typ 2 IgM

SUMMARY

[Well-Ag]–**Ab**–[AHIgM-HRP]–[TMB]–A$_{450}$

Assay type: EIA (non-competitive)
Detection: Colorimetric A$_{450}$
Format: Microtitre well, Ag coated
Sample type: Serum
Sample pre-treatment:
    None
Sample volume: 10 μl (+ 1 ml diluent)*
Number of tests: 96
Controls - standards run in assay:
    Controls: Neg (2), Pos (2)
Incubation:
    30 min (RT) + 30 min (RT) + 15 min (RT) (first two
        incubations on plate shaker)
Washes: 2

CONTENTS

Antibodies, antigens, labelled components:
    HSV-2 Ag bound to well
    Anti-human IgM Ab HRP conjugated
Substrate: TMB, H$_2$O$_2$
Controls - standards supplied:
    Controls: Neg and Pos (human serum)
Additional reagents:
    None
Special equipment required:
    None

INTERPRETATION

Comments on Interpretation:
    Classification of results is according to cut-off; no further
        testing
    Quantitative interpretation also available
No. of references: 0

NOTES

110337.0

*Samples assayed in duplicate

Herpes simplex virus (HSV-2)
ANTIBODY DETECTION (IgM)

Manufacturer: Melja Diagnostik GmbH
Cat. No./Trade name: HSV-E04/Herpes Simplex Virus Type 2 IgM EIA Kit

SUMMARY

[Well-Ag]–**Ab**–[AHIgM-HRP]–[TMB]–A$_{450}$

Assay type: EIA (non-competitive)
Detection: Colorimetric A$_{450}$
Format: Microtitre well, Ag coated
Sample type: Serum, plasma
Sample pre-treatment:
    None
Sample volume: 100 μl of 1:100 dilution x 2
Number of tests: 96
Controls - standards run in assay:
    Controls: low Pos (2), high Pos (2), Neg (2)
Incubation:
    1 hr (RT) + 30 min (RT) + 15 min (RT)
Washes: 2

CONTENTS

Antibodies, antigens, labelled components:
    HSV-2 Ag bound to well
    Anti-human IgM Ab HRP conjugated
Substrate: TMB
Controls - standards supplied:
    Controls: low Pos, high Pos and Neg
Additional reagents:
    None
Special equipment required:
    None

INTERPRETATION

Comments on Interpretation:
    Positive: > cut-off + 20%
    Negative: < cut-off - 20%
    A MELJA titre may be calculated from a single sample
        dilution
No. of references: 8

NOTES

110364.0

© KLUWER ACADEMIC PUBLISHERS 1994, ISSN 1381-5067

Herpes simplex virus (HSV-2)
ANTIBODY DETECTION (IgM)

Manufacturer: Melotec S.A.
Cat. No./Trade name: MH2M/MELOTEST HSV-2 IgM

SUMMARY

[Well-Ag]–**Ab**–[AHIgM-HRP]–[TMB]–A$_{450}$

Assay type: EIA (non-competitive)
Detection: Colorimetric A$_{450}$
Format: Microtitre well, Ag coated
Sample type: Serum, plasma
Sample pre-treatment:
  Incubation with absorbant 20 min (RT) to remove IgG
Sample volume: 5 µl (+195 µl diluent) x 2*
Number of tests: 96
Controls - standards run in assay:
  Controls: Neg (1), low Pos (2), high Pos (1)**
Incubation:
  20 min (RT) + 20 min (RT) + 10 min (RT)
Washes: 2

CONTENTS

Antibodies, antigens, labelled components:
  HSV-2 Ag bound to well
  Control coated well
  Anti-human IgM Ab HRP conjugated
Substrate: TMB, H$_2$O$_2$
Controls - standards supplied:
  Controls: Neg, low Pos, high Pos (human serum)
Additional reagents:
  None
Special equipment required:
  None

INTERPRETATION

Comments on interpretation:
  Equivocal: ratio of OD sample to low Pos control is within
    the range 0.9 to 1.1; retest fresh sample
  Repeatably equivocal: retest fresh sample in 1 week
No. of references: 9

NOTES

110132.0

*Samples and controls assayed simultaneously in antigen
  and control coated wells (control wells eliminate any antinuclear antibody interference not neutralised by the
  absorbant)

Herpes simplex virus (HSV-2)
ANTIBODY DETECTION (IgM)

Manufacturer: United Biotech Inc
Cat. No./Trade name: IA-404/MAGIWEL® HSV-2 IgM

SUMMARY

[Well-Ag]–**Ab**–[AHIgM-HRP]–[TMB]–A$_{450}$

Assay type: EIA (non-competitive)
Detection: Colorimetric A$_{450}$
Format: Microtitre well, Ag coated
Sample type: Serum
Sample pre-treatment:
  None
Sample volume: 100 µl of 1:101 dilution
Number of tests: 96
Controls - standards run in assay:
  Controls: Neg (1)
  Calibrator: (1)
Incubation:
  30 min (RT) + 30 min (RT) + 15 min (RT)
Washes: 2

CONTENTS

Antibodies, antigens, labelled components:
  HSV-2 Ag bound to well
  Anti-human IgM Ab (g) HRP conjugated
Substrate: TMB, H$_2$O$_2$
Controls - standards supplied:
  Controls: Neg
  Calibrator: IgM Pos (100 EU/ml)
Additional reagents:
  H$_2$SO$_4$
Special equipment required:
  None

INTERPRETATION

Comments on interpretation:
  Positive: ⩾ 100 EU/ml
No. of references: 5

NOTES

110501.0

Herpes simplex virus (HSV-2)
ANTIBODY DETECTION

Manufacturer: Incstar
Cat. No./Trade name: 1830/HSV-2 Fluoro Kit®

SUMMARY

[Slide-Ag]–**Ab**–[AHIg-FITC]–fluorescence

Assay type: Immunofluorescence assay (indirect)
Detection: Fluorescence microscopy
Format: Slide well, Ag coated
Sample type: Serum, plasma
Sample pre-treatment:
   None
Sample volume: 20 µl of 1:10 and 1:20 dilution*
Number of tests: 60, 120
Controls - standards run in assay:
   Controls: Neg (1), Pos (1)
Incubation:
   30 min (RT) + 30 min (RT)
Washes: 2

CONTENTS

Antibodies, antigens, labelled components:
   HSV-2 infected and uninfected tissue culture cells bound
      to slide wells
   Anti-human Ig Ab (g or sh) FITC conjugated
Substrate:
Controls - standards supplied:
   Controls: HSV 2 positive and negative (human serum)
Additional reagents:
   None
Special equipment required:
   None

INTERPRETATION

Comments on interpretation:
   Positive: ≥(1+) specific apple-green fluorescence of
      the nucleus and/or cytoplasm of at least 10% to 75%
      of the cells
No. of references: 14

NOTES

110277.0

*Previously screened positive sera should be titred to end-
   point
The assay may be run in parallel with the HSV-1 Fluoro Kit®

Herpes simplex virus (HSV-2)
ANTIBODY DETECTION (IgG)

Manufacturer: Bion Enterprises Ltd
**Cat. No./Trade name: HS2-G-60/Herpes Simplex Virus
Type 2 IgG**

SUMMARY

[Well-Ag]–**Ab**–[AHIgG-FITC]–fluorescence

Assay type: Immunofluorescence assay (indirect)
Detection: Fluorescence microscopy
Format: Slide well, Ag coated
Sample type: Serum
Sample pre-treatment:
   None
Sample volume: 50 µl (+450 µl diluent)
Number of tests: 60, 120
Controls - standards run in assay:
   Controls: Neg (1), Pos (1)
Incubation:
   30 min (RT) + 30 min (RT)
Washes: 2

CONTENTS

Antibodies, antigens, labelled components:
   HSV-2 (strain G) infected and uninfected diploid
      fibroblasts fixed to slide well
   Anti-human IgG Ab (g) FITC conjugated
Substrate:
Controls - standards supplied:
   Controls: Pos and Neg (human serum)
Additional reagents:
   None
Special equipment required:
   None

INTERPRETATION

Comments on interpretation:
   Positive: >(+1) grade fluorescence with well-defined
      nuclear inclusions and/or homogeneous nuclear and
      cytoplasmic fluorescence in 10-50% cells at dilution
      ≥1:10
   Serial dilutions (1:10-1:2560) tested for a quantitative
      assay
No. of references: 27

NOTES

110304.0

Herpes simplex virus (HSV-2)
ANTIBODY DETECTION (IgG)

Manufacturer: Gen Bio
Cat. No./Trade name: 1402 EB/Herpes 2 IgG Test Kit

SUMMARY

[Slide-Ag]–**Ab**–[AHIgG-FITC]–fluorescence

Assay type: Immunofluorescence assay (indirect)
Detection: Fluorescence microscopy
Format: Slide well, Ag coated
Sample type: Serum
Sample pre-treatment:
  None
Sample volume: 30 µl of 1:10 and 1:100 dilutions*
Number of tests: 100
Controls - standards run in assay:
  Controls: Neg (1), Pos (4) (serial dilutions 1:10 to 1:200)*
Incubation:
  30 min (37°C) + 30 min (37°C)
Washes: 2

CONTENTS

Antibodies, antigens, labelled components:
  HSV-2 infected and uninfected cells bound to slide well
  Anti-human IgG Ab (g) FITC conjugated
Substrate:
Controls - standards supplied:
  Controls: Neg and Pos (human serum)
Additional reagents:
  None
Special equipment required:
  None

INTERPRETATION

Comments on interpretation:
  Negative: no specific fluorescence at 1:10 dilution
  Positive: specific apple green cytoplasmic/nuclear
    fluorescence at intensity (1+) to (4+). The endpoint
    is considered to be the highest dilution showing a
    (2+) fluorescence in infected cells
  Antibody titre of samples may be obtained by testing
    further serial sample dilutions
  Non-specific reaction: fluorescence in infected and
    uninfected cells usually due to antinuclear antibody in
    test serum
No. of references: 11

NOTES

110375.0

*The choice of sample dilution and the number of control
  dilutions run is at the discretion of the user. The example
  given is suggested by the manufacturer

Herpes simplex virus (HSV-2)
ANTIBODY DETECTION (IgG)

Manufacturer: Schiapparelli Biosystems Inc
Cat. No./Trade name: 2600/VIRGO HSV-2 IgG IFA

SUMMARY

[Slide-Ag]–**Ab**–[AHIgG-FITC]–fluorescence

Assay type: Immunofluorescence assay (indirect)
Detection: Fluorescence microscopy
Format: Slide well, Ag coated
Sample type: Serum
Sample pre-treatment:
  None
Sample volume: 20 µl of 1:10 and 1:100 dilution
Number of tests: 96, 200
Controls - standards run in assay:
  Controls: Neg (1), Pos (1)
Incubation:
  30 min (RT) + 30 min (RT)
Washes: 2

CONTENTS

Antibodies, antigens, labelled components:
  HSV-2 infected and uninfected tissue culture cells bound
    to slide well
  Anti-human IgG Ab (g) FITC conjugated
Substrate:
Controls - standards supplied:
  Controls: Neg and Pos (human serum)
Additional reagents:
  None
Special equipment required:
  None

INTERPRETATION

Comments on interpretation:
  Positive: ≥(1+) specific apple green fluorescence at
    1:10 dilution or greater OR little or no fluorescence at
    1:10 but ≥(1+) at 1:100 dilution or greater
  Acute and convalescent sera should be tested together
    to diagnose recent or current infection
  Serial dilutions for quantitative assay
No. of references: 31

NOTES

110413.0

Herpes simplex virus (HSV-2)
ANTIBODY DETECTION (IgG)

Manufacturer: Zeus Scientific Inc
Cat. No./Trade name: 9101-10

SUMMARY

[Slide-Ag]–**Ab**–[AHIgG-FITC]–fluorescence

Assay type: Immunofluorescence assay (indirect)
Detection: Fluorescence microscopy
Format: Slide well, Ag coated
Sample type: Serum
Sample pre-treatment:
  None
Sample volume: 20 µl of 1:10 and 1:100 dilutions (for screening)*
Number of tests: 100
Controls - standards run in assay:
  Controls: Pos (1), Neg (1)
Incubation:
  30 min (RT) + 30 min (RT)
Washes: 2

CONTENTS

Antibodies, antigens, labelled components:
  HSV-2 infected substrate cells fixed to slide/well
  Anti-human IgG Ab (r or g) FITC conjugated**
Substrate:
Controls - standards supplied:
  Controls: Pos and Neg, human serum
Additional reagents:
  None
Special equipment required:
  None

INTERPRETATION

Comments on interpretation:
  Positive: (1+) to (4+) apple green fluorescence in the nucleus and/or cytoplasm of infected cells. Serum titre ≥ 1:10
No. of references: 13

NOTES

110295.0

*Positive sera are titred to end-point
**Anti-human IgM Ab-FITC conjugated is also available

Herpes simplex virus (HSV-2)
ANTIBODY DETECTION (IgM)

Manufacturer: Gen Bio
Cat. No./Trade name: 1502 EB/Herpes 2 IgM Test Kit

SUMMARY

[Slide-Ag]–**Ab**–[AHIgM-FITC]–fluorescence

Assay type: Immunofluorescence assay (indirect)
Detection: Fluorescence microscopy
Format: Slide well, Ag coated
Sample type: Serum
Sample pre-treatment:
  None
Sample volume: 30 µl serial dilutions 1:5 to 1:160*
Number of tests: 100
Controls - standards run in assay:
  Controls: Neg (1), Pos (5) (serial dilutions 1:10 to 1:160)*
Incubation:
  1 hr (37°C) + 30 min (37°C)
Washes: 2

CONTENTS

Antibodies, antigens, labelled components:
  HSV-2 infected and uninfected cells bound to slide well
  Anti-human IgM Ab (g) FITC conjugated
Substrate:
Controls - standards supplied:
  Controls: Neg and Pos (human serum)
Additional reagents:
  None
Special equipment required:
  None

INTERPRETATION

Comments on interpretation:
  Negative: no specific fluorescence at 1:5 dilution
  Positive: specific apple green cytoplasmic/nuclear fluorescence at intensity (1+) to (4+)
  Antibody titre of samples may be obtained by testing further serial sample dilutions
  Non-specific reaction: fluorescence in infected and uninfected cells usually due to antinuclear antibody in test serum
No. of references: 12

NOTES

110377.0

*The choice of sample dilution and the number of control dilutions run is at the discretion of the user. The example given is suggested by the manufacturer
It is recommended that HSV-IgG antibody testing be performed simultaneously with HSV-IgM antibody tests

Human immunodeficiency virus (HIV-1 and HIV-2) (Acquired immune deficiency syndrome; AIDS)

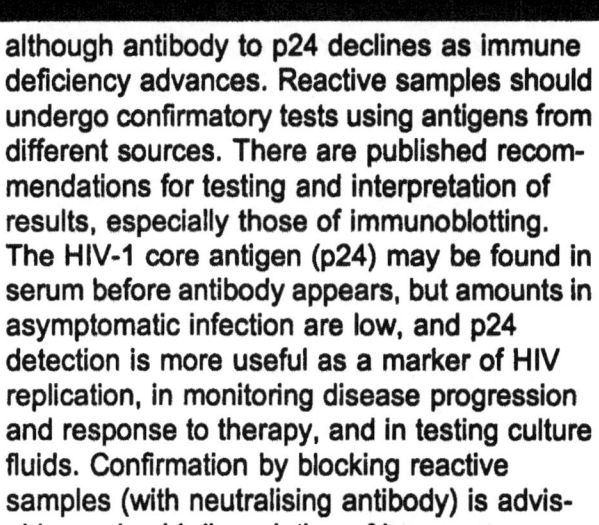

Natural history

Infection with human immunodeficiency virus type 1 occurs all over the world, whilst HIV-2 is prevalent in West Africa. A significant variant, subtype O of HIV-1, is found in West Central Africa. Infection is established by free virus or by infected cells in blood or body fluids, transmitted by sexual contact, injection of blood or untreated blood products, or from mother to infant. An initial mononucleosis-like illness occurs in some 40% of cases, followed by an asymptomatic period (clinical latency) varying from months to more than ten years before the development of AIDS. HIV is a retrovirus (sub-family: lentivirus) infecting CD4 + T lympho-cytes and other cells such as macrophages. These RNA viruses replicate by way of a DNA provirus integrated into the host cell genome. Activation of HIV-infected cells leads to new virus production, progressive decline in CD4 + cell count and significant deterioration of cellular immune function. AIDS is defined by the appearance of characteristic opportunist infections or tumours or, after childhood, a fall in CD4 + T lymphocyte count to below 200/µl (or < 14% of total lymphocytes), in someone Infected with HIV. AIDS appears within 5 years in 20% of infected individuals, while approximately one half develop AIDS within 10 years: mortality has been > 90% within 5 years of a diagnosis of AIDS. Prophylaxis against oppor-tunist infections and anti-retroviral therapy have a place in management of those infected with HIV.

Diagnosis and markers

Immunoassays for antibody are used in screening for HIV infection. Native and recombinant proteins and synthetic peptides in a variety of combinations now provide assays capable of detecting all classes of immunoglo-bulins early in infection. Structural antigens include the major core protein, p24 (p26 in HIV-2) from the *gag* gene; external membrane (envelope) glycoprotein, gp120 (gp125 in HIV-2) and transmembrane gp41 (gp36 in HIV-2) from the *env* gene. Antibody to precursor proteins gp160 or p55 is detectable when infected cell antigens are used. An antibody response to HIV usually develops in 2–12 weeks after exposure, by 6 months in > 95% of cases, and remains detectable throughout life, although antibody to p24 declines as immune deficiency advances. Reactive samples should undergo confirmatory tests using antigens from different sources. There are published recom-mendations for testing and interpretation of results, especially those of immunoblotting. The HIV-1 core antigen (p24) may be found in serum before antibody appears, but amounts in asymptomatic infection are low, and p24 detection is more useful as a marker of HIV replication, in monitoring disease progression and response to therapy, and in testing culture fluids. Confirmation by blocking reactive samples (with neutralising antibody) is advis-able, and acid dissociation of immune complexes may be required before antigen can be detected. Isolation of HIV is not widely available. Detection of viral nucleic acid by PCR has an increasing role in diagnosis of congenital or antibody-negative infection, in study of antiviral resistance, and in epidemiology.

Comment

Tests to detect infection with HIV are generally not applied without the informed consent of the individual. Current practice in donor screening is to use combined assays for antibody to HIV-1 and HIV-2. Initial screening of saliva, urine or eluted dried blood with an antibody-capture assay is useful in other settings. All antibody positive persons (over age 15 months) are persistently infected and are potential sources of infection.

Reference

Davey RT, Lane HC. Laboratory methods in the diagnosis and prognostic staging of infection with human immunodeficiency virus type 1. Reviews of Infectious Diseases. 1990;12:912–930.

© KLUWER ACADEMIC PUBLISHERS 1994, ISSN 1381-5067

Human immunodeficiency virus
ANTIGEN DETECTION

Manufacturer: Innogenetics SA
Cat. No./Trade name: /INNOTEST HIV-1/HIV-2 ANTIGEN

SUMMARY

[Well-PAb]–Ag–[Ab-HRP]–[TMB]–A_{450}

Assay type: EIA (non-competitive)
Detection: Colorimetric A_{450}
Format: Microtitre well, Ab coated
Sample type: Serum, plasma, cell culture supernatant (do not heat inactivate)
Sample pre-treatment:
    None
Sample volume: 200 μl
Number of tests: 96
Controls - standards run in assay:
    Controls: Neg (1), Pos (1) per microplate strip*
    For cell culture: run HIV-Neg cell culture supernatant as control
Incubation:
    a) 1 hr (37°C) + 1 hr (37°C) + 30 min (RT)
    b) 16 hr (RT) + 1 hr (37°C) + 30 min (RT)
Washes: 2

CONTENTS

Antibodies, antigens, labelled components:
    Anti-HIV PAb bound to well
    Anti-HIV Ab (h) HRP conjugated
Substrate: TMB, H_2O_2
Controls - standards supplied:
    Controls: Neg (human serum), Pos (rec p24 Ag)
Additional reagents:
    H_2SO_4
Special equipment required:
    None

INTERPRETATION

Comments on interpretation:
    Positive: ≥ cut-off repeatably and confirmed by neutralisation using INNOTEST HIV confirmatory reagents
    Semi-quantitative interpretation is available
No. of references: 5

NOTES

110039.0

*If more than one strip used, include at least 2 Neg and 2 Pos controls per stripholder

Human immunodeficiency virus
ANTIBODY DETECTION

Manufacturer: Organon Teknika NV
Cat. No./Trade name: 80197/Vironostika® HIV Core

SUMMARY

$$[\text{Well-MAb}]-[\text{Ag}] \begin{cases} \textbf{Ab} \\ [\text{MAb-HRP}] \end{cases} -[\text{TMB}]-A_{450}$$

Assay type: EIA (competitive)
Detection: Colorimetric A_{450}
Format: Microtitre well, Ab coated
Sample type: Serum, plasma
Sample pre-treatment:
    None
Sample volume: 100 μl
Number of tests: 192
Controls - standards run in assay:
    Controls:
    Neg (1), Pos (1) (one strip of 12 wells)
    Neg (2), Pos (2) (for two strips)
    Neg (3), Pos (3) (three or more strips)
Incubation:
    1 hr 30 min (37°C) + 30 min (RT)
Washes: 1

CONTENTS

Antibodies, antigens, labelled components:
    Anti-HIV (p24) MAb (m) bound to well
    HIV Ag
    Anti-HIV (p24) MAb (m) HRP conjugated
Substrate: TMB, H_2O_2
Controls - standards supplied:
    Controls: Neg and Pos (human serum)
Additional reagents:
    H_2SO_4
Special equipment required:
    None

INTERPRETATION

Comments on interpretation:
    Positive: ≤ cut-off repeatably
No. of references: 10

NOTES

110388.0

© KLUWER ACADEMIC PUBLISHERS 1994, ISSN 1381-5067

Human immunodeficiency virus
ANTIBODY DETECTION

Manufacturer: Abbott Laboratories
Cat. No./Trade name: 3A10/ABBOTT RECOMBINANT HIV-1/HIV-2 3RD GENERATION EIA

SUMMARY

[Bead-Ag]–**Ab**–[Ag-HRP]–[OPD]–A_{492}

Assay type: EIA (non-competitive)
Detection: Colorimetric A_{492}
Format: Reaction well, Ag coated bead
Sample type: Serum, plasma (do not heat inactivate)
Sample pre-treatment:
   None
Sample volume: 150 µl (+50 µl diluent)
Number of tests: 100, 1000
Controls - standards run in assay:
   Controls: Neg (3), Pos (2)
Incubation:
   a) Dynamic: 30 min (40°C) + 30 min (40°C) + 30 min (RT)
   b) Static: 2 hr (40°C) + 1 hr (40°C) + 30 min (RT)
Washes: 2

CONTENTS

Antibodies, antigens, labelled components:
   rec HIV-1 env and gag/HIV-2 env proteins bound to beads
   rec HIV-1 env and gag/HIV-2 env proteins HRP conjugated
Substrate: OPD, H_2O_2
Controls - standards supplied:
   Controls: Neg and Pos (human plasma)
Additional reagents:
   H_2SO_4
Special equipment required:
   Commander Dynamic Incubator required for Dynamic incubation (optional)

INTERPRETATION

Comments on interpretation:
   Positive: ≥ cut-off repeatably and confirmed by supplemental tests.
   If supplemental tests are indeterminate; retest a fresh specimen in 3-6 months
No. of references: 29

NOTES

110130.0

Human immunodeficiency virus
ANTIBODY DETECTION

Manufacturer: Behringwerke AG
Cat. No./Trade name: /OPUS® Anti-HIV 1 + 2 EIA

SUMMARY

[Glass-fibre-A/G]–**Ab**–[Ag-AP]–[4-MP]–fluorescence

Assay type: EIA (non-competitive)
Detection: Fluorometric
Format: Test module, protein A/G coated glass fibre
Sample type: Serum, plasma
Sample pre-treatment:
   None
Sample volume: 10 µl (min. fill level 100 µl)
Number of tests: 50
Controls - standards run in assay:
   Calibrators: Neg (3), Pos (6)
Incubation:
   Automated (23 min for first sample)
Washes: Automated

CONTENTS

Antibodies, antigens, labelled components:
   rec protein A/G bound to glass fibre
   HIV-1 (gp 41) and HIV-2 (gp 36) AP conjugated
Substrate: 4-MP
Controls - standards supplied:
   Calibrators: Neg (1); Pos (2) (HIV-1 and HIV-2 rabbit Abs in human serum)
Additional reagents:
   None
Special equipment required:
   OPUS® analyser, specimen cups and pipette tips

INTERPRETATION

Comments on interpretation:
   Results calculated automatically and classified according to cut-off
   Positive: Repeatably reactive and confirmed by supplemented test
No. of references: 16

NOTES

110148.0

© KLUWER ACADEMIC PUBLISHERS 1994, ISSN 1381-5067

Human immunodeficiency virus
ANTIBODY DETECTION

Manufacturer: Cambridge Biotech Corporation
Cat. No./Trade name: 96040/RECOMBIGEN® HIV-1/HIV-2 EIA

SUMMARY

[Well-Ag]–**Ab**–[AHIg-HRP]–[OPD]–A$_{490}$

Assay type: EIA (non-competitive)
Detection: Colorimetric A$_{490}$
Format: Microtitre well, Ag coated
Sample type: Serum, plasma
Sample pre-treatment:
　None
Sample volume: 15 µl (+300 µl diluent)*
Number of tests: 192
Controls - standards run in assay:
　Controls: Neg (2), HIV-1 Pos (3), HIV-2 Pos (2)
Incubation:
　1 hr (37°C) + 30 min (37°C) + 30 min (RT)
Washes: 2

CONTENTS

Antibodies, antigens, labelled components:
　rec HIV-1 (gp41, gp120, p24) and HIV-2 (gp41, gp120)
　　proteins bound to well
　Anti-human Ig Ab (g) HRP conjugated
Substrate: OPD, H$_2$O$_2$
Controls - standards supplied:
　Controls: Neg, HIV-1 Pos and HIV-2 Pos (human serum)
Additional reagents:
　H$_2$SO$_4$
Special equipment required:
　None

INTERPRETATION

Comments on interpretation:
　Positive: ≥cut-off repeatably and confirmed by
　　supplemental tests
No. of references: 20

NOTES

110653.0

*If using automatic diluter use 10 µl sample (+200 µl diluent)

Human immunodeficiency virus
ANTIBODY DETECTION

Manufacturer: Genetic Systems Corporation/Sanofi Diagnostics Pasteur
Cat. No./Trade name: 0230/GENETIC SYSTEMS® HIV-1/HIV-2 EIA

SUMMARY

[Well-Ag]–**Ab**–[AHIgG/IgM-HRP]–[TMB]–A$_{450}$

Assay type: EIA (non-competitive)
Detection: Colorimetric A$_{450}$
Format: Microtitre well, Ag coated
Sample type: Serum, plasma
Sample pre-treatment:
　None
Sample volume: 5 µl (+500 µl diluent)
Number of tests: 192, 960, 4800
Controls - standards run in assay:
　Controls: Neg (3), Pos HIV-1 (2), Pos HIV-2 (2)
Incubation:
　1 hr (37°C) + 1 hr (37°C) + 30 min (RT)
Washes: 2

CONTENTS

Antibodies, antigens, labelled components:
　HIV-1$_{LAV}$ Ag/HIV-2$_{ROD}$ Ag bound to well
　Anti-human IgG and IgM Ab (g) HRP conjugated
Substrate: TMB, H$_2$O$_2$
Controls - standards supplied:
　Controls: Neg, Pos (HIV-1) and Pos (HIV-2) (human
　　serum)
Additional reagents:
　None
Special equipment required:
　None

INTERPRETATION

Comments on interpretation:
　Positive: ≥cut-off repeatably and confirmed by more
　　specific supplemental tests (e.g. Western Blot,
　　radioimmunoprecipitation)
　When supplemental tests indeterminate; test further
　　sample 3-6 months later
No. of references: 25

NOTES

110040.0

© KLUWER ACADEMIC PUBLISHERS 1994, ISSN 1381-5067

Human immunodeficiency virus
ANTIBODY DETECTION

Manufacturer: Murex Diagnostics Limited
Cat. No./Trade name: VK54/55/Wellcozyme HIV 1+2

SUMMARY

[Well-Ag]–**Ab**–[Ag-AP]–[NADH-ampl]–A_{492}

Assay type: EIA (non-competitive, amplified)
Detection: Colorimetric A_{492}
Format: Microtitre well, Ag coated
Sample type: Serum, plasma (do not heat inactivate plasma samples)*
Sample pre-treatment:
  None
Sample volume: 25 µl
Number of tests: 96, 480
Controls - standards run in assay:
  Controls: Neg (4), anti-HIV-1 Pos (1), anti-HIV-2 Pos (1)
Incubation:
  30 min (37°C) + 30 min (37°C) + 20 min (37°C) + 10 min (RT)
Washes: 2

CONTENTS

Antibodies, antigens, labelled components:
  rec and syn HIV-1 (env + core) Ag and HIV-2 (env) Ag bound to wells
  rec and syn HIV-1 (env + core) Ag and HIV-2 (env) Ag AP conjugated
Substrate: NADP + amplifier
Controls - standards supplied:
  Controls: Neg, anti-HIV-1 Pos and anti-HIV-2 Pos (human serum)
Additional reagents:
  H_2SO_4
Special equipment required:
  Wellcozyme microwell plate washing system (optional)
  Wellcozyme microwell plate reader system (optional)

INTERPRETATION

Comments on interpretation:
  Positive: ≥ cut-off repeatably
  Further testing may be required to confirm original observations and to distinguish between HIV-1 and HIV-2
No. of references: 7

NOTES

110165.0

*Plasma samples collected in EDTA or sodium citrate may be tested

Human immunodeficiency virus
ANTIBODY DETECTION

Manufacturer: Murex Diagnostics Limited
Cat. No./Trade name: VK74/SUDS® HIV - 1+2 Test

SUMMARY

[Particle-Ag]–**Ab**–[AHIgM/IgG-AP]–[BCIP]–blue colour

Assay type: EIA (non-competitive)
Detection: Visual
Format: Test cartridge, Ag coated particles
Sample type: Serum, plasma
Sample pre-treatment:
  None
Sample volume: 50 µl
Number of tests: 30, 90
Controls - standards run in assay:
  Controls: Neg (1), Pos (1)*
Incubation:
  3 min (RT) + 3 min (RT) + 2 min (RT)
Washes: 2

CONTENTS

Antibodies, antigens, labelled components:
  HIV-1, HIV-2 bound to latex particles
  Anti-human IgG and IgM Ab (g) AP conjugated
Substrate: BCIP
Controls - standards supplied:
  Controls: Neg and Pos (human plasma or serum) (two outer circles with no reagents on bottom of cartridge act as integral procedure controls)
Additional reagents:
  None
Special equipment required:
  Wellcozyme microwell plate washing system (optional)
  Wellcozyme microwell plate reader system (optional)

INTERPRETATION

Comments on interpretation:
  Negative: no colour observed in central circle and white or light grey in outer circles
  Positive: blue colour observed in centre circle and white or light grey in outer circles repeatably
  Inconclusive: blue colour in one or both outer circles; retest
No. of references: 0

NOTES

110613.0

*Limit the number of cartridges to 12 in a single run
One positive and one negative control should be assayed at least once during a 24 hour period

Human immunodeficiency virus
ANTIBODY DETECTION

Manufacturer: Organon Teknika NV
Cat. No./Trade name: 80347/Vironostika® HIV Uni-Form II

SUMMARY

[Well-Ag]–**Ab**–[Ag-HRP]–[TMB]–$A_{450/660}$

Assay type: EIA (non-competitive)
Detection: Colorimetric $A_{450/660}$
Format: Microtitre well, Ag coated
Sample type: Serum, plasma
Sample pre-treatment:
  None
Sample volume: 50 µl (+100 µl diluent)
Number of tests: 192, 576
Controls - standards run in assay:
  Controls: Neg (3), Pos anti-HIV-1 (1)
  Optional: Pos anti-HIV-2 (1)
Incubation:
  1 hr (37°C) + 30 min (RT)
Washes: 1

CONTENTS

Antibodies, antigens, labelled components:
  rec HIV-1 (p24), viral HIV-1 (gp160) and syn HIV-2 (gp36 env) bound to well
  rec HIV-1 (p24), viral HIV-1 (gp160) and syn HIV-2 (gp36 env) HRP conjugated
Substrate: TMB, H_2O_2
Controls - standards supplied:
  Controls: Neg, Pos (anti-HIV-1), Pos (anti-HIV-2) (human serum)
Additional reagents:
  H_2SO_4
Special equipment required:
  None

INTERPRETATION

Comments on interpretation:
  For anti-HIV-1 and/or anti-HIV-2
  Positive: ≥ cut-off repeatably and confirmed by supplemental tests
No. of references: 3

NOTES

110548.0

Human immunodeficiency virus
ANTIBODY DETECTION

Manufacturer: Roche Diagnostic Systems
Cat. No./Trade name: 07 3448 9/COBAS CORE Anti-HIV-1/HIV-2 EIA

SUMMARY

[Bead-Ag]–**Ab**–[AHIg-HRP]–[TMB]–A_{450}

Assay type: EIA (non-competitive)
Detection: Colorimetric A_{450}
Format: Tube, Ag coated bead
Sample type: Serum or plasma (do not heat inactivate)
Sample pre-treatment:
  None
Sample volume: 25 µl (+250 µl diluent)
Number of tests: 100, 500
Controls - standards run in assay:
  Controls: Neg (1), Pos (3)
Incubation:
  20 min (37°C)* + 20 min (37°C)* + 20 min (RT)
Washes: 2

CONTENTS

Antibodies, antigens, labelled components:
  rec HIV Ags (HIV-1 env, HIV-1 core, HIV-2 env) bound to bead
  Anti-human Ig (g) HRP conjugated
Substrate: TMB, H_2O_2
Controls - standards supplied:
  Controls: Neg and Pos (human serum)
Additional reagents:
  Substrate (supplied as separate kit)
Special equipment required:
  Cobas® EIA shaking incubator, tube washer and photometer (optional)
  Cobas® Core automated analyser (optional)

INTERPRETATION

Comments on interpretation:
  Grey zone: within cut-off -15% and cut-off; retest to confirm
  Positive: ≥ cut-off; repeatably and confirmed by supplemental tests
No. of references: 15

NOTES

110305.0

*with shaking

© KLUWER ACADEMIC PUBLISHERS 1994, ISSN 1381-5067

Human immunodeficiency virus
ANTIBODY DETECTION

Manufacturer: Sanofi Diagnostics Pasteur
Cat. No./Trade name: 72266/GENELAVIA® MIXT

SUMMARY

[Well-Ag]–**Ab**–[AHIgG/IgM-POD]–[OPD]–$A_{492/620}$

Assay type: EIA (non-competitive)
Detection: Colorimetric $A_{492/620}$
Format: Microtitre well, Ag coated
Sample type: Serum, plasma
Sample pre-treatment:
    None
Sample volume: 20 µl (+80 µl diluent)
Number of tests: 96, 480
Controls - standards run in assay:
    Controls: Neg (1), Pos (1), cut-off (3)
Incubation:
    30 min (40°C) + 30 min (40°C) + 30 min (RT)
Washes: 2

CONTENTS

Antibodies, antigens, labelled components:
    HIV-1 and HIV-2 envelope glycoprotein antigens (gp41
        and gp36 and rec gp160) bound to well
    Anti-human IgG and IgM Ab (g) POD conjugated
Substrate: OPD
Controls - standards supplied:
    Controls: Neg, Pos, cut-off (human serum)
Additional reagents:
    None
Special equipment required:
    None

INTERPRETATION

Comments on interpretation:
    Equivocal: within cut-off and cut-off −10% range; retest to
        confirm
    Positive: ≥cut-off value repeatably and confirmed by
        Western Blot
No. of references: 21

NOTES

110261.0

Human immunodeficiency virus
ANTIBODY DETECTION

Manufacturer: Syva Company
Cat. No./Trade name: 8J219UL/MicroTrak® II HIV-1/
HIV-2 EIA

SUMMARY

[Well-Ag]–**Ab**–[AHIg-HRP]–[TMB]–$A_{450/630}$

Assay type: EIA (non-competitive)
Detection: Colorimetric $A_{450/630}$
Format: Microtitre well, Ag coated
Sample type: Serum, plasma
Sample pre-treatment:
    None
Sample volume: 100 µl of 1:21 dilution
Number of tests: 192
Controls - standards run in assay:
    Controls: Neg (2), HIV-1 Pos (3), HIV-2 Pos (2)
Incubation:
    1 hr (37°C) + 30 min (37°C) + 30 min (37°C)
Washes: 2

CONTENTS

Antibodies, antigens, labelled components:
    rec gp41, gp120 (HIV-1), gp41, gp120 (HIV-2), p24 (HIV-
        1) bound to well
    Anti-human Ig PAb (g) HRP conjugated
Substrate: TMB, H_2O_2
Controls - standards supplied:
    Controls: Neg, HIV-1 Pos, HIV-2 Pos (human serum)
Additional reagents:
    MicroTrak® II EIA Universal reagents (8K209UL)
Special equipment required:
    Syva MicroTrak® EIA autowasher and autoreader
    Syva Microtrak® XL system

INTERPRETATION

Comments on interpretation:
    Positive: ≥cut-off repeatably and confirmed by
        supplemental tests
No. of references: 20

NOTES

110518.0

© *KLUWER ACADEMIC PUBLISHERS 1994, ISSN 1381-5067*

Human immunodeficiency virus
ANTIBODY DETECTION

Manufacturer: United Biotech Inc
Cat. No./Trade name: /Anti-HIV-1 and -2 Kit

SUMMARY

[Well-Ag]–**Ab**–[AHIg-HRP]–[TMB]–A_{450}

Assay type: EIA (non-competitive)
Detection: Colorimetric A_{450}
Format: Microtitre well, Ag coated
Sample type: Serum, plasma
Sample pre-treatment:
    None
Sample volume: 200 µl of 1:40 dilution
Number of tests: 96
Controls - standards run in assay:
    Controls: Neg (2), Pos (2)
Incubation:
    30 min (37°C) + 30 min (37°C) + 10 min (RT)
Washes: 2

CONTENTS

Antibodies, antigens, labelled components:
    rec HIV-1 and HIV-2 Ag bound to well
    Anti-human Ig Ab HRP conjugated
Substrate: TMB
Controls - standards supplied:
    Controls: Neg and Pos
Additional reagents:
    None
Special equipment required:
    None

INTERPRETATION

Comments on interpretation:
    Positive: ⩾ cut-off repeatably; confirm in Western Blot
No. of references: 7

NOTES

110504.0

For research use only

Human immunodeficiency virus
ANTIBODY DETECTION (IgG)

Manufacturer: Abbott Laboratories
Cat. No./Trade name: IA80-24/ABBOTT RECOMBINANT HIV-1/HIV-2 EIA

SUMMARY

[Bead-Ag]–**Ab**–[AHIgG-HRP]–[OPD]–A_{492}

Assay type: EIA (non-competitive)
Detection: Colorimetric A_{492}
Format: Reaction well, Ag coated bead
Sample type: Serum, plasma (do not heat inactivate)
Sample pre-treatment:
    None
Sample volume: 10 µl (+ 400 µl diluent)
Number of tests: 100, 1000
Controls - standards run in assay:
    Controls: Neg (2), Pos (3)
Incubation:
    30 min (40°C) + 30 min (40°C) + 30 min (RT)
Washes: 2

CONTENTS

Antibodies, antigens, labelled components:
    rec proteins (E. coli) HIV-1 core and env, HIV-2 env
        bound to bead
    Anti-human IgG Ab (g) HRP conjugated
Substrate: OPD
Controls - standards supplied:
    Controls: Pos and Neg (human plasma)
Additional reagents:
    H_2SO_4
Special equipment required:
    None

INTERPRETATION

Comments on interpretation:
    Positive: ⩾ cut-off repeatably and confirmed by
        supplemental tests
    If supplemental tests are negative/indeterminate; test
        further specimen in 3-6 months
No. of references: 28

NOTES

110044.0

Human immunodeficiency virus
ANTIBODY DETECTION (IgG)

Manufacturer: Behringwerke AG
Cat. No./Trade name: OWRP/Enzygnost® Anti-HIV-1/HIV-2

SUMMARY

[Well-Ag]–**Ab**–[AHIgG-POD]–[TMB]–A_{450}

Assay type: EIA (non-competitive)
Detection: Colorimetric A_{450}
Format: Microtitre well, Ag coated
Sample type: Serum, plasma
Sample pre-treatment:
   None
Sample volume: 50 µl
Number of tests:
Controls - standards run in assay:
   Controls: Neg (4), Pos (2)
Incubation:
   30 min (37°C) + 30 min (37°C) + 30 min (RT)
Washes: 2 (+ plate pre-wash)

CONTENTS

Antibodies, antigens, labelled components:
   HIV env synthetic peptides (gp41, gp36) bound to well
   Anti-human IgG (r) FAb' POD conjugated
Substrate: TMB, H_2O_2
Controls - standards supplied:
   Controls: Neg and Pos (human serum)
Additional reagents:
   None
Special equipment required:
   Behring ELISA processor (optional)

INTERPRETATION

Comments on interpretation:
   Equivocal: within range of cut-off and cut-off -10%; retest in duplicate to confirm
   Positive: > cut-off repeatably and confirmed by supplemental tests
No. of references: 4

NOTES

110102.0

Human immunodeficiency virus
ANTIBODY DETECTION (IgG)

Manufacturer: Bio-Stat Diagnostics
Cat. No./Trade name: 851205/ELISA IgG Antibody Test

SUMMARY

[Well-Ag]–**Ab**–[AHIgG-AP]–[PNP]–A_{405}

Assay type: EIA (non-competitive)
Detection: Colorimetric A_{405}
Format: Microtitre well, Ag coated
Sample type: Serum (do not heat inactivate)
Sample pre-treatment:
   None
Sample volume: 10 µl (+400 µl diluent)
Number of tests: 96
Controls - standards run in assay:
   Controls: Neg (3), Pos (3)
Incubation:
   30 min (37°C) + 30 min (37°C) + 30 min (RT)
Washes: 2 (+ preliminary plate wash)

CONTENTS

Antibodies, antigens, labelled components:
   HIV-1 p18, p24, gp41, gp20 and HIV-2 gp36 syn peptides bound to wells
   Anti-human IgG Ab (sh) AP conjugated
Substrate: PNP
Controls - standards supplied:
   Controls: Neg and Pos
Additional reagents:
   None
Special equipment required:
   None

INTERPRETATION

Comments on interpretation:
   Borderline: between cut-off and cut-off −25%; retest
   Positive: ≥cut-off repeatably and confirmed by supplemental tests
   Visual interpretation is possible
No. of references: 0

NOTES

110092.0

© *KLUWER ACADEMIC PUBLISHERS 1994, ISSN 1381-5067*

Human immunodeficiency virus
ANTIBODY DETECTION (IgG)

Manufacturer: Bio-Stat Diagnostics
Cat. No./Trade name: 851403/DETECT HIV®

SUMMARY

[Well-Ag]–**Ab**–[AHIgG-HRP]–[TMB]–A$_{450}$

Assay type: EIA (non-competitive)
Detection: Colorimetric A$_{450}$
Format: Microtitre well, Ag coated
Sample type: Serum, plasma
Sample pre-treatment:
　None
Sample volume: 5 µl (+ 250 µl diluent)
Number of tests: 96
Controls - standards run in assay:
　Controls: Neg (3), Pos (2)
Incubation:
　30 min (RT) + 30 min (RT) + 30 min (RT)
Washes: 2

CONTENTS

Antibodies, antigens, labelled components:
　HIV-1, HIV-2 syn peptides bound to well
　Anti-human IgG Ab (g) HRP conjugated
Substrate: TMB
Controls - standards supplied:
　Controls: Neg and Pos
Additional reagents:
　None
Special equipment required:
　None

INTERPRETATION

Comments on interpretation:
　Classification of sample is according to cut-off; no further
　　testing
　Differentiate between HIV-1 and HIV-2 using BIO-STAT
　　SELECT-HIV® KIT
No. of references: 0

NOTES

110619.0

Human immunodeficiency virus
ANTIBODY DETECTION (IgG)

Manufacturer: Biochrom
**Cat. No./Trade name: D7651/BIOCHROM-HIV 1/2
ELISA**

SUMMARY

[Well-Ag]–**Ab**–[AHIgG-POD]–[TMB]–A$_{450}$

Assay type: EIA (non-competitive)
Detection: Colorimetric A$_{450}$
Format: Microtitre well, Ag coated
Sample type: Serum, plasma
Sample pre-treatment:
　None
Sample volume: 20 µl (+ 180 µl diluent)
Number of tests: 96
Controls - standards run in assay:
　Controls: Neg (3), Pos (1)
Incubation:
　30 min (37°C) + 30 min (37°C) + 30 min (RT)
Washes: 2 (+ preliminary plate wash)

CONTENTS

Antibodies, antigens, labelled components:
　HIV-1 (gp41 and gp120) and HIV-2 (gp36) bound to well
　Anti-human IgG PAb (sh) POD conjugated
Substrate: TMB
Controls - standards supplied:
　Controls: Pos and Neg (human serum)
Additional reagents:
　None
Special equipment required:
　None

INTERPRETATION

Comments on interpretation:
　Equivocal: within cut-off and cut-off –10%; retest to
　　confirm
　Positive: ≥ cut-off repeatably and confirmed by
　　supplemental tests
No. of references: None

NOTES

110309.0

© KLUWER ACADEMIC PUBLISHERS 1994, ISSN 1381-5067

Human immunodeficiency virus
ANTIBODY DETECTION (IgG)

Manufacturer: bioMerieux
Cat. No./Trade name: 30206/VIDAS HIV 1 + 2 (HIV)

SUMMARY

[Solid phase-Ag]–**Ab**–[AHIgG-AP]–[4-MP]–fluorescence

Assay type: EIA (non-competitive)
Detection: Fluorometric
Format: Solid phase receptacle (SPR), Ag coated reagent strip
Sample type: Serum, plasma
Sample pre-treatment:
    None
Sample volume: 100 µl
Number of tests: 60
Controls - standards run in assay:
    Controls: Neg (1), Pos (1)
    Standard: (1)*
Incubation:
    Automated - total time 40 minutes
Washes: Automated

CONTENTS

Antibodies, antigens, labelled components:
    Synthetic HIV-1 and HIV-2 peptides bound to solid phase
    Anti-human IgG MAb (m) AP conjugated
Substrate: 4-MP
Controls - standards supplied:
    Controls: Neg and Pos (human serum)
    Standard: Pos (human serum)
Additional reagents:
    None
Special equipment required:
    Vitek Immunodiagnostic assay system (VIDAS)

INTERPRETATION

Comments on interpretation:
    Sample reactivity is calculated automatically and
        classification is according to cut-off
    Equivocal: retest to confirm
    Positive and repeatably equivocal samples confirm by
        Western Blot
No. of references: 8

NOTES

110478.0

*Recalibrate with each new lot of reagents and every 14
    days

Human immunodeficiency virus
ANTIBODY DETECTION (IgG)

Manufacturer: Biotest Diagnostics
Cat. No./Trade name: 807004/BIOTEST Anti-HIV-1/2

SUMMARY

[Well-Ag]–**Ab**–[AHIgG-POD]–[OPD]–A_{492}

Assay type: EIA (non-competitive)
Detection: Colorimetric A_{492}
Format: Microtitre well, Ag coated
Sample type: Serum, plasma (do not heat inactivate)
Sample pre-treatment:
    None
Sample volume: a)10 µl (+ 200 µl diluent) in plate
    b)25 µl (+ 500 µl diluent) predilute in tubes
Number of tests: 96, 480
Controls - standards run in assay:
    Controls: Neg (2), Pos (2)
Incubation:
    a) 30 min (40°C) + 30 min (40°C) + 15 min (RT)
    b) 45 min (37°C) + 45 min (37°C) + 15 min (RT)*
    c) 1 hr (37°C) + 1 hr (40°C) + 15 min (RT)
Washes: 2

CONTENTS

Antibodies, antigens, labelled components:
    rec proteins HIV-1 (p24, gp41); HIV-2 (p35) bound to well
    Anti-human IgG MAb POD conjugated
Substrate: OPD
Controls - standards supplied:
    Controls: Neg and Pos (human plasma)
Additional reagents:
    H_2SO_4
Special equipment required:
    None

INTERPRETATION

Comments on interpretation:
    Grey area: values between cut-off and cut-off minus
        10%; retest to confirm
    Positive: ≥ cut-off repeatably and confirmed by
        supplemental test
No. of references: 0

NOTES

110179.0

*Alternative incubation using 37°C heating block

© KLUWER ACADEMIC PUBLISHERS 1994, ISSN 1381-5067

Human immunodeficiency virus
ANTIBODY DETECTION (IgG)

Manufacturer: Boehringer Mannheim
Cat. No./Trade name: 1489 798/Enzymun-Test® Anti-HIV 1+2

SUMMARY

[Tube-strept]–[Ag-biotin]–**Ab**–[AHFcγ-POD]–[ABTS]–A_{420}

Assay type: EIA (non-competitive)
Detection: Colorimetric A_{420}
Format: Tube, streptavidin coated
Sample type: Serum, plasma (do not heat inactivate)
Sample pre-treatment:
  None
Sample volume: 20 µl
Number of tests: 145
Controls - standards run in assay:
  Controls: Neg (3), Pos (3)
Incubation:
  1 hr (RT) + 1 hr (RT) + 1 hr (RT)
Washes: 2 (+ preliminary tube pre-wash)

CONTENTS

Antibodies, antigens, labelled components:
  HIV 1/2 antigens (rec p24, synthetic peptides from gp41, gp120, gp32) biotinylated
  Anti-human Fcγ PAb (sh) POD conjugated
Substrate: ABTS, H_2O_2
Controls - standards supplied:
  Controls: Neg (human serum), Pos (Ab in bovine serum)
Additional reagents:
  Substrate and streptavidin-coated tubes
Special equipment required:
  Automated Enzymun-Test Systems (optional)

INTERPRETATION

Comments on interpretation:
  Borderline: within cut-off and cut-off - 10%; retest to confirm
  Positive: ≥cut-off repeatably; confirm borderline and positive samples in complementary test
No. of references: 0

NOTES

110470.0

Human immunodeficiency virus
ANTIBODY DETECTION (IgG)

Manufacturer: Gamma SA
Cat. No./Trade name: /ELISA-Test for HIV antibodies

SUMMARY

[Well-Ag]–**Ab**–[AHIgG-AP]–[PNP]–A_{405}

Assay type: EIA (non-competitive)
Detection: Colorimetric A_{405}
Format: Microtitre well, Ag coated
Sample type: Serum, plasma (do not heat inactivate)
Sample pre-treatment:
  None
Sample volume: 50 µl (+50 µl diluent)
Number of tests: 96
Controls - standards run in assay:
  Controls: Neg (3), Pos (2)
Incubation:
  30 min (37°C) + 30 min (37°C) + 30 min (RT)
Washes: 2 (+ preliminary plate wash)

CONTENTS

Antibodies, antigens, labelled components:
  HIV syn peptides (gp41, gp36) and rec HIV Ag (p24 gag) bound to well
  Anti-human IgG Ab (sh) AP conjugated
Substrate: PNP
Controls - standards supplied:
  Controls: Neg and Pos (human serum
Additional reagents:
  None
Special equipment required:
  None

INTERPRETATION

Comments on interpretation:
  Equivocal: within cut-off and cut-off x0.9; retest
  Repeatably equivocal; retest using an alternative test system (e.g. Western Blot)
  Positive: ≥cut-off repeatably and confirmed by supplemental tests
No. of references: 0

NOTES

110585.0

© KLUWER ACADEMIC PUBLISHERS 1994, ISSN 1381-5067

Human immunodeficiency virus
ANTIBODY DETECTION (IgG)

Manufacturer: IFCI Clone Systems
Cat. No./Trade name: 07.1017/Human Immunodeficiency Virus HIV-1 and HIV-2 EIA

SUMMARY

[Well-Ag]–**Ab**–[AHIgG-HRP]–[TMB]–A_{450}

Assay type: EIA (non-competitive)
Detection: Colorimetric A_{450}
Format: Microtitre well, Ag coated
Sample type: Serum, plasma (do not heat inactivate)
Sample pre-treatment:
None
Sample volume: 5 µl (+250 µl diluent)
Number of tests: 96
Controls - standards run in assay:
Controls: Neg (3), Pos (2)
Incubation:
30 min (RT) + 30 min (RT) + 30 min (RT)
Washes: 2

CONTENTS

Antibodies, antigens, labelled components:
syn peptides HIV-1 and HIV-2 bound to well
Anti-human IgG Ab (g) HRP conjugated
Substrate: TMB, H_2O_2
Controls - standards supplied:
Controls: Neg and Pos (human serum)
Additional reagents:
None
Special equipment required:
None

INTERPRETATION

Comments on interpretation:
Positive: ⩾ cut-off repeatably and confirmed by supplemental tests (e.g. Western Blot or indirect immunofluorescence)
No. of references: 8

NOTES

110134.0

Human immunodeficiency virus
ANTIBODY DETECTION (IgG)

Manufacturer: Innogenetics SA
Cat. No./Trade name: /INNOTEST HIV-1/HIV-2 Ab s.p.

SUMMARY

[Well-Ag]–**Ab**–[AHIgG-HRP]–[TMB]–A_{450}

Assay type: EIA (non-competitive)
Detection: Colorimetric A_{450}
Format: Microtitre well, Ag coated
Sample type: Serum, plasma
Sample pre-treatment:
None
Sample volume: 10 µl (+100 µl diluent)
Number of tests: 96, 480
Controls - standards run in assay:
Controls: Neg (1), Pos (1), per microplate strip*
Incubation:
30 min (37°C) + 30 min (37°C) + 30 min (RT)
Washes: 2

CONTENTS

Antibodies, antigens, labelled components:
syn HIV-1 env Ag and HIV-2 env Ag bound to well
Anti-human IgG Ab (g) HRP conjugated
Substrate: TMB, H_2O_2
Controls - standards supplied:
Controls: Neg and Pos (human serum)
Additional reagents:
H_2SO_4
Special equipment required:
None

INTERPRETATION

Comments on interpretation:
Positive: ⩾ cut-off repeatably and confirmed by supplemental tests
No. of references: 11

NOTES

110038.0

*If more than one strip used include at least 2 Neg and 2 Pos controls per strip holder

© KLUWER ACADEMIC PUBLISHERS 1994, ISSN 1381-5067

Human immunodeficiency virus
ANTIBODY DETECTION (IgG)

Manufacturer: Murex Diagnostics Limited
Cat. No./Trade name: VK61/Wellcozyme HIV 1+2 GAC ELISA

SUMMARY

[Well-AHIgG]–**Ab**–[Ag-AP]–[NADP+ampl]–A_{492}

Assay type: EIA (non-competitive, amplified)
Detection: Colorimetric A_{490}
Format: Microtitre well, Ab coated
Sample type: Saliva, urine, whole blood
Sample pre-treatment:
   Dried bloodspots: elution 200 ml PBS (18 hr)
Sample volume: Saliva/urine 50 µl; blood spot eluates 10 µl (+90 µl diluent)
Number of tests: 96
Controls - standards run in assay:
   Controls: Neg (3), anti-HIV-1 Pos (1), anti-HIV-2 Pos (1)
Incubation:
   30 min (37°C) + 1 hr (37°C) + 20 min (37°C) + 10 min (RT)
Washes: 2

CONTENTS

Antibodies, antigens, labelled components:
   Anti-human IgG Ab (r) bound to well
   rec and syn HIV-1 (env and core) Ag and HIV-2 (env) Ag AP conjugated
Substrate: NADP + amplifier
Controls - standards supplied:
   Controls: Neg, anti-HIV-1 Pos and anti-HIV-2 Pos (human serum)
Additional reagents:
   H_2SO_4
Special equipment required:
   Wellcozyme microwell plate washing system (optional)
   Wellcozyme microwell plate reader (optional)

INTERPRETATION

Comments on interpretation:
   Positive: ≥cut-off repeatably and confirmed by supplemental testing of subsequent fresh sample by conventional serology
No. of references: 11

NOTES

110166.0

See manufacturer's notes on clinical use

Human immunodeficiency virus
ANTIBODY DETECTION (IgG)

Manufacturer: Ortho Diagnostic Systems
Cat. No./Trade name: /ORTHO® HIV-1/HIV-2 ELISA Test System

SUMMARY

[Well-Ag]–**Ab**–[AHIgG-HRP]–[OPD]–A_{490}

Assay type: EIA (non-competitive)
Detection: Colorimetric A_{490}
Format: Microtitre well, Ag coated
Sample type: Serum, plasma
Sample pre-treatment:
   None
Sample volume: 15 µl (+300 µl diluent)
Number of tests: 480
Controls - standards run in assay:
   Controls: Neg (3), Pos HIV-1 (1), Pos HIV-2 (1)
Incubation:
   1 hr (37°C) + 1 hr (37°C) + 30 min (RT)
Washes: 2

CONTENTS

Antibodies, antigens, labelled components:
   rec HIV-1 env Ag and syn HIV-2 env Ag bound to well
   Anti-human IgG MAb (m) HRP conjugated
Substrate: OPD, H_2O_2
Controls - standards supplied:
   Controls: Neg, Pos HIV-1, and Pos HIV-2 (human serum)
Additional reagents:
   H_2SO_4
Special equipment required:
   None

INTERPRETATION

Comments on interpretation:
   Positive: ≥cut-off repeatably and confirmed by supplemental tests
No. of references: 13

NOTES

110147.0

© *KLUWER ACADEMIC PUBLISHERS 1994, ISSN 1381-5067*

Human immunodeficiency virus
ANTIBODY DETECTION (IgG)

Manufacturer: Sorin Biomedica
Cat. No./Trade name: 3076/ETI-AB-HIV-1/2K

SUMMARY

[Well-Ag]–**Ab**–[AHIgG-HRP]–[TMB]–A_{450}

Assay type: EIA (non-competitive)
Detection: Colorimetric A_{450}
Format: Microtitre well, Ag coated
Sample type: Serum, plasma
Sample pre-treatment:
 None
Sample volume: 10 µl (+ 200 µl diluent)
Number of tests: 192
Controls - standards run in assay:
 Controls: Neg (3), Pos (2)
Incubation:
 30 min (37°C) + 30 min (37°C) + 30 min (RT)
Washes: 2

CONTENTS

Antibodies, antigens, labelled components:
 HIV-1 p24, HIV-1 gp41 and HIV-2 gp36 (rec) bound to well
 Anti-human IgG Ab (g) HRP conjugated
Substrate: TMB H_2O_2
Controls - standards supplied:
 Controls: Neg (human serum) and Pos (human plasma)
Additional reagents:
 None
Special equipment required:
 ETI system reader, washer and shaker/incubator (optional)

INTERPRETATION

Comments on interpretation:
 Positive: $\geq$ cut-off repeatably and confirmed by supplemental tests
No. of references: 8

NOTES

110101.0

Human immunodeficiency virus
ANTIBODY DETECTION

Manufacturer: Chembio Diagnostic Systems Inc
Cat. No./Trade name: HIV101/HIV1/2 STAT-PAK

SUMMARY

[Membrane-Ag]–**Ab**–[AHIg-dye]–rose band

Assay type: Immunochromatographic assay
Detection: Visual
Format: Testcard, Ag coated membrane
Sample type: Serum, plasma, blood
Sample pre-treatment:
 None
Sample volume: Serum, plasma: 1 drop* (+ 5 drops diluent)
 Blood: 2 drops (+ 5 drops diluent)
Number of tests: 20, 50
Controls - standards run in assay:
 Controls: Pos (1)** bought separately
 Integral control (1)
Incubation:
 Read result 10-15 min after adding diluent to sample window of test card
Washes:

CONTENTS

Antibodies, antigens, labelled components:
 syn HIV-1, HIV-2 Ag bound to membrane (test well)
 Anti-human Ig PAb dye conjugated (absorbent pad)
Substrate:
Controls - standards supplied:
 None
Additional reagents:
 Positive control (anti-HIV Ab (g)) is available separately from Chembio
Special equipment required:
 None

INTERPRETATION

Comments on interpretation:
 Negative: rose coloured band in control well, and no rose coloured band in test well
 Positive: rose coloured band in control window and rose coloured band in test window repeatably and confirmed by supplemental tests
 Inconclusive: no rose coloured band in control well. Test a fresh specimen or repeat if present specimen less than 1 hr old
No. of references: 3

NOTES

110603.0

*1 drop = 20 µl
**Pos control should be run at least once per day

© KLUWER ACADEMIC PUBLISHERS 1994, ISSN 1381-5067

Human immunodeficiency virus
ANTIBODY DETECTION

Manufacturer: Ortho Diagnostic Systems
Cat. No./Trade name: 771585-901/HIVCHEK® 1 + 2

SUMMARY

[Membrane-Ag]–**Ab**–[Protein A-gold conjugate]–red spot

Assay type: Immunoblot assay
Detection: Visual
Format: Test unit, Ag coated membrane
Sample type: Serum, plasma
Sample pre-treatment:
   None
Sample volume: 1 drop
Number of tests: 100
Controls - standards run in assay:
   Controls: Neg (1), weak Pos (1), strong Pos (1)*
Incubation:
   Read results within 10 min of completing assay
      procedure
Washes: 2

CONTENTS

Antibodies, antigens, labelled components:
   rec HIV-1 env and HIV-2 env proteins adsorbed to filter
      membrane
   Protein A-gold conjugate
Substrate:
Controls - standards supplied:
   Controls: Neg, weak Pos and strong Pos (human serum)
Additional reagents:
   None
Special equipment required:
   None

INTERPRETATION

Comments on interpretation:
   Positive: Red Spot on membrane; retest and test by
      supplemental tests to confirm and distinguish
      between HIV-1 and HIV-2
No. of references: 6

NOTES

110148.0

*Recommended to run controls each time samples are run

Human immunodeficiency virus
ANTIBODY DETECTION

Manufacturer: Savyon Diagnostics Ltd
Cat. No./Trade name: 380-01/HIVSAV 1 & 2 Rapid
SeroTest®

SUMMARY

[Membrane-Ag]–**Ab**–[colloidal gold conjugate]–red dot

Assay type: Immunoblot assay
Detection: Visual
Format: Test cartridge, Ag coated membrane
Sample type: Serum, plasma
Sample pre-treatment:
   None
Sample volume: 1 drop
Number of tests: 50
Controls - standards run in assay:
   Not specified
Incubation:
   Read results within 5 min of carrying out assay procedure
Washes: 2 applications of wash solution

CONTENTS

Antibodies, antigens, labelled components:
   HIV-1 Ag and HIV-2 Ag bound to membrane
   Colloidal gold conjugate
Substrate: Not specified
Controls - standards supplied:
   None
Additional reagents:
   None
Special equipment required:
   None

INTERPRETATION

Comments on interpretation:
   Negative: no red dot on inner circle of membrane or slight
      pink colouration
   Positive: red dot on inner circle of membrane
No. of references: 0

NOTES

110595.0

© KLUWER ACADEMIC PUBLISHERS 1994, ISSN 1381-5067

Human immunodeficiency virus
ANTIBODY DETECTION

Manufacturer: Agen Biomedical Ltd
Cat. No./Trade name: HSRKII/SimpliRED® HIV-1/HIV-2 ANTIBODY TEST

SUMMARY

[RBC]–[MAb–Ag]–**Ab**–agglutination

Assay type: Particle RBC agglutination assay*
Detection: Visual
Format: Agglutination tray, patient/donor RBC
Sample type: Whole blood, serum, plasma**
Sample pre-treatment:
  None
Sample volume: 10 µl x 2
Number of tests: 25, 100
Controls - standards run in assay:
  Controls: Neg (1), Pos (1)
Incubation:
  Total time 4 minutes
Washes: 0

CONTENTS

Antibodies, antigens, labelled components:
  Anti-RBC MAb - HIV gp 41 and HIV gp 36 syn peptide
    conjugate (binds to RBC during assay)
Substrate:
Controls - standards supplied:
  Controls: Neg and Pos
Additional reagents:
  None
Special equipment required:
  None

INTERPRETATION

Comments on interpretation:
  Negative: no agglutination in test well but agglutination
    after addition of Pos control reagent
  Positive: agglutination in test well, and no agglutination in
    control well repeatably
No. of references: 0

NOTES

110105.0

*In the assay, patient/donor RBC are coated with the MAb-
  syn peptide conjugate. This causes cross-linking and
  visible agglutination when HIV-1 Ag in the patient sample
  binds to the RBC + conjugate
**If using serum or plasma, whole blood from a donor must
  be added

Human immunodeficiency virus
ANTIBODY DETECTION

Manufacturer: Fujirebio
Cat. No./Trade name: /SERODIA® - HIV

SUMMARY

[Particle-Ag]–**Ab**–Agglutination

Assay type: Particle agglutination assay
Detection: Visual
Format: Microtitre well, Ag coated particles
Sample type: Serum, plasma
Sample pre-treatment:
  Sample absorption if unsensitized cells show (+)
    agglutination
Sample volume: 25 µl (+75 µl diluent)*
Number of tests: 220, 550
Controls - standards run in assay:
  Control: Pos (1)
Incubation:
  2 hour (RT)
Washes: 0

CONTENTS

Antibodies, antigens, labelled components:
  HIV Ag bound to gelatin particles
Substrate:
Controls - standards supplied:
  Controls: Pos (rabbit serum titre 1:128) and control
    unsensitized gelatin particles
Additional reagents:
  None
Special equipment required:
  None

INTERPRETATION

Comments on interpretation:
  Negative: (-)Agglutination at serum dilution 1:32
    (±)Agglutination regarded as Neg but should be
    further titrated for accurate interpretation
  Positive: (+)Agglutination at serum dilution 1:32 and
    showing (-)agglutination with control cells at serum
    dilution 1:16
No. of references: 0

NOTES

110199.0

This is a screening test
*Further dilutions are performed in the tray to give 1:32 final
  serum dilution
Control particles tested at 1:16 final serum dilution

© KLUWER ACADEMIC PUBLISHERS 1994, ISSN 1381-5067

Human immunodeficiency virus (HIV-1)
ANTIGEN DETECTION

Manufacturer: Abbott Laboratories
Cat. No./Trade name: 7042/ABBOTT HIVAG-1

SUMMARY

[Bead-Ab]–**Ag**–[Ab]–[ARIgG-HRP]–[OPD]–A$_{492}$

Assay type: EIA (non-competitive)
Detection: Colorimetric A$_{492}$
Format: Reaction well, Ab coated bead
Sample type: Serum, plasma, cell culture supernatant
Sample pre-treatment:
   None
Sample volume: 200 µl (+20 µl diluent)
Number of tests: 100
Controls - standards run in assay:
   For serum, plasma: Controls: Neg (3), Pos (2)
   For cell culture: Controls: Neg (6), Pos (2)
Incubation:
   16-20 hr (RT) + 4 hr (40°C) + 2 hr (40°C) + 30 min
     (RT)
Washes: 3

CONTENTS

Antibodies, antigens, labelled components:
   Anti-HIV-1 Ab (h) bound to bead
   Anti-HIV-1 Ab (r)
   Anti-rabbit IgG Ab (g) HRP conjugated
Substrate: OPD, H$_2$O$_2$
Controls - standards supplied:
   Controls: Neg (human plasma) and Pos
Additional reagents:
   H$_2$SO$_4$
   Cell culture Neg control (uninfected cell culture)
Special equipment required:
   None

INTERPRETATION

Comments on interpretation:
   Positive: ⩾cut-off repeatably and confirmed by
     supplemental testing with HIVAG-1 blocking antibody
     test (Abbott)
   For cell culture specimens; can retest second sample
     from same culture as alternative to Blocking Assay
No. of references: 36

NOTES

110128.0

HIV-1 antigen is a low sensitivity marker for HIV infection

Human immunodeficiency virus (HIV-1)
ANTIGEN DETECTION

Manufacturer: Coulter Corporation
Cat. No./Trade name: 6603698/COULTER® HIV-1 p24
Antigen Assay

SUMMARY

[Well-MAb]–**Ag**–[Ab-biotin]–[strept-HRP]–[TMB]–A$_{450}$

Assay type: EIA (non-competitive)
Detection: Colorimetric A$_{450}$
Format: Microtitre well, Ab coated
Sample type: Serum, plasma, tissue culture media
Sample pre-treatment:
   None
Sample volume: 200 µl
Number of tests: 96, 2400
Controls - standards run in assay:
   Controls: Neg (3), Pos (2)*
Incubation:
   1 hr (37°C) + 1 hr (37°C) + 30 min (37°C) + 30 min
     (RT)
Washes: 3

CONTENTS

Antibodies, antigens, labelled components:
   Anti-HIV core MAb (m) bound to well
   Anti-HIV Ab biotinylated
   Streptavidin HRP conjugated
Substrate: TMB
Controls - standards supplied:
   Controls: Neg (normal human serum) and Pos (normal
     human serum + 50 µl antigen reagent)
Additional reagents:
   HIV Neg control tissue culture media
Special equipment required:
   None

INTERPRETATION

Comments on interpretation:
   Borderline (not specified): repeat and if consistently
     borderline, retest a fresh sample 4 weeks later
   Positive: ⩾cut-off repeatably and confirmed by
     COULTER HIV-1 p24 Antigen Neutralisation Kit
No. of references: 8

NOTES

110625.0

For research purposes only
*For serum and plasma the Neg control is normal human
   serum
For tissue culture samples, the Neg control is tissue culture
   media

© KLUWER ACADEMIC PUBLISHERS 1994, ISSN 1381-5067

Human immunodeficiency virus (HIV-1)
ANTIGEN DETECTION

Manufacturer: Organon Teknika NV
Cat. No./Trade name: 59518/Vironostika® HIV-1 Antigen

SUMMARY

$$[Well-MAb]-\mathbf{Ag}-[Ab-HRP]-[TMB]-A_{450/630}$$

Assay type: EIA (non-competitive)
Detection: Colorimetric $A_{450/630}$
Format: Microtitre well, Ab coated
Sample type: Serum, plasma, cell culture supernatant
Sample pre-treatment:
Cell culture supernatant: centrifuge
Sample volume: 100 µl*
Number of tests: 192
Controls - standards run in assay:
Qualitative assay: Controls: Neg (3), Pos (1)
Semi-quantitative assay: Controls: Neg (4), Pos (2)
With supernatant: additional Neg cell culture controls (3)
Incubation:
1 hr (37°C) + 1 hr (37°C) + 30 min (RT)
Washes: 2

CONTENTS

Antibodies, antigens, labelled components:
Anti-HIV-1 (p24) core MAb (m) bound to well
Anti-HIV-1 Ab (h) HRP conjugated
Substrate: TMB, H_2O_2
Controls - standards supplied:
Controls: Neg and Pos (human serum)
Additional reagents:
HIV-1 neg for cell culture supernatant fluid
Special equipment required:
None

INTERPRETATION

Comments on interpretation:
Positive: ≥ cut-off repeatably and confirmed using
Vironostika® HIV-1 antigen neutralization system
Semi-quantitative procedure available
No. of references: 37

NOTES

110389.0

*Serial dilutions required for semi-quantitative test

Human immunodeficiency virus (HIV-1)
ANTIBODY DETECTION

Manufacturer: Behringwerke AG
Cat. No./Trade name: OWSA/Enzygnost® Anti-HIV-1

SUMMARY

$$[Well-Ag]\left\{\begin{matrix}\mathbf{Ab}\\ [Ab-POD]\end{matrix}\right.-[TMB]-A_{450}$$

Assay type: EIA (competitive)
Detection: Colorimetric A_{450}
Format: Microtitre well, Ag coated
Sample type: Serum, plasma
Sample pre-treatment:
None
Sample volume: 100 µl (+25 µl diluent)
Number of tests: 96
Controls - standards run in assay:
Controls: Neg (4), Pos (2)
Incubation:
1 hr (37°C) + 30 min (37°C) + 30 min (RT)
Washes: 1

CONTENTS

Antibodies, antigens, labelled components:
HIV Ag bound to well
Anti-HIV Ab (h) POD conjugated
Substrate: TMB, H_2O_2
Controls - standards supplied:
Controls: Neg and Pos (human serum)
Additional reagents:
None
Special equipment required:
Behring ELISA processor (optional)

INTERPRETATION

Comments on interpretation:
Equivocal: within cut-off and cut-off + 10%; retest to confirm
Positive: < cut-off repeatably; and confirmed by supplemental tests
No. of references: 4

NOTES

110460.0

© KLUWER ACADEMIC PUBLISHERS 1994, ISSN 1381-5067

Human immunodeficiency virus (HIV-1)
ANTIBODY DETECTION

Manufacturer: Coulter Corporation
Cat. No./Trade name: 6604526/COULTER® HIV-1 p24 Antibody Assay

SUMMARY

$$[\text{Well-MAb}] \genfrac{}{}{0pt}{}{\textbf{Ab}}{} \Big\rangle [Ag]–[Ab\text{-}biotin]–[strept\text{-}HRP]–[TMB]–A_{450}$$

Assay type: EIA (competitive)
Detection: Colorimetric A_{450}
Format: Microtitre well, Ab coated
Sample type: Serum, plasma
Sample pre-treatment:
  None
Sample volume: 200 µl
Number of tests: 96
Controls - standards run in assay:
  Controls: Neg* (3) normal human serum (2)
  Standards: (5)**
Incubation:
  1 hr (37°C) + 1 hr (37°C) + 30 min (37°C) + 30 min (RT)
Washes: 3

CONTENTS

Antibodies, antigens, labelled components:
  Anti-HIV p24 core MAb (m) bound to well
  HIV p24 Ag
  Anti-HIV p24 Ab (h) biotinylated
  Streptavidin HRP conjugated
Substrate: TMB
Controls - standards supplied:
  Controls: Normal human serum (acts as Ab Neg control on addition of HIV Ag reagent) and antibody reference reagent (dilutetd to form 5 standards)**
Additional reagents:
  Negative control tissue culture media
Special equipment required:
  None

INTERPRETATION

Comments on interpretation:
  Classification of results is according to cut-off; no further testing
No. of references: 8

NOTES

110624.0

For research purposes only
*The antibody negative control is normal human serum to which 50 µl of HIV Ag reagent has been added per well
**Serial dilutions are made of the antibody reference reagent (i.e. A–E titre 0.125–2 Units/ml) and each dilution in run in duplicate for the reference curve

Human immunodeficiency virus (HIV-1)
ANTIBODY DETECTION

Manufacturer: Murex Diagnostics Limited
Cat. No./Trade name: VK56/57/Wellcozyme HIV Recombinant

SUMMARY

$$[\text{Well-MAb} + \text{Ag}] \genfrac{}{}{0pt}{}{\textbf{Ab}}{[Ab\text{-}HRP]} \Big\{ –[TMB]–A_{492}$$

Assay type: EIA (competitive)
Detection: Colorimetric A_{450}
Format: Microtitre well coated with (Ag + Ab) complex
Sample type: Serum, plasma (may be heat inactivated if temperature ⩽56°C)
Sample pre-treatment:
  None
Sample volume: 50 µl
Number of tests: 96, 480
Controls - standards run in assay:
  Controls: Neg (2), low Pos (cut-off control) (3), high Pos (1)
Incubation:
  1 hr (37°C) + 20 min (RT)
Washes: 1

CONTENTS

Antibodies, antigens, labelled components:
  rec HIV-1 (core + env) Ag captured by anti-HIV-1 MAb (m) bound to well
  Anti-HIV-1 Ab (h) HRP conjugated
Substrate: TMB, H_2O_2
Controls - standards supplied:
  Controls: Neg, low Pos, high Pos (human serum)
Additional reagents:
  H_2SO_4
Special equipment required:
  Wellcozyme microwell plate washing system (optional)
  Wellcozyme microwell plate reader system (optional)

INTERPRETATION

Comments on interpretation:
  Positive: ⩽cut-off repeatably and confirmed by supplemental tests
No. of references: 10

NOTES

110168.0

Human immunodeficiency virus (HIV-1)
ANTIBODY DETECTION

Manufacturer: Abbott Laboratories
Cat. No./Trade name: 3A01/HIVAB p24 (rDNA)

SUMMARY

[Bead-Ag]–**Ab**–[Ag-HRP]–[OPD]–A_{492}

Assay type: EIA (non-competitive)
Detection: Colorimetric A_{492}
Format: Reaction well, Ag coated bead
Sample type: Serum, plasma
Sample pre-treatment:
  None
Sample volume: 50 µl (+ diluent). Dilution protocol according to expected titre*
Number of tests: 100, 500
Controls - standards run in assay:
  Calibrators: Neg (2), Pos (3)
Incubation:
  16-22 hr (RT) + 30 min (40°C) + 30 min (RT)
Washes: 2

CONTENTS

Antibodies, antigens, labelled components:
  rec HIV-1 p24 Ag bound to beads
  rec HIV-1 p24 Ag HRP conjugated
Substrate: OPD, H_2O_2
Controls - standards supplied:
  Calibrators: Neg (bovine serum), Pos (human serum)
Additional reagents:
  H_2SO_4
Special equipment required:
  None

INTERPRETATION

Comments on interpretation:
  Assay designed for semi-quantitative procedure with 3 dilution protocols
  Qualitative cut-off is applied to undiluted samples with titre <1 and no further testing is required
No. of references: 16

NOTES

110136.0

For research use only
Dilution protocols: (1) 1:5 through 1:3125; (2) 1:625 through 1:390625; (3) undiluted

Human immunodeficiency virus (HIV-1)
ANTIBODY DETECTION

Manufacturer: Genetic Systems Corporation/Sanofi Diagnostics Pasteur
Cat. No./Trade name: 0218/GENETIC SYSTEMS® LAV EIA

SUMMARY

[Well-Ag]–**Ab**–[AHIgG/IgM-HRP]–[TMP]–A_{450}

Assay type: EIA (non-competitive)
Detection: Colorimetric A_{450}
Format: Microtitre well, Ag coated
Sample type: Serum, plasma, whole blood
Sample pre-treatment:
  Dried blood spots: punch 1/4" disk, add 200 µl diluent, elute overnight (2-8°C)
Sample volume: Serum/plasma: 100 µl (of 1:401 dilution); eluted blood spot: 10 µl (+90 µl diluent)
Number of tests: 192, 960, 4800
Controls - standards run in assay:
  Controls: Neg (3), Pos (2)
Incubation:
  1 hr (37°C) + 1 hr (37°C) + 30 min (RT)
Washes: 2

CONTENTS

Antibodies, antigens, labelled components:
  HIV-1 Ag bound to well
  Anti-human IgM and IgG Ab (g) HRP conjugated
Substrate: TMB, H_2O_2
Controls - standards supplied:
  Controls: Neg and Pos (human serum)
Additional reagents:
  None
Special equipment required:
  None

INTERPRETATION

Comments on interpretation:
  Positive: ≥cut-off repeatably and confirmed by more specific supplemental test (e.g. Western Blot, radioimmunoprecipitation assay)
  When supplemental tests indeterminate; test further sample 3-6 months later
No. of references: 20

NOTES

110042.0

© KLUWER ACADEMIC PUBLISHERS 1994, ISSN 1381-5067

Human immunodeficiency virus (HIV-1)
ANTIBODY DETECTION

Manufacturer: Murex Diagnostics Limited
Cat. No./Trade name: VK60/Wellcozyme HIV-1 anti-p24

SUMMARY

[Well-Ag]–**Ab**–[Ag-AP]–[NADP-ampl]–A_{492}

Assay type: EIA (non-competitive, amplified)
Detection: Colorimetric A_{492}
Format: Microtitre well, Ag coated
Sample type: Serum, plasma (do not heat inactivate plasma samples)*
Sample pre-treatment:
 None
Sample volume: 25 µl
Number of tests: 96
Controls - standards run in assay:
 Controls: Neg (4), Pos (2)
Incubation:
 30 min (37°C) + 30 min (37°C) + 20 min (37°C) + 10 min (RT)
Washes: 2

CONTENTS

Antibodies, antigens, labelled components:
 rec HIV-1 core (p24) Ag bound to well
 rec HIV-1 core (p24) Ag AP conjugated
Substrate: NADP + amplifier
Controls - standards supplied:
 Controls: Neg and Pos (human serum)
Additional reagents:
 H_2SO_4
Special equipment required:
 Wellcozyme microwell plate washing system (optional)
 Wellcozyme microwell plate reader system (optional)

INTERPRETATION

Comments on interpretation:
 Classification of samples is according to cut-off; no further testing
 Antibody titre of samples may be obtained by testing serial sample dilutions
No. of references: 6

NOTES

110167.0

Not to be used for primary screening or as a confirmatory test: sole use is for investigating individuals confirmed as HIV Pos
*Plasma samples collected in EDTA or sodium citrate may also be used

Human immunodeficiency virus (HIV-1)
ANTIBODY DETECTION

Manufacturer: Sanofi Diagnostics Pasteur
Cat. No./Trade name: 72254/ELAVIA anti-P25*

SUMMARY

[Well-Ag]–**Ab**–[Ag-HRP]–[OPD]–$A_{492/620}$

Assay type: EIA (non-competitive)
Detection: Colorimetric $A_{492/620}$
Format: Microtitre well, Ag coated
Sample type: Serum, plasma
Sample pre-treatment:
 None
Sample volume: 100 µl of diluted sample**
Number of tests: 96
Controls - standards run in assay:
 Controls: Neg (2), Pos (2)
Incubation:
 Overnight (RT) + 1 hr (40°C) + 30 min (RT)
Washes: 2

CONTENTS

Antibodies, antigens, labelled components:
 rec HIV-1 p25 Ag bound to well
 rec HIV-1 p25 Ag HRP conjugated
Substrate: OPD
Controls - standards supplied:
 Controls: Neg and Pos (human serum)
Additional reagents:
 None
Special equipment required:
 None

INTERPRETATION

Comments on interpretation:
 This assay is used to access prognosis of asymptomatic seropositive subjects and subjects at ARC stage
No. of references: 8

NOTES

110671.0

*It is not for use as a diagnostic test for early detection of seroconversion
**(a)1:50 for seropositive, unknown clinical states;
(b) 1:2500 for seropositive high anti-P25;
(c) undiluted for seropositive, symptomatic

Human immunodeficiency virus (HIV-1)
ANTIBODY DETECTION (IgG)

Manufacturer: Abbott Laboratories
Cat. No./Trade name: 1458-24/ABBOTT RECOMBINANT HIV 1 EIA

SUMMARY

[Bead-Ag]—**Ab**—[AHIgG-HRP]—[OPD]—A_{492}

Assay type: EIA (non-competitive)
Detection: Colorimetric A_{492}
Format: Reaction well, Ag coated bead
Sample type: Serum, plasma (do not heat inactivate)
Sample pre-treatment:
    None
Sample volume: 10 µl (+400 µl diluent)
Number of tests: 100, 1000
Controls - standards run in assay:
    Controls: Neg (2), Pos (3)
Incubation:
    30 min (40°C) + 30 min (40°C) + 30 min (RT)
Washes: 2

CONTENTS

Antibodies, antigens, labelled components:
    rec HIV 1 Ag (env and core) bound to bead
    Anti-human IgG Ab (g) HRP conjugated
Substrate: OPD, H_2O_2
Controls - standards supplied:
    Controls: Neg and Pos (human plasma)
Additional reagents:
    H_2SO_4
Special equipment required:
    None

INTERPRETATION

Comments on interpretation:
    Positive: ≥ cut-off repeatably
No. of references: 14

NOTES

110135.0

Human immunodeficiency virus (HIV-1)
ANTIBODY DETECTION (IgG)

Manufacturer: Boehringer Mannheim
Cat. No./Trade name: 1373 412/Enzymun-Test® Anti-HIV-p24 Quantitative

SUMMARY

[Tube-strept]—[Ag-biotin]—**Ab**—[AHFcγ-POD]—[ABTS]—A_{420}

Assay type: EIA (non-competitive)
Detection: Colorimetric A_{420}
Format: Tube, streptavidin coated
Sample type: Serum, plasma (do not heat inactivate)
Sample pre-treatment:
    None
Sample volume: 10 µl*
Number of tests: 145
Controls - standards run in assay:
    Controls: Pos (1)
    Standards: (5)
Incubation:
    1 hr (RT) + 1 hr (RT) + 1 hr (RT)
Washes: 2 (+tube pre-wash)

CONTENTS

Antibodies, antigens, labelled components:
    HIV-1 Ag (rec p24) biotinylated
    Anti-human Fc γ PAb (sh) POD conjugated
Substrate: ABTS, H_2O_2
Controls - standards supplied:
    Controls: Pos (human serum)
    Standards: Set of 5 with defined EIA values (human serum)
Additional reagents:
    Substrate and streptavidin-coated tubes
Special equipment required:
    Automated Enzymun-Test Systems (optional)

INTERPRETATION

Comments on interpretation:
    This is a quantitative assay
No. of references: 0

NOTES

110471.0

*1:10 dilution may be necessary

© *KLUWER ACADEMIC PUBLISHERS 1994, ISSN 1381-5067*

Human immunodeficiency virus (HIV-1)
ANTIBODY DETECTION (IgG)

Manufacturer: Bouty Diagnostici
Cat. No./Trade name: 25300/BEIA SINT HIV 1

SUMMARY

[Well-Ag]–**Ab**–[AHIgG-HRP]–[OPD]–$A_{492/620}$

Assay type: EIA (non-competitive)
Detection: Colorimetric $A_{492/620}$
Format: Microtitre well, Ag coated
Sample type: Serum
Sample pre-treatment:
    None
Sample volume: 20 µl (+400 µl diluent) x 2*
Number of tests: 96
Controls - standards run in assay:
    Controls: Neg (2), cut-off (4)
Incubation:
    1 hr (37°C) + 30 min (37°C) + 15 min (RT)
Washes: 2

CONTENTS

Antibodies, antigens, labelled components:
    HIV-1 gp41 synthetic peptide bound to well
    Anti-human IgG PAb (g) HRP conjugated
Substrate: OPD, H_2O_2
Controls - standards supplied:
    Controls: Cut-off and Neg (human serum)
Additional reagents:
    None
Special equipment required:
    None

INTERPRETATION

Comments on interpretation:
    Positive: ≥cut-off repeatably in duplicate
No. of references: None

NOTES

110308.0

*Samples and controls run in duplicate

Human immunodeficiency virus (HIV-1)
ANTIBODY DETECTION

Manufacturer: Organon Teknika NV
Cat. No./Trade name: 72827/HIV-1 WESTERN BLOT

SUMMARY

[Strip-Ag]–**Ab**–[AHIg-HRP]–[substrate]–brown band

Assay type: Immunoblot assay
Detection: Visual
Format: Reaction tray, nitrocellulose strip, Ag coated
Sample type: Serum, plasma
Sample pre-treatment:
    None
Sample volume: 40 µl (+2 ml diluent)
Number of tests: 20
Controls - standards run in assay:
    Controls: Neg (1), low Pos (1), high Pos*
Incubation:
    a) 1 hr (RT) + 45 min (RT) + 10 min (RT)
    b) 6-24 hr (2-8°C) + 45 min (RT) + 10 min (RT)
Washes: 2

CONTENTS

Antibodies, antigens, labelled components:
    HIV-1 specific viral protein bands transblotted onto strips
    Protein bands are: env (gp160, gp120, gp41), pol (p65,
        p51, p31) and gag (p55, p24, p18)
    Anti-human Ig Ab (g) HRP conjugated
Substrate: Not specified
Controls - standards supplied:
    Controls: Neg, low Pos, and high Pos (human serum)
Additional reagents:
    None
Special equipment required:
    None

INTERPRETATION

Comments on interpretation:
    Negative: band reactivity is absent
    Positive: band reactivity must be present in at least two
        out of three major bands (gps 120/160, gp41, gp24)
    Intermediate: any band reactivity not meeting positive
        criteria
    (Band reactivity is defined by comparison to control
        strips)
No. of references: 12

NOTES

110547.0

*High Pos control is only essential with first run of every pack
    of strips

© KLUWER ACADEMIC PUBLISHERS 1994, ISSN 1381-5067

Human immunodeficiency virus (HIV-1)
ANTIBODY DETECTION

Manufacturer: Sorin Biomedica
Cat. No./Trade name: 2843/HIV-1 W.B. Set

SUMMARY

[Solid phase Ag]–**Ab**–[AHIgG-AP]–[BCIP]–visible band

Assay type: Immunoblot assay
Detection: Visual
Format: Well, Ag coated nitrocellulose strips
Sample type: Serum, heat inactivated
Sample pre-treatment:
None
Sample volume: 20 µl
Number of tests: 36
Controls - standards run in assay:
Controls: Neg (1), low Pos (1), high Pos (1)
Incubation:
a) 18-22 hr (RT) + 30 min (RT) + 15 min (RT)
b) 1 hr (RT) + 1 hr (RT) + 15 min (RT)
Washes: 3

CONTENTS

Antibodies, antigens, labelled components:
HIV proteins (p15, p24, gp41, p53, p55, p64, gp120 and gp 160 on nitrocellulose strips
Anti-human IgG Ab (g) AP conjugated
Substrate: BCIP
Controls - standards supplied:
Controls: Neg, low Pos and high Pos (human serum)
Additional reagents:
None
Special equipment required:
None

INTERPRETATION

Comments on interpretation:
Negative: Absence of protein bands
Positive: At least 3 bands: p24, p31 and gp41 or gp 120/160
For suspect positive and intermediate samples exact details are given in the package insert literature
No. of references: 13

NOTES

110244.0

*Pre-incubation of nitrocellulose strips in buffer for 15 min (on plate shaker) before assay

Human immunodeficiency virus (HIV-1)
ANTIBODY DETECTION (IgG)

Manufacturer: Sanofi Diagnostics Pasteur
Cat. No./Trade name: 72251/NEW LAV-BLOT I

SUMMARY

[Strip-Ag]–**Ab**–[AHIgG-AP]–[BCIP]–Visual band(s)

Assay type: Immunoblot assay
Detection: Visual
Format: Microcellulose strips, Ag coated
Sample type: Serum, plasma
Sample pre-treatment:
None
Sample volume: 20 µl (+2 ml diluent)
Number of tests: 18
Controls - standards run in assay:
Controls: Neg (1), Pos (1)
Incubation:
2 hr (RT) + 1 hr (RT) + approx 5 min (RT) - all with slow shaking
Washes: 3

CONTENTS

Antibodies, antigens, labelled components:
HIV-1 proteins separated by electrophoresis, bound to strip
Anti-human IgG Ab (g) AP conjugated
Substrate: BCIP
Controls - standards supplied:
Controls: Neg and Pos (human serum)
Additional reagents:
None
Special equipment required:
None

INTERPRETATION

Comments on interpretation:
Equivocal: a) 1 env ± gag ± pol bands;
b) gag + pol bands;
c) gag or pol bands only
Positive: 2 env ± gag ± pol bands
No. of references: 20

NOTES

110262.0

Human immunodeficiency virus (HIV-1 and HIV-2)
ANTIBODY DETECTION (IgG)

Manufacturer: Bio-Stat Diagnostics
Cat. No./Trade name: /851400/SELECT-HIV®

SUMMARY

[Well-Ag]–**Ab**–[AHIgG-HRP]–[TMB]–A_{450}

Assay type: EIA (non-competitive)
Detection: Colorimetric A_{450}
Format: Microtitre well, Ag coated
Sample type: Serum, plasma (do not heat inactivate)
Sample pre-treatment:
　None
Sample volume: 5 µl (+250 µl diluent)*
Number of tests: 192
Controls - standards run in assay:
　Controls: Neg (3), HIV-1 Pos (1), HIV-2 Pos (2)
Incubation:
　30 min (RT) + 30 min (RT) + 30 min (RT)
Washes: 2

CONTENTS

Antibodies, antigens, labelled components:
　HIV-1 syn peptide bound to well
　HIV-2 syn peptide bound to well
　Anti-human IgG Ab (g) HRP conjugated
Substrate: TMB
Controls - standards supplied:
　Controls: Neg, HIV-1 Pos, HIV-2 Pos
Additional reagents:
　None
Special equipment required:
　None

INTERPRETATION ❸

Comments on interpretation:
　Positive (HIV-1): > cut-off for HIV-1 and < cut-off for HIV-2
　Positive (HIV-2): > cut-off for HIV-2 and < cut-off for HIV-1
　If absorbance > cut-off for both HIV-1 and HIV-2, calculate binding ratio (BR), then:
　Positive (HIV-1): BR ⩽ 0.5
　Positive (HIV-2): BR ⩾ 2
　Positive (HIV-1 and HIV-2): BR < 2 and > 0.6
　Confirm all positives with supplemental tests
No. of references: 0

NOTES

110620.0

*Assay run in duplicate with HIV-1 and HIV-2 coated wells

Human immunodeficiency virus (HIV-1 and HIV-2)
ANTIBODY DETECTION (IgG)

Manufacturer: Innogenetics SA
Cat. No./Trade name: /INNO-LIA HIV-1/HIV-2 Ab

SUMMARY

[Strip-Ag]–**Ab**–[AHIgG-AP]–[BCIP]–colour

Assay type: Immunoblot assay
Detection: Visual
Format: Nylon strip, Ag coated
Sample type: Serum, plasma, saliva, whole blood
Sample pre-treatment:
　Blood spot: elute in 1 ml diluent
　Saliva: dilute 1:100, vortex to dissolve mucus, centrifuge
Sample volume: Serum, plasma, 10 µl (+ 1 ml diluent); blood, 1 drop
Number of tests: 20
Controls - standards run in assay:
　Controls: Neg (1), Pos (1), integral Pos controls in strip (4)
Incubation:
　1 hr (RT) + 30 min (RT) + 10-30 min (RT)*
Washes: 2

CONTENTS

Antibodies, antigens, labelled components:
　HIV-1 and HIV-2 rec and syn protein Ags** bound to nylon strips in discrete lines
　Anti-human IgG Ab (g) AP conjugated
Substrate: BCIP
Controls - standards supplied:
　Controls: Neg and Pos (human serum)
　4 integral strip controls: low cut-off, high cut-off, moderate Pos and high Pos
Additional reagents:
　None
Special equipment required:
　None

INTERPRETATION

Comments on interpretation:
　Negative: All HIV lines with negative rating
　Equivocal: reactivity but not meeting the Positive criteria
　Positive HIV-1: at least gp36 with min (1+) reactivity and p31 plus p24 or p17 with min (1+) reactivity
　Pos HIV-2: at least gp41 with min (1+) reactivity and gp41 neg
No. of references: None

NOTES

110212.0

*Overnight incubation for greater sensitivity
**HIV-1 Ags: p24, p17, gp41, p24
HIV-2 Ag: gp36

© *KLUWER ACADEMIC PUBLISHERS 1994, ISSN 1381-5067*

Human immunodeficiency virus (HIV-1 and HIV-2)
ANTIBODY DETECTION (IgG)

Manufacturer: Organon Teknika NV
Cat. No./Trade name: 80200/8032/LiaTek® HIV 1 + 2

SUMMARY

[Strip-Ag]–**Ab**–[AHIgG-AP]–[BCIP]–visible band

Assay type: Immunochromatographic assay
Detection: Visual/scanner
Format: Trough, Ag coated test strip
Sample type: Serum, plasma, whole blood, saliva
Sample pre-treatment:
  None
Sample volume: 10 μl (+ 1 ml diluent)
Number of tests: 20
Controls - standards run in assay:
  Controls: Neg (1), Pos (1)
  Integral controls: strong Pos (1), moderate Pos (1), low
    cut-off (1), high cut-off (1)
Incubation:
  1 hr (RT) + 30 min (RT) + 30 min (RT) + 10-30 min
    (RT)*
Washes: 2

CONTENTS

Antibodies, antigens, labelled components:
  Rec and syn HIV-1 (gp41, p31, p24, p17) and HIV-2
    (gp36) coated as discrete lines on test strip
  Anti-human IgG Ab (g) AP conjugated
Substrate: BCIP
Controls - standards supplied:
  Controls: Neg and Pos (human serum)
  Integral controls (human IgG and anti-human IgG (sh)
    coated on test strip)
Additional reagents:
  None
Special equipment required:
  None

INTERPRETATION

Comments on interpretation:
  Classification of samples and differential detection of
    HIV-1 and HIV-2 antibodies is according to band
    reactivity pattern (details given in pack insert)
  Semi-quantitative procedure is available
No. of references: 9

NOTES

110390.0

1st incubation may be 14-18 hr (RT)
All incubations and washes should be performed using an
  orbital shaker

Human immunodeficiency virus (HIV-2)
ANTIBODY DETECTION

Manufacturer: Behringwerke AG
Cat. No./Trade name: OWRB/Enzygnost® Anti-HIV-2

SUMMARY

[Well-Ag]–**Ab**–[Ag-POD]–[TMB]–A$_{450}$

Assay type: EIA (non-competitive)
Detection: Colorimetric A$_{450}$
Format: Microtitre well, Ag coated
Sample type: Serum, plasma
Sample pre-treatment:
  None
Sample volume: 100 μl (+ 25 μl diluent)
Number of tests: 96
Controls - standards run in assay:
  Controls: Neg (4), Pos (2)
Incubation:
  30 min (37°C) + 30 min (37°C) + 30 min (RT)
Washes: 2 (+ plate pre-wash)

CONTENTS

Antibodies, antigens, labelled components:
  HIV-2 gp36 peptide (env) bound to well
  HIV-2 peptide POD conjugated
Substrate: TMB, H$_2$O$_2$
Controls - standards supplied:
  Controls: Neg and Pos (human serum)
Additional reagents:
  None
Special equipment required:
  Behring ELISA processor (optional)

INTERPRETATION

Comments on interpretation:
  Equivocal: within cut-off and cut-off -10%; retest to
    confirm
  Positive: > cut-off repeatably; and confirmed by
    supplemental tests
No. of references: 4

NOTES

110461.0

Human immunodeficiency virus (HIV-2)
ANTIBODY DETECTION

Manufacturer: Genetic Systems Corporation/Sanofi Diagnostics Pasteur
Cat. No./Trade name: 0220/GENETIC SYSTEMS® HIV-2 EIA

SUMMARY

[Well-Ag]–**Ab**–[AHIgG/IgM-HRP]–[TMP]–A_{450}

Assay type: EIA (non-competitive)
Detection: Colorimetric A_{450}
Format: Microtitre well, Ag coated
Sample type: Serum, plasma
Sample pre-treatment:
　None
Sample volume: 100 µl (of a 1:401 dilution)
Number of tests: 192, 960, 4800
Controls - standards run in assay:
　Controls: Neg (3), Pos (2)
Incubation:
　1 hr (37°C) + 1 hr (37°C) + 30 min (RT)
Washes: 2

CONTENTS

Antibodies, antigens, labelled components:
　HIV-2$_{ROD}$ Ag bound to well
　Anti-human IgM and IgG Ab (g) HRP conjugated
Substrate: TMB
Controls - standards supplied:
　Controls: Neg and Pos (human serum)
Additional reagents:
　None
Special equipment required:
　None

INTERPRETATION

Comments on interpretation:
　Positive: ≥ cut-off repeatably and confirmed by more
　　specific supplemental test (e.g. Western Blot,
　　radioimmunoprecipitation assay)
　When supplemental tests indeterminate; test further
　　sample 3-6 months later
No. of references: 22

NOTES

110041.0

Human immunodeficiency virus (HIV-2)
ANTIBODY DETECTION (IgG)

Manufacturer: Cambridge Biotech Corporation
Cat. No./Trade name: 8055/CBC HIV-2 WESTERN BLOT KIT

SUMMARY

[Strip-Ag]–**Ab**–[AHIgG-biotin]–[avidin-HRP]–[substrate]–
visible bands

Assay type: Immunoblot assay
Detection: Visual
Format: Tray, Ag coated nitrocellulose strip
Sample type: Serum, plasma
Sample pre-treatment:
　None
Sample volume: 20 µl of 1:100 dilution
Number of tests: 27
Controls - standards run in assay:
　Controls: Neg (1), weak Pos (1), strong Pos (2)
Incubation:
　5 min (RT) + overnight (RT) + 1 hr (RT) + 1 hr (RT) +
　　6-10 min (RT)
Washes: 5

CONTENTS

Antibodies, antigens, labelled components:
　HIV-2 proteins transblotted in bands on nitrocellulose
　　strip
　Anti-human IgG Ab (g) biotinylated
　Avidin HRP conjugated
Substrate: 4-chloro-1-naphthol, H_2O_2
Controls - standards supplied:
　Controls: Neg, weak Pos and strong Pos (human serum)
Additional reagents:
　None
Special equipment required:
　None

INTERPRETATION

Comments on interpretation:
　Negative: no significant visible bands
　Positive: visible bands at gp105 and/or gp34 and/or p26
　　or p31 (or p68, 58, 55)
No. of references: 7

NOTES

110651.0

For investigational use only

© KLUWER ACADEMIC PUBLISHERS 1994, ISSN 1381-5067

Human immunodeficiency virus (HIV-2)
ANTIBODY DETECTION (IgG)

Manufacturer: Genetic Systems Corporation/Sanofi Diagnostics Pasteur
Cat. No./Trade name: 0421-48/GENETIC SYSTEMS® HIV-2 Western Blot

SUMMARY

[Strip-Ag]–**Ab**–[AHIgG-AP]–[BCIP]–visual band

Assay type: Immunoblot assay
Detection: Visual
Format: Reaction tray, nitrocellulose strips, Ag coated
Sample type: Serum, plasma
Sample pre-treatment:
None
Sample volume: 20 µl (+1 ml diluent)
Number of tests: 48
Controls - standards run in assay:
Controls: Neg (1), low Pos (1), high Pos (1)
Incubation:
1 hr (RT) + 45 min (RT) + 3 min (RT) + 5 min (RT)
Washes: 2

CONTENTS

Antibodies, antigens, labelled components:
Resolved HIV-2 protein bands (gp 140, gp105, gp36; p68, p56, p26, p16) transblotted onto nitrocellulose strips
Anti-human IgG Ab (g) AP conjugated
Substrate: BCIP
Controls - standards supplied:
Controls: Neg, low Pos, high Pos (human serum)
Additional reagents:
None
Special equipment required:
None

INTERPRETATION

Comments on interpretation:
By comparison with high Pos control p26 reaction:
Negative: no viral bands present
Indeterminate: viral bands do not meet criteria for Pos result; retest
Positive: at least two of the significant bands (gp 105, gp36; p26) are present
No. of references: 11

NOTES

110081.0

Human immunodeficiency virus (HIV-2)
ANTIBODY DETECTION (IgG)

Manufacturer: Sanofi Diagnostics Pasteur
Cat. No./Trade name: 72252/NEW LAV-BLOT II

SUMMARY

[Strip-Ag]–**Ab**–[AHIgG-AP]–[BCIP]–visible band

Assay type: Immunoblot assay
Detection: Visual
Format: Tray, nitrocellulose strip, Ag coated
Sample type: Serum, plasma (heat inactivated)
Sample pre-treatment:
None
Sample volume: 20 µl (+2 ml diluent)
Number of tests: 18
Controls - standards run in assay:
Controls: Neg (1), Pos (1) for each test run
Incubation:
5 min (RT) + 2 hr (RT) + 1 hr (RT) + 5 min (RT) all with slow shaking
Washes:

CONTENTS

Antibodies, antigens, labelled components:
HIV-2 viral proteins bound to nitrocellulose strips in specific bands
Anti-human IgG Ab (g) AP conjugated
Substrate: BICP
Controls - standards supplied:
Controls: Neg and Pos (human serum)
Additional reagents:
None
Special equipment required:
None

INTERPRETATION

Comments on interpretation:
Comparison of sample and Pos control strips identifies presence of env, gag and pol viral bands (blue violet) in patient serum
Positive: presence of env, gag and pol virus bands
Indeterminate: presence of env + gag, env + pol or gag or pol or env bands alone
Negative: no bands or unclassified bands. Further testing not specified
No. of references: 20

NOTES

110872.0

© KLUWER ACADEMIC PUBLISHERS 1994, ISSN 1381-5067

Human T-cell lymphotropic virus (Adult T-cell leukaemia)

Natural history

Infection with the human T-cell lymphotrophic virus type I is endemic in areas such as Southwest Japan, the Caribbean, Melanesia and parts of Africa, where it is carried in T lymphocytes by 5–15% of the population in certain regions. Seropositivity increases in adult women, with spread occurring by sexual transmission from men to women, spread in the opposite direction being less common. The other modes of transmission are by blood transfusion and from mother to infant. However this retrovirus (subfamily: oncovirus) is very cell-associated, free virus has low infectivity and transmission requires transfer of infected cells. Breast-feeding is the principal risk factor in transmission from mother to infant. Infection with HTLV-I is mainly asymptomatic, but associated with development of adult T-cell leukaemia/lymphoma (ATL) in 2–4% of carriers some 4–6 decades later. Infection acquired from blood transfusion may present with a chronic progressive myelopathy – tropical spastic paresis/HTLV-associated myelopathy (TSP/HAM) – in 1% some 2–3 years later. In endemic areas other diseases have been associated with HTLV-I infection, including chronic infective dermatitis and uveitis. In the rest of the world HTLV-I infection is unusual, although sporadic cases are found, mainly in patients with connections to the endemic regions. In Japan screening of blood donors has proved worthwhile, and screening in pregnancy of women from endemic countries allows for advice to avoid breast-feeding to be considered.

HTLV-II

HTLV-II was isolated soon after HTLV-I, but there is still no clear association with disease. Infection has been noted particularly in intravenous drug users, and their sexual partners, and found to be endemic in American Indians of North and Central America. Transmission is presumed to be very similar to that of HTLV-I.

Diagnosis and markers

Immunoassays for antibody to HTLV-I based on HTLV-I viral lysate detect antibody to structural proteins of the core (p19, p24) from the *gag* gene, and surface glycoproteins (gp46, gp61) from the *env* gene which have considerable cross-reactivity with those from HTLV-II. Improved sensitivity comes from inclusion of the recombinant common antigen gp21. Recombinant and synthetic type-specific antigens will differentiate antibody to the two viruses in most cases. Confirmation of reactive samples is accomplished by immunoblotting or radioimmunoprecipitation. Antibody levels are often high in TSP/HAM, and antibody is found in the cerebrospinal fluid in these cases. Antibody to the virus transactivating protein p40 from the *tax* gene has been associated with increased transmission of virus to infants or sexual partners. Human T-lymphotropic viruses can be isolated in cell culture, but this procedure is restricted to reference laboratories. Proviral DNA in peripheral blood mononuclear cells can be amplified by PCR for virus detection and discrimination between HTLV-I and HTLV-II.

Comment

Testing for HTLV should be accompanied by counselling and consent because of the implications of carriage. Advice to reduce transmission to partners or infants can be given, and carriers should be advised not to donate blood, tissues or organs.

Reference

Centers for Disease Control and Prevention and the U.S.P.H.S. Working Group. Guidelines for counselling persons infected with Human T-lymphotropic Virus type I (HTLV-I) and type II (HTLV-II). Annals of Internal Medicine. 1993;118:448–454.

Human T-cell lymphotropic virus
ANTIGEN DETECTION

Manufacturer: Coulter Corporation
Cat. No./Trade name: 6604416/COULTER® HTLV-I/II Antigen EIA Kit

SUMMARY

[Well-MAb]–**Ag**–[Ab-biotin]–[strept-HRP]–[TMB]–A_{450}

Assay type: EIA (non-competitive)
Detection: Colorimetric A_{450}
Format: Microtitre well, Ab coated
Sample type: Tissue culture media
Sample pre-treatment:
  None
Sample volume: 200 µl
Number of tests: 96
Controls - standards run in assay:
  Controls: Neg (3), Pos (2)*
Incubation:
  2 hr (37°C) + 1 hr (37°C) + 30 min (37°C) + 30 min
  (RT)
Washes: 3

CONTENTS

Antibodies, antigens, labelled components:
  Anti-HTLV-I, HTLV-II p24 MAb (m) bound to well
  Anti-HTLV-I, HTLV-II biotinylated
  Streptavidin HRP conjugated
Substrate: TMB
Controls - standards supplied:
  Controls: Pos (HTLV-I Ag reagent)
Additional reagents:
  Negative control tissue culture media
Special equipment required:
  None

INTERPRETATION

Comments on interpretation:
  Positive: ≥ cut-off repeatably
No. of references: 4

NOTES

110623.0

For research use only
*When testing tissue culture samples, 3 tissue culture
  controls from uninfected tissue culture samples must be
  assayed

Human T-cell lymphotropic virus
ANTIBODY DETECTION (IgG)

Manufacturer: Bio-Stat Diagnostics
Cat. No./Trade name: 851398/EIAgen HTLV-I and HTLV-II Comb Kit

SUMMARY

[Well-Ag]–**Ab**–[AHIgG-HRP]–[TMB]–A_{450}

Assay type: EIA (non-competitive)
Detection: Colorimetric A_{450}
Format: Microtitre well, Ag coated
Sample type: Serum, plasma (do not heat inactivate)
Sample pre-treatment:
  None
Sample volume: 5 µl (+ 250 µl diluent)
Number of tests: 96
Controls - standards run in assay:
  Controls: Neg (3), Pos (2)
Incubation:
  30 min (RT) + 30 min (RT) + 30 min (RT)
Washes: 2

CONTENTS

Antibodies, antigens, labelled components:
  HTLV-I and HTLV-II syn peptides bound to well
  Anti-human IgG Ab (g) HRP conjugated
Substrate: TMB
Controls - standards supplied:
  Controls: Neg and Pos
Additional reagents:
  None
Special equipment required:
  None

INTERPRETATION

Comments on interpretation:
  Positive: ≥ cut-off repeatably and confirmed by
    supplemental tests
  Use BIO-STAT SELECT - HTLV® KIT to differentiate
    between HTLV-I and HTLV-II
No. of references: 6

NOTES

110621.0

© KLUWER ACADEMIC PUBLISHERS 1994, ISSN 1381-5067

Human T-cell lymphotropic virus
ANTIBODY DETECTION (IgG)

Manufacturer: IFCI Clone Systems
Cat. No./Trade name: 07.1020/ElAgen HTLV-I and HTLV-II COMB Kit

SUMMARY

$[Well-Ag]-Ab-[AHIgG-HRP]-[TMB]-A_{450}$

Assay type: EIA (non-competitive)
Detection: Colorimetric A_{450}
Format: Microtitre well, Ag coated
Sample type: Serum, plasma (do not heat inactivate)
Sample pre-treatment:
    None
Sample volume: 5 µl (+250 µl diluent)
Number of tests: 192
Controls - standards run in assay:
    Controls: Neg (3), Pos (2)
Incubation:
    30 min (RT) + 30 min (RT) + 30 min (RT)
Washes: 2

CONTENTS

Antibodies, antigens, labelled components:
    syn peptides HTLV-I and HTLV-II bound to well
    Anti-human IgG Ab (g) HRP conjugated
Substrate: TMB, H_2O_2
Controls - standards supplied:
    Controls: Neg and Pos (human serum)
Additional reagents:
    None
Special equipment required:
    None

INTERPRETATION

Comments on interpretation:
    Positive: ≥ cut-off repeatably and confirmed by
    supplemental tests (e.g. Western Blot)
No. of references: 6

NOTES

110065.0

Human T-cell lymphotropic virus
ANTIBODY DETECTION (IgG)

Manufacturer: Murex Diagnostics Limited
Cat. No./Trade name: VK80/81/MUREX anti-HTLV I/II

SUMMARY

$[Well-Ag]-Ab-[AHIgG-AP]-[PNP]-A_{410}$

Assay type: EIA (non-competitive)
Detection: Colorimetric A_{410}
Format: Microtitre well, Ag coated
Sample type: Serum, plasma
Sample pre-treatment:
    None
Sample volume: 20 µl (+ 200 µl diluent)
Number of tests: 96, 480
Controls - standards run in assay:
    Controls: Neg (2), HTLV-1 Pos (3), HTLV-2 Pos (1)
Incubation:
    1 hr (37°C) + 30 min (37°C) + 30 min (37°C)
Washes: 2

CONTENTS

Antibodies, antigens, labelled components:
    HTLV-I Ag and rec env protein bound to well
    Anti-human IgG Ab (g) AP conjugated
Substrate: PNP
Controls - standards supplied:
    Controls: Neg, Pos (anti-HTLV-1), Pos (anti-HTLV-2)
    (human serum)
Additional reagents:
    H_2SO_4
Special equipment required:
    Wellcozyme microwell plate washing system (optional)
    Wellcozyme microwell plate reader system (optional)

INTERPRETATION

Comments on interpretation:
    Positive: ≥ cut-off repeatably
No. of references: 14

NOTES

110812.0

© KLUWER ACADEMIC PUBLISHERS 1994, ISSN 1381-5067

Human T-cell lymphotropic virus
ANTIBODY DETECTION (IgG)

Manufacturer: Roche Diagnostic Systems
Cat. No./Trade name: 07 3615 5/COBAS CORE Anti-HTLV-I/II EIA

SUMMARY

[Bead-Ag]–**Ab**–[AHIgG-HRP]–[TMB]–A$_{450}$

Assay type: EIA (non-competitive)
Detection: Colorimetric A$_{450}$
Format: Tube, Ag coated bead
Sample type: Serum or plasma (do not heat inactivate)
Sample pre-treatment:
   None
Sample volume: 25 µl (+250 µl diluent)
Number of tests: 100
Controls - standards run in assay:
   Controls: Neg (1), Pos (3)
Incubation:
   20 min (37°C) + 20 min (37°C) + 15 min (37°C) all with
      shaking
Washes: 2

CONTENTS

Antibodies, antigens, labelled components:
   rec HTLV-I env bound to beads
   Anti-human IgG (g) HRP conjugated
Substrate: TMB, H$_2$O$_2$
Controls - standards supplied:
   Controls: Neg and Pos (human serum)
Additional reagents:
   Substrate (supplied as separate kit)
Special equipment required:
   Cobas® EIA shaking incubator, tube washer and
      photometer (optional)
   Cobas® Core automated analyser (optional)

INTERPRETATION

Comments on interpretation:
   Positive: ≥ cut-off; repeatably and confirmed by
      supplemental tests
No. of references: 16

NOTES

110409.0

Human T-cell lymphotropic virus (HTLV-I)
ANTIBODY DETECTION

Manufacturer: Genetic Systems Corporation/Sanofi Diagnostics Pasteur
Cat. No./Trade name: 0240-02/GENETIC SYSTEMS® HTLV-I EIA

SUMMARY

[Well-Ag]–**Ab**–[AHIgG/IgM-HRP]–[TMP]–A$_{450}$

Assay type: EIA (non-competitive)
Detection: Colorimetric A$_{450}$
Format: Microtitre well, Ag coated
Sample type: Serum, plasma
Sample pre-treatment:
   None
Sample volume: 5 µl (+500 µl diluent)
Number of tests: 192, 960, 4800
Controls - standards run in assay:
   Controls: Neg (3), Pos (2)
Incubation:
   1 hr (37°C) + 1 hr (37°C) + 30 min (RT)
Washes: 2

CONTENTS

Antibodies, antigens, labelled components:
   HTLV-I Ag bound to well
   Anti-human IgM and IgG Ab (g) HRP conjugated
Substrate: TMB, H$_2$O$_2$
Controls - standards supplied:
   Controls: Neg and Pos (human serum)
Additional reagents:
   None
Special equipment required:
   None

INTERPRETATION

Comments on interpretation:
   Positive: ≥ cut-off repeatably and confirmed by more
      specific supplemental test (e.g. Western Blot,
      radioimmunoprecipitation assay)
   When supplemental tests indeterminate; test further
      sample 3-6 months later
No. of references: 25

NOTES

110082.0

© KLUWER ACADEMIC PUBLISHERS 1994, ISSN 1381-5067

Human T-cell lymphotropic virus (HTLV-I)
ANTIBODY DETECTION

Manufacturer: Organon Teknika NV
Cat. No./Trade name: 72820/Vironostika® HTLV-I Micro elisa system

SUMMARY

[Well-Ag]–**Ab**–[AHIg-HRP]–[OPD]–A_{490}

Assay type: EIA (non-competitive)
Detection: Colorimetric A_{490}
Format: Microtitre well, Ag coated
Sample type: Serum, plasma
Sample pre-treatment:
   None
Sample volume: 20 µl (+80 µl diluent)
Number of tests: 192, 576
Controls - standards run in assay:
   Controls: Neg (3), Pos (1)
Incubation:
   30 min (37°C) + 30 min (37°C) + 30 min (RT)
Washes: 2

CONTENTS

Antibodies, antigens, labelled components:
   HTLV-I Ag bound to well
   Anti-human Ig Ab (g) HRP conjugated
Substrate: OPD, H_2O_2
Controls - standards supplied:
   Controls: Neg and Pos (human serum)
Additional reagents:
   None
Special equipment required:
   None

INTERPRETATION

Comments on interpretation:
   Positive: ≥cut-off repeatably and confirmed by
      supplemental test (e.g. Western Blot or RIA)
No. of references: 13

NOTES

110546.0

Human T-cell lymphotropic virus (HTLV-I)
ANTIBODY DETECTION (IgG)

Manufacturer: Cambridge Biotech Corporation
Cat. No./Trade name: 8051/HTLV-I (p21 enhanced) WESTERN BLOT KIT

SUMMARY

[Strip-Ag]–**Ab**–[AHIgG-biotin]–[avidin-HRP]–[substrate]–
visible bands

Assay type: Immunoblot assay
Detection: Visual
Format: Tray, Ag coated nitrocellulose strip
Sample type: Serum, plasma
Sample pre-treatment:
   None
Sample volume: 20 µl of 1:100 dilution
Number of tests: 27
Controls - standards run in assay:
   Controls: Neg (1), Pos (1)
Incubation:
   5 min (RT) + overnight (RT) + 1 hr (RT) + 1 hr (RT) +
      3-10 min (RT)
Washes: 5

CONTENTS

Antibodies, antigens, labelled components:
   rec and viral HTLV-1 proteins transblotted in bands on
      nitrocellulose strips
   Anti-human IgG Ab (g) biotinylated
   Avidin HRP conjugated
Substrate: 4-chloro-1-naphthol, H_2O_2
Controls - standards supplied:
   Controls: Neg, HTLV-I Pos and HTLV-II Pos (human
      serum)
Additional reagents:
   None
Special equipment required:
   None

INTERPRETATION

Comments on interpretation:
   Negative: no significant visible bands
   Positive: visible bands at p24, gp46 or p21
   Intermediate: band pattern does not meet criteria for a
      Pos or Neg result
No. of references: 3

NOTES

110652.0

For research use only

© KLUWER ACADEMIC PUBLISHERS 1994, ISSN 1381-5067

Human T-cell lymphotropic virus (HTLV-I)
ANTIBODY DETECTION

Manufacturer: Fujirebio
Cat. No./Trade name: /SERODIA® HTLV-I

SUMMARY

[Particle-Ag]–**Ab**–Agglutination

Assay type: Particle agglutination assay
Detection: Visual
Format: Microtitre well, Ag coated particles
Sample type: Serum, plasma
Sample pre-treatment:
  Sample absorption if unsensitized cells show (+) agglutination
Sample volume: 25 µl (+25 µl diluent)*
Number of tests: 100, 220, 550
Controls - standards run in assay:
  Controls: Pos (1)
Incubation:
  2 hours (RT)
Washes: 0

CONTENTS

Antibodies, antigens, labelled components:
  HTLV-I Ag bound to gelatin particles
Substrate:
Controls - standards supplied:
  Controls: Pos (rabbit serum, titre 1:64)
  Control unsensitized gelatin particles
Additional reagents:
  None
Special equipment required:
  None

INTERPRETATION

Comments on Interpretation:
  Negative: (-)agglutination at serum dilution 1:16
    (±)agglutination regarded as neg but should be further titrated for accurate interpretation
  Positive: (+)agglutination at serum dilution 1:16 and showing (-)agglutination with control cells at serum dilution 1:8
No. of references: 0

NOTES

110202.0

This is a screening test
*Further dilutions are performed in the tray to give a 1:16 final serum dilution
Control particles tested at 1:8 final serum dilution

Human T-cell lymphotropic virus (HTLV-I and HTLV-II)
ANTIBODY DETECTION (IgG)

Manufacturer: Bio-Stat Diagnostics
Cat. No./Trade name: 851396/ElAgen SELECT® - HTLV

SUMMARY

[Well-Ag]–**Ab**–[AHIgG-HRP]–[TMB]–A$_{450}$

Assay type: EIA (non-competitive)
Detection: Colorimetric A$_{450}$
Format: Microtitre well, Ag coated
Sample type: Serum, plasma (do not heat inactivate)
Sample pre-treatment:
  None
Sample volume: 5 µl (+250 µl diluent)*
Number of tests: 192
Controls - standards run in assay:
  Controls: Neg (2), HTLV-I Pos (1), HTLV-II Pos (1)
Incubation:
  30 min (RT) + 30 min (RT) + 30 min (RT)
Washes: 2

CONTENTS

Antibodies, antigens, labelled components:
  HTLV-I syn peptide bound to well
  HTLV-II syn peptide bound to well
  Anti-human IgG Ab (g) HRP conjugated
Substrate: TMB
Controls - standards supplied:
  Controls: Neg, HTLV-I Pos, HTLV-II Pos
Additional reagents:
  None
Special equipment required:
  None

INTERPRETATION

Comments on Interpretation:
  Positive HTLV-I: > cut-off for HTLV-1 and < cut-off for HTLV-II
  Positive HTLV-II: > cut-off for HTLV-II and < cut-off for HTLV-I
  If absorbance > cut-off for both HTLV-I and HTLV-II calculate binding ration (BR) then:
  Positive HTLV-I: BR ⩽0.5
  Positive HTLV-II: BR ⩾2
  Positive HTLV-I and HTLV-II: BR <2 and >0.5
  Confirm all positives with supplemental tests
No. of references: None

NOTES

110622.0

*Assay is run in duplicate with HTLV-I and HTLV-II coated wells

Human T-cell lymphotropic virus (HTLV-I and HTLV-II)
ANTIBODY DETECTION (IgG)

Manufacturer: IFCI Clone Systems
Cat. No./Trade name: 07.1021/ElAgen HTLV-I and HTLV-II DIFF Kit

SUMMARY

[Well-Ag]–**Ab**–[AHIgG-HRP]–[TMB]–A_{450}

Assay type: EIA (non-competitive)
Detection: Colorimetric A_{450}
Format: Microtitre well, Ag coated
Sample type: Serum, plasma (do not heat inactivate)
Sample pre-treatment:
   None
Sample volume: 5 µl (+250 µl diluent)*
Number of tests: 192
Controls - standards run in assay:
   Controls: Neg (3), Pos HTLV-I (1), Pos HTLV-II (1)*
Incubation:
   30 min (RT) + 30 min (RT) + 30 min (RT)
Washes: 2

CONTENTS

Antibodies, antigens, labelled components:
   HTLV-I (syn peptide) bound to well
   HTLV-II (syn peptide) bound to well
   Anti-human IgG Ab (g) HRP conjugated
Substrate: TMB, H_2O_2
Controls - standards supplied:
   Controls: Neg, HTLV-I Pos, HTLV-II Pos (human serum)
Additional reagents:
   None
Special equipment required:
   None

INTERPRETATION

Comments on interpretation:
   Classification of samples is according to cut-off for anti-HTLV-I antibody or anti-HTLV-II antibody
   Typing of samples reactive for both antibodies is determined by the binding ratio (BR)
   Samples with BR within <2 and >0.5 are untypable
   Confirm repeatably reactive samples with supplemental tests
No. of references: 6

NOTES

110064.0

*Samples and controls both assayed in duplicate in separate HTLV-I and HTLV-II coated microtitre wells

© KLUWER ACADEMIC PUBLISHERS 1994, ISSN 1381-5067

Neisseria gonorrhoeae (Gonorrhoea)

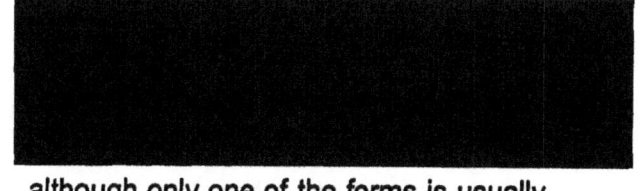

Natural history

Gonorrhoea is an infection of the mucosal surfaces of the genitourinary tract and is mainly transmitted by sexual intercourse. In men an acute purulent urethritis usually develops after an incubation period of about 3–5 days. In women a precise incubation period is difficult to determine as approximately 70% or more of infections may cause no symptoms. Although the urethra is invariably involved in hetero-sexual men, in homosexually acquired infection the urethra is involved in only around 50% of cases with the rectum and throat also infected in 25–50%: the throat is involved in around 10–15% of heterosexual cases. In women the cervix is infected in 85–90% of cases and the rectum in 25–50%. In about 10% of untreated cases, infection spreads to the endometrium and fallopian tubes giving rise to pelvic inflammatory disease. In less than 1% of untreated cases systemic spread gives rise to disseminated gonococcal infection charac-terised clinically by arthritis with or without skin lesions. Gonococcal conjunctivitis of the new-born is now rare in developed countries.

Diagnosis and markers

Antibody detection tests are unreliable in the diagnosis of gonorrhoea. This is due to a combination of factors including: marked antigenic heterogeneity between different strains of gonococci; cross-reactivity between certain gonococcal and meningococcal anti-gens, the mucosal nature of gonococcal infection; and the high rate of pharyngeal colonisation with meningococci. A presumptive diagnosis of gonorrhoea can be made in over 90% of men and about 50% of women by finding Gram-negative diplococci within poly-morphonuclear leucocytes on a Gram stained smear of genital secretions. Culture on selective media followed by screening for oxidase-positive Gram-negative diplococci which are then confirmed as gonococci by biochemical and/or immunological tests re-mains the mainstay of diagnosis and is essential for sites other than the urethra or cervix. The immunological tests used in confirmation utilise monoclonal antibodies reactive with epitopes on protein I (Pr I), the major gonococcal outer membrane protein. Protein I is present in two forms, PrIA and PrIB,

although only one of the forms is usually present on a given gonococcal strain. In order to detect the wide spectrum of antigenic types of gonococci (over 20 PrIA and over 30 PrIB serovariants) the best results are obtained when separate pools of PrIA and PrIB reagents are used. Because of the fastidious nature of *N. gonorrhoeae* there are problems in transporting specimens to the laboratory. These factors make non-cultural tests an attractive alternative. Unfortunately the mono-clonal antibody tests used in culture confirma-tion are not sufficiently sensitive to detect the small numbers of organisms (approx. 100/ml) that may be found in infected secretions. Currently direct antigen detection tests to detect gonococci in patient exudates tend to utilise polyclonal antibodies and are subject to cross-reactions which limit their utility, particu-larly in low prevalence populations. Recently, tests based on nucleic acid hybridisation and the polymerase chain reaction (PCR) have been introduced for the detection of gonococci in patient exudates.

Comment

In assessing the utility of methods for identifying gonococci it is important to be aware of the spectrum of neisserial colonisation at a given site. Because meningococci are gener-ally found much more frequently in the pharynx that at ano-genital sites, a low level of cross-reactivity can considerably reduce the positive predictive value when testing pharyngeal specimens. The same problem occurs to a less extent in male rectal specimens where meningococci also comprise a significant proportion of the Gram-negative cocci isolated on selective media. Whenever direct antigen detection tests are used it is important to confirm positive reactions by optimum culture procedures in order that antibiotic susceptibility testing can be performed.

References

Britigan BE, Cohen MS, Sparling PF. Gono-coccal infection: a model of molecular patho-genesis. New England Journal of Medicine. 1985;312:1683–1694.

Ison CA. Laboratory methods in genitourinary medicine. Methods of diagnosing gonorrhoea. Genitourinary Medicine. 1990;66:453–459.

Neisseria gonorrhoeae
ANTIGEN DETECTION

Manufacturer: Abbott Laboratories
Cat. No./Trade name: 6502/GONOZYME®
DIAGNOSTIC KIT

SUMMARY

[Bead-Gonozyme]–**Ag**–[Ab]–[ARIgG-HRP]–[OPD]–A_{492}

Assay type: EIA (non-competitive)
Detection: Colorimetric A_{492}
Format: Reaction well, GONOZYME® coated bead
Sample type: Swabs: urethral (male), endocervical*
Sample pre-treatment:
  Swab + 1 ml diluent (2 min), vortex
Sample volume: 200 µl of treated sample
Number of tests: 100
Controls - standards run in assay:
  Controls: Neg (3), Pos (1)
Incubation:
  45 min (37°C) + 45 min (37°C) + 45 min (37°C) + 30
    min (RT)
Washes: 3

CONTENTS

Antibodies, antigens, labelled components:
  GONOZYME® bound to bead
  Anti-N. gonorrhoeae Ab (r)
  Anti-rabbit IgG Ab (g) HRP conjugated
Substrate: OPD, H_2O_2
Controls - standards supplied:
  Controls: Neg and Pos
Additional reagents:
  H_2SO_2
Special equipment required:
  None

INTERPRETATION

Comments on interpretation:
  Males: Positive: ⩾cut-off
  Females: Positive: ⩾cut-off and confirmed by
    supplemental test (e.g. culture, sugar fermentation,
    etc.)
No. of references: 18

NOTES

110303.0

*Use only STD-EZE (female), STD-PEN (male) swabs
  provided

Neisseria gonorrhoeae
ANTIGEN DETECTION

Manufacturer: Syva Company
Cat. No./Trade name: 8H559/MicroTrak® Neisseria
gonorrhoeae culture confirmation test

SUMMARY

[Slide]–**Ag**–[MAb-FITC]–fluorescence

Assay type: Immunofluorescence assay (direct)
Detection: Fluorescence microscopy
Format: Slide well, specimen coated
Sample type: Plate-cultured colonies
Sample pre-treatment:
  Heat fix air-dried smear
Sample volume:
Number of tests: 85
Controls - standards run in assay:
  Controls: Neg (1), Pos (1)
Incubation:
  15 min (37°C)
Washes: 1

CONTENTS

Antibodies, antigens, labelled components:
  Anti-N. gonorrhoeae MAbs (m) FITC conjugated
Substrate:
Controls - standards supplied:
  None
Additional reagents:
  Pos and Neg microscope slide well controls
Special equipment required:
  None

INTERPRETATION

Comments on interpretation:
  Positive: fluorescent staining of intact diplococci
No. of references: 10

NOTES

110522.0

Neisseria gonorrhoeae
ANTIGEN DETECTION

Manufacturer: Becton Dickinson
Cat. No./Trade name: 4344000/GonoGen®

SUMMARY

[Staph-MAb]–**Ag**–agglutination

Assay type: Particle agglutination assay (coagglutination)
Detection: Visual
Format: Ab coated staphylococci (test done on slide)
Sample type: Colony from a clinical sample grown on selective enriched medium
Sample pre-treatment:
    Colony sample resuspended in distilled water, heated (100°C, 10 min), and vortexed
Sample volume: 1 drop x 2*
Number of tests: 50, 125
Controls - standards run in assay:
    Controls: Pos (1), Neg (1)
Incubation:
    2 min (RT)
Washes: None

CONTENTS

Antibodies, antigens, labelled components:
    Anti-N. gonorrhoeae protein I Ags MAbs (m) bound to staphylococcal cells
    Normal rabbit IgG bound to staphylococcal cells (control cells)
Substrate:
Controls - standards supplied:
    Controls: Positive and negative
Additional reagents:
    None
Special equipment required:
    None

INTERPRETATION

Comments on interpretation:
    Positive: agglutination of Ab coated staphylococcal cells within 2 minutes
No. of references: 8

NOTES

110366.0

*Sample tested in parallel on Ab coated and control staphylococcal cells

Neisseria gonorrhoeae
ANTIGEN DETECTION

Manufacturer: Boule Diagnostics AB
Cat. No./Trade name: 10-6461-12/Phadebact®
Monoclonal GC OMNI Test

SUMMARY

[Staph-MAb]–**Ag**–coagglutination

Assay type: Particle agglutination assay (coagglutination)
Detection: Visual
Format: Ab coated staphylococci (test done on slide)
Sample type: Colony from primary plate culture (incubated at 37°C for 16-24 hr)*
Sample pre-treatment:
    Suspend colonies in saline, heat for at least 5 min (100°C), cool
Sample volume: 1 drop of prepared suspension x 2**
Number of tests: 50
Controls - standards run in assay:
    Controls: Neg (1), Pos as required
Incubation:
    Results read within 1 min of mixing reagents and sample
Washes:

CONTENTS

Antibodies, antigens, labelled components:
    Anti-N gonorrhoeae (proteins IA and IB) MAb (m) bound to staphylococci (OMNI REAGENT)
    Non-immunised rabbit Ig Ab bound to staphylococci (Neg control reagent)
Substrate:
Controls - standards supplied:
    Controls: Neg (Neg control reagent)
Additional reagents:
    Phadebact® GC Positive Control Kit bought separately for quality control
Special equipment required:
    Disposable slides

INTERPRETATION

Comments on interpretation:
    Positive: coagglutination of test sample with OMNI reagent and no agglutination with Neg control reagent
No. of references: 8

NOTES

110564.0

*Clinical samples are from any part of the body where viable organisms are present, in transport medium and inoculated onto plate culture
**Sample tested in parallel will gonococcal OMNI reagent and Neg control reagent

Neisseria gonorrhoeae
ANTIGEN DETECTION

Manufacturer: Boule Diagnostics AB
Cat. No./Trade name: /Phadebact® Monoclonal GC Test

SUMMARY

[Staph-MAb]–Ag–coagglutination

Assay type: Particle agglutination assay
(coagglutination)
Detection: Visual
Format: Ab coated staphylococci (test done on slide)
Sample type: Colony from primary plate culture (incubated at 37°C for 16-24 hr)*
Sample pre-treatment:
Suspend colonies in saline, boil 5 min, cool
Sample volume: 1 drop x 2**
Number of tests: 50
Controls - standards run in assay:
Controls: Pos as required
Incubation:
Result read within 1 min of mixing reagents and sample
Washes: 0

CONTENTS

Antibodies, antigens, labelled components:
Anti-N. gonorrhoeae (protein IA) MAbs (m) bound to staphylococci (WI Gonococcal reagent)
Anti-N. gonorrhoeae (protein IB) MAb (m) bound to staphylococci (WII/III Gonococcal reagent)
Substrate:
Controls - standards supplied:
None
Additional reagents:
Phadebact® GC Positive Controls bought separately for quality control purposes
Special equipment required:
Disposable slide

INTERPRETATION

Comments on interpretation:
Negative: no agglutination with WI or WII/III reagents
Positive: agglutination with either WI or WII/III reagents indicates appropriate serogroup
Agglutination with both reagents due to the presence of both serogroups is rare
No. of references: 8

NOTES

110584.0

*Clinical specimens are from any part of the body where viable organisms are present, in transport medium and innoculated onto plate culture
**Sample tested simultaneously with WI reagent and WII/III reagent on slide

Neisseria gonorrhoeae
ANTIGEN DETECTION

Manufacturer: Meridian Diagnostics Inc
Cat. No./Trade name: 202050/MERITEC® GC

SUMMARY

[Staph-MAb]–Ag–coagglutination

Assay type: Particle agglutination assay
(coagglutination)
Detection: Visual
Format: Ab coated staphylococci (test done on card)
Sample type: N. gonorrhoeae culture (≤48 hrs old preferred)
Sample pre-treatment:
Suspend colonies in 0.5 ml purified water; heat 10 min (100°C); cool; vortex
Sample volume: 1 drop of test suspension x 2
Number of tests: 50
Controls - standards run in assay:
Controls: Neg (1), Pos (1)*
Incubation:
0
Washes: 0

CONTENTS

Antibodies, antigens, labelled components:
Anti-N. gonorrhoeae (protein I serotypes) MAbs adsorbed to staphylococci
Substrate:
Controls - standards supplied:
Controls: Neg (non-human immunoglobulin, adsorbed to staphylococci), Pos (N. gonorrhoeae, various serotypes)
Additional reagents:
None
Special equipment required:
None

INTERPRETATION

Comments on interpretation:
Indeterminant: similar agglutination with test and Staphylococcus control reagent; retest with larger innoculum
Repeatably indeterminant; retest using alternative procedure
Positive: stronger agglutination with test then Staphylococcus control reagent
No. of references: 11

NOTES

110153.0

*Neg control run with each test suspension
Pos control run once per day

© KLUWER ACADEMIC PUBLISHERS 1994, ISSN 1381-5067

Neisseria gonorrhoeae
ANTIBODY DETECTION

Manufacturer: Alfa Biotech
Cat. No./Trade name: 05770322/GONORRHOEA
Agglutinotest® TETRAKIT

SUMMARY

[Particle-Ag]–**Ab**–agglutination

Assay type: Particle agglutination assay
Detection: Visual
Format: Slide, latex particles Ag coated
Sample type: Serum
Sample pre-treatment:
Heat sera for 30 min at 56°C in a waterbath before testing.
Sample volume: 1 drop*
Number of tests: 50
Controls - standards run in assay:
Controls: Neg (1), Pos (1)
Incubation:
Read results 5 min after mixing sample and latex Ag reagent
Washes: 0

CONTENTS

Antibodies, antigens, labelled components:
N. gonorrhoeae Ag bound to latex particles
Substrate:
Controls - standards supplied:
Controls: Neg and Pos (serum)
False positive control (absorbant solution of N. sicca and G. glava extract)
Additional reagents:
None
Special equipment required:
None

INTERPRETATION

Comments on interpretation:
Positive: visible agglutination within 5 min and confirmed by visible agglutination on repeat testing using absorbent solution
Negative: no agglutination or preliminary agglutination not confirmed when test is repeated using absorbent solution
No. of references: 4

NOTES

110667.0

*Serial dilutions of test serum are used for the quantitative test

Streptococcus beta-haemolytic group B (*Streptococcus agalactiae*)

Natural history

Group B beta-haemolytic streptococci (GBS) are found in the genital and gastrointestinal tracts of approximately 25% of healthy adults. Whilst GBS rarely may cause genital tract infection and post-partum septicaemia they are a major cause of bacteraemia and other invasive infection in the newborn within the first few days of life. Dense vaginal colonization seems to make transmission more likely while prematurity and a prolonged labour after rupture of the membranes are important risk factors. Although carriage rates in pregnant women range from 10 to 30%, and the transmission rate from colonised mother to infant may be as high as 70%, invasive infections develop only in about 1% of colonised babies. The reported incidence of GBS disease ranges from 1 to 5 per 1000 live births with a fatality rate ranging from 20 to 80%. Two different types of illness, 'early onset' and 'late onset' have been described. The early onset disease, although septicaemic in type, may also be meningitic, whereas the late onset disease is almost always meningitic. Early onset disease may occur within five days of birth, but usually within the first 24–36 hours and is caused by the transmission of GBS from mother to infant either in utero or during delivery. There is a close association between early onset infection and maternal complications, particularly premature labour and a prolonged period between rupture of the membranes and delivery. Late onset disease usually presents after the tenth day of life as a purulent meningitis and is usually a result of nosocomial transmission. The mortality rate, 15 to 20%, is lower than in early onset disease. Group A beta-haemolytic strains (*Streptococcus pyogenes*) are responsible for the majority of human infections including tonsillitis and skin infections such as impetigo. Spreading cellulitis is the classical skin involvement.

Diagnosis and markers

GBS can be detected by identifying the organisms after conventional culture or by detecting antigen from patient swabs or body fluids. Immunological tests are widely used in both approaches. Serological subdivision of the haemolytic streptococci exploits differences in the group specific polysaccharide antigens in the cell wall (Lancefield grouping). There are 20 Lancefield groups identified by sequential letters A–H and K–V. For epidemiological purposes GBS may be sub-divided into seven serotypes on the basis of four carbohydrate antigens and the presence or absence of protein antigens. Tests to detect GBS use either monoclonal or polyclonal antibody against the group B polysaccharide antigen and may or may not require a chemical or enzymatic extraction of the carbohydrate antigen from the streptococcal cell. When the clinical situation suggests GBS infection these tests can be used on vaginal swabs and on a variety of body fluids (e.g. urine, serum, CSF) to detect or exclude GBS. When testing cultured beta-haemolytic streptococci it is normal to test the organisms against a range of individual reagents each containing specific antibody against one of the main Lancefield group antigens (e.g. A, B, C, D, F, G).

Comments

Conventional culture and identification usually takes between 24 and 48 hours and is therefore most useful in screening and in confirming positive antigen detection results. Direct detection of antigen is best suited to the identification of GBS carriers early in labour, or to identify GBS infection in neonates when the clinical situation raises the possibility of such infection. Criteria for screening and selection for intrapartum chemoprophylaxis vary considerably.

References

Editorial. Prevention of early onset Group B streptococcal infection in the newborn. Lancet. 1984;i:1056–1057.

Ross PW. Ecology of Group B streptococci. In: Skinner FA, Quesnel LB (eds). Streptococci. London, Academic Press 1978.

Streptococcus beta-haemolytic group B
ANTIGEN DETECTION

Manufacturer: Binax
Cat. No./Trade name: E320.000/Equate Strep B

SUMMARY

[Tube-Ab]–**Ag**–[Ab-HRP]–[TMB]–colour

Assay type: EIA (non-competitive)
Detection: Visual
Format: Tube, Ab coated
Sample type: Swabs: (vaginal, cervical)*
Sample pre-treatment:
    None (sample extraction is incorporated into the assay)
Sample volume:
Number of tests: 20,80
Controls - standards run in assay:
    Controls: Neg (1), Pos (1)
Incubation:
    1 min (RT) + 10 min (RT) + 5 min (RT)
Washes: 1

CONTENTS

Antibodies, antigens, labelled components:
    Anti-GBS Ab (r) bound to tube
    Anti-GBS Ab (r) HRP conjugated
Substrate: TMB, H_2O_2
Controls - standards supplied:
    Controls: Pos
Additional reagents:
    None
Special equipment required:
    None

INTERPRETATION

Comments on interpretation:
    Negative: colourless
    Positive: blue colour
No. of references: 8

NOTES

110210.0

*Swabs are supplied. Certain types are unsuitable

Streptococcus beta-haemolytic group B
ANTIGEN DETECTION

Manufacturer: Hybritech
Cat. No./Trade name: 4520BE/ICON® STREP B

SUMMARY

[Membrane-Ab]–**Ag**–[Ab-AP]–[Substrate]–Purple spot

Assay type: EIA (non-competitive)
Detection: Visual
Format: Test cylinder, Ab coated filter membrane
Sample type: Vaginal and cervical swabs, infant urine, cell culture colony swab*
Sample pre-treatment:
    Extraction of swab (reagents provided), incubate 1-5 min (RT)
Sample volume: Total extracted volume
Number of tests: 24
Controls - standards run in assay:
    Integral controls: Neg (1), Pos (1), on filter
    Batch controls: Neg (1), Pos (1)
Incubation:
    2 min (RT) + 2 min (RT)
Washes: 2

CONTENTS

Antibodies, antigens, labelled components:
    Anti-GBS Ab (r) bound to filter membrane
    Anti-GBS Ab (r) AP conjugated
Substrate: Not specified
Controls - standards supplied:
    Integral controls: Neg and Pos on filter
    Batch controls: Pos (contains extracted Group B streptococcus antigen), Neg (sterile swabs)
Additional reagents:
    None
Special equipment required:
    None

INTERPRETATION

Comments on interpretation:
    Positive: Circular purple spot in the patient result zone
No. of references: 7

NOTES

110078.0

*Kit can be used as a confirmatory test for specimens cultured on blood agar plates
All specimens require special swabs provided with kit or swabs with dacron or rayon tips
Transport medium containing gelatin agar or charcoal should not be used

© *KLUWER ACADEMIC PUBLISHERS 1994, ISSN 1381-5067*

Streptococcus beta-haemolytic group B
ANTIGEN DETECTION

Manufacturer: VEDA-LAB
Cat. No./Trade name: /STREP-B-CHECK-1

SUMMARY

[Membrane-Ab]–**Ag**–[MAb-gold]–pink line

Assay type: Immunochromatographic assay
Detection: Visual
Format: Test slide unit, Ab coated membrane
Sample type: Vaginal swabs*
Sample pre-treatment:
    Extraction of swabs with reagents provided, incubate 2-5 min (RT)
Sample volume: 200 µl
Number of tests: 20
Controls - standards run in assay:
    Controls: Integral reagent control (1)
Incubation:
    Result read 5-10 min after addition of patient sample to slide unit
Washes: NA

CONTENTS

Antibodies, antigens, labelled components:
    Anti-GBS PAb bound to membrane (test window)
    Anti-murine Ig Ab (g) bound to membrane (reagent control window)
    Anti-GBS MAb colloidal gold labelled (in absorbent pad)
Substrate:
Controls - standards supplied:
    Integral reagent control bound to membrane
Additional reagents:
    None
Special equipment required:
    None

INTERPRETATION

Comments on interpretation:
    Negative: pink line in control window, no line in test window
    Inconclusive: no line in control window; repeat with fresh unit using same or fresh sample
    Positive: pink line in control window and test window
No. of references: 5

NOTES

110360.0

*Special swabs and transport tubes provided with kit

Streptococcus beta-haemolytic group B
ANTIGEN DETECTION

Manufacturer: Becton Dickinson
Cat. No./Trade name: 352/Directigen® Group B Strep

SUMMARY

[Latex-MAb]–**Ag**–agglutination

Assay type: Particle agglutination assay
Detection: Visual
Format: Ab coated latex (test done on slide)
Sample type: Serum, urine, CSF
Sample pre-treatment:
    CSF - none
    Serum and unconcentrated urine - heat (100°C, 5 min), centrifuge and dilute 1:1
Sample volume: 50 µl pretreated sample x 2*
Number of tests: 30
Controls - standards run in assay:
    Controls: Pos (1), Neg (1) x 2*
Incubation:
    10 min (RT) with rotation
Washes: None

CONTENTS

Antibodies, antigens, labelled components:
    Anti-GBS MAb (m) bound to latex
    Murine Ig bound to latex (control latex)
Substrate:
Controls - standards supplied:
    Controls: Pos and Neg Ag controls
Additional reagents:
    None
Special equipment required:
    None

INTERPRETATION

Comments on interpretation:
    Positive: agglutination only in the anti-GBS coated latex suspension
No. of references: 4

NOTES

110365.0

*Ab-coated and control latex run in parallel

Streptococcus beta-haemolytic group B
ANTIGEN DETECTION

Manufacturer: Boule Diagnostics AB
Cat. No./Trade name: /Phadebact® Strep B Test

SUMMARY

[Staph-Ab]–**Ag**–coagglutination

Assay type: Particle agglutination assay (coagglutination)
Detection: Visual
Format: Ab coated staphylococci (test done on slide)
Sample type: GBS colony from primary plate culture or from broth culture*
Sample pre-treatment:
None
Sample volume: 1-5 colonies x 2**
Number of tests: 100
Controls - standards run in assay:
Controls: Neg (1), Pos as required
Incubation:
Result read within 1 min of mixing reagents and sample
Washes: 0

CONTENTS

Antibodies, antigens, labelled components:
Anti-GBS Ab (r) bound to staphylococci
Substrate:
Controls - standards supplied:
Controls: Phadebact® Neg control reagent
Additional reagents:
Phadebact® Strep Positive controls (separate vials from groups A, B, C, D, F and G)
Special equipment required:
Disposable slides

INTERPRETATION

Comments on interpretation:
Positive: coagglutination of test sample with anti-GBS reagent and no agglutination with Neg control reagent
No. of references: 18

NOTES

110566.0

*Clinical specimens are from any part of the body where viable organs are present, in transport medium and innoculated into broth
**Sample tested in parallel with anti-GBS reagent and Neg control reagent

Streptococcus beta-haemolytic group B
ANTIGEN DETECTION

Manufacturer: Dako A/S
Cat. No./Trade name: K019/DAKO Group B Streptococcus Serotyping Test

SUMMARY

[Strep-Ab]–**Ag**–agglutination

Assay type: Particle agglutination assay (coagglutination)
Detection: Visual
Format: Ab coated GBS (test done on plate)*
Sample type: GBS overnight plate culture
Sample pre-treatment:
None
Sample volume: Several colonies (2-3 μl) x 6*
Number of tests: 30
Controls - standards run in assay:
Controls: Pos (1)
Incubation:
None
Washes: 0

CONTENTS

Antibodies, antigens, labelled components:
Anti-GBS Ab (r) to types Ia, Ib, II, III, IV, V bound to inactivated group G streptococci (6 separate reagents)
Substrate:
Controls - standards supplied:
Controls: Pos (group B streptococci, type III)
Additional reagents:
None
Special equipment required:
None

INTERPRETATION

Comments on interpretation:
Positive: visible agglutination within 2 mins with 1 of the 6 reagents indicating serotype
No. of references: 1

NOTES

110045.0

*Test consists of 6 samples per patient applied to 6 numbered rings on test plate, performed with 6 separate (GBS-Ab) reagents containing 1 of the 6 serotypes

© *KLUWER ACADEMIC PUBLISHERS 1994, ISSN 1381-5067*

Streptococcus beta-haemolytic group B
ANTIGEN DETECTION

Manufacturer: Meridian Diagnostics Inc
Cat. No./Trade name: 200360/MERITEC-Strep

SUMMARY

[Staph-Ab]–**Ag**–coagglutination

Assay type: Particle agglutination assay (coagglutination)
Detection: Visual
Format: Ab coated staphylococci (test done on slide)
Sample type: GBS culture (primary plate colony) or 4 hr or 18-24 hr broth subcultures
Sample pre-treatment:
   None
Sample volume: 1 colony or 1 drop of broth culture x 2*
Number of tests: 60
Controls - standards run in assay:
   Controls: Pos (1)**, Neg (1)
Incubation:
   3 minutes
Washes: 0

CONTENTS

Antibodies, antigens, labelled components:
   Anti-GBS PAb (r) bound to staphylococci
   Non-human Ig bound to staphylococci (non-immune CoA reagent)
Substrate:
Controls - standards supplied:
   Controls: Pos
Additional reagents:
   None
Special equipment required:
   None

INTERPRETATION

Comments on interpretation:
   Positive: (+) agglutination
No. of references: 20

NOTES

110154.0

*Parallel test run with non-immune Co-A reagents
**Pos control tested once every day

Streptococcus beta-haemolytic group B
ANTIGEN DETECTION

Manufacturer: Murex Diagnostics Limited
Cat. No./Trade name: ZL20/Wellcogen Strep B

SUMMARY

[Latex-Ab]–**Ag**–agglutination

Assay type: Particle agglutination assay
Detection: Visual
Format: Ab coated latex (test done on reaction card)
Sample type: Body fluids, blood culture
Sample pre-treatment:
   CSF and urine: heat (5 min)
   Serum: Add EDTA and heat (5 min)
   Blood culture: Centrifuge, test supernatant
Sample volume: 40 µl (one drop) x 2*
Number of tests: 30
Controls - standards run in assay:
   Controls: Control latex (1), Pos (1)**
Incubation:
   Read result within 3 min of mixing reagents
Washes:

CONTENTS

Antibodies, antigens, labelled components:
   Anti-GBS Ab (r) bound to latex particles
Substrate:
Controls - standards supplied:
   Controls: Pos (polyvalent Ag); Control latex particles (coated with non-immune rabbit globulins)
Additional reagents:
   None
Special equipment required:
   None

INTERPRETATION

Comments on interpretation:
   Positive: agglutination within 3 min
   Non-interpretable result: agglutination of control latex; retest after clarifying the sample
No. of references: 8

NOTES

110174.0

*Samples tested in parallel with test and control latex particle reagents
**Positive control is used from time to time to check performance

---

Streptococcus beta-haemolytic group B
ANTIGEN DETECTION

Manufacturer: Omega Diagnostics Ltd
Cat. No./Trade name: OD014-L/AVISTREP

SUMMARY

[Latex-Ab]–**Ag**–agglutination

Assay type: Particle agglutination assay
Detection: Visual
Format: Ab coated latex (test done on card)
Sample type: Streptococcal culture (primary plate or pure subculture on solid or liquid media)
Sample pre-treatment:
   Plate: add colonies to extraction enzyme
   Liquid: add 0.1 ml to extraction enzyme
Sample volume: 1 drop
Number of tests: 50
Controls - standards run in assay:
   Controls: Pos (1)
Incubation:
   10 min (37°C)
Washes: 0

CONTENTS

Antibodies, antigens, labelled components:
   Anti-GBS Ab (r) bound to latex particles*
Substrate:
Controls - standards supplied:
   Controls: Pos (polyvalent for strep groups A, B, C, D, F, G)
Additional reagents:
   Extraction enzyme
Special equipment required:
   None

INTERPRETATION

Comments on interpretation:
   Positive: agglutination in appropriate circle on test card in 1 min
No. of references: None

NOTES

110046.0

*Kit contains latex suspensions with Abs to strep groups A, C, D, F, G in addition to group B and is designed to be performed for all groups simultaneously

Streptococcus beta-haemolytic group B
ANTIGEN DETECTION

Manufacturer: Orion Diagnostica
Cat. No./Trade name: D350/D366/STREP B
ENRICHMENT BROTH AND LATEX TEST

SUMMARY

[Latex treated]–**Ag**–agglutination

Assay type: Particle agglutination assay
Detection: Visual
Format: Treated latex (test done on card)
Sample type: Vaginal swab
Sample pre-treatment:
   Place swab in enrichment broth, incubate 5-7 hr (37°C), vortex
Sample volume: 25 µl
Number of tests: 40
Controls - standards run in assay:
   Controls: Pos (1); Stage II: control latex (1)
Incubation:
   Read results within 2 min of mixing reagents
Washes:

CONTENTS

Antibodies, antigens, labelled components:
   GBS latex reagent (treated latex particles)
Substrate:
Controls - standards supplied:
   Controls: control latex reagent, Pos
Additional reagents:
   None
Special equipment required:
   None

INTERPRETATION

Comments on interpretation:
   Stage I Negative: no agglutination in 2 min
   Stage I Positive: agglutination within 2 min; heat and retest with Strep B latex reagent and control latex reagent for stage II of assay
   Stage II Positive: agglutination within 2 min
No. of references: 9

NOTES

110097.0

Assay performed in 2 stages. Stage I screens out clear negatives and does not involve control latex reagent. Stage II confirms positives from stage I using Strep B latex reagent and control latex

© KLUWER ACADEMIC PUBLISHERS 1994, ISSN 1381-5067

Streptococcus beta-haemolytic group B
ANTIGEN DETECTION

Manufacturer: PRO-LAB Diagnostics
Cat. No./Trade name: PL050/PROLEX® Strep Kit

SUMMARY

[Latex-Ab]–**Ag**–agglutination

Assay type: Particle agglutination assay
Detection: Visual
Format: Ab coated latex (test done on card)
Sample type: Colony from culture plate (18-24 hr)
Sample pre-treatment:
Extraction using reagents provided, incubate 2 min (RT), vortex 10-15 sec
Sample volume: 1 drop (x 6: one per circle per Strep group)
Number of tests: 60
Controls - standards run in assay:
Controls: Pos (1), Pos (known specific strain) (1), Neg (1)
Incubation:
0
Washes: 0

CONTENTS

Antibodies, antigens, labelled components:
Group specific immunoglobulins (r) bound to latex particles (6 separate reagents for gps A, B, C, D, F, G)
Substrate:
Controls - standards supplied:
Controls: Pos (polyvalent extract representing Ag from Strep groups A, B, C, D, F, G). Neg (normal saline, bought separately)
Additional reagents:
Extract from known strain for additional Pos control
Special equipment required:
None

INTERPRETATION

Comments on interpretation:
Negative: no agglutination
Positive: strong agglutination with only one of the latex reagents indicates specific Strep group
No. of references: 11

NOTES

110331.0

Streptococcus beta-haemolytic group B
ANTIGEN DETECTION

Manufacturer: Shield Diagnostics
Cat. No./Trade name: FSTR110-160/Streptococcal Grouping Kit

SUMMARY

[Latex-Ab]–**Ag**–agglutination

Assay type: Particle agglutination assay
Detection: Visual
Format: Ab coated latex (test done on card)
Sample type: Colony from plate culture, or 4-18 hr broth
Sample pre-treatment:
Culture: mix 2-4 colonies with extraction enzyme
Broth: 1 drop of broth mixed with extraction enzyme; incubate 10-15 min
Sample volume: 1 drop of prepared suspension
Number of tests: 50
Controls - standards run in assay:
Controls: Pos (1)
Incubation:
1 min (RT)
Washes:

CONTENTS

Antibodies, antigens, labelled components:
Anti-GBS Ab bound to latex particle
Substrate:
Controls - standards supplied:
Controls: Pos (polyvalent with extract from all groups A-G)
Additional reagents:
None
Special equipment required:
None

INTERPRETATION

Comments on interpretation:
Negative: no agglutination
Positive for GBS; agglutination of sample extract with Group B latex reagent
No. of references: 4

NOTES

110581.0

© **KLUWER ACADEMIC PUBLISHERS 1994, ISSN 1381-5067**

Streptococcus beta-haemolytic group B
ANTIGEN DETECTION

Manufacturer: Unipath Limited
Cat. No./Trade name: /Streptococcal grouping kit

SUMMARY

[Latex-Ab]–**Ag**–agglutination

Assay type: Particle agglutination assay
Detection: Visual
Format: Ab coated latex (test done on card)
Sample type: Overnight streptococcal culture on a blood agar plate
Sample pre-treatment:
Extraction of 2-5 test colonies in enzyme reagent 10 min (37°C)
Sample volume: 1 drop
Number of tests:
Controls - standards run in assay:
Control: Pos (1)
Incubation:
Agglutination visible within 30 seconds
Washes: 0

CONTENTS

Antibodies, antigens, labelled components:
Latex particles coated with antibody to Strep. groups A, B, C, D, F and G
Substrate:
Controls - standards supplied:
Controls: Pos (polyvalent for groups A, B, C, D, F and G)
Additional reagents:
None
Special equipment required:
None

INTERPRETATION

Comments on Interpretation:
Negative: no agglutination
Positive: agglutination with one grouping within approx. 30 sec
No. of references: 7

NOTES

110211.0

Treponema pallidum sub-species pallidum (Syphilis)

Natural history

Syphilis is spread principally by sexual intercourse and is a venereal disease: it may be acquired congenitally and by blood transfusion. The incubation period is 9–90 days. The organisms penetrate mucous membranes or abraded skin where they multiply locally as well as disseminating via the lymphatic and circulatory systems. Infection is systemic from the onset and is characterised by periods of latency, often in excess of 20 years. In the early infectious stage, moist mucocutaneous lesions occur, particularly on the genitalia. If untreated the lesions tend to heal and the disease becomes 'hidden' or latent. The latent or non-infectious stage (greater than two years duration) may persist for decades without producing obvious clinical changes. A proportion of patients (30–40%) will unpredictably develop active involvement of the cardio-vascular system, the central nervous system, or localised gummatous destructive lesions.

Diagnosis and markers

T. pallidum cannot be cultured in vitro. Diagnosis depends on demonstrating *T. pallidum* in the serous exudate from the depth of early lesions and/or antibodies in the serum. Organisms in lesions are demonstrated by dark ground microscopy, immunofluorescence staining or antigen detected by EIA. Antibodies can be detected by a variety of methods using tests based on non-treponemal antigen (cardiolipin) or *T. pallidum* antigen derived from rabbit testes. Cardiolipin antigen tests may be negative in late infection and can be used to monitor efficacy of treatment. *T. pallidum* antigen tests are sensitive at all stages of infection and remain positive after treatment. During natural infection antibodies can be detected to more than 20 polypeptide antigens. There are no specific markers used in routine serological tests: a monoclonal antibody reactive with a 47–48 kD pathogen specific surface antigen is used in antigen detection. The spectrum and intensity of the antibody response increases throughout the primary and secondary stages and declines thereafter. By the time clinical symptoms are present IgG invariably accompanies IgM. Specific IgM indicates active (or recently treated) infection but may disappear in about half of cases of late and latent infection without treatment intervention. Whilst a positive IgM test substantiates the need for treatment a negative test cannot be used to exclude the need for treatment in late infection. Cloned antigen tests are a recent development; an EIA based on the 44,000 Mdal pathogen specific antigen TmpA is available commercially.

Comment

Traditionally the diagnosis of syphilis depends on dual testing. Sera are screened by cardiolipin and/or specific tests and positive reactions confirmed by another method. The FTA-ABS is the standard confirmatory test. Cardiolipin tests are insensitive in screening for latent infection. Detection of latent infection is important as treatment will prevent the occurrence of late stage disease. As syphilis may mimic a variety of dermatological, medical and surgical conditions serological testing is widespread. Screening of antenatal patients and blood donors is performed to prevent congenital and transfusion-acquired syphilis respectively. Detection of primary infection depends upon a high index of clinical suspicion; a proportion (10–15%) of cases will be seronegative.

Note

Infection with the following pathogenic treponemes produces infections that are serologically indistinguishable from syphilis: *T. pallidum* subspecies *pertenue* (yaws); *T. pallidum* 'subspecies' *endemicum* (non-venereal endemic syphilis); *T. carateum* (pinta).

References

Norris SJ (and the *Treponema pallidum* Polypeptide Research Group). Polypeptides of *Treponema pallidum*: progress toward understanding their structural, functional, and immunologic roles. Microbiological Reviews. 1993;57:750–779.

Young H. Syphilis: new diagnostic directions (editorial). International Journal of STD & AIDS. 1992;3:391–413.

Treponema pallidum
ANTIBODY DETECTION

Manufacturer: Behringwerke AG
Cat. No./Trade name: OWVO/Enzygnost® Syphilis

SUMMARY

$$[\text{Well-Ag}]\genfrac{(}{}{0pt}{}{\text{Ab}}{[\text{Ab-POD}]}\!-\![\text{TMB}]\!-\!A_{450}$$

Assay type: EIA (competitive)
Detection: Colorimetric A_{450}
Format: Microtitre well, Ag coated
Sample type: Serum, plasma
Sample pre-treatment:
    None
Sample volume: 25 µl
Number of tests: 192
Controls - standards run in assay:
    Controls: Neg (4), Pos (2)
Incubation:
    1 hr 10 min (37°C) + 30 min (RT)
Washes: 1

CONTENTS

Antibodies, antigens, labelled components:
    T. pallidum Ag bound to well
    Anti-T. pallidum (human) POD conjugated
Substrate: TMB, H_2O_2
Controls - standards supplied:
    Controls: Neg and Pos (human serum)
Additional reagents:
    None
Special equipment required:
    Behring ELISA processor (optional)

INTERPRETATION

Comments on interpretation:
    Equivocal: sample absorbance within the range (O.D.
        Neg control x 0.6) and (O.D. Neg control x 0.7); retest
        to confirm
No. of references: 12

NOTES

110459.0

Treponema pallidum
ANTIBODY DETECTION

Manufacturer: Diesse
Cat. No./Trade name: 91052/ENZYWELL SYPHILIS SCREEN

SUMMARY

$$[\text{Well-Ag}]\genfrac{(}{}{0pt}{}{\text{Ab}}{[\text{Ab-POD}]}\!-\![\text{TMB}]\!-\!A_{450}$$

Assay type: EIA (competitive)
Detection: Colorimetric A_{450}
Format: Microtitre well, Ag coated
Sample type: Serum, plasma
Sample pre-treatment:
    None
Sample volume: 30 µl
Number of tests: 192
Controls - standards run in assay:
    Calibrator: (2)
Incubation:
    1 hr 30 min (37°C) + 15 min (RT)
Washes: 1

CONTENTS

Antibodies, antigens, labelled components:
    T. pallidum Ag bound to well
    Anti-Treponema pallidum IgG Ab POD conjugated
Substrate: TMB, H_2O_2
Controls - standards supplied:
    Calibrator (bovine serum)
Additional reagents:
    None
Special equipment required:
    None

INTERPRETATION

Comments on interpretation:
    Classification of samples is according to cut-off; no
        further testing
    Semiquantitative procedure available
No. of references: 6

NOTES

110598.0

© *KLUWER ACADEMIC PUBLISHERS 1994, ISSN 1381-5067*

Treponema pallidum
ANTIBODY DETECTION

Manufacturer: Biologische Analysensystem GmbH
Cat. No./Trade name: 3645/BAG-Tp-EIA

SUMMARY

[Well-Ag]–Ab–[AHIgG/IgM-HRP]–[OPD]–A_{492}

Assay type: EIA (non-competitive)
Detection: Colorimetric A_{492}
Format: Microtitre well, Ag coated
Sample type: Serum
Sample pre-treatment:
　None
Sample volume: 5 µl (+ 1 ml diluent)
Number of tests: 96
Controls - standards run in assay:
　Controls: Neg (1), Cut-off (2), Pos (1)
Incubation:
　1 hr (RT) + 1 hr (RT) + 30 min (RT)
Washes: 2 (+ preliminary plate wash)

CONTENTS

Antibodies, antigens, labelled components:
　T. pallidum bound to well
　Anti-human IgG/IgM Ab HRP conjugated
Substrate: OPD
Controls - standards supplied:
　Controls: Neg, Pos and cut-off (human)
Additional reagents:
　None
Special equipment required:
　None

INTERPRETATION

Comments on interpretation:
　Equivocal: within cut-off ± 10%; retest or use another
　　test system
No. of references: 0

NOTES

110206.0

Treponema pallidum
ANTIBODY DETECTION

Manufacturer: Euro-Diagnostica B.V.
Cat. No./Trade name: /Recombinant DNA derived Treponema Pallidum Ig EIA

SUMMARY

[Well-Ag]–Ab–[AHIg-HRP]–[TMB]–A_{450}

Assay type: EIA (non-competitive)
Detection: Colorimetric A_{450}
Format: Microtitre well, Ag coated
Sample type: Serum, plasma (do not heat inactivate)
Sample pre-treatment:
　None
Sample volume: 5 µl (+ 100 µl diluent)
Number of tests: 96
Controls - standards run in assay:
　Controls: Neg (3), Pos (3)
Incubation:
　1 hr (37°C) + 1 hr (37°C) + 30 min (RT)
Washes: 2

CONTENTS

Antibodies, antigens, labelled components:
　rec TmpA Ag bound to wells
　Anti-human Ig Ab HRP conjugated
Substrate: TMB
Controls - standards supplied:
　Controls: Neg and Pos (human serum)
Additional reagents:
　None
Special equipment required:
　None

INTERPRETATION

Comments on interpretation:
　Equivocal: between cut-off x 1 and cut-off x 2; retest to
　　confirm
No. of references: 0

NOTES

110100.0

For research use only

Treponema pallidum
ANTIBODY DETECTION

Manufacturer: Shield Diagnostics
Cat. No./Trade name: PC009/SYPH-GM

SUMMARY

[Well-Ag]–**Ab**–[AHIgG/IgM-POD]–[TMB]–A_{450}

Assay type: EIA (non-competitive)
Detection: Colorimetric A_{450}
Format: Microtitre well, Ag coated
Sample type: Serum
Sample pre-treatment:
   None
Sample volume: 100 µl (of a 1:200 dilution)
Number of tests: 96
Controls - standards run in assay:
   Controls: Neg (1), Low Pos (2), High Pos (1)
Incubation:
   1 hr (37°C) + 30 min (37°C) + 10 min (RT)
Washes: 2

CONTENTS

Antibodies, antigens, labelled components:
   T. pallidum Ag bound to well
   Anti-human IgM and IgG Ab (g) POD conjugated
Substrate: TMB
Controls - standards supplied:
   Controls: Neg, Low Pos, High Pos (human serum)
Additional reagents:
   None
Special equipment required:
   None

INTERPRETATION

Comments on interpretation:
   Equivocal: antibody index(ratio of test: low positive
      control absorbance) between 0.9 and 1.1; retest
   Repeatably equivocal: test fresh patient sample
No. of references: 4

NOTES

110083.0

Treponema pallidum
ANTIBODY DETECTION (IgG)

Manufacturer: ADI Diagnostics
Cat. No./Trade name: /VISUWELL® REAGIN

SUMMARY

[Well-Ag]–**Ab**–[AHIgG-urease]–[substrate]–A_{620}

Assay type: EIA (non-competitive)
Detection: Colorimetric A_{620}
Format: Microtitre well, Ag coated
Sample type: Serum, plasma (do not heat inactivate)
Sample pre-treatment:
   None
Sample volume: Qualitative: 50 µl
   Quantitative 100 µl
Number of tests: 480, 960
Controls - standards run in assay:
   Controls: Neg (1), Pos (1)
Incubation:
   30 min (RT) + 20 min (RT) + 10 min (RT)*
Washes: 2

CONTENTS

Antibodies, antigens, labelled components:
   Reagin Ag bound to well
   Anti-human IgG PAb (r) urease conjugated
Substrate: Not specified
Controls - standards supplied:
   Controls: Neg and Pos (human serum)
Additional reagents:
   None
Special equipment required:
   None

INTERPRETATION

Comments on interpretation:
   Qualitative: positive ≥ cut-off repeatably
   Quantitative: the titre of the sample is the highest dilution
      where absorbance ≥ cut-off
   Visual interpretation is possible
No. of references: 3

NOTES

110614.0

*The third incubation of 10 min maximises sensitivity and an
alternative third incubation of 5 min optimises specificity
for use in blood banks/plasmapheresis centres

© KLUWER ACADEMIC PUBLISHERS 1994, ISSN 1381-5067

Treponema pallidum
ANTIBODY DETECTION (IgG)

Manufacturer: ADI Diagnostics
Cat. No./Trade name: VISUWELL® Syphilis Antibody

SUMMARY

[Well-Ag]–**Ab**–[AHIgG-POD]–[TMB]–A_{450}

Assay type: EIA (non-competitive)
Detection: Colorimetric A_{450}
Format: Microtitre well, Ag coated
Sample type: Serum (do not heat inactivate)
Sample pre-treatment:
    None
Sample volume: 100 μl
Number of tests: 192, 960
Controls - standards run in assay:
    Controls: Neg (3), Pos (2)
Incubation:
    30 min (37°C) + 30 min (37°C) + 30 min (RT)
Washes: 2

CONTENTS

Antibodies, antigens, labelled components:
    rec 47 kDA protein bound to well
    Anti-human IgG MAb (r) POD conjugated
Substrate: TMB
Controls - standards supplied:
    Controls: Neg and Pos (human serum)
Additional reagents:
    None
Special equipment required:
    None

INTERPRETATION

Comments on interpretation:
    Qualitative: positive ≥ cut-off repeatably
No. of references: 7

NOTES

110656.0

Treponema pallidum
ANTIBODY DETECTION (IgG)

Manufacturer: Centocor Inc
Cat. No./Trade name: M411/CAPTIA® Syphilis - G

SUMMARY

[Well-Ag]–**Ab**–[AHIgG-biotin + strept-HRP]–[TMB]–A_{450}

Assay type: EIA (non-competitive)
Detection: Colorimetric A_{450}
Format: Microtitre well, Ag coated
Sample type: Serum
Sample pre-treatment:
    None
Sample volume: 5 μl (+100 μl diluent)
Number of tests: 96
Controls - standards run in assay:
    Controls: Neg (1), low Pos (2), Pos (1)
Incubation:
    1 hr (37°C) + 1 hr (37°C) + 30 min (RT)
Washes: 2

CONTENTS

Antibodies, antigens, labelled components:
    T. pallidum Ag bound to well
    Anti-human IgG MAb biotinylated
    Streptavidin HRP conjugated
Substrate: TMB, H_2O_2
Controls - standards supplied:
    Controls: Neg, low Pos, high Pos (human serum)
Additional reagents:
    H_2SO_4
Special equipment required:
    None

INTERPRETATION

Comments on interpretation:
    Equivocal: within cut-off ±10%; retest to confirm
    Positive: ≥ cut-off +10% repeatably
No. of references: 3

NOTES

110085.0

© *KLUWER ACADEMIC PUBLISHERS 1994, ISSN 1381-5067*

Treponema pallidum
ANTIBODY DETECTION (IgG)

Manufacturer: Clark Laboratories
Cat. No./Trade name: /CLARK Treponema Pallidum IgG

SUMMARY

[Well-Ag]–**Ab**–[AHIgG-HRP]–[TMB]–A_{450}

Assay type: EIA (non-competitive)
Detection: Colorimetric A_{450}
Format: Microtitre well, Ag coated
Sample type: Serum
Sample pre-treatment:
  Sample absorption to decrease competitive spirochete and reagin antibodies: 10 μl + 200 μl sorbent
Sample volume: 100 μl sorbent diluted sample (x2)
Number of tests: 96
Controls - standards run in assay:
  Controls: Neg (2), Pos (2)
  Calibrator: (2)
Incubation:
  20 min (RT) + 20 min (RT) + 10 min (RT)
Washes: 2

CONTENTS

Antibodies, antigens, labelled components:
  T. pallidum Ag bound to well
  Anti-human IgG PAb (g) HRP conjugated
Substrate: TMB, H_2O_2
Controls - standards supplied:
  Controls: Pos and Neg (human serum or plasma)
  Calibrator: (1) human serum or plasma with assigned value
Additional reagents:
  H_2SO_4
Special equipment required:
  None

INTERPRETATION

Comments on interpretation:
  Sample absorbances are converted to ISR values
  Equivocal: ISR 0.90-1.10: retest to confirm
  Positive: ISR >1.10
No. of references: 6

NOTES

110674.0

Treponema pallidum
ANTIBODY DETECTION (IgG)

Manufacturer: IFCI Clone Systems
Cat. No./Trade name: OD.1012D/EIAgen Treponema Pallidum

SUMMARY

[Well-Ag]–**Ab**–[AHIgG-POD]–[TMB]–A_{450}

Assay type: EIA (non-competitive)
Detection: Colorimetric A_{450}
Format: Microtitre well, Ag coated
Sample type: Serum
Sample pre-treatment:
  None
Sample volume: 10 μl (+ 1 ml diluent)*
Number of tests: 96
Controls - standards run in assay:
  Controls: Neg (2), Pos (2), cut-off control (3)
Incubation:
  45 min (37°C) + 45 min (37°C) + 15 min (RT)
Washes: 2

CONTENTS

Antibodies, antigens, labelled components:
  T. pallidum Ag bound to well
  Anti-human IgG MAb POD conjugated
Substrate: TMB, H_2O_2
Controls - standards supplied:
  Controls: Neg, Pos and cut-off control (sera)
Additional reagents:
  None
Special equipment required:
  None

INTERPRETATION

Comments on interpretation:
  Equivocal: within cut-off ±10%; retest to confirm
  Repeatably equivocal: retest fresh specimen
No. of references: 0

NOTES

110096.0

*Duplicate testing of sample is recommended

© KLUWER ACADEMIC PUBLISHERS 1994, ISSN 1381-5067

Treponema pallidum
ANTIBODY DETECTION (IgG)

Manufacturer: International Immunodiagnostics
Cat. No./Trade name: 590-048/VISUWELL® REAGIN

SUMMARY

[Well-Ag]–**Ab**–[AHIgG-urease]–[substrate]–A_{620}

Assay type: EIA (non-competitive)
Detection: Colorimetric A_{620}
Format: Microtitre well, Ag coated
Sample type: Serum, plasma (do not heat inactivate)
Sample pre-treatment:
    None
Sample volume: Qualitative: 50 µl
    Quantitative: 100 µl
Number of tests: 480, 960
Controls - standards run in assay:
    Conrols: Neg (1), Pos (1)
Incubation:
    30 min (RT) + 20 min (RT) + 10 min (RT)
Washes: 2

CONTENTS

Antibodies, antigens, labelled components:
    Reagin Ag bound to well
    Anti-human IgG PAb (r) urease conjugated
Substrate: Not specified
Controls - standards supplied:
    Controls: Neg and Pos (human serum)
Additional reagents:
    None
Special equipment required:
    None

INTERPRETATION

Comments on interpretation:
    Qualitative: Positive: ≥ cut-off repeatably
    Quantitative: the titre of the sample is the highest dilution
        where absorbance ≥ cut-off
    Visual interpretation is possible
No. of references: 3

NOTES

110615.0

Treponema pallidum
ANTIBODY DETECTION (IgG)

Manufacturer: Menarini Diagnostics
Cat. No./Trade name: M6288/HF Treponema IgG

SUMMARY

[Well-Ag]–**Ab**–[AHIgG-POD]–[TMB]–A_{450}

Assay type: EIA (non-competitive)
Detection: Colorimetric A_{450}
Format: Microtitre well, Ag coated
Sample type: Serum
Sample pre-treatment:
    None
Sample volume: 100 µl (of a 1:101 dilution)
Number of tests: 96
Controls - standards run in assay:
    Controls: Neg (1), Pos (1), cut-off (1)
Incubation:
    45 min (37°C) + 45 min (37°C) + 15 min (RT)
Washes: 2

CONTENTS

Antibodies, antigens, labelled components:
    T. pallidum Ag bound to well
    Anti-human IgG MAb POD conjugated
Substrate: TMB, H_2O_2
Controls - standards supplied:
    Controls: Neg, Pos and cut-off (serum)
Additional reagents:
    None
Special equipment required:
    Not specified

INTERPRETATION

Comments on interpretation:
    Not specified
No. of references: 0

NOTES

110352.0

© *KLUWER ACADEMIC PUBLISHERS 1994, ISSN 1381-5067*

Treponema pallidum
ANTIBODY DETECTION (IgG)

Manufacturer: Omega Diagnostics Ltd
Cat. No./Trade name: OD 087/Syphilis IgG EIA

SUMMARY

[Well-Ag]–**Ab**–[AHIgG-HRP]–[TMB]–A_{450}

Assay type: EIA (non-competitive)
Detection: Colorimetric A_{450}
Format: Microtitre well, Ag coated
Sample type: Serum
Sample pre-treatment:
 None
Sample volume: 10 µl (+ 490 µl diluent)
Number of tests: 96, 960
Controls - standards run in assay:
 Controls: Neg (1), low Pos (2), high Pos (1)
Incubation:
 1 hr (37°C) + 30 min (37°C) + 15 min (37°C)
Washes: 2

CONTENTS

Antibodies, antigens, labelled components:
 T. pallidum Ag bound to well
 Anti-human IgG Ab HRP conjugated
Substrate: TMB
Controls - standards supplied:
 Controls: Neg, low Pos and high Pos (serum)
Additional reagents:
 None
Special equipment required:
 None

INTERPRETATION

Comments on interpretation:
 Equivocal: cut-off ± 10%; retest to confirm
No. of references: 3

NOTES

110618.0

Treponema pallidum
ANTIBODY DETECTION (IgM)

Manufacturer: Centocor Inc
Cat. No./Trade name: M410/CAPTIA® Syphillis - M

SUMMARY

[Well-AHIgM]–**Ab**–[Ag + MAb-biotin + strept-HRP]–
[TMB]–A_{450}

Assay type: EIA (non-competitive)
Detection: Colorimetric A_{450}
Format: Microtitre well, Ab coated
Sample type: Serum
Sample pre-treatment:
 None
Sample volume: 5 µl (+ 250 µl diluent)
Number of tests: 96
Controls - standards run in assay:
 Controls: Neg (1), low Pos (2), Pos (1)
Incubation:
 1 hr (37°C) + 1 hr (37°C) + 30 min (RT)
Washes: 2

CONTENTS

Antibodies, antigens, labelled components:
 Anti-human IgM Ab (r) bound to well
 T. pallidum Ag
 Anti-*T. pallidum* MAb biotinylated
 Streptavidin HRP conjugated
Substrate: TMB, H_2O_2
Controls - standards supplied:
 Controls: Neg, low Pos, high Pos (human serum)
Additional reagents:
 H_2SO_4
Special equipment required:
 None

INTERPRETATION

Comments on interpretation:
 Equivocal: within cut-off ± 10%; retest to confirm
 Repeatably equivocal: retest fresh sample
No. of references: 12

NOTES

110084.0

© KLUWER ACADEMIC PUBLISHERS 1994, ISSN 1381-5067

Treponema pallidum
ANTIBODY DETECTION (IgM)

Manufacturer: Fujirebio
Cat. No./Trade name: /Imzyne M - TP

SUMMARY

[Bead-Ag]–Ab–[AHIgM-HRP]–[ABTS]–A_{420}

Assay type: EIA (non-competitive)
Detection: Colorimetric A_{420}
Format: Tube, Ag coated bead
Sample type: Serum
Sample pre-treatment:
    None
Sample volume: 5 µl (+400 µl diluent)
Number of tests: 22
Controls - standards run in assay:
    Controls: Pos (2)
Incubation:
    2 hr (37°C) + 1 hr (37°C) + 1 hr (37°C)
Washes: 2

CONTENTS

Antibodies, antigens, labelled components:
    T. pallidum Ag bound to beads
    Anti-human IgM Ab (r) HRP conjugated
Substrate: ABTS
Controls - standards supplied:
    Controls: Pos (human serum) (titre = 1 unit)
Additional reagents:
    None
Special equipment required:
    None

INTERPRETATION

Comments on interpretation:
    Negative: unit value ≤0.9 units
    Inconclusive: unit value 1.0 - 1.2 units
    Positive: unit value ≥1.3 units
No. of references: 13

NOTES

110325.0

Treponema pallidum
ANTIBODY DETECTION (IgM)

Manufacturer: IFCI Clone Systems
Cat. No./Trade name: 08.1021D/EIAgen Treponema Pallidum IgM

SUMMARY

[Well-AHIgM]–Ab–[Ag+MAb-POD]–[TMB]–A_{450}

Assay type: EIA (non-competitive)
Detection: Colorimetric A_{450}
Format: Microtitre well, Ab coated
Sample type: Serum
Sample pre-treatment:
    None
Sample volume: 10 µl (+1 ml diluent)*
Number of tests: 96
Controls - standards run in assay:
    Controls: Neg (2), Pos (2), cut-off control (3)
Incubation:
    45 min (37°C) + 45 min (37°C) + 15 min (RT)
Washes: 2

CONTENTS

Antibodies, antigens, labelled components:
    Anti-human IgM MAb bound to well
    T. pallidum Ag
    Anti-T. pallidum MAb POD conjugated
Substrate: TMB, H_2O_2
Controls - standards supplied:
    Controls: Neg, Pos and cut-off control (serum)
Additional reagents:
    None
Special equipment required:
    None

INTERPRETATION

Comments on interpretation:
    Equivocal: within cut-off ±10%; retest to confirm
    Repeatably equivocal: retest fresh specimen
No. of references: 0

NOTES

110095.0

*Duplicate testing of sample is recommended

© KLUWER ACADEMIC PUBLISHERS 1994, ISSN 1381-5067

Treponema pallidum
ANTIBODY DETECTION (IgM)

Manufacturer: Menarini Diagnostics
Cat. No./Trade name: M6239/HF Treponema IgM

SUMMARY

[Well-AHIgM]–**Ab**–[Ag + MAb-POD]–[TMB]–A_{450}

Assay type: EIA (non-competitive)
Detection: Colorimetric A_{450}
Format: Microtitre well, Ab coated
Sample type: Serum
Sample pre-treatment:
    Optional: serum absorption using IgM Confirmation Kit (M6350) to eliminate interfering factors
Sample volume: 100 µl (of a 1:101 dilution)
Number of tests: 96
Controls - standards run in assay:
    Controls: Neg (1), Pos (1), cut-off (1)
Incubation:
    45 min (37°C) + 45 min (37°C) + 15 min (RT)
Washes: 2

CONTENTS

Antibodies, antigens, labelled components:
    Anti-human IgM MAb bound to well
    T. pallidum Ag
    Anti-T. pallidum MAb POD conjugated
Substrate: TMB, H_2O_2
Controls - standards supplied:
    Controls: Neg, Pos and cut-off (serum)
Additional reagents:
    None
Special equipment required:
    Not specified

INTERPRETATION

Comments on Interpretation:
    Not specified
No. of references: 0

NOTES

110353.0

Treponema pallidum
ANTIBODY DETECTION (IgG)

Manufacturer: Diagast Laboratories
Cat. No./Trade name: 69135N/BLOTSYPH KIT

SUMMARY

[Strip-Ag]–**Ab**–[AHIgG-HRP]–[4-chloronaphthol]–
            blue band

Assay type: Immunoblot assay
Detection: Visual
Format: Membrane strip, Ag coated
Sample type: Serum
Sample pre-treatment:
    None
Sample volume: 100 µl (+2.0 ml diluent)
Number of tests: 16
Controls - standards run in assay:
    Controls: Pos (1)
Incubation:
    2 hr (RT) + 1 hr (RT) + 30 min (RT)
Washes: 3

CONTENTS

Antibodies, antigens, labelled components:
    T. pallidum Ag bound to strip
    Anti-human IgG Ab peroxidase conjugated
Substrate: 4-chloronaphthol
Controls - standards supplied:
    Control: Pos
Additional reagents:
    None
Special equipment required:
    None

INTERPRETATION

Comments on Interpretation:
    Positive: dark blue band. The position of the bands correspond to the proteins described in the reference chart
No. of references: 1

NOTES

110675.0

For research use only

© KLUWER ACADEMIC PUBLISHERS 1994, ISSN 1381-5067

Treponema pallidum
ANTIBODY DETECTION

Manufacturer: bioMerieux
Cat. No./Trade name: 7568 1/Trepo-spot IF

SUMMARY

[Slide-Ag]–**Ab**–[AHIg-FITC]–fluorescence

Assay type: Immunofluorescence assay (indirect)
Detection: Fluorescence microscopy
Format: Slide well, Ag coated
Sample type: Serum
Sample pre-treatment:
All test sera are diluted (1:5) with sorbent to remove non-specific antibodies
All control sera are diluted (1:5) with sorbent and with PBS
Sample volume: 10 µl of pretreated sample
Number of tests: 100
Controls - standards run in assay:
Controls: Neg (2)*, Pos (2), non-specific (2)
Incubation:
30 min (37°C) + 30 min (37°C)
Washes: 2

CONTENTS

Antibodies, antigens, labelled components:
T. pallidum bound to slide
Anti-human Ig PAb (g) FITC conjugated
Substrate:
Controls - standards supplied:
Controls: Reactive control serum (human) and non-specific control serum (human; with non-specific treponemal antibodies)
Additional reagents:
A negative control serum
Special equipment required:
None

INTERPRETATION

Comments on interpretation:
Negative: <(1+) fluorescence
Positive: (1+) to (4+) green fluorescence
No. of references: None

NOTES

110543.0

*The negative, positive and non-specific control sera are tested in duplicate (a) diluted in PBS and (b) diluted in sorbent

Treponema pallidum
ANTIBODY DETECTION

Manufacturer: Diagast Laboratories
Cat. No./Trade name: 69128R/SYPHIX-GAM

SUMMARY

[Slide well-Ag]–**Ab**–[AHIgG,A,M-FITC]–fluorescence

Assay type: Immunofluorescence assay (indirect)
Detection: Fluorescence microscopy
Format: Slide well, Ag coated
Sample type: Serum, CSF
Sample pre-treatment:
Sample absorption: 20 µl + 80 µl sorbent
Sample volume: 20 µl sorbent treated sample
Number of tests: 10
Controls - standards run in assay:
Controls: Pos (1), non-specific reactive (1)
Incubation:
30 min (RT) + 10 min (37°C)
Washes: 2

CONTENTS

Antibodies, antigens, labelled components:
T. pallidum Ag bound to slide well
Anti-human IgG,A,M, Ab FITC conjugated
Substrate:
Controls - standards supplied:
Controls: Positive and reactive non-specific
Additional reagents:
None
Special equipment required:
None

INTERPRETATION

Comments on interpretation:
Positive: Varying degrees of green fluorescence (2+ to 4+)
Serial dilutions are tested for a quantitative assay
No. of references: None

NOTES

110876.0

Treponema pallidum
ANTIBODY DETECTION

Manufacturer: Sanofi Diagnostics Pasteur
Cat. No./Trade name: 63557*/SYPHILAM

SUMMARY

[Slide-Ag]–**Ab**–[AHIg-FITC]–fluorescence

Assay type: Immunofluorescence assay (indirect)
Detection: Fluorescence microscopy
Format: Slide well, Ag coated
Sample type: Serum (heat inactivated)
Sample pre-treatment:
 Samples and controls diluted 1:5 with sorbent, incubate 5 min
Sample volume: 20 μl of 1:5 dilution**
Number of tests: 120
Controls - standards run in assay:
 Controls: Neg (1), Pos (1)
Incubation:
 30 min (37°C) + 30 min (37°C)
Washes: 2

CONTENTS

Antibodies, antigens, labelled components:
 T. pallidum bound to slide well
 Anti-human Ig Ab FITC conjugated (code 74511)
Substrate:
Controls - standards supplied:
 Controls: Pos (human serum) (Code 76751)
Additional reagents:
 Sorbent Neg human serum
Special equipment required:
 None

INTERPRETATION

Comments on interpretation:
 Positive: ⩾(1+) green fluorescence of T. pallidum
No. of references: 5

NOTES

110257.0

*Component parts bought separately
**Previously screened positive sera should be titred to endpoint

Treponema pallidum
ANTIBODY DETECTION (IgG)

Manufacturer: Amico Laboratories Inc
Cat. No./Trade name: FT001/FTA-ABS Test Kit

SUMMARY

[Slide-Ag]–**Ab**–[AHIgG-FITC]–fluorescence

Assay type: Immunofluorescence assay (indirect)
Detection: Fluorescence microscopy
Format: Slide well, Ag coated
Sample type: Serum
Sample pre-treatment:
 Heat sample 30 min (56°C). Dilute sample: 1 drop (+4 drops sorbant)
Sample volume: 1 drop of diluted sample
Number of tests: 100
Controls - standards run in assay:
 Controls: Neg (1), Pos (1)
Incubation:
 30 min (37°C) + 30 min (37°C)
Washes: 1

CONTENTS

Antibodies, antigens, labelled components:
 T. pallidum Ag bound to slide well
 Anti-human IgG Ab FITC conjugated
Substrate:
Controls - standards supplied:
 Controls: Neg and Pos (slides)
Additional reagents:
 None
Special equipment required:
 None

INTERPRETATION

Comments on interpretation:
 Negative: no fluorescence seen
 Borderline: <(+1) fluorescence; repeat and report repeatably <(+1) as borderline result
 Positive: (+1) fluorescence repeatably or (+2) to (+4) fluorescence with no retest required
No. of references: 6

NOTES

110579.0

© KLUWER ACADEMIC PUBLISHERS 1994, ISSN 1381-5067

Treponema pallidum
ANTIBODY DETECTION (IgG)

Manufacturer: Mast Diagnostics Ltd
Cat. No./Trade name: IF401/MASTAFLUOR-FTA-ABS

SUMMARY

[Slide-Ag]–Ab–[AHIgG-FITC]–fluorescence

Assay type: Immunofluorescence assay (indirect)
Detection: Fluorescence microscopy
Format: Slide well, Ag coated
Sample type: Serum
Sample pre-treatment:
Heat inactivate all sera and controls (56°C, 30 min). All test sera are diluted (1:5) with sorbent to remove non-specific antibodies
The reactive and non-specific controls are diluted (1:5) with sorbent and with PBS. Treated samples are incubated (37°C, 30 min)
Sample volume: 20 µl pretreated sample
Number of tests: 100
Controls - standards run in assay:
Controls: Reactive (2)*, non-specific (2), sorbent (1), PBS (1)
Incubation:
30 min (37°C) + 30 min (37°C)
Washes: 2

CONTENTS

Antibodies, antigens, labelled components:
T. pallidum bound to slide
Anti-human IgG Ab FITC conjugated
Substrate:
Controls - standards supplied:
Controls: Reactive control (human) and non-specific control (human; with non-specific treponemal antibodies)
Additional reagents:
None
Special equipment required:
None

INTERPRETATION

Comments on interpretation:
Negative: <(+1) fluorescence and no treponema seen on dark field examination
Borderline: (+/-) fluorescence; retest to confirm
Positive: >(+1) fluorescence
No. of references: None

NOTES

110542.0

*The reactive and non-specific controls are tested in duplicate: (a) diluted in PBS and (b) diluted in sorbent

Treponema pallidum
ANTIBODY DETECTION (IgG)

Manufacturer: Schiapparelli Biosystems Inc
Cat. No./Trade name: 2300/VIRGO FTA-ABS IgG IFA

SUMMARY

[Slide-Ag]–Ab–[AHIgG-FITC]–fluorescence

Assay type: Immunofluorescence assay (indirect)
Detection: Fluorescence microscopy
Format: Slide well, Ag coated
Sample type: Serum
Sample pre-treatment:
Heat 30 min (56°C) and cool.
Removal of non-specific Ab: dilute 25 µl sample in 100 µl sorbent, 15 min (RT)
Sample volume: 20 µl of 1:5 dilution
Number of tests: 60, 200
Controls - standards run in assay:
Controls: Neg (4), Pos (3)
Incubation:
30 min (37°C) + 30 min (37°C)
Washes: 2

CONTENTS

Antibodies, antigens, labelled components:
T. pallidum organisms bound to slide
Anti-human IgG Ab (r) FITC conjugated
Substrate:
Controls - standards supplied:
Controls: Neg and Pos (human serum)
Additional reagents:
None
Special equipment required:
None

INTERPRETATION

Comments on interpretation:
Equivocal: (1+) specific apple green fluorescence repeatably: retest 1-2 weeks later to confirm
Positive: >(1+) specific apple green fluorescence repeatably
No. of references: 40

NOTES

110417.0

This test is not intended for routine use or screening

Treponema pallidum
ANTIBODY DETECTION (IgG)

Manufacturer: Zeus Scientific Inc
Cat. No./Trade name: 7001DS/FTA-ABS DOUBLE STAIN TEST SYSTEM

SUMMARY

[Slide-Ag] $\Big\langle$ Ab–[AHIgG-RITC]–red fluorescence

[Ab-FITC]–green fluorescence

Assay type: Immunofluorescence assay (indirect)
Detection: Fluorescence microscopy
Format: Slide well, Ag coated
Sample type: Serum
Sample pre-treatment:
Heat sera for 30 min (56°C). Previously heated sera must be reheated at least 10 min prior to retesting
Sample volume: 50 μl (+200 μl sorbent)
Number of tests: Not specified
Controls - standards run in assay:
Controls: Reactive (2), Minimal Reactive (2), Non-Specific (2)*
Incubation:
30 min (37°C) + 30 min (37°C) + 20 min (37°C)
Washes: 3

CONTENTS

Antibodies, antigens, labelled components:
T. pallidum Ag fixed to slide well
Anti-human IgG Ab RITC labelled
Anti-T. pallidum Ab FITC labelled
Substrate:
Controls - standards supplied:
Controls: Reactive and non-specific (minimal reactive control is a PBS dilution of reactive control)
Additional reagents:
T. pallidum antigen suspension (for optional preparation of FTA-ABS DS antigen smears)
Special equipment required:
None

INTERPRETATION

Comments on interpretation:
Negative: <(1+) red fluorescence with green staining due to anti-T. pallidum Ab FITC label
Equivocal: (1+) red fluorescence; retest to confirm
Positive: >(1+) red fluorescence repeatably
No. of references: 19

NOTES

110662.0

*Controls are tested in duplicate (a) diluted in PBS and (b) diluted in sorbent

Treponema pallidum
ANTIBODY DETECTION (IgM)

Manufacturer: Sanofi Diagnostics Pasteur
Cat. No./Trade name: 63557*/SYPHILAM

SUMMARY

[Slide-Ag]–Ab–[AHIgM-FITC]–fluorescence

Assay type: Immunofluorescence assay (indirect)
Detection: Fluorescence microscopy
Format: Slide well, Ag coated
Sample type: Serum (heat inactivated)
Sample pre-treatment:
Samples and controls diluted 1:5 with sorbent, incubate 5 min
Sample volume: 20 μl of 1:5 dilution**
Number of tests: 120
Controls - standards run in assay:
Controls: Neg (1), Pos (1)
Incubation:
30 min (37°C) + 30 min (37°C)
Washes: 2

CONTENTS

Antibodies, antigens, labelled components:
T. pallidum bound to slide well
Anti-human IgM Ab FITC conjugated (Code 74591)
Substrate:
Controls - standards supplied:
Controls: Pos (human serum) (Code 76751)
Additional reagents:
Sorbent Neg human serum
Special equipment required:
None

INTERPRETATION

Comments on interpretation:
Positive: ≥(1+) green fluorescence
No. of references: 5

NOTES

110495.0

*Component parts bought separately
**Previously screened positive sera should be titred to end-point

© KLUWER ACADEMIC PUBLISHERS 1994, ISSN 1381-5067

Urinary tract infection bacterial pathogens
ANTIBODY DETECTION

Manufacturer: Shield Diagnostics
Cat. No./Trade name: FUTI 200/URISTAT UTI IgA/IgG ELISA

SUMMARY

[Well-Ag]–**Ab**–[AHIgG/IgA-AP]–[PMP]–A$_{550/585}$

Assay type: EIA (non-competitive)
Detection: Colorimetric A$_{540/565}$
Format: Microtitre well, Ag coated
Sample type: Urine
Sample pre-treatment:
   None
Sample volume: 100 µl
Number of tests: 96
Controls - standards run in assay:
   Controls: Low Pos (2), high Pos (2)
Incubation:
   15 min (RT) + 15 min (RT) + 15 min (RT)
Washes: 2

CONTENTS

Antibodies, antigens, labelled components:
   Bacterial antigens (E. coli, Prot. mirabilis, Kleb. pneumoniae, Staph. saprophyticus, Ps. aeruginosa, Cit freundi and Strep. faecalis) bound to well
   Anti-human IgG and IgA MAb (m) AP conjugated
Substrate: PMP
Controls - standards supplied:
   Controls: Low Pos and high Pos (positive for specific antibodies to UTI bacterial pathogens)
Additional reagents:
   None
Special equipment required:
   None

INTERPRETATION

Comments on Interpretation:
   Positive: Ratio of sample: low positive control absorbance > 1.0
No. of references: None

NOTES

110582.0

The kit tests simultaneously for one or more bacterial pathogens causing UTI (E. coli, Prot. mirabilis, Kleb. pneumoniae, Staph. saprophyticus, Ps. aeruginosa, Cit. freundi and Strep. faecalis)

LIST OF MANUFACTURERS AND DISTRIBUTORS

Abbott Laboratories

Corporate
Abbott Laboratories
Diagnostics Division
Abbott Park
North Chicago, IL 60064
USA
Tel: +1-312-937-6100

By region
AUSTRALIA
Abbott Australasia Pty Ltd
Diagnostics Division
PO Box 394
North Ryde
New South Wales 2113
Australia
Tel: +61-2-8881111
Fax: +61-2-8873948

AUSTRIA
Abbott GmbH
Diagnostics Division
Diefenbachgasse 35
1150 Vienna
Austria
Tel: +43-1-89124
Fax: +43-1-8941747

BELGIUM
Abbott SA
Diagnostics Division
Rue du Bosquet 2
1348 Ottognies-
Louvain-la-Neuve
Belgium
Tel: +32-10-475311
Fax: +32-10-475334

CANADA
Abbott Laboratories Ltd
Diagnostics Division
7115 Milcreek Drive
Mississauga
Ontario, L5N 3R3
Canada
Tel: +1-416-858-2450
Fax: +1-416-858-2462

DENMARK
Abbott A/S
Diagnostics Division
Bygstubben 16
Troeroed
2950 Vedbaek
Denmark
Tel: +45-42-894452
Fax: +45-42-890132

FRANCE
Laboratoires Abbott
Division Diagnostic
12 rue de la Couture
Silic 203
94518 Rungis Cedex
France
Tel: +33-1-45602500
Fax: +33-1-45600498

GERMANY
Abbott Diagnostic Products
GmbH
Max-Planck-Ring 2
65205 Wiesbaden-

Delkenheim
Germany
Tel: +49-61-2250101
Fax: +49-61-22501244
Telex: 4182 598

GREECE
Abbott Laboratories (Hellas)
SA
Diagnostics Division
194 Syngrou Ave
Athens
Greece
Tel: +30-1-9519019
Fax: +30-1-9592790

HONG KONG
Abbott Laboratories Ltd
Unit No. 3005, 30/F
West Tower, Shun Tak Centre
200 Connaught Road
Hong Kong
Tel: +852-5490019
Fax: +852-8580498

IRELAND
Abbott Laboratories Ireland
Ltd
70 Broomhill Road
Tallaght
Dublin 24
Ireland
Tel: +353-16-517388
Fax: +353-16-517765

ITALY
Abbott SpA
Divisione Diagnostici
Via Mar della Ciria 262
00144 Rome
Italy
Tel: +39-6-529911
Fax: +39-6-52991436

JAPAN
Dainabot Co Ltd
33 Mori Building 6th floor
8-21 Toranomon 3-chome
Minato-ku
Tokyo 105
Japan
Tel: +81-3-34379441
Fax: +81-3-34379367

MEXICO
Abbott Laboratories de
Mexico SA
Diagnostics Division
Apartado Postal No 44-983
Mexico 03100, D.F.
Mexico
Tel: +52-5-7264600
Fax: +52-5-7264644

NETHERLANDS
Abbott NV
Maalderij 21
1185 ZB Amstelveen
Netherlands
Tel: +31-20-5454540
Fax: +31-20-6402231

NEW ZEALAND
Abbott Laboratories (NZ) Ltd
Diagnostics Division
148 Harris Road
PO Box 58-611
Greenmount, Auckland

New Zealand
Tel: +64-9-2749886
Fax: +64-9-2746633

PHILIPPINES
Abbott Laboratories (Phils)
Inc
POB 29
Commercial Center
Makati
Metro Manila
Philippines
Tel: +63-2-6318471
Fax: +63-2-6318488

PORTUGAL
ABBOTT Laboratorios Ltd
Apartado 20/Alfragide
2700 Amadora
Portugal
Tel: +351-1-4712575
Fax: +351-1-4712725

PUERTO RICO
Abbott Laboratories
Diagnostics Division
PO Box 4706
Carolina 00628
Puerto Rico
Tel: +1-809-7623366
Fax: +1-809-7505454

SINGAPORE
Abbott Laboratories Private
Ltd
GPO Box 1016
Singapore 9020
Singapore
Tel: +65-2788343
Fax: +65-2708873

SOUTH AFRICA
Abbott LABS South Africa
(Pty) Ltd
Diagnostics Division
PO Box 1616
Johannesburg 2000
South Africa
Tel: +27-11-4941957
Fax: +27-11-4943041

SPAIN
Abbott Cientifica SA
Costa Brava, 13
28034 Madrid
Spain
Tel: +34-1-3373400
Fax: +34-1-7349664

SWEDEN
Abbott AB
Diagnostics Division
PO Box 1074
164 21 Kista-Stockholm
Sweden
Tel: +46-8-7036700
Fax: +46-8-7527123

SWITZERLAND
Abbott AG
Diagnostics Division
Gewerbestrasee 5
6330 Cham/Zug
Switzerland
Tel: +41-42-444400
Fax: +41-42-415140

UNITED KINGDOM
Abbott Diagnostics
Abbott House
Norden Road
Maidenhead
Berkshire, SL6 4XF
United Kingdom
Tel: +44-628-784041
Fax: +44-628-644205

USA
Abbott Laboratories
Diagnostics Division
1921 Hurd
PO Box 152020
Irving
TX 75015-2020
USA
Tel: +1-214-518-6000

Abbott Laboratories
Diagnostics Division
Abbott Park
North Chicago, IL 60064
USA
Tel: +1-312-937-6100

Abbott Laboratories
Diagnostics Division
820 Mission St
South Pasadena, CA 91030
USA
Tel: +1-818-440-0700

ADI Diagnostics Inc

Corporate
ADI Diagnostics Inc
30 Meridian Road
Rexdale, Ontario
M9W 4Z7
Canada
Tel: +1-416-674-0863
Fax: +1-416-674-2992

Agen Biomedical Ltd

Corporate
Agen Biomedical Ltd
PO Box 391
Acacia Ridge
Queensland 4110
Australia
Tel: +61-7-2736266
Fax: +61-7-2736224

By region
AUSTRALIA
Agen Biomedical Ltd
PO Box 391
Acacia Ridge
Queensland 4110
Australia
Tel: +61-7-2736266
Fax: +61-7-2736224

USA
AGEN Inc
20 Waterview Boulevard
Parsippany, NJ 07054
USA
Tel: +1-201-335-8535
Fax: +1-201-335-8155

Alfa Biotech

Corporate

Alfa Biotech
Viale Sarca 223
20126 Milan
Italy
Tel: +39-2-661381
Fax: +39-2-66138443

Amico Laboratories Inc

Corporate

Amico Laboratories Inc
PO Box 90203
5012 Illinois Avenue
Nashville, TN 37209
USA
Tel: +1-615-385-3114
Fax: +1-615-385-3114

Baxter Diagnostics Inc

Corporate

Baxter Diagnostics Inc
Stratus Immunochemistry
10 555 West Flagler
Miami, FL 33174
USA
Tel: +1-305-222-6686
Fax: +1-305-222-6200

By region

AUSTRALIA
Baxter Healthcare Pty Ltd
PO Box 88
Toongabbie
New South Wales 2146
Australia
Tel: +61-2-6889111
Fax: +61-2-6889123

BELGIUM
Baxter World Trade SA
Baxter SA
Rue Colonel Bourg, 105B
1140 Brussels
Belgium
Tel: +32-2-7411711
Fax: +32-2-7322381

FRANCE
Baxter SA
Avenue Louis-Pasteur
Boite Postale 56
78311 Maurepas Cedex
France
Tel: +33-1-34615050
Fax: +33-1-34615008

GERMANY
Baxter Deutschland GmbH
Edisonstrasse 3
85716 Unterschleissheim
Germany
Tel: +49-89-317010
Fax: +49-89-31701-177

ITALY
Baxter SpA
Via Lampedusa 11/A

20141 Milan
Italy
Tel: +39-2-89501732
Fax: +39-2-89527222

JAPAN
Baxter Limited, Sales Office
Sankaido Building
9-13 Alasaka 1-chome
Minato-ku
Tokyo 107
Japan
Tel: +81-3-32376627
Fax: +81-3-35057811

NETHERLANDS
Baxter BV
PO Box 1536
3600 BM Maarssem
Netherlands
Tel: +31-30-468911
Fax: +31-30-411755

NORWAY
Baxter A/S
Gjerdrumsvei 10B
0486 Oslo 4
Norway
Tel: +47-2-184101
Fax: +47-2-184109

SPAIN
Baxter SA
Calle Solsones, No. 2, Bajo
Local 7
08820 El Prat de Llobregat
Barcelona
Spain
Tel: +34-3-4787162
Fax: +34-3-4787109

SWITZERLAND
Baxter AG
BonnStrasse
CH-3186 Dudingen
Switzerland
Tel: +41-37-438111
Fax: +41-37-438960

UNITED KINGDOM
B.M. Browne (UK) Ltd
9 Commerce Park
Brunel Road
Theale, Reading
RG7 4AB
United Kingdom
Tel: +44-0734-305333
Fax: +44-0734-305111

USA
Baxter Diagnostics Inc.
Stratus Immunochemistry
10 555, West Flagler
Miami, FL 33174
USA
Tel: +1-305-222-6200
Fax: +1-305-222-6686

Becton Dickinson Immuno-diagnostics

Corporate

Becton Dickinson
Immunodiagnostics
Mountain View Avenue

Orangeburg, NY 10962-1294
USA
Tel: +1-914-359-2700
Fax: +1-415-966-8914

By region

BELGIUM
Becton Dickinson Benelux NV
Denderstraat 24
POB 13
9440 Erembodegem-Aalst
Belgium
Tel: +32-53-720550
Fax: +32-53-720549
Telex: 12337

CANADA
Becton Dickinson Canada
2464 South Sheridan Way
Mississauga, Ontario
L5J 2M8
Canada
Tel: +1-416-822-4820
Fax: +1-416-822-2644

FRANCE
Becton Dickinson Europe
Headquarters
5 Chemin Des Sources - BP 37
38241 Meylan Cedex
France
Tel: +33-76908035
Fax: +33-76416464
Telex: 980640

Becton Dickinson France SA
11 Rue Aristide Berges
38800 Le Point de Claix
France
Tel: +33-76683707
Fax: +33-76683693
Telex: 980156

Beckton Dickinson Middle
East and Africa Operations
5, Chemin des Sources - BP 37
38241 Meylan Cedex
France
Tel: +33-76908035
Fax: +33-76411577
Telex: 980640

GERMANY
Becton Dickinson GmBH
Postfach 10 16 29
69006 Heidelberg
Germany
Tel: +49-6221-305288
Fax: +49-6221-303708
Telex: 461534

GREECE
Becton Dickinson Greece
EPE
36A Ionias Street
17456 Alimos Athens
Greece
Tel: +30-1-9933800
Fax: +30-1-9934494

ITALY
Becton Dickinson Italia SpA
Via Caldera 21
20153 Milan
Italy

Tel: +39-2-482401
Fax: +39-2-48204775
Telex: 353565

NETHERLANDS
Becton Dickinson BV
Mon Plaisir 87B
Postbus 514
4870 AM Etten-Leur
Netherlands
Tel: +31-1608-37720
Fax: +31-1608-14133
Telex: 74328

SPAIN
Becton Dickinson Espana SA
Apartado Correos 31091
28080 Madrid
Spain
Tel: +34-1-8418311
Fax: +34-1-8418139
Telex: 46018

SWEDEN
Becton Dickinson AB
Kilabergsudgen B
Box 32045
126 11 Hagersten
Sweden
Tel: +46-8-7753070
Fax: +46-8-6450808
Telex: 11786

SWITZERLAND
Becton Dickinson AG
PO Box
4002 Basel
Switzerland
Tel: +41-61-3225717
Fax: +41-61-3225830
Telex: 964784

UNITED ARAB EMIRATES
Becton Dickinson Arab
Peninsula Operations
c/o City Pharmacy - PO Box 4831
Dubai
United Arab Emirates
Tel: +971-4-379525
Fax: +971-4-379551
Telex: 46260

UNITED KINGDOM
Becton Dickinson UK Ltd
Between Towns Road
Cowley
Oxford, OX4 3LY
United Kingdom
Tel: +44-0865-748844
Fax: +44-0865-781627
Telex: 837438

USA
Becton Dickinson
Immunodiagnostics
Mountain View Avenue
Orangeburg, NY 10962-1294
USA
Tel: +1-914-359-2700
Fax: +1-415-966-8914

Behringwerke AG

Corporate

Behringwerke AG

Postfach 1140
35001 Marburg
Germany
Tel: +49-6421-390
Fax: +49-6421-66064
Telex: 48232001

By region
ANTILLES
Curacao Pharmacal Company
NV
Ontarioweg 8
Salinja Curacao, NA
PO Box 252
Willemstad
Curacao
Antilles
Fax: +599-9-614819
Telex: 1256

ARGENTINA
Merck Quimica Argentina
SAIC
Behring Diagnosticos
Artilleros 2436
1428 Buenos Aires
Argentina
Tel: +54-1-7886558
Fax: +54-1-7883365

AUSTRALIA
Behring Diagnostics Australia
Pty Ltd
103 Vanessa St. Kingsgrove
2208
Locked Mail Bag 200
Kingsgrove
NSW 2208
Australia
Tel: +61-2-5541600
Fax: +61-2-5024256

AUSTRIA
Behring Institut GmbH
Altmannsdorfer Str 104
1127 Vienna
Austria
Tel: +43-1-80101
Telex: 133701

BAHAMAS
Lowe's Pharmacy Ltd
PO Box N-7504
Nassau
Bahamas
Tel: +1-809-3228006
Telex: 20477

BAHRAIN
Bahrain Pharmacy & General
Store
PO Box 403
Bahrain
Tel: +973-53491/255506
Fax: +973-275195
Telex: 8979

BANGLADESH
Hoechst Bangladesh Co. Ltd
PO Box 534
133 Kakrail
New Bailey Road
Dhaka 1000
Bangladesh
Tel: +880-2834928
Fax: +880-2-834902
Telex: 632253

BARBADOS, W INDIES
Collins Ltd
PO Box 203
28 Broad Street
Bridgetown
Barbados, W Indies
Tel: +1-809-4249182
Fax: +1-809-4264246
Telex: 2595

BELGIUM
Hoechst Belgium SA
Chaussee de Charleroi 111-
113
1060 Brussels
Belgium
Tel: +32-2-5364111
Fax: +32-2-5334265
Telex: 21396

BOLIVIA
Corimex Ltda
Calle Goita 135
La Paz
Bolivia
Tel: +591-2-359337
Fax: +591-2-391230
Telex: 3508

BRAZIL
Hoechst do Brasil
Quimica e Farmaceutica SA
Setor Diagnosticos Behring
Av. das Nacoes Unidas
18.001
8 Andar - Sala 801
CEP 04795 Sao Paulo
Brazil
Tel: +55-11-5257893
Fax: +55-11-5257895
Telex: 1170501

BULGARIA
Hoechst Handelsvertreting
Pionerski Pat No. 2
1618 Sofia
Bulgaria
Tel: +359-2-550119
Fax: +359-2-550116
Telex: 22060

CANADA
Hoechst Roussel Canada Inc
4045 Cote Vertu
Montreal
Quebec H4R ZE8
Canada
Tel: +1-514-333-3605
Fax: +1-514-333-3769

CHILE
Merck Quimica Chilens Ltd
Casilla 4232
Santiago de Chile
Chile
Tel: +56-2-2381160
Fax: +56-2-2383527
Telex: 440197

COLOMBIA
Merck Colombia SA
Apartado Aereo 9896
Bogota, D.E.
Colombia
Tel: +57-1-2907855
Fax: +57-1-2628881
Telex: 41405

COSTA RICA
Hoechst Costa Rica SA
Diagnosticos Behring
Apartado 10158
1000 San Jose
Costa Rica
Tel: +506-334722
Fax: +506-228221
Telex: 2111

CROATIA
Behring Institut GmbH
Altmannsdorfer Str 104
1121 Vienna
Austria
Tel: +43-1-80101
Telex: 133701

CZECH REPUBLIC
Behring Institut GmbH
Altmannsdorfer Str 104
1121 Vienna
Austria
Tel: +43-1-80101
Telex: 133701

DENMARK
Hoechst Danmark A/S
Islevdalveij 110
2610 Rodovre
Denmark
Tel: +45-44888227
Fax: +45-44888352
Telex: 35366

DOMINICAN REPUBLIC
Hoechst Dominicana SA
Apartado Postal 830
Zona Postal 1
Santo Domingo
Dominican Republic
Tel: +1809-5302988
Fax: +1809-5302976
Telex: 3460305

ECUADOR
Merck Ecuador CA
Avda America 1735
Casilla 17-01-2574
Quito
Ecuador
Tel: +593-2-562703
Fax: +593-2-651150
Telex: 2252

EGYPT
Hoechst Orient SAA
PO Box 1486
3 Sharia El Massaneh
(Zeitoun)
Cairo
Egypt
Tel: +20-2-2575840
Fax: +20-2-694755
Telex: 02331

EL SALVADOR
Quimica Hoechst de El
Salvador SA
Km 9,5 carre. al Puerto de la
Libertad
Nuevo San Salvador
El Salvador
Tel: +503-780533
Fax: +503-780909
Telex: 20143

FINLAND
Oy Hoechst Fennica Ab
Postbox 237
00101 Helsinki 10
Finland
Tel: +35-80-8705721
Fax: +35-80-8709812
Telex: 12-4801

FRANCE
Tour Roussel Hoechst
1 Terrasse Bellini
92800 Puteaux
France

Behring Diagnostics
Division de la S.a.p.b.,
Hoechst-Behring
260, Avenue Napoleon
Bonaparte
92504 Rueil Malmaison
France
Tel: +33-1-47082661
Fax: +33-1-47082661
Telex: 631183

GERMANY
Behringwerke AG
PO Box 1212
65835 Liederbach
Germany
Tel: +49-69-34020
Fax: +49-69-303834
Telex: 416853

Behringwerke AG
Postfach 1140
35001 Marburg
Germany
Tel: +49-6421-390
Fax: +49-6421-66064
Telex: 48232001

GREECE
Hoechst Hellas AG
Pharma Division
10240 Athens
Greece
Tel: +30-1-809395
Fax: +30-1-8071577
Telex: 0215890

GUATEMALA
Quimica Hoechst de
Guatemala SA
Diagnosticos Behring
Apartado 155
km 15.5 Carretera Roosevelt
Guatemala City
Guatemala
Tel: +502-2-910011/15
Fax: +502-2-954016
Telex: 5946

GUYANA
Guyana Pharmaceutical Corp
Ltd
PO Box 160
La Penitence
Demerara
Guyana
Tel: +592-632815
Telex: 2203

HONG KONG
Hoechst China Ltd
23/F Shell Tower
Times Square, 1 Matheson

St.
Causeway Bay
Hong Kong
Tel: +852-5068333
Fax: +852-5062537

HUNGARY
Hoechst AG
Magyarorszagi kepviselet
Bajcsy-Zs ut. 12
1051 Budapest
Hungary
Tel: +36-1-179011
Fax: +36-1-182822
Telex: 225975

INDIA
E Merck (India) Ltd
Atus House
87 Dr Annie Besant Road,
Worli
Bombay 400018
India
Tel: +91-22-4922855
Fax: +91-22-4950354

INDONESIA
PT Mensa Binasukses
Pulo Bueran Kav. DD 1A
Jakarta Indust. Est.
Pulgadung
Jakarta 13939
Indonesia
Tel: +62-21-4601950
Fax: +62-21-4601953

IRELAND
Hoechst Ireland Ltd
Cookstown
Tallaght
Dublin 24
Ireland
Tel: +353-1-511544
Fax: +353-1-596068
Telex: 25158

ISRAEL
Chemipharm Ltd
43 Brodelzky Street
PO Box 17025
Tel Aviv 61170
Israel
Tel: +972-3-6422031
Fax: +972-3-6428762
Telex: 342204

ITALY
Istituto Behring SpA
Sistemi Diagnostici
Sede di Milano
Piazzale Stefano Turr 5
20149 Milan
Italy
Tel: +39-2-31071
Fax: +39-2-31072828
Telex: 320165

JAMAICA, W INDIES
HD Hopwood & Company Ltd
PO Box 165
3 Cari ftd. Ave
Kingston 11
Jamaica, W Indies
Tel: +1-809-92384816
Fax: +1-809-9236351
Telex: 2122

JAPAN
Hoechst Japan Ltd
10-16 Akasaka 8-chome
Pharma Division
Toyko 107
Japan
Tel: +81-3-4795111
Fax: +81-3-4791524
Telex: 242-2342

JORDAN
Salim Sabbagh Sons
Company
PO Box 346
Amman
Jordan
Tel: +962-6-6623158
Fax: +962-6-627376
Telex: 21529

KENYA
Hoechst East Africa Ltd
PO Box 30467
Nairobi
Kenya
Tel: +254-2-557744
Fax: +254-2-545837
Telex: 24031

KOREA
Han-Dok Remedia Ind. C., Ltd
Kangnam PO Box 1560
Seoul 135-615
Korea
Tel: +82-2-5275114
Fax: +82-2-5275002

KUWAIT
Yusuf Ibrahim Alghanim & Co.
W.L.L.
PO Box 435
13005 Safat
Kuwait
Tel: +965-5812148
Fax: +965-5844954
Telex: 23607

LEBANON
Union Pharmacy
PO Box 113-5461
Beyrouth
Lebanon
Telex: 21665/20680

MALAYSIA
Hoechst Malaysia SDN, BHD
12th Floor, Wisma,
Damansara
Jalan Semantan
PO Box 10540
Kuala Lumpur
Malaysia
Tel: +60-3-2549100
Fax: +60-3-2559420
Telex: 30370

MEXICO
Quimica Hoechst de Mexico
SA de CV
Direccion Farma Agro-Vet
Div. Behring Diagnostika
Tecoyotitla 412
Deleg. Alvaro Obregon
01050 Mexico DF
Mexico
Tel: +52-5-6612987
Fax: +52-5-6611612

NETHERLANDS
Hoechst Holland NV
Postbus 12987
1100 AZ Amsterdam
Netherlands
Tel: +31-20-5908514
Fax: +31-20-6910412
Telex: 12051

NEW ZEALAND
Hoechst New Zealand Ltd
CPO Box 67
21-39 Jellicoe Road
Panmure
Auckland
New Zealand
Tel: +64-9-5700700
Fax: +64-9-5709511
Telex: 2338

NIGERIA
Nigerian Hoechst plc
Pharma Division
Plot 144, Oba Akran Avenue
PO Box 261
Ikeja, Lagos
Nigeria
Tel: +234-1-900130/9
Fax: +234-1-964474
Telex: 26381

NORWAY
Norske Hoechst A/S
Okemveien 145
PO Box 177 Okern
0509 Oslo 5
Norway
Tel: +47-2-22727513
Fax: +47-2-22631828
Telex: 71744

OMAN
Muscat Pharmacy
PO Box 438
Muscat
Oman
Tel: +968-722297/702542
Fax: +968-795202
Telex: 8361

PAKISTAN
Progressive Medicals Ltd
415 Muhammadi House
1.1 Chundrigar Road
Karachi
Pakistan
Tel: +92-21-2402601
Fax: +92-21-2414323
Telex: 2603

PARAGUAY
C.E.I.S.A.
Casilla Correo 427
Asuncion
Paraguay
Tel: +595-21-490-25113

PERU
Merck Peruana SA
Avda. Monterrico Chico
Cuadra 2,
Urb. Santa Teresa
Lima 33
Peru
Tel: +51-14-499523
Fax: +51-14-499480

PHILIPPINES
Zuellig Pharma Corporation
PO Box 604
Manila
Philippines
Tel: +63-2-8191561
Fax: +63-2-7610138

POLAND
Hoechst Polska Sp. z.o.o.
ul. Stawki 2, 25 pietro
PO Box 15
00 950 Warsaw
Poland
Tel: +48-2-6353332
Fax: +48-2-6351546
Telex: 812298

PORTUGAL
Hoechst Portuguesa SA
Pharma Division
Apartado 6
2726 Mem Martins Codex
Portugal
Tel: +351-1-9212160
Fax: +351-1-3556762
Telex: 16380

QATAR
Doha Drug Store
PO Box 3331
Doha
Qatar
Tel: +974-426201
Fax: +974-423484
Telex: 4234

ROMANIA
Hoechst AG
Reprezentanta Tehnica
Hotel Bucuresti
Str. Luterana 2-4, Scara D2
Etaj 7, Ap. 19/20
Bukarest
Romania
Tel: +40-1-3125340
Fax: +40-1-3120075
Telex: 11646

RUSSIA
Hoechst
Pharma Moscow
Trjochprudnyj per 11/13
Moscow
Russia
Tel: +7-095-9236001
Fax: +7-095-2002206
Telex: 413138

SAUDI ARABIA
Fuad Al Fadhli
Trading Establishment
PO Box 3506
Riyadh
Saudi Arabia
Tel: +966-1-4550807
Fax: +966-1-4543356
Telex: 400071

SINGAPORE
Hoechst Singapore Pte Ltd
Tanjong Pagar
PO Box 102
Singapore
Tel: +65-2257227
Fax: +65-2257228
Telex: 21662

© KLUWER ACADEMIC PUBLISHERS 1994, ISSN 1381-5067

SLOVAKIA
Behring Institut GmbH
Altmannsdorfer Str 104
1127 Vienna
Austria
Tel: +43-1-80101
Telex: 133701

SLOVENIA
Behring Institut GmbH
Altmannsdorfer Str 104
1127 Vienna
Austria
Tel: +43-1-80101
Telex: 133701

SOUTH AFRICA
Novistan Ltd Behring
Diagnostics
326 Mark Street
Waltloo, Pretoria 0001
South Africa
Tel: +27-12-835372
Fax: +27-12-834121
Telex: 4-25879

SPAIN
Hoechst Iberica SA
Airbau 197-199
08021 Barcelona
Spain
Tel: +34-3-34198438
Fax: +34-3-34198256
Telex: 53160/52496

SRI LANKA
Hoechst (Ceylon) Company
Ltd
PO Box 1127
114 Ward Place
Colombo 8
Sri Lanka
Tel: +94-1-547620
Fax: +94-1-699006
Telex: 21648

SWEDEN
Svenska Hoechst AB
Box 42026
126 12 Stockholm 42
Sweden
Tel: +46-8-7757104
Fax: +46-8-198014
Telex: 10456

SWITZERLAND
Hoechst Pharma AG
Behring Abteilung
Postbox 8048
8048 Zurich
Switzerland
Tel: +41-1-4342627
Fax: +41-1-4318463
Telex: 822189

SYRIA
Tabasch Commerce
PO Box 1323
Aleppo
Syria
Fax: +963-21-235821

TAIWAN
Cheng Hsin Medical Supply
Co. Ltd
3th Fl, 50 Chang Av E. Rd
Section 1
Taipei

Taiwan
Tel: +886-2-5118022
Fax: +886-2-5118026

THAILAND
Hoechst Thai Limited
PO Box 1495
Bangkok
Thailand
Tel: +66-2-23329818
Fax: +66-2-2368155
Telex: 82312

TRINIDAD, W INDIES
Alstons Marketing Company
Ltd
PO Box 1256, Port of Spain
Uriah Butler Highway
Chaguanas
Trinidad, W Indies
Tel: +1809-6712713/20
Fax: +1809-6712857
Telex: 22284

TURKEY
Turk Hoechst Sanayi ve
Ticaret AS
Davutpasa Cad. No. 145
Topkapi 34020
Istanbul
Turkey
Tel: +90-1-5679500
Fax: +90-1-5679532
Telex: 30315/30316

UNITED ARAB EMIRATE
Al Ittihad Pharmacy Co.
PO Box 602
Abu Dhabi
United Arab Emirates
Tel: +971-2-211600
Fax: +971-2-211535
Telex: 22386

Al Ittihad Drug Store
PO Box 5374
Dubai
United Arab Emirates
Tel: +971-6-594585
Fax: +971-6-596490
Telex: 68292

Hoechst Consulting
Arabian Gulf Office
PO Box 2326
Dubai
United Arab Emirates
Tel: +971-4-221153/54
Telex: 47155

UNITED KINGDOM
Behring, A Division of
Hoechst UK Ltd
Hoechst House
50 Salisbury Road
PO Box 18
Hounslow
Middlesex, TW4 6JH
United Kingdom
Tel: +44-081-5707712
Fax: +44-081-5694834
Telex: 23284

URUGUAY
EMOL SA
Colon 1563, Of. 001
C.C. 6632
Montevideo

Uruguay
Tel: +598-2-962444
Fax: +598-2-963611
Telex: 23933

USA
Behring Diagnostics Inc
141 University Avenue
Westwood, MA 02090
USA
Tel: +1-617-320-3000
Fax: +1-617-320-3193

VENEZUELA
Laboratorios Geminis SRL
Apartado Postal 61290
Caracas 1060-A
Venezuela
Tel: +58-2-2621897
Fax: +58-2-335011
Telex: 27839

YUGOSLAVIA
Jugohemija
Farmacija
General Zdanova 31
11000 Belgrade
Yugoslavia
Tel: +38-11-341140
Fax: +38-11-331674
Telex: 11390

ZIMBABWE
Hoechst Zimbabwe (Pvt) Ltd
PO Box 3229
Harare
Zimbabwe
Tel: +263-4-700063
Fax: +263-4-704987
Telex: 26076

Binax Inc.

Corporate
Binax Inc.
217 Read Street
Portland, ME 04103
USA
Tel: +1-207-772-3988
Fax: +1-207-871-5751

Biochrom KG

Corporate
Biochrom KG
POB 46 0309
12213 Berlin
Germany
Tel: +49-30-77990642
Fax: +49-30-7710012

Biodata SpA (see Serono)

Corporate
Biodata SpA (see Serono)

Biokit

Corporate
Biokit
Llissa d'Amunt

08186 Barcelona
Spain
Tel: +34-3-8414250

BAG - Biologische Analysensystem GmbH

Corporate
BAG - Biologische
Analysensystem GmbH
Amstgerichtstrasse 1-5
35423 Lich
Germany
Tel: +49-6404-925-0
Fax: +49-6404-62554

---

bioMerieux sa

Corporate
bioMerieux sa
Marcy-L'Etoile 69280
France
Tel: +33-78872000
Fax: +33-78872090
Telex: 330 967

By region
AUSTRALIA
bioMerieux Vitek-Australia Pty
Ltd
Unit 1/6 Gladstone Road
Castle Hill, NSW 2154
Australia
Tel: +61-2-8911232

AUSTRIA
bioMerieux Osterreich
Lamezanstrasse 17
PO Box 124
1232 Vienna
Austria
Tel: +43-1677371
Fax: +43-167737133

BELGIUM
bioMerieux Benelux sa
Victor-Hugostraat 215
1040 Brussels
Belgium
Tel: +32-2-7365949
Fax: +32-2-7335597
Telex: 61909

BRAZIL
Biolab
Estrada do Mapua 491
Jacarepagua
22713 Rio de Janerio
Brazil
Tel: +55-21-4455454
Fax: +55-21-3426099
Telex: 2131211

CANADA
API produits de laboratoire/
bioMerieux Canada Inc
8114-B Route
Transcanadienne
Saint-Laurent Quebec, H4S
1M5
Canada
Tel: +1-514-3367-321
Fax: +1-514-3366-450

© KLUWER ACADEMIC PUBLISHERS 1994, ISSN 1381-5067

CHILE
bioMerieux Chile SA
Av. Ricardo Lyon 1899
Providencia/Casilla 2291
Santiago de Chile
Chile
Tel: +56-22514047
Fax: +56-22091604

FRANCE
bioMerieux sa
Marcy-L'Etoile 69280
France
Tel: +33-78872000
Fax: +33-78872090
Telex: 330 967

GERMANY
bioMerieux Deutschland
    GmbH
Weberstrasse 8
72633 Nurtingen
Germany
Tel: +49-702-230070
Fax: +49-702-236110
Telex: 7267414

HONG KONG
bioMerieux Vitek
8/F Parkview Commercial
    Building
9-11 Shelter St. Causeway
    Bay
Hong Kong
Tel: +852-8906067
Fax: +852-8955174

ITALY
bioMerieux Italia srl
Via G Moscati 9
00168 Rome
Italy
Tel: +39-6-3050208
Fax: +39-6-3050079
Telex: 625458

JAPAN
bioMerieux Japon Ltd
Yanagisawa bldg
14-12 Hirakawacho 2-chome
Chiyoda-ku
Tokyo 102
Japan
Tel: +81-3-5210-3221
Fax: +81-3-5210-3150

KOREA
bioMerieux Korea Office
Suit 1012 Samhung Bldg.,
    705-9
Yuksam-Dong, Kangnam-ku
Seoul
Korea
Tel: +850-25628260/1
Fax: +850-25658262

MEXICO
bioMerieux Mexico
Av. Cuauhtemoc n.1338 of
    404A
Delegacion Benito Juarez
C.P. 03310 Mexico, DF
Mexico
Tel: +52-5-56057957
Fax: +52-5-56040243

NETHERLANDS
bioMerieux Benelux BV

Bruistensingel 620
5232 AJ's Hertogenbosch
Pays-Bas
Netherlands
Tel: +31-73-144592
Fax: +31-73-139930
Telex: 50029

POLAND
bioMerieux Polska Sp zo.o
ul. Zelazna 68
00866 Warsaw
Poland
Tel: +48-2-39120313
Fax: +48-2-39120313

PORTUGAL
bioMerieux Portugal
Calcada de Santa Catarina
9-C r/c Dto
Cruz Quebrada - 1495 Lisbon
Portugal
Tel: +351-1-4150278
Fax: +351-1-4150118

SPAIN
bioMerieux sa
Manuel Tovar 36
Madrid 28034
Spain
Tel: +34-1-3581142
Fax: +34-1-3580629
Telex: 46620

SWEDEN
Jean-Francoise Fougere
Triolab
PO Box 2109
43102 Molndal
Sweden
Tel: +46-31819650
Fax: +46-31169908

SWITZERLAND
bioMerieux sa
51 avenue Blanc
1202 Geneva
Switzerland
Tel: +41-22-7325760
Fax: +41-22-7388842

UNITED KINGDOM
bioMerieux UK Ltd
Grafton Way
Basingstoke
Hampshire, RG22 6HY
United Kingdom
Tel: +44-0256-461881
Fax: +44-0256-816863
Telex: 858055

USA
Vitek Systems
595 Anglum Drive
Hazelwood
Missouri 63042-2395
USA
Tel: +1-314-731-8500
Fax: +1-314-731-8800

Vitek Systems
1022 Hingham Street
02370 Rockland, MA
USA
Tel: +1-617-871-4442
Fax: +1-617-871-3470

Bion Enterprises Ltd

Corporate
Bion Enterprises Ltd
674 Busse Highway
Park Ridge, IL 60068
USA
Tel: +1-708-692-9333
Fax: +1-708-692-4747

Bio-Stat Ltd

Corporate
Bio-Stat Ltd
Bio-Stat House
Pepper Road, Hazel Grove
Stockport, SK7 5BW
United Kingdom
Tel: +44-061-483-5884
Fax: +44-061-483-5778

Biotest AG

Corporate
Biotest AG
Landsteinerstrasse 5
63303 Dreieich
Germany
Tel: +49-6103-8010
Fax: +49-6103-801130
Telex: 4 185 429

By region
AUSTRIA
Biotest Pharmazeutika GmbH
Einsiedlergasse 58
1053 Vienna
Austria
Tel: +43-1-5451561
Fax: +43-1-545156137
Telex: 134 644

BENELUX
NV Biotest Seralc SA
Weiveldlaan 41, bus 31
1930 Zaventem
Belgium
Tel: +32-2-7257560
Fax: +32-2-7257598

CYPRUS
Cyprus Pharmaceutical Org.
    Ltd
Papaellina House
35 King Paul 1 Street
PO Box 1005
Nicosia 136
Cyprus
Tel: +357-2-443140
Fax: +357-2-365136
Telex: 2 417

CZECHOSLOVAKIA
Merck Spol.
Slavetinska 26
19000 Prague 9 - Klanovice
Czechoslovakia
Tel: +42-2-7882063
Fax: +42-2-7881203

DENMARK
Meda S/A

Dynamovej 11
2730 Herlev
Denmark
Tel: +45-42844211
Fax: +45-845199
Telex: 35 289

Struers A/S
Valhojs Alle 176
2610 Redovre/Copenhagen
Denmark
Tel: +45-708090
Fax: +45-721320
Telex: 19 625

FRANCE
Biotest S.a.r.l.
Zone Industrielle Centre
80 Rue Helene Boucher
78530 Buc
France
Tel: +33-1-39202080
Fax: +33-1-39202081
Telex: 696229

GERMANY
Biotest AG
Landsteinerstrasse 5
63303 Dreieich
Germany
Tel: +49-6103-8010
Fax: +49-6103-801130
Telex: 4 185 429

HUNGARY
Biotest Ungam
Dobsinai Utca 6/B
1124 Budapest
Hungary
Tel: +36-1-1561697
Fax: +36-1-1561697

ITALY
Biotest S.r.l.
Via Leonardo da Vinci, 43
20090 Trezzano sul Naviglio
Italy
Tel: +39-2-48401818
Fax: +39-2-48402068
Telex: 315 453

JAPAN
Biotest Japan Liason Office
Cuatro Mita Building
Mita 4-1-4 Minato-ku
Tokyo 108
Japan
Tel: +81-3-52321654
Fax: +81-3-52321655

SWITZERLAND
Biotest (Schweiz) AG
Bahnhofstr. 18
5504 Othmarsingen
Switzerland
Tel: +41-64-562770
Fax: +41-64-562750

UNITED KINGDOM
Biotest (UK) Ltd
Unit 21A
Monkspath Business Park
Highlands Road
Shirley, Solihull
West Midlands
B90 4NZ
United Kingdom
Tel: +44-021-7333393

Fax: +44-021-7333066
Telex: 335 745

USA
Biotest Diagnostics Corp
66 Ford Road, Suite 131
Denville, NJ 07834
USA
Tel: +1-201-625-1300
Fax: +1-201-625-9454

BioWhittaker Inc

Corporate
BioWhittaker Inc
PO Box 127
Walkersville
USA
Tel: +1-301-8987025
Fax: +1-301-8458291

Boehringer Mannheim GmbH

Corporate
Boehringer Mannheim GmbH
Sandhofer Strasse 116
68305 Mannheim
Germany
Tel: +49-621-7590
Fax: +49-621-7592890
Telex: 462420

By region
ARGENTINA
Boehringer Mannheim
Argentina SAClel
Viamonte 2213/15
1056 Buenos Aires
Argentina

AUSTRALIA
Boehringer Mannheim
Australia Pty Ltd
PO Box 955
31 Victoria Avenue
Castle Hill
New South Wales 2154
Australia

AUSTRIA
Boehringer Mannheim GmbH
Wien
Engelhorngasse 3
1210 Vienna
Austria
Tel: +43-222-27787
Fax: +43-222-8712

BELGIUM
Boehringer Mannheim
Belgium
Ave des Croix de Guerre 90
1120 Brussels
Belgium
Tel: +32-2-2474747
Fax: +32-2-2474680

CANADA
Boehringer Mannheim
Canada Ltd
201 Armand-Frappier Blvd
Laval
Quebec, H7V 4AZ

Canada
Tel: +1-514-686-7050
Fax: +1-514-686-7559

CHILE
Boehringer Mannheim de
Chile Ltda
Calderon 43
Casilla de Correo 16 408
Santiago 9
Chile

FRANCE
Boehringer Mannheim France
SA
2 Ave du Vercors
BP 59
38242 Meylan Cedex
France

GERMANY
Boehringer Mannheim GmbH
Sandhofer Strasse 116
68305 Mannheim
Germany
Tel: +49-621-7590
Fax: +49-621-7592890
Telex: 462420

GUATEMALA
Boehringer Mannheim de
Guatemala SA
Oficina Regional de Centro
America y Republica
Dominicana
2A Avenida 2-67, Zona 10
Apartado Postal 1675
Guatemala

INDIA
Boehringer Mannheim India
Ltd
54A Mathuradas Vissanji
Road
Chakala, Andheri (East)
Bombay 400093
India

ITALY
Boehringer Mannheim Italia
SpA
Via San Uguzzone 5
21026 Milan
Italy

JAPAN
Boehringer Mannheim Japan
KK
10-11 Toranomon, 3-chome
Minato-ku
Tokyo 105
Japan

MEXICO
Farmaceuticos Lakeside SA
de CV
Huizaches 25
Coo. Rancho Los Colorines
14386 Mexico DF
Mexico

NETHERLANDS
Boehringer Mannheim BV
Postbus 1007
1300 BA Almere
Netherlands

NEW ZEALAND
Boehringer Mannheim NZ Ltd
PO Box 62-089
15 Rakino Way
Mt Wellington
Auckland
New Zealand

PORTUGAL
Laboratorios Boehringer
Mannheim de Portugal Lda
Rua Diogo do Couto
1-B, Apartado 46
2795 Linda-A-Velha
Portugal

PUERTO RICO
Boehringer Mannheim Puerto
Rico Inc
Punto Oro Industrial Park
Box 7021/Marginal Road
Ponce 00731
Puerto Rico

SINGAPORE
Boehringer Mannheim (Far
East) Pte Ltd
7th Storey Inchcape House
450-452 Alexandra Rd
Singapore 0511
Singapore

SOUTH AFRICA
Boehringer Mannheim (South
Africa) Pty Ltd
PO Box 1927
259 Kent Avenue
Randburg 2125
South Africa

SPAIN
Boehringer Mannheim SA
Copernico 660 y 61-63
Apartado 5052
08006 Barcelona
Spain

SWEDEN
Boehringer Mannheim
Scandinavia AB
Box 147
Karlsbodavagen 30
161 26 Bromma
Sweden

SWITZERLAND
Boehringer Mannheim
(Schweiz) AG
Industriestrasse
6343 Rotkreuz
Switzerland

UNITED KINGDOM
Boehringer Mannheim UK
(Pharmaceuticals) Ltd
Simpson Parkway
Kirkton Campus
Livingston
W Lothian, EH54 7BH
United Kingdom

Boehringer Mannheim UK Ltd
(Diagnostic &
Biochemicals) Ltd
Bell Lane
Lewes
E Sussex, BN7 1LG
United Kingdom

URUGUAY
Boehringer Mannheim
Uruguay SA
Bv Gral Artigas 1436
11600 Montivideo
Uruguay

USA
Boehringer Mannheim Corp
9115 Hague Rd
Indianapolis, IN 46250-0457
USA

De Puy Inc
PO Box 988
700 Orthopaedic Drive
Warsaw, IN 46581-0988
USA

Boehringer Mannheim
Pharmaceuticals Corp
15204 Omega Drive
Rockville, MD 20850-3241
USA

Microgenics Corporation
2380A Bisso Lane
Concord, CA 94520
USA

ZAIRE
Pharmakina SARL
BP 122
Cyangugu/Rwanda
Zaire

Boule Diagnostics AB

Corporate
Boule Diagnostics AB
Lunastigen 3
14144 Huddinge
Sweden
Tel: +46-8-7460035
Fax: +46-8-7468496

Bouty SpA

Corporate
Bouty SpA
Viale Casiraghi 471
20099 Seston San Giovanni
Milan
Italy
Tel: +39-2-262891
Fax: +39-2-26221305

Cambridge Biotech Corporation

Corporate
Cambridge Biotech
Corporation
365 Plantation Street
Worcester, MA 01605
USA
Tel: +1-508-797-5777
Fax: +1-508-791-0224

By region
IRELAND
Cambridge Biotech Ltd

Mervue Industrial Estate
Galway
Ireland
Tel: +353-91-757534
Fax: +353-91-752551

USA
Cambridge Biotech
  Corporation
365 Plantation Street
Worcester, MA 01605
USA
Tel: +1-508-797-5777
Fax: +1-508-791-0224

Cellabs Pty Ltd

Corporate
Cellabs Pty Ltd
Unit 7, 27 Dale Street
PO Box 421
Brookvale
New South Wales 2100
Australia
Tel: +61-2-9050133
Fax: +61-2-9056426

Centocor

Corporate
Centocor
200 Great Valley Parkway
Malvern
PA 19355-1307
USA
Tel: +1-215-889-4666
Fax: +1-215-889-4666

By region
AUSTRALIA
Immuno Diagnostics
c/o Palk Freight
12 Ewan Street
Mascot
New South Wales 2020
Australia

FRANCE
CIS Bioindustries
CIS Bio International
BP No. 32
91192 Gif-Sur-Yvette Cedex
France

GERMANY
BYK Sangtec
c/o Manfred Borchardt
  Luftfract
Frankfurt Int. Airport
Frankfurt
Germany

Buecker
Hermann Hesse Strasse 56
55127 Mainz
Germany

Boehringer Mannheim GmbH
c/o Rhenus Customs Brokers
Frankfurt Int. Airport
Frankfurt
Germany

ITALY
Sorin Biomedica SpA

c/o Mr Baldazzi, Broker
Turin Airport
Turin
Italy

Ares Serono Diag.
Rinaldo Rinaldi/Fiumicino Arpt
For Ares Serono Diag.
  Biodata
via Tiburtina Valeria KM
  19600
Guidonia Monticelio
Rome
Italy

Medical Systems SpA
c/o G Damiano, Agent
Cristoforo Columbia Airport
Genoa
Italy

JAPAN
Toray Fuji Bionics, Inc.
11-12 Kitimachi 1 Chrome
Nerima-ku
Tokyo 176
Japan

SPAIN
Izasa SA
Consigned to Munoz Y
  Cabrero
C Balmes 49
08001 Barcelona
Spain

SWITZERLAND
Hoffman La-Roche
Diagnostic Division
Department DIA/T, Building
  203
4002 Basle
Switzerland

Sorin Switzerland
Pretorio 13 Sugano
6901
Switzerland

USA
Centocor
200 Great Valley Parkway
Malvern
PA 19355-1307
USA
Tel: +1-215-889-4666
Fax: +1-215-889-4666

Hybritech Inc.
7330 Carroll Road
San Diego, CA 92121
USA

Abbott Diagnostics
Skokie Warehouse Building,
  K-2
Route 41 & 22nd Street
North Chicago, IL 60064
USA

Amersham Corporation
2636 South Clearbrook
Arlington Heights
IL 60005
USA

Chembio
Diagnostic Systems
Inc

Corporate
Chembio Diagnostic Systems
  Inc
3661 Horse Block Road
Medford, NY 11763
USA
Tel: +1-516-924-1135
Fax: +1-561-924-6033

Chimica
Diagnostica

Corporate
Chimica Diagnostica
Via Nicola d'Apulia 15
21025 Milan
Italy

By region
CROATIA
Chrono Poduzece SPO
Tijardoviceva 14
58000 Split
Croatia
Tel: +38-58-364664
Fax: +38-58-364901

FRANCE
Labinter SA
15 rue du Quattre Septembre
13100 Aix-en-Provence
Cedex 01
France
Tel: +33-42384858
Fax: +33-42276801

ITALY
Chimica Diagnostica
via Nicola d'Apulia 15
20125 Milan
Italy
Tel: +39-2-2896742
Fax: +39-2-2896779

JORDAN
Jordan Lab. Equipment Est.
Al-Sayegh Center, 1st Floor
Al-Abdali
Amman
Jordan
Tel: +962-6-615470
Fax: +962-6-601846

PORTUGAL
Rosalina Carvalho
Importacao e Distribuicao de
  Equipaamentos e Reagentes
  Lab.
Av. dos Missionarios 62
2735 Cacem
Portugal
Tel: +351-1-9143318
Fax: +351-1-9143318

SAUDI ARABIA
Mada Al-Saudi
Olyah Prince Sultan Bin
  Abdulaziz St.
Behind Arab National Bank
PO Box 9671

Riyadh 11433
Saudi Arabia
Tel: +966-1-4640652
Fax: +966-1-4647379

SPAIN
Coulter Cientifica SA
Poligono Industrial 2
La Fuensanta, Parcela 11
28936 Mostoles (Madrid)
Spain
Tel: +34-91-6453011
Fax: +34-91-6455690

SRI LANKA
Asiri Hospitals Ltd
181 Kirula Road
Colombo 5
Sri Lanka
Tel: +94-1-500608
Fax: +94-1-698315

TURKEY
AB Medikal
Sanayi ve Ticaret Ltd
Mecidiye Koy Cad 24/2
Istanbul
Turkey
Tel: +90-1-2244470
Fax: +90-1-2249767

Clark Laboratories

Corporate
Clark Laboratories
PO Box 1059
Jamestown, NY 14702-1059
USA
Tel: +1-716-483-3851
Fax: +1-716-488-1990

Coulter Electronics
Ltd

Corporate
Coulter Electronics Ltd
Northwell Drive
Luton, Beds
LU3 3RH
United Kingdom
Fax: +44-524-490390
Telex: 825074

DAKO A/S

Corporate
DAKO A/S
Produktionsvej 42
Postbox 1359
2600 Glostrup
Denmark
Tel: +45-44920044
Fax: +45-42841822
Telex: 35128

By region
ARGENTINA
Chemetron Latinoamericana
  SA
Junin 262
PB 1 Capital Federal
1026 Buenos Aires
Argentina

Tel: +54-1-9538918
Fax: +54-1-9538918
Telex: 9900

AUSTRALIA
Bio Scientific Pty Ltd
PO Box 78
28 Monroe Avenue
Kirrawee
Gymea
New South Wales 2227
Australia
Tel: +61-2-5212177
Fax: +61-2-5423037

AUSTRIA
Bender and Co GmbH
Dr. Boehringergasse 5-11
PO Box 103
1121 Vienna
Austria
Tel: +43-1-801050
Fax: +43-1-80105488
Telex: 132430

BELGIUM
Prosan bvba sprl
Maurits Sabbestraat 67
9050 Gentbrugge
Belgium
Tel: +32-91-313704
Fax: +32-91-319898

BRAZIL
Embrabio-Empressa
 Brasileira de Biotechnologia
 Ltda
Rua Apinages 1.081
05017 Sao Paulo/Sp
Brazil
Tel: +55-11-2625511
Fax: +55-11-2630272
Telex: 035970

CANADA
Dimension Laboratories Inc.
12 Falconer Drive, Unit 4
Mississauga
Ontario L5N 3L9
Canada
Tel: +1-416-858-8510
Fax: +1-416-858-8801

CHILE
PROLAB
Vergara 24
Oficina 908
Casilla 3645
Santiago
Chile
Tel: +56-2-6987215
Fax: +56-2-6989617

COSTA RICA

Laboratorios Zeiedon SA
Apartado Postal 5236-1000
San Jose
Costa Rica
Tel: +506-353959
Fax: +506-351275

CYPRUS
Medisell Co. Ltd
55A Limassol Avenue
PO Box 8318
Nicosia
Cyprus

Tel: +357-2-311362
Fax: +357-2-494300

DENMARK
DAKO A/S
Produktionsvej 42
Postbox 1359
2600 Glostrup
Denmark
Tel: +45-44920044
Fax: +45-42841822
Telex: 35128

ECUADOR
Proveedores Para
 Laboratorios C, Ltda
Edificio-Pro-Lab.
Luis Urdaneta Y Ave
del Ejercito
Guayaquil
Ecuador
Tel: +593-4-281943
Fax: +593-4-285953
Telex: 42985

EGYPT
LAB TECHNOLOGY
4 Leith Ben Saad Str.
PO Box 5959
Heliopolis West 113351
Cairo
Egypt
Tel: +20-2-2351785
Fax: +20-2-2428366
Telex: 22127

FINLAND
COFACTOR
Suomen biotekniikka Oy
Kavallinmaki 13
02700 Kauniainen
Finland
Tel: +358-0-594822
Fax: +358-0-594864

Soumen biotekniikka Oy
 Cofactor
Kavallinmaki 13
02700 Kauniainen
Finland

FRANCE
DAKO SA
2 rue Albert Einstein
BP 149
78196 Trappes Cedex
France
Tel: +33-30500050
Fax: +33-30500011
Telex: 695029

GERMANY
DAKO Diagnostika GmbH
Am Stadtrand
22047 Hamburg
Germany
Tel: +49-40-6937026
Fax: +49-40-6952741

GREECE
Ange M. Calliphronas
4 Evripidou Street
10559 Athens
Greece
Tel: +30-1-3213272
Fax: +30-1-3218871

HONG KONG
China South Technology Ltd
Rm 1303-4, 13/F, Remex
Centre
42 Wong Chuh Hang Road
Hong Kong
Tel: +852-5528339
Fax: +852-5526883

INDIA
J Mitra & Bros. Pvt. Ltd
A-180, Okhla
Industrial Area, Phase 1
Okhla
New Delhi 110020
India
Tel: +91-11-6818971
Fax: +91-11-6818970
Telex: 031-75314

INDONESIA
PT DWI Marga Sakti
J1 Kemuning No. 17
Tomang Raya
PO Box 4129 Jkt
Jakarta Barat
Indonesia
Tel: +62-21-597102
Fax: +62-21-591286

IRAN
Eskan Teb Tech. Co.
6 Business Section, ESKAN
Buildings
Mirdamad Avenue
PO Box 19395
1836 Teheran
Iran
Tel: +98-21-8087602
Fax: +98-21-4279491
Telex: 214158

ISRAEL
Tzamal Ltd
21 Gonen Street
PO Box 3064
Kiryat Matalon
Petac Tiqva
Israel
Tel: +972-3-9240288
Fax: +972-3-9240259
Telex: 381542

ITALY
DAKO SpA
Via G. Fantoli 21/17
20138 Milan
Italy
Tel: +39-2-58011221
Fax: +39-2-504778

JAPAN
DAKO Japan Co. Ltd
Hiraoka Building
Nishinotouin-higashiiru
Shijo-dori, Shimogyo-ku
Kyoto 600
Japan
Tel: +81-75-2113655
Fax: +81-75-2111755

KOREA
Fine Chemical Co. Ltd
Garden Tower Building, Rm
No. 1103
98-78 Wun Ni-Dong, Jong Ro-
Go
KPO Box 1260

Seoul
Korea
Tel: +82-2-7447859
Fax: +82-2-7445281

KUWAIT
WARBA Medical Supplies Co.
Nakib Building, 4th Floor
Abu Bakir Street, Al Jiblah
PO Box 26267
13123 Safat
Kuwait
Tel: +965-2426939
Fax: +965-2429482
Telex: 44470

MALAYSIA
General Scientific Co. Sdn.
 Bhd
No. 7 Jalan 222
Section 51 A
46100 Petaling Jaya
Selangor Darul Ehsan
Malaysia
Tel: +60-3-7575433
Fax: +60-3-7571768
Telex: 374431

MALTA
Michele Perssso Ltd
Catalunya Building, Psaila
 Street
B'Kara
Malta
Tel: +356-492191
Fax: +356-482593

MEXICO
Dostym SA de CV
J.GPE. Montenegro No. 2325
Col. Arcos Sur.
CP 44150
Guadalajara
Jalisco
Mexico
Tel: +52-36-6153385
Fax: +52-36-5236153513
Telex: 683226

NETHERLANDS
ITK diagnostics bv
Johan Enschedeweg 13
1422 DR Uithoom
Netherlands
Tel: +31-2975-68893
Fax: +31-2975-63458

NEW ZEALAND
Med-Bio Enterprises Ltd
PO Box 33-135
Barrington, Christchurch
New Zealand
Tel: +64-3-3381020
Fax: +64-3-3380028

NORWAY
Bio-Test A/S
Idrettsveien 2
PO Box 66
1580 Rygge
Norway
Tel: +47-69261777
Fax: +47-69261760

OMAN
Mustafa & Tawad Trading Co.
 LLC
S & I Dept.

PO Box 4918
Ruwi
Oman
Tel: +968-709955
Fax: +968-54005

PANAMA
Importador DMD SA
Apartado 8556 Calle 31
Esto No. 1-95
Panama
Tel: +507-270537/251247
Fax: +507-271246

PARAGUAY
Dr Ruben A Sosky
Calidad, Mexico 923
Ascuncion
Paraguay
Tel: +595-21-447680
Fax: +595-21-447392

PERU
Representaciones Atlanta SA
Av. Republica de Panama
NRO 465
Callao 1
Peru
Tel: +51-14-652421
Fax: +51-14-654833

PHILIPPINES
Levin's International Corp.
3rd Floor R. Syjuco Building
993 E. Delos Santos Ave
cor. Bansalangin St, Diliman
Qeuzon City
Philippines
Tel: +63-2-974475/2
Fax: +63-2-984841

POLAND
ALAB sp. 20.0
Ul. Pasteura 3
02-093 Warsaw
Poland
Tel: +48-2-6598571
Fax: +48-2-6582059

PORTUGAL
Labometer LDA
Rua Duque de Palmela No.
30, 1-G
1200 Lisbon
Portugal
Tel: +351-1-537284
Fax: +351-1-3525066
Telex: 18489

SAUDI ARABIA
Medical Business Centre,
MBC
PO Box 189
Jeddah 21411
Saudi Arabia
Tel: +966-2-6421437
Fax: +966-2-6442502

SINGAPORE
Lab Essentials (S) Pte Ltd
108 Pasir Panjang Road
#02-02, Amcol Warehouse
Singapore 0511
Singapore
Tel: +65-4794009
Fax: +65-4790013

SOUTH AFRICA
Southern Cross
Biotechnology (Pty) Ltd
PO Box 23681
Claremont 7735
South Africa
Tel: +27-21-615166
Fax: +27-21-617734

SPAIN
Atom SA
Passeig d'Amunt 18
08024 Barcelona
Spain
Tel: +34-3-2847904
Fax: +34-3-2108255
Telex: 51227

SWEDEN
DAKOPATTS AB
Box 13
72521 Alosjo
Sweden
Tel: +46-8-996000
Fax: +46-8-996065

SWITZERLAND
IG-Instrumenten Gesellschaft
AG
Raffelstrasse 32
8045 Zurich
Switzerland
Tel: +41-1-4613311
Fax: +41-1-4613001
Telex: 813432

Lablink
PO Box 178
8059 Zurich
Switzerland

THAILAND
Science Tech. Co. Ltd
321/43 Nanglinchee Road
Chongnondsee
Yannawa
Bangkok 10120
Thailand
Tel: +66-2-2854101-3
Fax: +66-2-2854856
Telex: 82731

TURKEY
Hayat Corporation Inc.
Millet Cad. Renk Apt. No 75
Kat:4 D-8
34280 Findilezade
Istanbul
Turkey
Tel: +90-1-5879887
Fax: +90-1-5879402

UNITED ARAB EMIRATES
Al-Zahrawi Medical
PO Box No. 5973
Dubai
United Arab Emirates
Tel: +971-4-622728
Fax: +971-4-625506

UNITED KINGDOM
DAKO Ltd
16 Manor Courtyard
Hughenden Avenue
High Wycombe
Bucks, HP13 5RE
United Kingdom
Tel: +44-0494-452016

Fax: +44-0494-441553

DAKO Diagnostics Ltd
Denmark House
Angel Drove
Ely, Cambridgeshire
CA7 4ET
United Kingdom
Tel: +44-0353-669911
Fax: +44-0353-668989

URUGUAY
Poliuruguay srl
Avda Uruguay 1771
Montevideo
Uruguay
Tel: +598-2-402365
Fax: +598-2-409017

USA
DAKO Corporation
6392 Via Real
Carpinteria, CA 93013
USA
Tel: +1-805-566-6655
Fax: +1-805-566-6688
Telex: 658481

ZIMBABWE
National Diagnostics Ltd
PO Box 3535
Harare
Zimbabwe
Tel: +263-4-791615
Fax: +263-4-728055

Diagast Laboratories

Corporate
Diagast Laboratories
59 Rue de Trevise
BP 2034
59014 Lille Cedex
France
Tel: +33-20526800
Fax: +33-20520610

Diamedix Corporation

Corporate
Diamedix Corporation
2140 North Miami Avenue
Miami, FL 33127
USA
Tel: +1-305-324-2300
Fax: +1-305-324-2395

Diesse Srl

Corporate
Diesse Srl
50020 Sanbuca
Firenze
Italy
Tel: +39-55-8071371
Fax: +39-55-8071373

E. Merck

Corporate
E. Merck
Diagnostics Division
Frankfurter Strasse 250
64293 Darmstadt
Germany
Tel: +49-6151-720
Fax: +49-6151-722000

By region
ARGENTINA
Merck Quimica Argentina
SAIC
Casilla correo 1442
1000 Buenos Aires
Argentina
Tel: +54-1-5510027
Fax: +54-1-112135
Telex: 21733

AUSTRALIA
Merck Pty
207 Colchester Road
Kilsyth
Victoria 3137
Australia
Tel: +61-2-7285855
Fax: +61-2-7281351
Telex: 33596

AUSTRIA
Merck Gesellschaft m.b.H.
Zimbagasse 5
Postfach 700
1147 Vienna
Austria
Tel: +43-1-9716110
Fax: +43-1-975560
Telex: 133188

BANGLADESH
GA Traders Ltd
PO Box 3430
16, Motijheel Commercial
Area
Dhaka 2100
Bangladesh
Tel: +880-227299/236187
Fax: +880-2863472

BELGIUM
Merck Belgolabo NV-SA
Brusselsesteenweg 288
3090 Overijse
Belgium
Tel: +32-6-890711
Fax: +32-6-879120
Telex: 23807

BOLIVIA
Corimex Ltda
Calle Goitia 135
Cajon Postal 4788
La Paz
Bolivia
Tel: +591-320216
Fax: +591-391230
Telex: 3508

BRAZIL
Quimitra
Comercio e Industria SA
Caixa Postal 70556
22741 Rio de Janeiro
Brazil

Tel: +55-21-3424646
Fax: +55-21-3421263
Telex: 2123792

BURMA
Inspection & Agency Corp.
Agency Division
PO Box 404
No. 383 Mahanbandoola
  Street
Rangoon
Burma
Tel: +95-1-76045/73169
Telex: 21215

CANADA
BDH Inc.
350 Evans Avenue
Toronto
Ontario M8Z 1K5
Canada
Tel: +1-416-255-8521
Fax: +1-416-255-7453
Telex: 6967678

CHILE
Merck Quimica Chilena Soc.
  Lda.
Francisco de Paulo Taforo
  1981
Casilla 4232
Santiago de Chile
Chile
Tel: +56-2-381160
Fax: +56-2-383527
Telex: 440197

CHINA
Jebsen & Co. Ltd
China Trade Division, EMO-
  Dept.
Prince's Building, 23rd Floor
GPO Box 97
Hongkong
Tel: +852-8437978
Fax: +852-681742
Telex: 73221

COLOMBIA
Merck Colombia SA
Apartado Aereo 9896
Bogota 6 DE
Colombia
Tel: +57-1-2907855
Fax: +57-1-2628881
Telex: 41405

COSTA RICA
Cooperation Cefa SA
Apartado 10300
San Jose de Costa Rica
Costa Rica
Tel: +506-322122/203040
Fax: +506-327125
Telex: 2557

CYPRUS
Markides & Vouros Ltd
PO Box 2002
5A + B Pargas Street
Nicosia
Cyprus
Tel: +357-2-475121/464193
Fax: +357-2-457158
Telex: 2939

CZECHOSLOVAKIA
Merck Spol sro

Slawetinska 26
1900 Prague-Klanovice
Czechoslovakia
Tel: +42-8-7881203

DENMARK
Merck Denmark AS
Skodsborgvej 48
2830 Virum
Denmark
Tel: +45-42856622
Fax: +45-45831224

ECUADOR
Merck Ecuador CA
Casilla 1701 2574
Quito
Ecuador
Tel: +593-2-561150
Fax: +593-2-562703
Telex: 22252

EGYPT
Akhnaton Trading &
  Representation
12 Muntazeh Street
Zamalek
PO Box 1002
Cairo
Egypt
Tel: +20-2-3404945
Fax: +20-2-3412677
Telex: 93882

EL SALVADOR
Merck El Salvador SA
Apartado Postal 2039
11 Avenida Norte Bis 513
San Salvador
El Salvador
Tel: +503-228381
Fax: +503-211277

FINLAND
Merck Oy
Niittysillantie 5 D
02200 Espoo
Finland
Tel: +358-0-4521644
Fax: +358-0-426811
Telex: 123348

FRANCE
Laboratoires Merck Clevenot
  SA
Division Laboratoire
5/9 Rue Anquetil
94736 Nogent sur Marne
France
Tel: +33-43945400
Fax: +33-48765815
Telex: 261374

Merck Clevenot SA
Division Laboratoire
5/9 rue Anquetil
94731 Nogent-sur-Marne
France
Tel: +33-43945400
Fax: +33-48765786
Telex: 261374

GERMANY
E. Merck
Diagnostics Division
Frankfurter Strasse 250
64293 Darmstadt
Germany

Tel: +49-6151-720
Fax: +49-6151-722000

GREECE
Merck-Hellas GmbH
PO Box 72545
16410 Argyroupoli
Greece
Tel: +30-9929944
Fax: +30-9953214
Telex: 216101

GUATEMALA
Merck Centroamericana SA
Apartado postal 1651
Ciudad de Guatemala
Guatemala
Tel: +502-2-922111
Fax: +502-2-941543
Telex: 5110

HONDURAS
Drogueria Paysen
SA de CV
Apartado 252
Tegucigalpa
Honduras
Tel: +504-325010/325251
Fax: +504-311110
Telex: 1111

HUNGARY
Merck Kft
Keteli Karoly 15/b
1024 Budapest
Hungary
Tel: +36-1-358166
Fax: +36-1-158562

INDIA
E. Merck India Ltd
87 Dr Annie Besant Road
PO Box 16554
Bombay 400018
India
Tel: +91-22-4922855
Fax: +91-22-4922354

INDONESIA
PT Multiredjeki Kita
Jalan Raya Gedong Desa No.
  8
Pasar Rebo
Jakarta Timur 13760
PO Box 4387
Jakarta 10001
Indonesia
Tel: +62-21-8402091/94
Fax: +62-21-8402095
Telex: 4-8472

IRAN
Merck Trading AG
PO Box 15745/653
Tehran
Iran
Tel: +98-21-890116
Fax: +98-21-890116
Telex: 212282

IRELAND
Norman Lauder Ltd
Dunfirth
Butterfield Avenue
Rathfarnham
Dublin 14
Ireland
Tel: +353-1-932643

Fax: +353-1-931606
Telex: 93392

ISRAEL
Mercury Chemical Agencies
  Ltd
7 Hasharoshet St.
PO Box 6
Ramat Hasharon 47100
Israel
Tel: +972-5-401215
Fax: +972-5-408403
Telex: 341302

ITALY
Bracco Industria Chimica SpA
Via E. Folli 50
20134 Milan
Italy
Tel: +39-2-21771
Fax: +39-2-26410678
Telex: 311185

IVORY COAST
Societe Polychimie
01-BP 3907
Abidjan 01
Republic de Cote d'Ivoire
Ivory Coast
Tel: +225-355667/357688
Fax: +225-351385
Telex: 439298

JAPAN
Kanto Chemical Co. Inc
2-8 Nihombashi-Honcho-3-
  chome
Chuo-ku
Tokyo 103
Japan
Tel: +81-3-2706500
Fax: +81-3-6690823
Telex: 2223446

Merck Japan Ltd
ARCO Tower, 5F
8-1 Shimomeguro 1-chome
Meguro-ku
Tokyo 153
Japan
Tel: +81-3-54344722
Fax: +81-3-54344706
Telex: 2226868

JORDAN
Henry Marroum & Sons
Prince Mohammed Street
PO Box 589
Amman
Jordan
Tel: +962-6-623523
Fax: +962-6-638088

KOREA
Merck Korea Ltd
Yeong-Dong
PO Box 312
Seoul
Korea
Tel: +82-2-5555964
Fax: +82-2-5571440
Telex: 26803

KUWAIT
Bader Sultan & Bros. Co. Ltd
6th Ring Road
PO Box 867
13009 Safat

Kuwait
Tel: +965-4332566
Fax: +965-4334217

MALAYSIA
Merck (Malaysia) SDN BHD
No. 25 Jalan 2/71
Taman Tun Dr., Ismail
60000 Kuala Lumpur
Malaysia
Tel: +60-7-178922
Fax: +60-7-178925

MEXICO
Merck-Mexico SA
Apartado 8619
Mexico DF 06000
Mexico
Tel: +52-5-7269015
Fax: +52-5-3590759
Telex: 1761818

MONACO/ALGERIA
Merck Clevenot SA
Division Laboratoire
5/9, rue Anquetil
94731 Nogent-sur-Marne
France
Tel: +33-43945400
Fax: +33-48765815
Telex: 261374

NETHERLANDS
E. Merck Netherland BV
Basisweg 34
Postbus 8198
1005 AD Amsterdam
Netherlands
Tel: +31-20-5811511
Fax: +31-20-6149694
Telex: 14382

NEW ZEALAND
BDH Chemicals Ltd
PO Box 1246
Palmerston North
New Zealand
Tel: +64-6-3582038
Fax: +64-6-3567311

NICARAGUA
Comercial Genie Penalba SA
Apartado 694
Managua DN
Nicaragua
Tel: +505-2-26120/22808
Fax: +505-2-25473
Telex: 1330

NORWAY
Merck AS
Postboks 51 Ellingsrudaasen
1006 Oslo 10
Norway
Tel: +47-2-321150
Fax: +47-2-305244
Telex: 77413

PAKISTAN
AD Marker (Pvt) Ltd
D-7 Shaheed-e-Millat Road
PO Box 2027
Karachi 8
Pakistan
Tel: +92-21-449031
Fax: +92-21-4559221
Telex: 25280 or 24166

PARAGUAY
Vincente Scavone & CIA
CEISA
Casilla de Correo 427
Asuncion
Paraguay
Tel: +595-21-490251
Fax: +595-21-494704
Telex: 44165

PERU
Merck Peruana SA
Casilla 4331
Lima 1
Peru
Tel: +51-14-620142
Fax: +51-14-620298

PHILIPPINES
Merck Inc.
PO Box 1799
Makati 1299
Metro Manila
Philippines
Tel: +63-2-8185860
Fax: +63-2-8103024
Telex: 66371

POLAND
E. Merck
Oddzial w Warszawie
Ul. Prozna 12 A
00950 Warsaw
Poland
Tel: +48-22-205923
Fax: +48-22-205923

PORTUGAL
Merck Portuguesa Lda
Apartado 3185
1304 Lisbon Codex
Portugal
Tel: +351-1-3621434
Fax: +351-1-3621445
Telex: 63916

SAUDI ARABIA
Al-Jeel Medical & Trading Co.
PO Box 5012
Riyadh 11422
Saudi Arabia
Tel: +966-1-4041717
Fax: +966-1-4059052
Telex: 401723

Almura's
PO Box 10735
Riyadh 11443
Saudi Arabia
Tel: +966-1-4652916
Fax: +966-1-4644981
Telex: 5405406

SENEGAL
Societe Polychimie SA
Boite Postale 284
Dakar
Republic du Senegal
Tel: +221-323348
Fax: +221-320125
Telex: 550

SINGAPORE
All Eight Marketing Services
Pte Ltd
BK-212 Hongkong Street 21
03-343 Singapore 1953
Singapore

Tel: +65-2886388
Fax: +65-2849805
Telex: 55461

FE Zuellig (Trading) Pty Ltd
421 Tagore Avenue
PO Box 725
9014 Singapore
Singapore
Tel: +65-4598832
Fax: +65-4582706
Telex: 21750

SOUTH AFRICA
Merck Laboratory Supplies
PO Box 1998
Midrand 1685
South Africa
Tel: +27-11-3151100
Fax: +27-11-3151353
Telex: 424534

SPAIN
Igoda SA
Depart. Diagnosticos
Apartados 47
08100 Mollet del Valles
Barcelona
Spain
Tel: +34-3-5705750
Fax: +34-3-5701656
Telex: 94180

SWEDEN
E. Merck AB
Kungsgatan 65
111 22 Stockholm
Sweden
Tel: +46-8-202114
Fax: +46-8-245594
Telex: 10677

SWITZERLAND
E. Merck (Schweiz) AG
Witikoner Str. 15
Postfach 213
8029 Zurich
Switzerland
Tel: +41-1-559233
Fax: +41-1-559958
Telex: 816135

SYRIA
Droguerie Syrie
Antranik Kaprielian
Boite Postale 5441
Aleppo
Syria
Tel: +963-21-220277
Telex: 331078

TAIWAN
Merck Taiwan Ltd
3. FL, No. 34 Min Chuen West
Road
PO Box 681058
Taipei
Taiwan
Tel: +886-2-5219331
Fax: +886-2-5367734
Telex: 21787

THAILAND
Merck Ltd
PO Box 128
Pratunam Post Office
Bangkok 10409
Thailand

Tel: +66-2-3080218
Fax: +66-2-3080218

TURKEY
Alfred Paluka & Co.
PO Box 532
Istanbul-Karakoy
Turkey
Tel: +90-1-451246/47
Fax: +90-1-524458
Telex: 24971

UNITED ARAB EMIRATES
Gulf Drug Establishment
PO Box 3264
Dubai
United Arab Emirates
Tel: +971-4-20512
Fax: +971-4-22267
Telex: 46553

UNITED KINGDOM
Merck Ltd
Merck House
Poole
Dorset, BH15 1TD
United Kingdom
Tel: +44-0202-669700
Fax: +44-0202-665599
Telex: 41186

URUGUAY
Quimica Oriental SA
Casilla de correo 1443
Montevideo
Uruguay
Tel: +598-2-250627
Fax: +598-2-253334
Telex: 23045

USA
EM Diagnostics Systems Inc.
480 Democrat Road
Gibbstown, NY 08027
USA
Tel: +1-609-423-6300
Fax: +1-609-423-0671

VENEZUELA
Merck SA
Apartado 2020
Caracas 1010 A
Venezuela
Tel: +58-2-213455
Fax: +58-2-217164
Telex: 25236

Euro-Diagnostica

Corporate
Euro-Diagnostica
PO Box 2820
7303 GC Apeldoorn
Netherlands
Tel: +31-55-422433
Fax: +31-55-425017

By region
BELGIUM
Innogenetics SA
Kronenburgstraat 45 - 9th
Floor
2000 Antwerpen
Belgium

Organon Teknika Int'l

Veedijk 58
2300 Turnhout
Belgium

CANADA
Immunocorp Sciences Inc
5800 Royalmount
Montreal
Quebec, H4P 1K5
Canada
Tel: +1-514-733-3000
Fax: +1-514-733-1212

FRANCE
Unipath SA
6 route de Paisy
Boite Postale 13
69572 Dardilly Cedex
France
Tel: +33-78351731
Fax: +33-78660376

GERMANY
Laboserv GmbH
Am Zollstock 2
35392 Giessen
Germany
Tel: +49-641-2674
Fax: +49-641-28535

GREECE
Biodiagnostics
8 Thetidos Street
11528 Athens
Greece
Tel: +30-1-7211185
Fax: +30-1-7214227

Biodynamics SA
Alexandras Avenue & 62
Koniari St.
11521 Athens
Greece
Tel: +30-1-6449421
Fax: +30-1-6442266

ITALY
IFCI Clone Systems Spa
Via Del Fornacial 24
40129 Bologna
Italy
Tel: +39-51-326267
Fax: +39-51-323136

Tema Ricerca Srl
Via della Repubblica 20
40068 Dan Lazaro di Savena
Bologna
Italy
Tel: +39-51-454324
Fax: +39-51-464685

SWEDEN
Euro-Diagnostica AB
Box 30561
200 62 Malmo
Sweden

SWITZERLAND
Bio Science AG
Gerliswillstrasse 43
6020 Emmenbruche
Switzerland
Tel: +41-41-555075
Fax: +41-41-558322

TURKEY
Hayat Lab. Maix

Sanavi ve Ticaret AS
Millet cadessi Renk Ap 76/4
D8
34280 Findikzade Istanbul
Turkey

UNITED KINGDOM
Euro-Path Ltd
Union Hill
Stratton Bude
Cornwall, EX23 9BL
United Kingdom
Tel: +44-0288-353686
Fax: +44-0288-352866

Eurogenetics NV

Corporate
Eurogenetics NV
Transportstraat 4
3980 Tessenderlo
Belgium
Tel: +32-13-668830
Fax: +32-13-664749
Telex: 39112

By region
BENELUX
Eurogenetics NV
Transportstraat 4
3980 Tessenderlo
Belgium
Tel: +32-13-668830
Fax: +32-13-664749
Telex: 39112

FRANCE
Eurogenetics France
Technoparc
2 rue Leonard di Vinci
45072 Orleans la Source
Cedex 2
France
Tel: +33-38697878
Fax: +33-38635900

GERMANY
Eurogenetics Deutschland
Steucon-Center III
Mergenthalerallee 79-81
65760 Eschborn/Ts
Germany
Tel: +49-6196-470405
Fax: +49-6196-470407

ITALY
Eurogenetics Italia
Corso Susa 299
10098 Rivoli-Torino
Italy
Tel: +39-11-9550333
Fax: +39-11-9550329

SWITZERLAND
ES Genetics
Fanghofli 14
6014 Littau-Luzern
Switzerland
Tel: +41-41-574480
Fax: +41-41-575064

UNITED KINGDOM
Eurogenetics UK Ltd
111-113 Waldegrave Road
Teddington, TW11 8LL
United Kingdom

Tel: +44-081-977-0166
Fax: +44-081-943-9493

Fujirebio America Inc

Corporate
Fujirebio America Inc
30 Two Bridges Road
Suite 250
Fairfield, NJ 07004
USA
Tel: +1-201-227-8888
Fax: +1-201-227-8585

Gamma SA

Corporate
Gamma SA
Parc de Recherches du Sart
Tilman
Rues des Chasseurs
Ardennais
Belgium
Tel: +32-41-674784
Fax: +32-41-674784

Gen Bio Inc

Corporate
Gen Bio Inc
Technical Service
15222 Avenue of Science
San Diego, CA 92128
USA
Tel: +1-619-892-9300
Fax: +1-619-892-9400

Genetic Systems Corporation

Corporate
Genetic Systems Corporation
3005 First Avenue
Seattle
Washington 98121
USA
Tel: +1-206-861-5062

Gull Laboratories Inc

Corporate
Gull Laboratories Inc
1011 East 4800 South
Salt Lake City, UT 84117
USA

Human GmbH

Corporate
Human GmbH
Silberbachstrasse 9
65232 Taunusstein
Germany
Tel: +49-6128-875-266
Fax: +49-6128-875100

Hybritech Europe SA

Corporate
Hybritech Europe SA
Parc Scientifique du Sart
Tilman
Allee des Noisetiers 12
4031 Liege
Belgium
Tel: +32-41-677000
Fax: +32-41-676210
Telex: 42208

By region
AUSTRALIA
Hybritech Division
Eli Lilly Australia
112 Wharf Road
West Ryde
New South Wales 2114
Australia
Tel: +61-2-8745377
Fax: +61-2-8746970
Telex: 24280

BELGIUM
Hybritech Europe SA
Parc Scientifique du Sart
Tilman
Allee des Noisetiers 12
4031 Liege
Belgium
Tel: +32-41-677000
Fax: +32-41-676210
Telex: 42208

CANADA
Hybritech Division
Eli Lilly Canada Inc
3650 Danforth Avenue
Scarborough
Ontario M1N 2E8
Canada
Tel: +1-416-694-3221
Fax: +1-416-699-7252
Telex: 25132

FRANCE
Hybritech France
Div Diag de Lilly France SA
BP 119
78192 Trappes Cedex
France
Tel: +33-1-30663336
Fax: +33-1-30661173
Telex: 695439

GERMANY
Hybritech GmbH
Emil-Hoffmann-Str 7a
50996 Koln
Germany
Tel: +49-2236-61051/4
Fax: +49-2236-68325
Telex: 8881869

ITALY
Hybritech
Div. Diag. della
Eli Lilly Italia SpA
Via A. Gramsci 733
50019 Sesto Fiorentino
Italy
Tel: +39-55-42571
Fax: +39-55-4257285

Telex: 570194

NETHERLANDS
Hybritech Nederland
Diag. Div. van Eli Lilly
Nederland bv
Raadstede 15
3431 HA Nieuwegein
Netherlands
Tel: +31-3402-79711
Fax: +31-3402-46554

SPAIN
Hybritech SA
POB 585
28080 Madrid
Spain
Tel: +34-1-6534500
Fax: +34-1-6235251
Telex: 22269

USA
Hybritech Inc
PO Box 269006
San Diego
CA 92196-9006
USA
Tel: +1-619-455-6700
Fax: +1-619-4534124
Telex: 188974

IBL Gesellschaft fur Immunchemie und Immunbiologie mbH

Corporate
IBL Gesellschaft fur
Immunchemie und
Immunbiologie mbH
Flughafenstrasse 52a
Airport Center, Haus C
22335 Hamburg
Germany
Tel: +49-40-5328910
Fax: +49-40-52389111

IFCI CloneSystems SpA

Corporate
IFCI CloneSystems SpA
Sede e Stabilimento
Via Magnanelli 2
40033 Casalecchio di Reno
Bologna
Italy
Tel: +39-51-575326
Fax: +39-51-592738

By region
ITALY
IFCI CloneSystems SpA
Sede e Stabilimento
Via Magnanelli 2
40033 Casalecchio di Reno
Bologna
Italy
Tel: +39-51-575326
Fax: +39-51-592738

SPAIN
IFCI Clone Systems Espana
Plaza de La Torre 7 - 4 Planta

08006 Barcelona
Spain
Tel: +34-3-2375932
Fax: +34-3-4158300

Incstar Corporation

Corporate
Incstar Corporation
PO Box 285
1990 Industrial Boulevard
Stillwater, MN 55082
USA
Tel: +1-612-439-9710
Fax: +1-612-779-7847
Telex: 02 6879023

By region
ARGENTINA
International Link SA
Conesa 2556
Buenos Aires 1428
Argentina
Tel: +54-1-5432310
Fax: +54-1-5413923
Telex: 18234

AUSTRALIA
Pacific Diagnostics
8 Murdoch Circuit
Acacia Ridge
Queensland 4110
Camperdown
Australia
Tel: +61-7-2737111
Fax: +61-7-2737122

AUSTRIA
Dipl Ing Zoltan Szabo GmbH
Kalbeckgasse 5
1180 Vienna
Austria
Tel: +43-222-471572
Fax: +43-222-47157220
Telex: 116667

BELGIUM
Sorin Biomedica SA
Rue de la Grenouillette 200F
Waterranonkelstraat 200F
1130 Brussels
Belgium
Tel: +32-2-2454020
Fax: +32-2-2454067
Telex: 21972

BRAZIL
Fergo Prod. Hosp. Ltda
Rua Tenente Costa 135
20771 Rio de Janeiro
Brazil
Tel: +55-21-5813445
Fax: +55-21-2816293

Labcare do Brasil Produtos
Hospitalares Ltda
Rua Dom Luiz de Braganca
80 Bairro de Mirandopolis
CEP 04050 Sao Paulo
Brazil
Tel: +55-11-5777955
Fax: +55-11-2766567

Pro-Cirurgica Produtos
Cirurgicos Ltda
Rua Dr Ramiro D'Avila Nr. 44

Porto Alegre - CEP 90.620
Brazil
Tel: +55-512-238775
Fax: +55-512-230125

CANADA
Incstar Corporation
PO Box 285
1990 Industrial Boulevard
Stillwater, MN 55082
USA
Tel: +1-800-328-1428
Fax: +1-612-779-7847

CHILE
Farmanuclear Ltda
Santa Filomena 91
Santiago
Chile
Tel: +56-2-775042
Fax: +56-2-378862
Telex: 346082

CZECHOSLOVAKIA
DRG-CSFR
Vicnovska 16
62800 Brno
Czechoslovakia
Tel: +42-5-746800
Fax: +42-5-746739

DENMARK
Biotech IgG Aps
Godthabsvaenget 14A
2000 Frederiksberg
Denmark
Tel: +45-31193011
Fax: +45-31190350

EASTERN EUROPE
DRG International Inc
1167 Route 22 East
Mountainside, NJ 07092
USA
Tel: +1-809-233-2075
Fax: +1-809-233-0758
Telex: 178110

ECUADOR
Commercial Mersal
Italia 344
PO Box 1135
Quito
Ecuador
Tel: +593-2-524936
Fax: +593-2-561976
Telex: 22298

EGYPT
Gamma Trade Company
PO Box 12655
61 El Mohandsin
Cairo
Egypt
Tel: +20-2-480997
Fax: +20-2-3492687
Telex: 20983

FINLAND
Oy Tamro AB/APTA
Rajatorpantie 41B
01640 Vantaa
Finland
Tel: +358-0-852011
Fax: +358-0-85201770

FRANCE
Sorin France SA

Parc de haute technologie
Antony 2
9 rue Georges Besse
Antony 92160
France
Tel: +33-1-46665611
Fax: +33-1-46661463
Telex: 632381 SORIN F

GERMANY
SORIN-Deutschland
Optizstrasse 10
40470 Dusseldorf
Germany
Tel: +49-211-6180316
Fax: +49-211-6180319

Sorin Biomedica Deutschland
AG
Opitzstrasse 10
40470 Dusseldorf
Germany
Tel: +49-211-618031113
Fax: +49-211-6180319
Telex: 8587842

GREECE
Achilles Phillipas
88 Michala Kopoulou Street
Athens 28
Greece
Tel: +30-1-7754379
Fax: +30-1-7758356
Telex: 225495

HONG KONG
Science International
Corporation
14/F Gee Tuck Building
16-20 Bonham Strang East
Sheung Wan
Hong Kong
Tel: +852-5437442
Fax: +852-5414089

INDIA
Ezra Brothers
Mustafa Building, 4th Floor
Sir P.M. Road
Fort, Bombay
India
Tel: +91-22-286-0975
Fax: +91-22-204-3098

ISRAEL
Pharmatope Ltd
3 Basel St
Kiriat Arich
Petach Tikvah
Israel
Tel: +972-3-9230048
Fax: +972-3-9232549
Telex: 341148

ITALY
SORIN-Italy
Via Crescentino
13040 VC Saluggia
Italy
Tel: +39-161-4871
Fax: +39-161-487396
Telex: 200064

JAPAN
Baxter Ltd
Sankaido Bldg
1-9-13 Akasaka
Minato-Ku

Tokyo 107
Japan
Tel: +81-3-5057831
Fax: +81-3-5057820

KOREA
New Korea Industrial Co Ltd
819-3 Yeok San-Dong
Kang Nam-ku
Seoul
Korea
Tel: +82-2-552-2531
Fax: +82-2-557-0763

MALAYSIA/PHILLIPINES
Singapore Biotech PTE LTD
12 Science Park Drive
02-01/03/04 The Mendel
Singapore Science Park
Singapore 0511
Singapore
Tel: +65-7791919
Fax: +65-7791112

MEXICO
Empresa Medica
Internacional SA
Fuentes Brontantes
31 Col Portales
Mexico City
CP 03570
Mexico
Tel: +52-5-5395524
Fax: +52-5-5326274
Telex: 1764326

NETHERLANDS
SORIN Biomedica
Zekeringstraat 48
1014 BT Amsterdam
Netherlands
Tel: +31-20-827856
Fax: +31-20-846741

NEW ZEALAND
Pacific Diagnostics
PO Box 18062
Glen Innes
Auckland
New Zealand
Tel: +64-9-5213100
Fax: +64-9-5213117

POLAND
DRG Technical Support
Office
ul Nowogrodzka 48/8
00-695 Warsaw
Poland
Tel: +48-22-293329
Fax: +48-22-293329

RUSSIA
DRG International Inc
V/O Sovincentr
Firm "Inpred"
Krasnopresnenskaya nab 12
Moscow 123610
Russia
Tel: +7-095-253-1094
Fax: +7-095-253-1082
Telex: 411813

SOUTH AFRICA
Ridge Diagnostics
PO Box 1216
Randpark Ridge
Johannesburg 2156

South Africa
Tel: +27-11-4651430/1
Fax: +27-11-4651454

SPAIN
SORIN Espana SA
Dr Esquerdo 70
28007 Madrid
Spain
Tel: +34-1-4096655
Fax: +34-1-4097763

SWEDEN
Karo Bio Diagnostics AB
Lunastigen 3
141 44 Huddinge
Sweden
Tel: +46-8-7460990
Fax: +46-8-7468496

SWITZERLAND
DRG AG
Altmoosstr 86
8157 Dielsdorf/Zuric
Switzerland
Tel: +41-1-8533626
Fax: +41-1-8532707

TAIWAN
New Scientific Equipment Co
Ltd
PO Box 33-022
11F-1 32 Kungyuan Rd
Taipei 10039
Taiwan
Tel: +886-2-3315260
Fax: +886-2-3116283

TURKEY
Aksen Import - Export Mktg
Co Ltd
PK 475 Kizilay
Ankara
Turkey
Tel: +90-4-229 7147
Fax: +90-4-2314191
Telex: 44388

UNITED KINGDOM
Incstar Ltd
Charles House
Toutley Rd
Wokingham
Berkshire, RG11 5QN
United Kingdom
Tel: +44-0734-772693
Fax: +44-0734-792061

USA
Incstar Corporation
PO Box 285
1990 Industrial Boulevard
Stillwater, MN 55082
USA
Tel: +1-612-439-9710
Fax: +1-612-779-7847
Telex: 02 6879023

YUGOSLAVIA
METALKA/DRG International
Inc
Dalmatinova 2
Ljubljana 61000
Yugoslavia
Tel: +38-62-25991
Fax: +38-62-212175
Telex: 33125

Innogenetics

Corporate
Innogenetics
Canadastraat 21
Haven 1009
2070 Zwijndrecht
Belgium
Tel: +32-3-2523711
Fax: +32-3-2523799
Telex: 32248

By region
AUSTRALIA
Churchill Diagnostics
Suite 1, 5 Ridge Street
North Sidney
Australia
Tel: +61-2-9593512
Fax: +61-2-9593404

AUSTRIA
Bender Medsystems GmbH
Dr. Boehringergasse 5
PO Box 103
1121 Vienna
Austria
Tel: +43-222-801050
Fax: +43-222-8040823

BELGIUM
Innogenetics
Canadastraat 21
Haven 1009
2070 Zwijndrecht
Belgium
Tel: +32-3-2523799
Fax: +32-3-2523799
Telex: 32248

CZECHOSLOVAKIA
APR Spol
Za Skalkou 14
14700 Prague 4
Czechoslovakia
Tel: +42-2-4638096

DENMARK
Nota Bene
PO Box 76
Nivaapark 7
2990 Nivaa
Denmark
Tel: +45-422-49041
Fax: +45-422-49301

FINLAND
Immuno Diag Oy
Markulantie 4
Box 342
131 31 Hameenlinna
Finland
Tel: +35-81-722758
Fax: +35-81-722039

FRANCE
InGeN
Sogaris 203
94654 Rungis Cedex
France
Tel: +33-1-46871142
Fax: +33-1-46871231

GERMANY
Medipro
Hohwiesenweg 51

68775 Ketsch
Germany
Tel: +49-620-263448
Fax: +49-620-264661

Bibby Dunn
Zurheiden 6
53567 Asbach
Germany
Tel: +49-268-343306
Fax: +49-268-342776

GREECE
Omikron
Tagmatarchou Plessa 29
17674 Kalithea
Greece
Tel: +30-1-9428106
Fax: +30-1-9425166

INDIA
Lupin
C.S.T. Road 159
Kalina
Santa Cruz East
Bombay 400098
India
Tel: +91-22-6124050
Fax: +91-22-6114008

ISRAEL
Pharmatope
3 Basel Street
POB 3962
49130 Kiriat Arie
Israel
Tel: +972-3-92300489
Fax: +972-3-9232549

ITALY
Nuclear Laser Medicine
Cascina Conighetto
20090 Settala (Milan)
Italy
Tel: +39-2-9589673
Fax: +39-2-9589158

MIDDLE EAST
Scitech Med
Science Park Drive 12, #04-01
0511 Singapore
Singapore
Tel: +65-7796638
Fax: +65-7793784

NETHERLANDS
Innogenetics
Toernoolveld 126
6525 C Nijmeghen
Netherlands
Tel: +31-805-28826
Fax: +31-805-40090

SPAIN
Ingelheim Diagnostica y
Tecnologia SA
Pau Alcover 31-33
08017 Barcelona
Spain
Tel: +34-9-4045220
Fax: +34-9-4045485

SWEDEN
Dakopatts AB
Box 13
S-125 21 Alvsjo
Sweden

Tel: +46-899-6000
Fax: +46-899-6065

SWITZERLAND
Endotell
Hasselstrasse 25
4103 Bottmingen
Switzerland
Tel: +41-61-4010787
Fax: +41-61-4010793

UNITED ARAB EMIRATES
Unimed
Akarlya (old) East Entrance
Siteen Street
Al Malaz Riyadh
United Arab Emirates

UNITED KINGDOM
Serotec
Bankside Station Field
  Industrial Estate
Oxford
OX5 1JD
United Kingdom
Tel: +44-867-579941
Fax: +44-867-53899

Mercia
Broadford Park
Guildford, Surrey
GU4 8EW
United Kingdom
Tel: +44-483-505255
Fax: +44-483-574822

VENEZUELA
Lab. Geminis
Calle La Joya Edif Cosmos
Ap. 61290
1060A Caracas
Venezuela
Tel: +58-2-613393
Fax: +58-2-335011

International Immuno-Diagnostics

Corporate
International Immuno-
Diagnostics
1155 Chess Drive #121
Foster City, CA 94404
USA
Tel: +1-415-345-9518
Fax: +1-415-578-1810

International Mycoplasma

Corporate
International Mycoplasma
BP 705
83030 Toulon, Cedex 9
France
Tel: +33-94885500
Fax: +33-94885505

Kodak Clinical Diagnostics Ltd

Corporate
Kodak Clinical Diagnostics Ltd
Mandeville House
62 The Broadway
Amersham
Bucks, HP7 0HJ
United Kingdom
Tel: +44-0494-431717
Fax: +44-0494-431165
Telex: 83447

By region
AUSTRALIA
Amersham Australia Pty Ltd
PO Box 99
North Ryde
New South Wales 2113
Australia
Tel: +61-2-8882288

BELGIUM
Amersham Belgium SA/NV
Rue Saint-Lambertstraat 135
1200 Brussels
Belgium
Tel: +32-2-7700075

CANADA
Kodak Canada Inc
3500 Eglinton Avenue West
Toronto
Ontario M6M 1V3
Canada
Tel: +1-416-761-4399
Fax: +1-416-766-5814

DENMARK
Amersham Denmark ApS
Blokken 11
3460 Birkerod
Denmark
Tel: +45-820222

FRANCE
Kodak Diagnostic SA
6 Ave du Canada
BP 232
91943 Les Ulis Cedex
France
Tel: +33-1-69865300
Fax: +33-1-64460464

GERMANY
Kodak Diagnostik
  (Deutschland) GmbH
Mascheroder Weg 1b
38124 Braunschweig
Germany
Tel: +49-531-2010

ITALY
Kodak Diagnostici Srl
Via le Matteotii 62
20092 Cinisello B
Milan
Italy
Tel: +39-2-660281
Fax: +39-2-66028765

JAPAN
Amersham Medical Ltd
Tokyo Toyama Kaikan
1-3-101 Hakusan 5-chome

Bunkyo-Ku
Tokyo 112
Japan
Tel: +81-3-38180216

NETHERLANDS
Amersham Nederland BV
Amerikastraat 3a
5232 BE Hertogenbosch
Netherlands
Tel: +31-73-418525

NORWAY
Kodak Norge A/S
Trollasvelen 6
1410 Kolbotn
Norway
Tel: +47-20-818181
Fax: +47-20-800612

UNITED KINGDOM
Kodak Clinical Diagnostics Ltd
Mandeville House
62 The Broadway
Amersham
Bucks, HP7 0HJ
United Kingdom
Tel: +44-0494-431717
Fax: +44-0494-431165

USA
Clinical Products Division
Eastman Kodak Company
Rochester, NY 14650
USA

Laboratoire Eurobio

Corporate
Laboratoire Eurobio
2a Courtaboef
7 Avenue de Scandanavia
Les Ulis, Cedex B 91953
France
Tel: +33-69079477
Fax: +33-69079534

Labsystems Oy

Corporate
Labsystems Oy
PO Box 8
00880 Helsinki
Finland
Finland
Fax: +358-0-7557610

Mast Immunosystems

Corporate
Mast Immunosystems
630 Clyde Court
Mountain View, CA 94043
USA
Tel: +1-415-961-5501
Fax: +1-415-969-2745

medac GmbH

Corporate
medac GmbH
Diagnostic Division
Fehlandtstrasse 3
20354 Hamburg
Germany
Tel: +49-40-3509020
Fax: +49-40-35090261

Melja Diagnostik GmbH

Corporate
Melja Diagnostik GmbH
Lilienthalstrasse 25
Unternehmenspark
34123 Kassel
Germany
Tel: +49-561-571577/8
Fax: +49-561-571636

Melotec SA

Corporate
Melotec SA
Parc Tecnologic
08290 Cerdanyola
Barcelona
Spain
Tel: +34-3-5820166
Fax: +34-3-5801438

Menarini Diagnostics

Corporate
Menarini Diagnostics
Via Sette Santi 3
50131 Firenze
Italy
Tel: +39-55-56801
Fax: +39-55-5680216

Meridian Diagnostics Inc

Corporate
Meridian Diagnostics Inc
3471 River Mills Drive
Cincinnati, OH 45244
USA
Tel: +1-513-271-3700
Fax: +1-513-271-0124

By region
ITALY
Meridian Diagnostics Europe,
  Srl
Via G. Strobino 4
PO Box 33
20025 Legnano
Milan
Italy
Tel: +39-2-544178
Fax: +39-2-544178

USA
Meridian Diagnostics Inc

© KLUWER ACADEMIC PUBLISHERS 1994, ISSN 1381-5067

3471 River Mills Drive
Cincinnati, OH 45244
USA
Tel: +1-513-271-3700
Fax: +1-513-271-0124

Mitsui Pharmaceuticals Inc.

Corporate
Mitsui Pharmaceuticals Inc.
12-2, Nihonbashi 3-chome
Chuo-ku
Tokyo 103
Japan
Tel: +81-3-32744711
Fax: +81-3-32744670

By region
JAPAN
Mitsui Pharmaceuticals Inc.
Diagnostics and Instrument Division
5-12, Iwamoto-cho 3-chome
Chiyoda-ku
Tokyo 101
Japan
Tel: +81-3-38645591
Fax: +81-3-38649732

Mitsui Pharmaceuticals Inc.
12-2, Nihonbashi 3-chome
Chuo-ku
Tokyo 103
Japan
Tel: +81-3-32744711
Fax: +81-3-32744670

Murex Diagnostics Ltd

Corporate
Murex Diagnostics Ltd
Central Road
Temple Hill
Dartford, Kent
DA1 5LR
United Kingdom
Tel: +44-322-277711
Fax: +44-322-282572

Omega Diagnostics Ltd

Corporate
Omega Diagnostics Ltd
Alloa Business Centre
Whins Road
Alloa, FK10 3SA
United Kingdom
Tel: +44-0259-217315
Fax: +44-0259-723251

Organon Teknika nv

Corporate
Organon Teknika nv
AKZO

Veedijk 58
2300 Turnhout
Belgium
Tel: +32-14-404040
Fax: +32-14-421600

Orion Corporation, Orion Diagnostica

Corporate
Orion Corporation, Orion Diagnostica
PO Box 83
02101 Espoo
Finland
Tel: +358-0-4291
Fax: +358-0-4292794

By region
FINLAND
Orion Corporation, Orion Diagnostica
PO Box 83
02101 Espoo
Finland
Tel: +358-0-4291
Fax: +358-0-4292794

Orion Corporation, Orion Diagnostica
PO Box 425
20101 Turku
Finland
Tel: +358-21-662011
Fax: +358-21-662546

NORWAY
Orion Diagnostica as
Postboks 321
1371 Asker
Norway
Tel: +47-66904675
Fax: +47-66904788

SWEDEN
Orion Diagnostica AB
Radhuset
S-619 00 Trosa
Sweden
Tel: +46-156-13260
Fax: +46-156-17355

USA
Orion Diagnostica Inc
PO Box 218
Somerset, NJ 08875-0218
USA
Tel: +1-908-246-3366
Fax: +1-908-246-0570

Ortho Diagnostic Systems Ltd

Corporate
Ortho Diagnostic Systems Ltd
Enterprise House
Station Road
Loudwater
High Wycombe, Bucks
HP10 9UF
United Kingdom
Tel: +44-0494-442211
Fax: +44-0494-461006

PRO-LAB Diagnostics

Corporate
PRO-LAB Diagnostics
10a Croft Business Park
Thursby Road
Bromborough, Wirral
Merseyside
United Kingdom
Tel: +051-334-0230
Fax: +051-334-0216

Radim

Corporate
Radim
Via del Mare, 125
00040 Pomezia
Rome
Italy
Tel: +39-6-9108364
Fax: +39-6-9106128

By region
BELGIUM
Radim SA
Parc Scientifique du Sart-Tilman
Avenue Pre Aily 10
4031 Angleur (Liege)
Belgium
Tel: +32-41-674464
Fax: +32-41-670063

ITALY
Radim
Via del Mare, 125
00040 Pomezia
Roma
Italy
Tel: +39-6-9108364
Fax: +39-6-9106128

SEAC srl
Via di Prato, 72/74
50041 Calenzano-Prato (FI)
Italy
Tel: +39-55-8877469
Fax: +39-55-8877771

SPAIN
Radim Iberica SA
C. Lepanto, 339
Bajos, Local 7
08025 Barcelona
Spain
Tel: +34-3-4333921
Fax: +34-3-4333796

Randox Laboratories Ltd

Corporate
Randox Laboratories Ltd
Ardmore, Diamond Road
Crumlin, Co. Antrim
BT29 4QY
Northern Ireland
Tel: +44-849-422413
Fax: +44-849-452912

By region
FRANCE
Randox Laboratoire Ltd
BP 434 Garonor
93617 Aulnay Sous Bois Cedex
France
Tel: +33-1-48657617
Fax: +33-1-48659821

NORTHERN IRELAND
Randox Laboratories Ltd
Ardmore, Diamond Road
Crumlin, Co. Antrim
BT29 4QY
Northern Ireland
Tel: +44-849-422413
Fax: +44-849-452912

PORTUGAL
Irlandox Laboratorios
Quimica Analitica Limitada
Rua Agnostinho
De Jesus E Sousa 258
4000 Porto
Portugal
Tel: +351-25104278
Fax: +351-2580200

F. Hoffmann-La Roche Ltd

Corporate
F. Hoffmann-La Roche Ltd
Roche Diagnostic Systems
4002 Basel
Switzerland
Tel: +41-61-6888726
Fax: +41-61-6814135

By region
AUSTRALIA
Roche Diagnostic Systems
Unit C1, 1-3 Rodborough Road
French Forest
New South Wales 2086
Australia
Tel: +61-2-9758150
Fax: +61-2-9755254

BENELUX
Produits Roche SA
75 Rue Dante
1070 Brussels
Belgium
Tel: +32-2-5258211
Fax: +32-2-5258201

BRAZIL
Produtos Roche Quimicos e Farmaceuticos SA
Caixa Postal 6364
01000 Sao Paulo SP
Brazil
Tel: +55-11-8693322
Fax: +55-11-8698877

CANADA
Hoffmann-La Roche Ltd
2455 Meadowpine Boulevard
Mississauga
Ontario L5N 6L7
Canada
Tel: +1-416-542-5555
Fax: +1-416-542-5649

EASTERN EUROPE
Hoffmann-La Roche Wien
  GmbH
Postfach 70
1103 Vienna
Austria
Tel: +43-222-781604
Fax: +43-222-781604253

FRANCE
Produits Roche SA
52 Boulevard du Parc
92521 Neuilly sur Seine
France
Tel: +33-1-46405000
Fax: +33-1-46405292

GERMANY
Hoffmann-La Roche AG
79639 Grenzach-Wyhlen
Germany
Tel: +49-7624-140
Fax: +49-7624-1019

ITALY
Dr G Minola
Prodotti Roche SpA
Piazza Durante 11
20131 Milan
Italy
Tel: +39-2-28841
Fax: +39-2-2884585

JAPAN
Nippon Roche KK
6th Floor, Shin-Onarimon
  Bldg
6-17-19, Shinbashi, Minato-ku
Tokyo 105
Japan
Tel: +81-3-54701707
Fax: +81-3-54701720

NEW ZEALAND
Roche Products (New
  Zealand) Ltd
PO Box 12-492
Penrose, Auckland
New Zealand
Tel: +64-9-640029
Fax: +64-9-640020

PORTUGAL
Roche Farmaceutica Quimica
  Lda
Estrada Nacional 249-1
2700 Amadora
Portugal
Tel: +351-1-4184565
Fax: +351-1-4186677

RUSSIA
DIAplus
Nauchny proezd, 8
Moscow 117246
Russia
Tel: +7-095-332-6440
Fax: +7-095-332-6557

SCANDINAVIA
Roche A/S
Industriholmen 59
2650 Hvidovre-Copenhagen
Denmark
Tel: +45-31787211
Fax: +45-3187215

SOUTH AFRICA
Roche Products (Pty) Ltd
PO Box 4589
Johannesburg 2000
South Africa
Tel: +27-11-9745335
Fax: +27-11-3922338

SOUTH EAST ASIA
Roche (Malaysia) SDN. BHD.
PO Box 1067
Jalan Semangat
46870 Petaling Jaya Selangor
Malaysia
Tel: +60-261-1100
Fax: +60-262-3808

SPAIN
Productos Roche SA
Apartado de Correos 1.157
28080 Madrid
Spain
Tel: +34-1-2086240
Fax: +34-1-2084442

SWITZERLAND
F. Hoffmann-La Roche Ltd
Roche Diagnostic Systems
4002 Basel
Switzerland
Tel: +41-61-6888726
Fax: +41-61-6814135

UNITED KINGDOM
Roche Products Ltd
Roche Diagnostic Systems
PO Box 8
Welwyn Garden City
Herts, AL7 3AY
United Kingdom
Tel: +44-0707-366000
Fax: +44-0707-373556

USA
Hoffmann-La Roche Inc
Roche Diagnostic Systems
  Inc
1080 US Highway 202
Branchburg, NJ 08876
USA
Tel: +1-908-253-7652
Fax: +1-908-253-7200

**Sanofi Diagnostics
Pasteur, Inc**

Corporate
Sanofi Diagnostics Pasteur,
  Inc
1000 Lake Hazeltine Drive
Chaska, MN 55318-1084
USA
Tel: +1-612-448-4848
Fax: +1-612-368-1110

By region
AUSTRALIA
Sanofi Diagnostics Pasteur
4th floor Clyde House
140 Arthur Street
North Sydney
New South Wales 2060
Australia
Tel: +61-2-9575515
Fax: +61-2-9290364

AUSTRIA
Sanofi Diagnostics Pasteur H.
  GmbH
Ameisgasse 31, 4/5
1140 Vienna
Austria
Tel: +43-222-8941290
Fax: +43-222-8941299

BELGIUM
Sanofi Diagnostics Pasteur
  NV
Woudstraat 25
3600 Genk
Belgium
Tel: +32-89-384292
Fax: +32-89-384392
Telex: 38087

CANADA
Sanofi Diagnostics Pasteur
2403 Guenette Street
Montreal
Quebec, H4R 2E9
Canada
Tel: +1-514-334-4372
Fax: +1-514-334-4415

FRANCE
Diagnostics Pasteur
3 Blvd Raymond Poincare
92430 Marnes la Coquette
France
Tel: +33-1-47956140
Fax: +33-1-47956141

GERMANY
Sanofi Diagnostics Pasteur
  GmbH
Sasbacher Strasse 5
79111 Freiburg
Germany
Tel: +49-761-490510
Fax: +49-761-4905199

ITALY
Sanofi Diagnostics Pasteur
Via Carbonera 2
20137 Milan
Italy
Tel: +39-2-739419
Fax: +39-2-57404678

JAPAN
Sanofi Fujirebio Diagnostics
Marumasu Shonjuku Bldg 7/8
  F
24.20 Shonjuku 6 - chome
Shinjuku-ku
Tokyo 160
Japan
Tel: +81-3-52720203
Fax: +81-3-52720215

MEXICO
Sanofi Diagnostics Pasteur
  SA
Av Periferico sur 6677 2nd
  Floor
Col Ejidos de Tepepan
Deleg Xochimilco
Mexico 16018
Mexico

NETHERLANDS
Sanofi Diagnostics Pasteur
  BV
Govert van Wijnkade 48

3144 EG Maassluis
Netherlands
Tel: +31-18-9917555
Fax: +31-18-9914555

PORTUGAL
Sanofi Diagnostics Pasteur
  Lda
Rua Artilharia UM, 63 - r/c
1200 Lisbon
Portugal
Tel: +351-1-3806008
Fax: +351-1-3806099

SPAIN
Sanofi Diagnostics Pasteur
  SA
Calle Jarama
28002 Madrid
Spain
Tel: +34-1-5630100
Fax: +34-1-5644383

SWITZERLAND
Sanofi Diagnostics Pasteur
  SA
Zuchwillerstrasse 41
PO Box 420
4501 Solothurn
Switzerland
Tel: +41-65-234151
Fax: +41-65234153

THAILAND
Sanofi Pacific Diagnostics
IFCT Building 9th Floor
1770 New Petchbury Road
Bangkok 10310
Thailand
Tel: +66-2-2548070
Fax: +66-2-2548060

UNITED KINGDOM
Sanofi Diagnostics Pasteur
  Ltd
PO Box 209
3 Rhodes Way
Watford, Hertfordshire
WD2 4QE
United Kingdom
Tel: +44-0923-212212
Fax: +44-0923-243001

USA
Sanofi Diagnostics Pasteur,
  Inc
1000 Lake Hazeltine Drive
Chaska, MN 55318-1084
USA
Tel: +1-612-448-4848
Fax: +1-612-368-1110

Genetic Systems
6565 185th Avenue North
  East
Redmond, WA 98052
USA
Tel: +1-206-881-8300
Fax: +1-206-861-5010

**Savyon/Omni
Triage Medical Ltd**

Corporate
Savyon/Omni Triage Medical
  Ltd

131 Tranmere Road
London, SW18 3QP
United Kingdom
Tel: +071-737-7781
Fax: +071-738-4473

Schlapparelli Biosystems BV

Corporate
Schiapparelli Biosystems BV
Pompmolenlaan 24
3447 GK Woerden
The Netherlands
Tel: +31-3480-87300
Fax: +31-3480-33000

Shield Diagnostics

Corporate
Shield Diagnostics
Technology Park
Dundee, DD2 1SW
United Kingdom
Tel: +0382-561000
Fax: +0382-561056

Sigma Chemical Company

Corporate
Sigma Chemical Company
PO Box 14508
St Louis, MO 63178
USA
Tel: +1-314-771-5750
Fax: +1-314-771-5757

By region
AUSTRALIA
Sigma-Aldrich Pty Ltd
Unit 2, 10 Anella Avenue
Castle Hill, NSW 2154
Australia
Tel: +61-2-899-9977
Fax: +61-2-899-9742

BELGIUM
Sigma Chemie
Bd. Lambermontlaan 140B6
1030 Brussels
Belgium
Tel: +32-3-8991301
Fax: +32-3-8991311

BRAZIL
Sigma-Aldrich Chemical
   Representocoes Ltda
Rua Sabara, 566 - Conj. 53
01239-010 Sao Paulo, SP
Brazil
Tel: +55-11-2311866
Fax: +55-11-2579079

CZECHOSLOVAKIA
Sigma-Aldrich sro
Krizikova 27
180 00 Prague 8
Czechoslovakia
Tel: +42-2-2366973
Fax: +42-2-2364141

FRANCE
Sigma Chimi S.a.r.l.
L'Isle d'Abeau Chesnes
BP 701
38070 St Quentin Fallavier
Cedex
France
Tel: +33-74822800
Fax: +33-74956808
Telex: 308215

GERMANY
Sigma Chemie GmbH
Grunwalder Weg 30
82041 Deisenhofen
Germany
Tel: +49-89-61301
Fax: +49-89-6135135
Telex: 528252

INDIA
Sigma-Aldrich Corporation
B-4/158 Safdarjung Enclave
New Delhi 110 029
India
Tel: +91-11-671175

ITALY
Sigma Chimica
Via Gallarate 154
20151 Milan
Italy
Tel: +39-2-33417-30
Fax: +39-2-38010737

SPAIN
Sigma Quimica
Apt. Correos 161
28100 Alcobendas
Madrid
Spain
Tel: +34-1-6619977
Fax: +34-1-6619642
Telex: 22189

SWITZERLAND
Sigma Chemie
PO Box 260
9470 Buchs
Switzerland
Telex: 855282

UNITED KINGDOM
Sigma Chemical Co. Ltd
Fancy Road
Poole
Dorset, BH17 7NH
United Kingdom
Tel: +44-0202-733114
Fax: +44-0202-715460

USA
Sigma Chemical Company
PO Box 14508
St Louis, MO 63178
USA
Tel: +1-314-771-5750
Fax: +1-314-771-5757

Scanlab Oy
Elsktracity, 4Krs
Yrityskeskus Dio
Tykistonkatu 2-4
20520 Turku
Finland
Tel: +358-21-63757729
Fax: +358-21-6375729

Sorin Biomedica

Corporate
Sorin Biomedica
Via Crescentino
13040 Saluggia
Italy
Tel: +39-161-4871
Fax: +39-161-487545

By region
ARGENTINA
Tecnogam
Avanida Cordoba 950
Piso 13
1054 Buenos Aires
Argentina
Tel: +54-1-3935041
Fax: +54-1-3935068

AUSTRALIA
CSL
45 Poplar Road
Parkville 3052
Victoria
Australia
Tel: +61-3-3891911
Fax: +61-3-3891646

AUSTRIA
Biomedica
   Handelsgesellschaft GmbH
Divischgasse 4
1210 Vienna
Austria
Tel: +43-222-393527
Fax: +43-222-3901361

BRAZIL
Sorin Biomedica Industrial
Rua Robert Bosch 130
Parque Industrial Tomas
   Edison
01141 Sao Paulo
Brazil
Tel: +55-11-8263377
Fax: +55-11-673873

EGYPT
Clinilab
127 Mohammed Farid Street
Cairo
Egypt
Tel: +20-2-3919397
Fax: +20-2-3915247

GREECE
Diachel
Sp. Merkouri 78 & Alkimachou
   1
11634 Athens
Greece
Tel: +30-1-7235523
Fax: +30-1-7219874

INDIA
Ranbaxy Laboratories
10th Floor, Devika Tower
6 Nehru Place
New Delhi 110019
India
Tel: +91-11-6437078
Fax: +91-11-6430633

ITALY
Sorin Biomedica

Via Crescentino
13040 Saluggia
Italy
Tel: +39-161-4871
Fax: +39-161-487545

JORDAN
Burgan Drugstores
PO Box 773
Amman
Jordan
Tel: +962-6-699170
Fax: +962-6-699171

KOREA
Boo Kyung
CPO Box 426
Seoul
Korea
Tel: +82-2-7483331
Fax: +82-2-7845123

LEBANON
Medek SARL
St Joseph Hospital Street
St Joseph Pharmacy Building
Beirut
Lebanon
Tel: +961-1-881042/898147

MALAYSIA
MD Products & Services SDN
   BHD
35A Jalan 1/76, Desa Pandan
Off Jalan Kampung Pandan
55100 Kuala Lumpur
Malaysia
Tel: +60-3-9862939
Fax: +60-3-9862935

NORWAY
Dan Meszanski AS
Holstsgate 6
PO Box 4324
Torshov
Oslo 4
Norway
Tel: +47-2-370788
Fax: +47-2-379585

OMAN
Muscat Pharmacy
PO Box 438
Muscat
Oman
Tel: +968-794501
Fax: +968-795202

PAKISTAN
Scherzo Agencies
1st Floor, Madina Market
32 Abkari Road
La Hore 2
Pakistan
Tel: +92-42-324626
Fax: +92-42-306299

PORTUGAL
Isoder
Rua dos Lusiades, 5-5
Letra H
1300 Lisbon
Portugal
Tel: +351-1-3647208
Fax: +351-1-3638788

SAUDI ARABIA
Al Salehia Medical Est.

PO Box 991
Riyadh 11421
Saudi Arabia
Tel: +966-1-4633205
Fax: +966-1-4634362

SWEDEN
Karo Bio Diagnostics
Lunastigen 3
141 44 Huddinge
Sweden
Tel: +46-8-7460990
Fax: +46-8-7468496

SWITZERLAND
Sodiag
via Locarno 76
6616 Losone
Switzerland
Tel: +41-93-350363
Fax: +41-93-350364

THAILAND
Rapport
4/631 Sahakom Klongkum
Soi 26
Sukhaphiban 2 Rd
Bangkapi
Bangkok 10240
Thailand
Tel: +66-2-3746977/6978
Fax: +66-2-3745312

TURKEY
Gokham Laboratuvar AS
1440 Solkak
No. 4 Alsancak
Izmir 35220
Turkey
Tel: +90-51-220055
Fax: +90-51-636904

Duzen Industry & Foreign
Trade Co. Ltd
Necatlbey Caddesi 88/8
Ankara
Turkey
Tel: +90-4-2298025/9323
Fax: +90-4-2300940

UNITED ARAB EMIRATES
Emirates Medical Co.
PO Box 1286
Ahmed Saif Bei Hasa Bldg
(opposite Dubai Police HQ)
Dubai Sharajah Road
Deira, Dubai
United Arab Emirates
Tel: +971-4-662319
Fax: +971-4-692774

VENEZUELA
Clini-kit srl
Edif. Alpha
Calle Republica Dominicane
Piso 3, Locale 4
Boleita Sur
Caracas 1070
Venezuela
Tel: +58-2-2392858
Fax: +58-2-2398905

Stellar Bio Systems Inc

Corporate
Stellar Bio Systems Inc
9075 Guildford Road
Columbia
USA
Tel: +1-410-381-8550
Fax: +1-410-381-8984

Nippon-Syntex KK
Tokyo Tatemono Shibuya
Bldg
9-9 Shibuya 3-Chome
Shibuya-ku
Tokyo 150
Japan
Tel: +81-3-37971480
Fax: +81-3-37975830

Syva Company

Corporate
Syva Company
3403 Yerba Buena Road
PO Box 49013
San Jose
CA 95161-9013
USA
Tel: +1-408-239-2000
Fax: +1-408-239-2552

By region
ARGENTINA
Quimica Erovne SA
Av. Cordoba 2552
1120 Buenos Aires
Argentina
Tel: +54-1-9619636
Fax: +54-1-9611504
Telex: 18479

AUSTRALIA
Syva Australia
2nd Floor, 66-68 Victoria
Road
Drummoyne
New South Wales 2047
Australia
Tel: +61-2-7198599
Fax: +61-2-7198867

AUSTRIA
Merck GmbH
5 Zimbagasse
1147 Vienna
Austria
Tel: +43-222-971611
Fax: +43-222-975560
Telex: 133188

BELGIUM
Syva Belgium
rue de Geneve 10
Genevestraat
bte 11 bus
1140 Brussels
Belgium
Tel: +32-2-7364040
Fax: +32-2-7335597
Telex: 61909

BRAZIL
Quimitra Comercio E Industria

Quimica SA
Estrada dos Bandeirantes,
1099
22710 Rio de Janeiro
Brazil
Tel: +55-21-3424646
Fax: +55-21-3421263
Telex: 2123792

CHILE
Merck Quimica Chilena Soc.
Ltda
Francisco de Paula
Taforo 1981
Santiago de Chile
Chile
Tel: +56-2-255797
Fax: +56-2-2383527
Telex: 440197

COLOMBIA
Merck Colombia SA
Departamento de Diagnostica
Cra 65 No. 10-95
Bogota, DE 6
Colombia
Tel: +57-1-2907855
Fax: +57-1-2628881
Telex: 41405

DENMARK
Syva Diagnostika APS (Syva
Denmark)
Christianshusvej 181
2970 Hoersholm
Denmark
Tel: +45-45766500
Fax: +45-45768611
Telex: 37214

ECUADOR SA
Comercial Mersal Cia Ltda
Italia 344
Edificio Artes Medicas
Piso 1
Quito
Ecuador SA
Tel: +593-2-524936
Fax: +593-2-504571
Telex: 2298

FINLAND
Oy Tamro AB/APTA Dept
Ruosilantie 14
00390 Helsinki
Finland
Tel: +358-0-54011
Fax: +358-0-545505
Telex: 125856

FRANCE
Syva France
Miniparc de Dardilly - Chemin
du Jubin
BP 63
69573 Dardilly Cedex
France
Tel: +33-78661155
Fax: +33-78475676
Telex: 900340

GERMANY
Syva Diagnostica GmbH
Aisfelder Strasse 6
64289 Darmstadt
Germany
Tel: +49-6151-74011
Fax: +49-6151-710210

Telex: 4197169

GUAM
Plus Marketing Medical
Systems
970 South Marine Drive
Suite 10-333
Tamuning
Guam 96911
Guam
Tel: +671-6469207/5907
Fax: +671-6469223
Telex: 7216555

HONG KONG
Science International
Corporation
14th Floor, Gee Tuck Building
16-20 Bonham Strand East
Hong Kong
Tel: +852-5437442
Fax: +852-5414089
Telex: 60285

INDONESIA
PT Labtechindo Perkasa
Scientific
Komplex Perkantoran Duta
Merlin
Blok E-17
Jalan Gajah Mada No. 3-5
Jakarta 10130
Indonesia
Tel: +62-21-3804674
Fax: +62-21-364929
Telex: 44522

ITALY
Bracco SpA
Via Egidio Folli, 50
20134 Milano
Italy
Tel: +39-2-21771
Fax: +39-2-2155169
Telex: 311183

KOREA
Dongbang Healthcare
Products Co. Ltd
3rd Floor, Unicom Building
140-17 Samseong-Dong
Gangnam-ku
Seoul
Korea
Tel: +82-2-5520781
Fax: +82-2-5557791
Telex: 25706

MALAYSIA
General Scientific Co. Sdn.
Bhd
No 7, Jalan 222
Section 51A
46100 Petaling Jaya
Selangor Darul Ehsan
Malaysia
Tel: +60-3-7575433
Fax: +60-3-7571768
Telex: 37443

MEXICO
Syntex SA de CV
Division Diagnostica
Paseo de la Reforma 2822
Mexico DF 11910
Mexico
Tel: +52-5-5703333
Fax: +52-5-5701325

Telex: 1771173

NETHERLANDS
E. Merck Nederland BV
Basisweg 34
1043 AP Amsterdam
Netherlands
Tel: +31-20-5811511
Fax: +31-20-149694
Telex: 14382

NEW ZEALAND
Syntex Laboratories (NZ) Ltd
(Syva Division)
5 Wall Place
Linden, Wellington
New Zealand
Tel: +64-4-325163
Fax: +64-4-4791687
Telex: 32005

NORWAY
Syva Norge AS
Storgata 16
2000 Lillestroem
Norway
Tel: +47-6-814580
Fax: +47-6-817890
Telex: 76510

PANAMA
Executive Marketing
Corporation
Avenida Paical, No. 30
Urbanizacion Industrial
Panama
Tel: +507-360114
Fax: +507-361820
Telex: 3483

PARAGUAY
G & T Scientific srl
25 de Mayo 1316
Asuncion
Paraguay
Tel: +595-21-23158
Fax: +595-21-23158
Telex: 743

PERU
Merck Peruana SA
Casilla 4331
Lima 1
Peru
Tel: +51-14-620142
Fax: +51-14-620298

PHILIPPINES
Dakila Trading Company
208 Pilar Street
Mandaluyong
Rizal
Philippines
Tel: +63-2-707511
Fax: +63-2-7210739

PORTUGAL
Ortho Diagnostic Systems
A Johnson & Johnson
Company
Rua Humberto Madeira 2
Valejas
2745 Queluz
Portugal
Tel: +351-1-4355171
Fax: +351-1-4354807
Telex: 43880

PUERTO RICO
Isla Lab Products Corporation
GPO Box 361810
San Juan 00936-1810
Puerto Rico
Tel: +1809-7922222
Fax: +1809-7814462

SINGAPORE
General Scientific Co. Sdn.
Bhd
1296 Lorong 1, Toa Payoh
#03-01, Siong Hoe
Warehouse
Singapore 123
Singapore
Tel: +65-2584377
Fax: +65-2586969
Telex: 39373

SPAIN
Syntex Latino SA
Gran Via Carlos III, 86 3a
planta
Barcelona 28
Spain
Tel: +34-3-4110409
Fax: +34-3-3391691
Telex: 54139

SWEDEN
Syva Scandinavia, Syntex
Diagnostics AB
Jaegerhorns Vaeg 6
141 70 Huddinge
Sweden
Tel: +46-8-7405880
Fax: +46-8-7109177
Telex: 10905

SWITZERLAND
E. Merck (Schweitz) AG
Diagnostics Department
Froebelstrasse 22
8029 Zurich
Switzerland
Tel: +41-1-559233
Fax: +41-1-559958
Telex: 816135

TAIWAN
Kaisers Medical Corporation
Pharmaceutical and Medical
Division
7th Floor, 23, Sec. 1
Chang An E. Road
Taipei 104
Taiwan
Tel: +886-2-5641681
Fax: +886-2-5610289
Telex: 11654

THAILAND
KV Scientific Co. Ltd
136 Nares Road
Bangrak
Bangkok 10500
Thailand
Tel: +66-2-2343188
Fax: +66-2-2381264
Telex: 20737

UNITED KINGDOM
Syva Europe
Syntex House
St Ives Road
Maidenhead

Berks, SL6 1RD
United Kingdom
Tel: +44-0628-777808
Fax: +44-0628-75321

Syva UK
23/25 Marlow Road
Maidenhead
Berks, SL6 7AA
United Kingdom
Tel: +44-0628-70969
Fax: +44-0628-773448

URUGUAY
Gustavo E. Arias
J.H. y Reissig 963
11200 Montevideo
Uruguay
Tel: +598-2-406430
Fax: +598-2-405065

USA
Syva Company
3403 Yerba Buena Road
PO Box 49013
San Jose
CA 95161-9013
USA
Tel: +1-408-239-2000
Fax: +1-408-239-2552

VENEZUELA
Merck SA
Av. PPAL.URB Lebrun
Ed. COFASA, Petare
Caracas 1010 A
Venezuela
Tel: +2-213455
Fax: +2-217164
Telex: 25236

Unipath Ltd

Corporate
Unipath Ltd
Wade Road
Basingstoke, Hampshire
RG24 8PW
United Kingdom
Tel: +44-0256-841144
Fax: +44-0256-463388

By region
AUSTRALIA
Oxoid Australia Pty Ltd
West Heidelberg
PO Box 220
Melbourne, Victoria 3081
Australia
Tel: +61-3-4581311
Fax: +61-3-4584759

FRANCE
Unipath SA
6 route de Paisy, BP 13
69572 Dardilly Cedex
France
Tel: +33-78351731
Fax: +33-78660376

GERMANY
Unipath GmbH
Am Lippeglacis 6-8
46483 Wesel
Germany

Tel: +49-281-1520
Fax: +49-281-1521

ITALY
Unipath SpA
Via Montenero 180
20024 Garbagnate
Milanese, Milan
Italy
Tel: +39-2-9955651
Fax: +39-2-9958260

NORTH AMERICA
Unipath Inc
217 Colonnade Road,
Nepean
Ontario, K2E 7K3
Canada
Tel: +1-613-226-1318
Fax: +1-613-226-3728

SPAIN
Unipath Espana SA
Via de los Poblados 10
Nave 3-13
Madrid 28033
Spain
Tel: +34-1-7642554
Telex: 45670

UNITED KINGDOM
Unipath Ltd
Wade Road
Basingstoke, Hampshire
RG24 8PW
United Kingdom
Tel: +44-0256-841144
Fax: +44-0256-463388

United Biotech Inc

Corporate
United Biotech Inc
110-C Pioneer Way
Mountain View, CA 94041
USA
Tel: +1-415-961-2910
Fax: +1-415-961-0766

Veda Laboratoire

Corporate
Veda Laboratoire
Siege Social
18 Rue Nicolas Appert
61000 Alencon
France
Tel: +33-33275625
Fax: +33-33277060

Zeus Scientific Inc

Corporate
Zeus Scientific Inc
PO Box 38
Raritan, NJ 08869
USA
Tel: +1-201-526-3744
Fax: +1-201-526-2058

INDEX BY MANUFACTURER, ASSAY TYPE, ANTIBODY/ANTIGEN DETECTION AND MICROORGANISM

Abbott Laboratories
EIA (competitive)
Antibody detection
Hepatitis A virus - 79
Hepatitis B virus (core antigen) - 95
Hepatitis B virus (core antigen) - 95
Hepatitis B virus (e antigen) - 128
Hepatitis B virus (e antigen) - 128
Hepatitis D virus - 177
EIA (non-competitive)
Antibody detection
Hepatitis B virus (surface antigen) - 157
Human immunodeficiency virus - 241
Human immunodeficiency virus (HIV-1) - 259
Antibody detection (IgG)
Human immunodeficiency virus - 246
Human immunodeficiency virus (HIV-1) - 261
Antibody detection (IgM)
Hepatitis A virus - 85
Hepatitis B virus (core antigen) - 105
Hepatitis B virus (core antigen) - 105
Antigen detection
Chlamydia trachomatis - 2
Hepatitis B virus (e antigen) - 118
Hepatitis B virus (e antigen) - 118
Hepatitis B virus (surface antigen) - 137
Hepatitis B virus (surface antigen) - 138
Human immunodeficiency virus (HIV-1) - 256
Neisseria gonorrhoeae - 276
RIA (competitive)
Antibody detection
Hepatitis A virus - 91
Hepatitis B virus (core antigen) - 115
RIA (non-competitive)
Antibody detection (IgM)
Hepatitis A virus - 92
Hepatitis B virus (core antigen) - 116

ADI Diagnostics
EIA (competitive)
Antibody detection
Hepatitis A virus - 80
Hepatitis B virus (core antigen) - 96
Hepatitis B virus (e antigen) - 129
EIA (non-competitive)
Antibody detection
Hepatitis B virus (surface antigen) - 157
Antibody detection (IgG)
Treponema pallidum - 291
Treponema pallidum - 292
Antibody detection (IgM)
Hepatitis A virus - 85
Hepatitis B virus (core antigen) - 106
Antigen detection
Hepatitis B virus (e antigen) - 119
Hepatitis B virus (surface antigen) - 138

Agen Biomedical Ltd
Particle RBC agglutination assay
Antibody detection
Human immunodeficiency virus - 255
Antigen detection
Hepatitis B virus (surface antigen) - 154

Alfa Biotech
Particle agglutination assay
Antibody detection
Neisseria gonorrhoeae - 279

Amico Laboratories Inc
EIA (non-competitive)
Antibody detection (IgG)
Chlamydia - 18
Cytomegalovirus - 34
Hepatitis A virus - 84
Herpes simplex virus - 188
Antibody detection (IgM)

Chlamydia - 24
Cytomegalovirus - 53
Hepatitis A virus - 86
Herpes simplex virus - 191
Immunofluorescence assay (indirect)
Antibody detection (IgG)
Chlamydia trachomatis - 27
Cytomegalovirus - 72
Herpes simplex virus - 198
Treponema pallidum - 299
Antibody detection (IgM)
Chlamydia trachomatis - 28
Cytomegalovirus - 75
Herpes simplex virus - 198

Baxter Diagnostics Inc (Bartels Division)
EIA (non-competitive)
Antibody detection (IgG)
Cytomegalovirus - 35
Herpes simplex virus (HSV-2) - 221
Antibody detection (IgM)
Cytomegalovirus - 53
Herpes simplex virus (HSV-1) - 208
Antigen detection
Chlamydia trachomatis - 2
Immunofluorescence assay (direct)
Antigen detection
Chlamydia trachomatis - 11
Herpes simplex virus - 187
Herpes simplex virus (HSV-1 and HSV-2) - 217
Immunofluorescence assay (indirect)
Antigen detection
Cytomegalovirus - 30
Cytomegalovirus - 30

Becton Dickinson
Particle agglutination assay
Antibody detection
Cytomegalovirus - 77
Antigen detection
Neisseria gonorrhoeae - 277
Streptococcus beta-haemolytic group B - 282

Behringwerke AG
EIA (competitive)
Antibody detection
Hepatitis B virus (core antigen) - 96
Hepatitis B virus (e antigen) - 129
Human immunodeficiency virus (HIV-1) - 257
Treponema pallidum - 289
EIA (non-competitive)
Antibody detection
Cytomegalovirus - 33
Hepatitis B virus (surface antigen) - 158
Human immunodeficiency virus - 241
Human immunodeficiency virus (HIV-2) - 265
Antibody detection (IgG)
Cytomegalovirus - 35
Herpes simplex virus - 188
Human immunodeficiency virus - 247
Antibody detection (IgG and/or IgM)
Cytomegalovirus - 52
Antibody detection (IgM)
Cytomegalovirus - 54
Hepatitis B virus (core antigen) - 106
Herpes simplex virus - 191
Antigen detection
Chlamydia (C. trachomatis, C. psittaci, C. pneumoniae) - 3
Hepatitis B virus (e antigen) - 119
Hepatitis B virus (surface antigen) - 139

Binax
EIA (non-competitive)
Antigen detection
Streptococcus beta-haemolytic group B - 281

Bio-Stat Diagnostics
EIA (non-competitive)
Antibody detection (IgG)
Cytomegalovirus - 36
Herpes simplex virus (HSV-2) - 222
Human immunodeficiency virus - 247
Human immunodeficiency virus - 248
Human immunodeficiency virus (HIV-1 and HIV-2) - 264
Human T-cell lymphotropic virus - 269
Human T-cell lymphotropic virus (HTLV-I and HTLV-II) - 273
Antibody detection (IgM)
Cytomegalovirus - 54
Herpes simplex virus - 192
Antigen detection
Herpes simplex virus (HSV-1) - 199
Herpes simplex virus (HSV-2) - 221

Biochrom
EIA (non-competitive)
Antibody detection (IgG)
Human immunodeficiency virus - 248

BIOKIT SA
EIA (non-competitive)
Antigen detection
Hepatitis B virus (surface antigen) - 139

Biologische Analysensystem GmbH
EIA (non-competitive)
Antibody detection
Treponema pallidum - 290
Antibody detection (IgG)
Cytomegalovirus - 36
Herpes simplex virus (HSV-1) - 200
Herpes simplex virus (HSV-2) - 222
Antibody detection (IgM)
Herpes simplex virus (HSV-1) - 209
Herpes simplex virus (HSV-2) - 231

Biologische Analysensytem GmbH
EIA (non-competitive)
Antibody detection (IgA)
Chlamydia trachomatis - 15
Antibody detection (IgG)
Chlamydia trachomatis - 18
Antibody detection (IgM)
Chlamydia trachomatis - 24
Cytomegalovirus - 55

bioMerieux
EIA (competitive)
Antibody detection
Hepatitis B virus (core antigen) - 97
EIA (non-competitive)
Antibody detection (IgG)
Cytomegalovirus - 37
Human immunodeficiency virus - 249
Antibody detection (IgM)
Cytomegalovirus - 55
Hepatitis A virus - 86
Hepatitis B virus (core antigen) - 107
Antigen detection
Chlamydia - 3
Hepatitis B virus (surface antigen) - 140
Immunofluorescence assay (indirect)
Antibody detection
Chlamydia trachomatis - 26
Treponema pallidum - 298

Bion Enterprises Ltd
Immunofluorescence assay (indirect)
Antibody detection (IgG)
Cytomegalovirus - 72
Herpes simplex virus (HSV-1) - 214
Herpes simplex virus (HSV-2) - 236

Biotest Diagnostics
EIA (non-competitive)
Antibody detection (IgG)
Cytomegalovirus - 37
Human immunodeficiency virus - 249
Antigen detection
Hepatitis B virus (surface antigen) - 140

Biowhittaker
EIA (non-competitive)
Antibody detection (IgG)
Chlamydia trachomatis - 19
Cytomegalovirus - 38
Cytomegalovirus - 38
Herpes simplex virus - 189
Herpes simplex virus - 189
Herpes simplex virus (HSV-1 and HSV-2) - 219
Herpes simplex virus (HSV-1 and HSV-2) - 219
Immunofluorescence assay (indirect)
Antibody detection (IgG)
Cytomegalovirus - 73
Herpes simplex virus (HSV-1) - 214

Boehringer Mannheim
EIA (competitive)
Antibody detection
Hepatitis A virus - 80
Hepatitis B virus (core antigen) - 97
Hepatitis B virus (e antigen) - 130
EIA (non-competitive)
Antibody detection
Hepatitis B virus (surface antigen) - 158
Antibody detection (IgG)
Hepatitis C virus - 169
Human immunodeficiency virus - 250
Human immunodeficiency virus (HIV-1) - 261
Antibody detection (IgM)
Hepatitis A virus - 87
Hepatitis B virus (core antigen) - 107
Antigen detection
Hepatitis B virus (e antigen) - 120
Hepatitis B virus (surface antigen) - 141

Boule Diagnostics AB
EIA (non-competitive)
Antigen detection
Chlamydia trachomatis (and C. psittaci) - 4
Particle agglutination assay (coagglutination)
Antigen detection
Neisseria gonorrhoeae - 277
Neisseria gonorrhoeae - 278
Streptococcus beta-haemolytic group B - 283

Bouty Diagnostici
EIA (non-competitive)
Antibody detection (IgG)
Cytomegalovirus - 39
Human immunodeficiency virus (HIV-1) - 262
Antibody detection (IgM)
Cytomegalovirus - 56

Cambridge Biotech Corporation
EIA (competitive)
Antibody detection
Hepatitis D virus - 177

EIA (non-competitive)
Antibody detection
Human immunodeficiency virus - 242
Antibody detection (IgG)
Herpes simplex virus (HSV-1) - 200
Herpes simplex virus (HSV-2) - 223
Antibody detection (IgM)
Hepatitis D virus - 180
Herpes simplex virus (HSV-1) - 209
Herpes simplex virus (HSV-2) - 232
Antigen detection
Hepatitis D virus - 174
Immunoblot assay
Antibody detection (IgG)
Human immunodeficiency virus (HIV-2) - 266
Human T-cell lymphotropic virus (HTLV-I) - 272

Cellabs Pty Ltd
EIA (non-competitive)
Antigen detection
Chlamydia trachomatis - 4
Immunofluorescence assay (direct)
Antigen detection
Chlamydia trachomatis - 12

Centocor Inc
EIA (competitive)
Antibody detection
Cytomegalovirus - 32
EIA (non-competitive)
Antibody detection (IgG)
Treponema pallidum - 292
Antibody detection (IgM)
Cytomegalovirus - 56
Treponema pallidum - 295

Chembio Diagnostic Systems Inc
Immunochromatographic assay
Antibody detection
Human immunodeficiency virus - 253
Antigen detection
Hepatitis B virus (surface antigen) - 152
Immunochromatographic assay
Antigen detection
Chlamydia trachomatis - 10

Chimica Diagnostica
EIA (non-competitive)
Antibody detection (IgG)
Cytomegalovirus - 39
Herpes simplex virus (HSV-1) - 201
Herpes simplex virus (HSV-2) - 223
Antibody detection (IgM)
Cytomegalovirus - 57
Herpes simplex virus (HSV-1) - 210
Herpes simplex virus (HSV-2) - 232

Clark Laboratories
EIA (non-competitive)
Antibody detection (IgG)
Treponema pallidum - 293

Coulter Corporation
EIA (competitive)
Antibody detection
Human immunodeficiency virus (HIV-1) - 258
EIA (non-competitive)
Antigen detection
Human immunodeficiency virus (HIV-1) - 256
Human T-cell lymphotropic virus - 269

Dako A/S
EIA (non-competitive, amplified)
Antigen detection
Chlamydia trachomatis - 5
Herpes simplex virus - 185

Immunofluorescence assay (direct)
Antigen detection
Chlamydia trachomatis - 12
Herpes simplex virus (HSV-1 and HSV-2) - 217
Particle agglutination assay (coagglutination)
Antigen detection
Streptococcus beta-haemolytic group B - 283

Diagast Laboratories
EIA (non-competitive)
Antibody detection (IgG)
Cytomegalovirus - 40
Immunoblot assay
Antibody detection (IgG)
Treponema pallidum - 297
Immunofluorescence assay (indirect)
Antibody detection
Treponema pallidum - 298

Diamedix Corporation
EIA (non-competitive)
Antibody detection (IgG)
Cytomegalovirus - 40
Herpes simplex virus (HSV-1) - 201
Herpes simplex virus (HSV-2) - 224
Antibody detection (IgM)
Cytomegalovirus - 57

Diesse
EIA (competitive)
Antibody detection
Cytomegalovirus - 32
Treponema pallidum - 289

E. Merck
EIA (non-competitive)
Antibody detection (IgG)
Chlamydia - 19
Cytomegalovirus - 41
Herpes simplex virus (HSV-1) - 202
Herpes simplex virus (HSV-2) - 224
Antibody detection (IgM)
Cytomegalovirus - 58
Herpes simplex virus - 192

E. Merck/Biotrol
EIA (non-competitive)
Antibody detection (IgG)
Chlamydia trachomatis (and C. psittaci) - 20

Euro-Diagnostica B.V.
EIA (non-competitive)
Antibody detection
Treponema pallidum - 290

Eurogenetics
EIA (non-competitive)
Antibody detection (IgA)
Chlamydia trachomatis - 16
Antibody detection (IgG)
Chlamydia trachomatis - 20
Cytomegalovirus - 41
Herpes simplex virus (HSV-1) - 202
Herpes simplex virus (HSV-2) - 225
Antibody detection (IgM)
Cytomegalovirus - 58
Herpes simplex virus - 193

Fujirebio
EIA (non-competitive)
Antibody detection (IgM)
Treponema pallidum - 296
Particle agglutination assay
Antibody detection
Human immunodeficiency virus - 255
Human T-cell lymphotropic virus (HTLV-I) - 273

Gamma SA
EIA (non-competitive)
Antibody detection (IgG)
Cytomegalovirus - 42
Cytomegalovirus - 42
Herpes simplex virus (HSV-1) - 203
Herpes simplex virus (HSV-2) - 225
Human immunodeficiency virus - 250
Antibody detection (IgG and/or IgM)
Cytomegalovirus - 52
Antibody detection (IgM)
Cytomegalovirus - 59
Herpes simplex virus - 193

Gen Bio
Immunoblot assay
Antibody detection (IgG)
Cytomegalovirus - 70
Cytomegalovirus - 70
Herpes simplex virus - 196
Herpes simplex virus - 197
Immunofluorescence assay (indirect)
Antibody detection (IgG)
Cytomegalovirus - 73
Herpes simplex virus (HSV-1) - 215
Herpes simplex virus (HSV-2) - 237
Antibody detection (IgM)
Cytomegalovirus - 76
Herpes simplex virus (HSV-1) - 216
Herpes simplex virus (HSV-2) - 238

Genetic Systems Corporation/ Sanofi Diagnostics Pasteur
EIA (non-competitive)
Antibody detection
Human immunodeficiency virus - 242
Human immunodeficiency virus (HIV-1) - 259
Human immunodeficiency virus (HIV-2) - 266
Human T-cell lymphotropic virus (HTLV-I) - 271
Antigen detection
Hepatitis B virus (surface antigen) - 141
Immunoblot assay
Antibody detection (IgG)
Human immunodeficiency virus (HIV-2) - 267

Gull Laboratories
EIA (non-competitive)
Antibody detection (IgG)
Cytomegalovirus - 43
Herpes simplex virus (HSV-2) - 226
Antibody detection (IgM)
Cytomegalovirus - 59
Herpes simplex virus (HSV-1) - 210
Herpes simplex virus (HSV-2) - 233
Immunofluorescence assay (indirect)
Antibody detection
Cytomegalovirus - 71
Herpes simplex virus - 197
Antibody detection (IgM)
Cytomegalovirus - 76
Herpes simplex virus - 199

Human GmbH
EIA (non-competitive)
Antibody detection (IgG)
Cytomegalovirus - 43
Herpes simplex virus (HSV-1) - 203
Herpes simplex virus (HSV-2) - 226
Antibody detection (IgM)
Cytomegalovirus - 60
Herpes simplex virus - 194
Antigen detection
Hepatitis B virus (surface antigen) - 142
Particle agglutination assay
Antigen detection
Hepatitis B virus (surface antigen) - 154

Hybritech
EIA (non-competitive)
Antigen detection
Streptococcus beta-haemolytic group B - 281

IFCI Clone Systems
EIA (competitive)
Antibody detection
Hepatitis B virus (core antigen) - 98
Hepatitis B virus (e antigen) - 130
EIA (non-competitive)
Antibody detection (IgG)
Cytomegalovirus - 44
Human immunodeficiency virus - 251
Human T-cell lymphotropic virus - 270
Human T-cell lymphotropic virus (HTLV-I and HTLV-II) - 274
Treponema pallidum - 293
Antibody detection (IgM)
Cytomegalovirus - 60
Hepatitis B virus (core antigen) - 108
Treponema pallidum - 296
Antigen detection
Hepatitis B virus (e antigen) - 120

Immunobiological Laboratories
EIA (non-competitive)
Antibody detection (IgG)
Herpes simplex virus (HSV-1) - 204
Herpes simplex virus (HSV-2) - 227
Antibody detection (IgM)
Herpes simplex virus (HSV-1) - 211
Herpes simplex virus (HSV-2) - 233

Incstar
EIA (non-competitive)
Antibody detection (IgG)
Cytomegalovirus - 44
Herpes simplex virus (HSV-1) - 204
Herpes simplex virus (HSV-2) - 227
Antibody detection (IgM)
Cytomegalovirus - 61
Immunofluorescence assay (indirect)
Antibody detection
Chlamydia trachomatis - 27
Cytomegalovirus - 71
Herpes simplex virus (HSV-1) - 213
Herpes simplex virus (HSV-2) - 236

Innogenetics SA
EIA (non-competitive)
Antibody detection (IgG)
Hepatitis C virus - 169
Human immunodeficiency virus - 251
Antigen detection
Human immunodeficiency virus - 240
Immunoblot assay
Antibody detection
Hepatitis C virus - 172
Antibody detection (IgG)
Human immunodeficiency virus (HIV-1 and HIV-2) - 264

International Immunodiagnostics
EIA (non-competitive)
Antibody detection (IgG)
Cytomegalovirus - 45
Herpes simplex virus (HSV-1) - 205
Herpes simplex virus (HSV-2) - 228
Treponema pallidum - 294
Antibody detection (IgM)
Cytomegalovirus - 61
Herpes simplex virus (HSV-1) - 211
Herpes simplex virus (HSV-2) - 234

International Mycoplasma
EIA (non-competitive)
Antigen detection
Chlamydia trachomatis - 5

Kodak Clinical Diagnostics
EIA (non-competitive)
Antigen detection
Chlamydia trachomatis - 6
Herpes simplex virus - 185
Luminometric immunoassay (competitive)
Antibody detection
Hepatitis B virus (core antigen) - 114
Luminometric immunoassay (non-competitive)
Antibody detection
Hepatitis B virus (surface antigen) - 166
Antibody detection (IgM)
Hepatitis A virus - 91
Hepatitis B virus (core antigen) - 114
Antigen and antibody detection
Hepatitis B virus (e antigen) - 127
Hepatitis B virus (surface antigen) - 153

Laboratoire Eurobio
EIA (competitive)
Antibody detection
Hepatitis A virus - 81
EIA (non-competitive)
Antibody detection (IgG)
Cytomegalovirus - 45
Herpes simplex virus - 190
Antibody detection (IgM)
Cytomegalovirus - 62
Hepatitis A virus - 87
Herpes simplex virus - 194

Labsystems Oy
EIA (competitive)
Antibody detection
Hepatitis B virus (core antigen) - 98
EIA (non-competitive)
Antibody detection (IgG)
Chlamydia trachomatis - 21
Cytomegalovirus - 46
Antibody detection (IgM)
Cytomegalovirus - 62
Hepatitis B virus (core antigen) - 108
Antigen detection
Chlamydia trachomatis - 6
Hepatitis B virus (surface antigen) - 142

Mast Diagnostics Ltd
EIA (non-competitive)
Antigen detection
Chlamydia trachomatis - 7
Immunofluorescence assay (indirect)
Antibody detection (IgG)
Treponema pallidum - 300

Medac Diagnostika
EIA (non-competitive)
Antibody detection (IgA)
Chlamydia trachomatis - 16
Antibody detection (IgG)
Chlamydia trachomatis - 21
Cytomegalovirus - 46
Antibody detection (IgM)
Chlamydia trachomatis - 25
Cytomegalovirus - 63

Melja Diagnostik GmbH
EIA (non-competitive)
Antibody detection (IgG)
Herpes simplex virus (HSV-1) - 205
Herpes simplex virus (HSV-2) - 228
Antibody detection (IgM)
Herpes simplex virus (HSV-1) - 212
Herpes simplex virus (HSV-2) - 234

Melotec S.A.
EIA (competitive)
Antibody detection
Hepatitis B virus (core antigen) - 99
Hepatitis B virus (e antigen) - 131

EIA (non-competitive)
Antibody detection
   Hepatitis B virus (surface antigen) - 159
Antibody detection (IgG)
   Chlamydia trachomatis - 22
   Cytomegalovirus - 47
   Hepatitis C virus - 170
   Herpes simplex virus (HSV-1) - 206
   Herpes simplex virus (HSV-2) - 229
Antibody detection (IgM)
   Cytomegalovirus - 63
   Herpes simplex virus (HSV-1) - 212
   Herpes simplex virus (HSV-2) - 235
Antigen detection
   Hepatitis B virus (e antigen) - 121
   Hepatitis B virus (surface antigen) - 143
   Hepatitis B virus (surface antigen) - 143

Menarini Diagnostics
EIA (non-competitive)
Antibody detection (IgG)
   Chlamydia trachomatis - 22
   Cytomegalovirus - 47
   Herpes simplex virus - 190
   Treponema pallidum - 294
Antibody detection (IgM)
   Cytomegalovirus - 64
   Herpes simplex virus - 195
   Treponema pallidum - 297

Meridian Diagnostics Inc
Particle agglutination assay (coagglutination)
Antigen detection
   Neisseria gonorrhoeae - 278
   Streptococcus beta-haemolytic group B - 284

Mitsui Pharmaceuticals Inc
EIA (non-competitive)
Antibody detection
   Hepatitis B virus (surface antigen) - 159
Antigen detection
   Hepatitis B virus (surface antigen) - 144

Murex Diagnostics Limited
EIA (competitive)
Antibody detection
   Hepatitis A virus - 81
   Hepatitis B virus (core antigen) - 99
   Hepatitis D virus - 178
   Human immunodeficiency virus (HIV-1) - 258
EIA (non-competitive, amplified)
Antibody detection
   Hepatitis B virus (surface antigen) - 160
   Human immunodeficiency virus - 243
   Human immunodeficiency virus - 243
   Human immunodeficiency virus (HIV-1) - 260
Antibody detection (IgG)
   Cytomegalovirus - 48
   Hepatitis C virus - 170
   Human immunodeficiency virus - 252
   Human T-cell lymphotropic virus - 270
Antibody detection (IgM)
   Cytomegalovirus - 64
   Hepatitis A virus - 88
   Hepatitis B virus (core antigen) - 109
   Hepatitis D virus - 181
Antigen detection
   Chlamydia trachomatis - 7
   Hepatitis B virus (e antigen) - 127
   Hepatitis B virus (surface antigen) - 144
   Hepatitis B virus (surface antigen) - 145
   Hepatitis D virus - 174
   Herpes simplex virus - 186

Particle agglutination assay
Antigen detection
   Streptococcus beta-haemolytic group B - 284

Omega Diagnostics Ltd
EIA (non-competitive)
Antibody detection (IgG)
   Treponema pallidum - 295
Antigen detection
   Hepatitis B virus (surface antigen) - 145
Particle agglutination assay
Antigen detection
   Hepatitis B virus (surface antigen) - 155
   Streptococcus beta-haemolytic group B - 285

Organon Teknika NV
EIA (competitive)
Antibody detection
   Hepatitis A virus - 82
   Hepatitis B virus (core antigen) - 100
   Hepatitis B virus (core antigen) - 100
   Hepatitis B virus (e antigen) - 131
   Hepatitis D virus - 178
   Human immunodeficiency virus - 240
EIA (non-competitive)
Antibody detection
   Hepatitis B virus (surface antigen) - 160
   Human immunodeficiency virus - 244
   Human T-cell lymphotropic virus (HTLV-I) - 272
Antibody detection (IgM)
   Cytomegalovirus - 65
   Hepatitis A virus - 88
   Hepatitis B virus (core antigen) - 109
Antigen detection
   Hepatitis A virus - 79
   Hepatitis B virus (e antigen) - 121
   Hepatitis B virus (surface antigen) - 146
   Hepatitis B virus (surface antigen) - 146
   Hepatitis D virus - 175
   Human immunodeficiency virus (HIV-1) - 257
Immunoblot assay
Antibody detection
   Human immunodeficiency virus (HIV-1) - 262
Immunochromatographic assay
Antibody detection (IgG)
   Human immunodeficiency virus (HIV-1 and HIV-2) - 265

Orion Diagnostica
Immunofluorescence assay (direct)
Antigen detection
   Chlamydia trachomatis - 13
Particle agglutination assay
Antigen detection
   Streptococcus beta-haemolytic group B - 285

Ortho Diagnostic Systems
EIA (non-competitive)
Antibody detection (IgG)
   Human immunodeficiency virus - 252
Immunoblot assay
Antibody detection
   Human immunodeficiency virus - 254

PRO-LAB Diagnostics
Particle agglutination assay
Antigen detection
   Streptococcus beta-haemolytic group B - 286

Radim
EIA (competitive)
Antibody detection
   Hepatitis B virus (core antigen) - 101
   Hepatitis B virus (e antigen) - 132

EIA (non-competitive)
Antibody detection (IgA)
   Chlamydia - 17
Antibody detection (IgG)
   Chlamydia - 23
   Cytomegalovirus - 48
   Herpes simplex virus (HSV-1) - 206
   Herpes simplex virus (HSV-2) - 229
Antibody detection (IgM)
   Cytomegalovirus - 65
   Hepatitis B virus (core antigen) - 110
   Herpes simplex virus - 195
Antigen detection
   Hepatitis B virus (e antigen) - 122
   Hepatitis B virus (surface antigen) - 147
RIA (competitive)
Antibody detection
   Hepatitis B virus (core antigen) - 115
   Hepatitis B virus (e antigen) - 136
RIA (non-competitive)
Antibody detection
   Hepatitis B virus (surface antigen) - 166
Antibody detection (IgM)
   Hepatitis B virus (core antigen) - 117
Antigen detection
   Hepatitis B virus (e antigen) - 126
   Hepatitis B virus (surface antigen) - 156

Randox Laboratories Ltd
EIA (competitive)
Antibody detection
   Hepatitis B virus (core antigen) - 101
   Hepatitis B virus (e antigen) - 132
EIA (non-competitive)
Antibody detection
   Hepatitis B virus (surface antigen) - 161
Antibody detection (IgM)
   Hepatitis B virus (core antigen) - 110
Antigen detection
   Hepatitis B virus (e antigen) - 122
   Hepatitis B virus (surface antigen) - 147

Roche Diagnostic Systems
EIA (competitive)
Antibody detection
   Hepatitis A virus - 82
   Hepatitis B virus (core antigen) - 102
   Hepatitis B virus (e antigen) - 133
EIA (non-competitive)
Antibody detection
   Hepatitis B virus (surface antigen) - 161
   Hepatitis B virus (surface antigen) - 162
   Human immunodeficiency virus - 244
Antibody detection (IgG)
   Cytomegalovirus - 49
   Human T-cell lymphotropic virus - 271
Antibody detection (IgM)
   Cytomegalovirus - 66
   Hepatitis A virus - 89
   Hepatitis B virus (core antigen) - 111
Antigen detection
   Hepatitis B virus (surface antigen) - 148

Sanofi Diagnostics Pasteur
EIA (competitive)
Antibody detection
   Cytomegalovirus - 33
   Hepatitis B virus (core antigen) - 102
   Hepatitis B virus (e antigen) - 133
   Hepatitis D virus - 179
EIA (non-competitive)
Antibody detection
   Hepatitis B virus (surface antigen) - 162
   Human immunodeficiency virus - 245
   Human immunodeficiency virus (HIV-1) - 260
Antibody detection (IgG)
   Hepatitis C virus - 171

Antibody detection (IgM)
  Hepatitis B virus (core antigen) - 111
  Hepatitis D virus - 181
Antigen detection
  Chlamydia (C. trachomatis, C. psittaci, C. pneumoniae) - 8
  Hepatitis B virus (e antigen) - 123
  Hepatitis B virus (surface antigen) - 148
  Hepatitis D virus - 175
Immunoblot assay
Antibody detection (IgG)
  Human immunodeficiency virus (HIV-1) - 263
  Human immunodeficiency virus (HIV-2) - 267
Immunofluorescence assay (indirect)
Antibody detection
  Treponema pallidum - 299
Antibody detection (IgM)
  Treponema pallidum - 301
Antigen detection
  Cytomegalovirus - 31

Savyon Diagnostics Ltd
EIA (non-competitive)
Antibody detection
  Chlamydia trachomatis - 15
Antibody detection (IgA)
  Cytomegalovirus - 34
Antibody detection (IgM)
  Chlamydia trachomatis - 25
  Chlamydia trachomatis - 26
  Cytomegalovirus - 66
Antigen detection
  Herpes simplex virus - 186
Immunoblot assay
Antibody detection
  Human immunodeficiency virus - 254
Immunochromatographic assay
Antigen detection
  Chlamydia trachomatis - 10
  Hepatitis B virus (surface antigen) - 153

Schiapparelli Biosystems Inc
EIA (competitive)
Antibody detection
  Hepatitis A virus - 83
  Hepatitis B virus (core antigen) - 103
  Hepatitis B virus (e antigen) - 134
EIA (non-competitive)
Antibody detection
  Hepatitis B virus (surface antigen) - 163
Antibody detection (IgA)
  Chlamydia trachomatis - 17
Antibody detection (IgG)
  Chlamydia trachomatis - 23
  Cytomegalovirus - 49
  Herpes simplex virus (HSV-1) - 207
  Herpes simplex virus (HSV-2) - 230
Antibody detection (IgM)
  Cytomegalovirus - 67
  Hepatitis A virus - 89
  Hepatitis B virus (core antigen) - 112
  Herpes simplex virus - 196
Antigen detection
  Hepatitis B virus (e antigen) - 123
  Hepatitis B virus (surface antigen) - 149
Immunofluorescence assay (indirect)
Antibody detection (IgG)
  Chlamydia trachomatis - 28
  Cytomegalovirus - 74
  Herpes simplex virus (HSV-1) - 215
  Herpes simplex virus (HSV-2) - 237
  Treponema pallidum - 300
Antibody detection (IgM)
  Cytomegalovirus - 77

Shield Diagnostics
EIA (non-competitive)
Antibody detection
  Treponema pallidum - 291
  Urinary tract infection bacterial pathogens - 302
Antigen detection
  Chlamydia trachomatis - 8
Immunofluorescence assay (direct)
Antigen detection
  Chlamydia trachomatis - 13
Particle agglutination assay
Antigen detection
  Streptococcus beta-haemolytic group B - 286

Sigma Diagnostics
EIA (non-competitive)
Antibody detection (IgG)
  Cytomegalovirus - 50
  Herpes simplex virus (HSV-1) - 207
  Herpes simplex virus (HSV-2) - 230
Antibody detection (IgM)
  Cytomegalovirus - 67
  Cytomegalovirus - 68
Antigen detection
  Chlamydia trachomatis - 9

Sorin Biomedica
EIA (competitive)
Antibody detection
  Hepatitis A virus - 83
  Hepatitis B virus (core antigen) - 103
  Hepatitis B virus (core antigen) - 104
  Hepatitis B virus (e antigen) - 134
  Hepatitis B virus (e antigen) - 135
  Hepatitis D virus - 179
  Hepatitis D virus - 180
EIA (non-competitive)
Antibody detection
  Hepatitis B virus (surface antigen) - 163
  Hepatitis B virus (surface antigen) - 164
  Hepatitis B virus (surface antigen) - 164
Antibody detection (IgG)
  Cytomegalovirus - 50
  Hepatitis C virus - 171
  Human immunodeficiency virus - 253
Antibody detection (IgM)
  Cytomegalovirus - 68
  Hepatitis A virus - 90
  Hepatitis B virus (core antigen) - 112
  Hepatitis B virus (core antigen) - 113
  Hepatitis D virus - 182
Antigen detection
  Hepatitis B virus (e antigen) - 124
  Hepatitis B virus (e antigen) - 124
  Hepatitis B virus (surface antigen) - 149
  Hepatitis B virus (surface antigen) - 150
  Hepatitis B virus (surface antigen) - 150
  Hepatitis D virus - 176
Immunoblot assay
Antibody detection
  Human immunodeficiency virus (HIV-1) - 263
RIA (competitive)
Antibody detection
  Hepatitis A virus - 92
  Hepatitis B virus (core antigen) - 116
  Hepatitis B virus (e antigen) - 137
  Hepatitis D virus - 182
RIA (non-competitive)
Antibody detection
  Hepatitis B virus (surface antigen) - 167
Antibody detection (IgM)
  Hepatitis A virus - 93
  Hepatitis B virus (core antigen) - 117
  Hepatitis D virus - 183
Antigen detection
  Hepatitis B virus (e antigen) - 126

Hepatitis B virus (surface antigen) - 156
Hepatitis D virus - 176

Stellar Bio Systems Inc
Immunofluorescence assay (indirect)
Antibody detection (IgG)
  Cytomegalovirus - 74

Syva Company
EIA (competitive)
Antibody detection
  Hepatitis A virus - 84
  Hepatitis B virus (core antigen) - 104
  Hepatitis B virus (e antigen) - 135
EIA (non-competitive)
Antibody detection
  Hepatitis B virus (surface antigen) - 165
  Human immunodeficiency virus - 245
Antibody detection (IgM)
  Hepatitis A virus - 90
  Hepatitis B virus (core antigen) - 113
Antigen detection
  Chlamydia trachomatis - 9
  Hepatitis B virus (e antigen) - 125
  Hepatitis B virus (surface antigen) - 151
Immunofluorescence assay (direct)
Antigen detection
  Chlamydia trachomatis - 14
  Chlamydia trachomatis - 14
  Herpes simplex virus - 187
  Herpes simplex virus (HSV-1 and HSV-2) - 218
  Herpes simplex virus (HSV-1 and HSV-2) - 218
  Neisseria gonorrhoeae - 276
Immunofluorescence assay (indirect)
Antigen detection
  Cytomegalovirus - 31

Unipath Limited
Immunochromatographic assay
Antigen detection
  Chlamydia trachomatis - 11
Particle agglutination assay
Antigen detection
  Streptococcus beta-haemolytic group B - 287

United Biotech Inc
EIA (non-competitive)
Antibody detection
  Human immunodeficiency virus - 246
Antibody detection (IgG)
  Cytomegalovirus - 51
  Herpes simplex virus (HSV-1) - 208
  Herpes simplex virus (HSV-2) - 231
Antibody detection (IgM)
  Cytomegalovirus - 69
  Herpes simplex virus (HSV-1) - 213
  Herpes simplex virus (HSV-2) - 235
Antigen detection
  Hepatitis B virus (surface antigen) - 151

VEDA-LAB
EIA (competitive)
Antibody detection
  Hepatitis B virus (core antigen) - 104
  Hepatitis B virus (e antigen) - 136
EIA (non-competitive)
Antibody detection
  Hepatitis B virus (surface antigen) - 165
Antigen detection
  Hepatitis B virus (e antigen) - 125
  Hepatitis B virus (surface antigen) - 152
Immunochromatographic assay
Antigen detection
  Streptococcus beta-haemolytic group B - 282

© *KLUWER ACADEMIC PUBLISHERS 1994, ISSN*

Particle agglutination assay
  Antigen detection
    Hepatitis B virus (surface antigen) - 155

Zeus Scientific Inc
EIA (non-competitive)
  Antibody detection (IgG)
    Cytomegalovirus - 51

Herpes simplex virus (HSV-1 and HSV-2) - 220
Antibody detection (IgM)
  Cytomegalovirus - 69
  Herpes simplex virus (HSV-1 and HSV-2) - 220

Immunofluorescence assay (indirect)
  Antibody detection (IgG)
    Cytomegalovirus - 75
    Herpes simplex virus (HSV-1) - 216
    Herpes simplex virus (HSV-2) - 238
    Treponema pallidum - 301

INDEX BY ASSAY TYPE, MICROORGANISM, ANTIGEN/ANTIBODY DETECTION AND MANUFACTURER

© *KLUWER ACADEMIC PUBLISHERS 1994, ISSN*

Herpes simplex virus (HSV-2)
Antibody detection
Incstar - 236
Antibody detection (IgG)
Bion Enterprises Ltd - 236
Gen Bio - 237
Schiapparelli Biosystems Inc - 237
Zeus Scientific Inc - 238
Antibody detection (IgM)
Gen Bio - 238
Treponema pallidum
Antibody detection
bioMerieux - 298
Diagast Laboratories - 298
Sanofi Diagnostics Pasteur - 299
Antibody detection (IgG)
Amico Laboratories Inc - 299
Mast Diagnostics Ltd - 300
Schiapparelli Biosystems Inc - 300
Zeus Scientific Inc - 301
Antibody detection (IgM)
Sanofi Diagnostics Pasteur - 301

Luminometric immunoassay (competitive)
Hepatitis B virus (core antigen)
Antibody detection
Kodak Clinical Diagnostics - 114

Luminometric immunoassay (non-competitive)
Hepatitis A virus
Antibody detection (IgM)
Kodak Clinical Diagnostics - 91
Hepatitis B virus (core antigen)
Antibody detection (IgM)
Kodak Clinical Diagnostics - 114
Hepatitis B virus (e antigen)
Antigen and antibody detection
Kodak Clinical Diagnostics - 127
Hepatitis B virus (surface antigen)
Antibody detection
Kodak Clinical Diagnostics - 166
Antigen detection

Kodak Clinical Diagnostics - 153

Particle agglutination assay
Cytomegalovirus
Antibody detection
Becton Dickinson - 77
Hepatitis B virus (surface antigen)
Antigen detection
Agen Biomedical Ltd - 154
Human GmbH - 154
Omega Diagnostics Ltd - 155
VEDA-LAB - 155
Human immunodeficiency virus
Antibody detection
Agen Biomedical Ltd - 255
Fujirebio - 255
Human T-cell lymphotropic virus (HTLV-I)
Antibody detection
Fujirebio - 273
Neisseria gonorrhoeae
Antibody detection
Alfa Biotech - 279
Antigen detection
Becton Dickinson - 277
Boule Diagnostics AB - 277
Boule Diagnostics AB - 278
Meridian Diagnostics Inc - 278
Streptococcus beta-haemolytic group B
Antigen detection
Becton Dickinson - 282
Boule Diagnostics AB - 283
Dako A/S - 283
Meridian Diagnostics Inc - 284
Murex Diagnostics Limited - 284
Omega Diagnostics Ltd - 285
Orion Diagnostica - 285
PRO-LAB Diagnostics - 286
Shield Diagnostics - 286
Unipath Limited - 287

RIA (competitive)
Hepatitis A virus
Antibody detection
Abbott Laboratories - 91

Sorin Biomedica - 92
Hepatitis B virus (core antigen)
Antibody detection
Abbott Laboratories - 115
Radim - 115
Sorin Biomedica - 116
Hepatitis B virus (e antigen)
Antibody detection
Radim - 136
Sorin Biomedica - 137
Hepatitis D virus
Antibody detection
Sorin Biomedica - 182

RIA (non-competitive)
Hepatitis A virus
Antibody detection (IgM)
Abbott Laboratories - 92
Sorin Biomedica - 93
Hepatitis B virus (core antigen)
Antibody detection (IgM)
Abbott Laboratories - 116
Radim - 117
Sorin Biomedica - 117
Hepatitis B virus (e antigen)
Antigen detection
Radim - 126
Sorin Biomedica - 126
Hepatitis B virus (surface antigen)
Antibody detection
Radim - 166
Sorin Biomedica - 167
Antigen detection
Radim - 156
Sorin Biomedica - 156
Hepatitis D virus
Antibody detection (IgM)
Sorin Biomedica - 183
Antigen detection
Sorin Biomedica - 176

© KLUWER ACADEMIC PUBLISHERS 1994, ISSN 1

GPSR Compliance

*The European Union's (EU) General Product Safety Regulation (GPSR)
is a set of rules that requires consumer products to be safe and our
obligations to ensure this.*

*If you have any concerns about our products, you can contact us on
ProductSafety@springernature.com*

In case Publisher is established outside the EU, the EU authorized
representative is:

Springer Nature Customer Service Center GmbH
Europaplatz 3
69115 Heidelberg, Germany

Batch number: 09625569

Printed by Printforce, the Netherlands